EMERGENCY NURSING

Books of Related Interest

Cummings: Quick Reference of Common Emergency Drugs, 1983, 0-471-87703-4

Fought: Psychosocial Nursing Care of the Emergency Patient, 1984, 0-471-87562-7

Harmon: Nursing Care of the Adult Trauma Patient, 1985, 0-471-88793-5

Howe: The Handbook of Nursing, 1984, 0-471-89524-5

Loebl: The Nurse's Drug Handbook, Third Edition, 1983, 0-471-09660-1

EMERGENCY NURSING
A Guide to Comprehensive Care

Edited by

Janet Gren Parker, R.N., M.S.

Assistant Director
Ambulatory Nursing
Assistant Professor
Medical-Surgical Nursing
Vanderbilt University
Nashville, Tennessee

A WILEY MEDICAL PUBLICATION
JOHN WILEY & SONS
New York • Chichester • Brisbane • Toronto • Singapore

Copyright © 1984 by John Wiley & Sons, Inc.

All rights reserved. Published simultaneously in Canada.

Reproduction or translation of any part of this
work beyond that permitted by Sections 107 or 108
of the 1976 United States Copyright Act without the
permission of the copyright owner is unlawful. Requests
for permission or further information should be addressed
to the Permissions Department, John Wiley & Sons, Inc.

Library of Congress Cataloging in Publication Data:

Main entry under title:
 Emergency nursing.

 (A Wiley medical publication)
 Includes index.
 1. Emergency nursing.   I. Parker, Janet Gren.
II. Series.   [DNLM: 1. Emergencies—Nursing.
WY 154 E523]

RT120.E4E474 1984   610.73′61   84-11971
ISBN 0-471-09907-4

Printed in the United States of America

10 9 8 7 6 5 4 3 2 1

*To the Vanderbilt Emergency Service Staff and John,
who have been extremely supportive and understanding
throughout this endeavor*

Contributors

Pamela W. Bourg, R.N., M.S., C.E.N.
Emergency Medical Services, Nursing Supervisor
Denver General Hospital
Assistant Clinical Professor
University of Colorado School of Nursing
Denver, Colorado

Marilyn K. Bourn, R.N., B.S.N., C.E.N.
Paramedic Field Coordinator
Swedish Medical Center
Englewood, Colorado

Cathy Bremer, R.N., M.S.
Formerly Clinical Nurse Specialist, Surgical Nursing
Cook County Hospital
Chicago, Illinois

Molly P. Bronaugh, R.N., M.S.N.
Formerly Coordinator of Paramedic Program
University of Tennessee
Nashville, Tennessee

Mary Ann Brown, R.N., M.S., C.N.M.
Private Practice, Nurse Midwife
Atlanta, Georgia

P. Howard Cummings, R.N., Ed.D., C.E.N.
Assistant Professor of Nursing
East Carolina University
Greenville, North Carolina

Sally Pahnke Cummings, R.N., M.S.N.
Assistant Professor of Nursing
East Carolina University
Greenville, North Carolina

Nancy Stephens Donatelli, R.N., M.S., C.E.N.
Coordinator, Educational Services
Shenango Valley Osteopathic Hospital
Farrell, Pennsylvania

Elizabeth G. Estrada, R.N., M.S.
President, Health Care Network, Inc.
San Francisco, California

Denise A. Gornick, R.N.
Emergency Medical Services, Staff Nurse
Denver General Hospital
Denver, Colorado

Nancy L. Griffith, R.N., M.S.N.
Assistant Professor
University of Nebraska College of Nursing
Omaha, Nebraska

Judy Stoner Halpern, R.N., M.S., C.E.N.
Clinical Nurse Specialist
Trauma and Emergency Center
Bronson Methodist Hospital
Kalamazoo, Michigan

Dorothy M. Kellmer, R.N., M.S.
Assistant Professor
Intercollegiate Center for Nursing Education
Spokane, Washington

Barbara Knezevich, R.N., M.S., C.E.N.
Staff Nurse, Intensive Care Unit
Mercy Hospital and Medical Center
Chicago, Illinois

Mitzi M. Lamberth, R.N., B.S.N., C.E.N.
Nurse Coordinator, Emergency Services
Vanderbilt University Hospital
Nashville, Tennessee

Judith "Ski" Lower, R.N., C.C.R.N., C.N.R.N., B.S.N.
Head Nurse, Neurosciences Critical Care Unit
Johns Hopkins Hospital
Baltimore, Maryland

Susan K. MacArthur, R.N., M.S.N., C.C.R.N.
Clinical Specialist CCIC
The Mt. Sinai Medical Center
Cleveland, Ohio

CONTRIBUTORS

Margaret E. Moser, R.N., B.S., C.E.N.
Staff Development Instructor
The Moses H. Cone Memorial Hospital
Greensboro, North Carolina

Janet Gren Parker, R.N., M.S.
Assistant Director
Ambulatory Nursing
Assistant Professor
Medical-Surgical Nursing
Vanderbilt University
Nashville, Tennessee

Nancy L. Parrish, R.N., M.S.N.
Trauma Nurse Coordinator
Baptist Hospital
Pensacola, Florida

Carol Beth Pulliam, R.N., M.S.N.
Clinical Nurse Specialist
Vanderbilt University Hospital
Nashville, Tennessee

Christina A. Ronshausen, R.N., M.S., N.S.
Assistant Professor of Nursing
University of Texas School of Nursing
Galveston, Texas

June D. Thompson, R.N., M.S.
Assistant Professor
The University of Texas Health Science Center
Houston, Texas

Ann M. Van Hoff, R.N., M.S.N.
Assistant Professor
University of Nebraska College of Nursing
Omaha, Nebraska

Debbie Van Meter, R.N., M.N., C.E.N.
Unit Director, Emergency Department
Children's Hospital
New Orleans, Louisiana

Judy Jo Wells-Mackie, R.N., M.S.
Westcliffe, Colorado

Preface

Emergency nursing is now a recognized speciality that requires unique knowledge and skills. Consequently, this book analyzes multiple aspects of emergency nursing care that might be rendered in an active emergency department.

Emergency Nursing: A Guide to Comprehensive Care can be used as a reference book by practicing emergency nurses. It can also be used as a nursing textbook to help guide students in their struggle to comprehend emergency nursing.

The first four chapters discuss the role of both the emergency department and the emergency nurse within the health care system. Topics discussed include legal aspects of the specialty and general concepts applicable to the subsequent clinical chapters.

The unique organization of the 26 clinical chapters reflects the usual process of patient flow in the emergency department setting. This process begins with the triage action (assessment). The triage process includes the initial history, a brief physical assessment, the development of the nursing diagnosis, and the plan of action. The next step in the process, enacting the plan of action, requires knowledge necessary to care for the patient and skills necessary to implement the plan of care. The last step relates to patient education and includes the various aspects of teaching, as well as actual patient discharge instructions.

Each clinical chapter, therefore, is unique in organization. Each chapter reviews the care of emergency department patients from their initial presentation in the department to their eventual admission to the hospital or discharge from the department.

The last section of the book, which relates to the interface between emergency nursing and the community, includes discussions on disaster planning and the future of emergency nursing.

I would like to acknowledge formally the help and support of all contributors. Everyone involved is dedicated to the advancement and improvement of emergency nursing. Michael Butler, my illustrator, also deserves a kind acknowledgment for his diligence in preparing the illustrations for this book.

This is a *nursing* book written by nurses dedicated to upgrading and improving the profession to provide the quality of care expected by the general public. It is my aspiration that this book will play a valuable role in the daily practice of every emergency nurse.

Janet Gren Parker

Contents

PART I AN OVERVIEW OF EMERGENCY NURSING

1 **Introduction to Emergency Department Nursing** 3
   Janet Gren Parker

2 **Psychological Factors in the Emergency Department** 11
   Elizabeth G. Estrada

3 **Legal Issues in the Emergency Department** 23
   Nancy Stephens Donatelli

4 **Triage: Concept and Format** 39
   Janet Gren Parker

PART II NURSING CARE OF SELECTED EMERGENCIES

5 **Airway Problems** 53
   Janet Gren Parker

6 **Coma** 69
   Janet Gren Parker

7 **A Respiratory Emergency** 83
   Christina A. Ronshausen

8 **Congestive Heart Failure, Pulmonary Edema, or Pulmonary Embolus** 103
   Nancy L. Parrish

9 **An Upper Respiratory Infection, Croup, or Epiglottitis** 125
   Debbie Van Meter

10 **Angina, Myocardial Infarction, or Cardiogenic Shock** 143
   Molly P. Bronaugh

11 **Cardiopulmonary Arrest** 171
   Judy Stoner Halpern

12 **Cardiac Dysrhythmias** 189
    Susan K. MacArthur

13 **Thrombus, Embolus, Hypertensive Crisis, or Cerebrovascular Accident** 211
    Carol Beth Pulliam

14 **Abdominal Pain** 235
    Barbara Knezevich

15 **Epigastric Pain** 253
    Barbara Knezevich

16 **Minor Wounds and Bites** 271
    Dorothy M. Kellmer

17 **Orthopedic Trauma** 303
    Ann M. Van Hoff
    Nancy L. Griffith

18 **Facial Trauma** 331
    Judy Jo Wells-Mackie

19 **A Burn Injury** 347
    Janet Gren Parker

20 **Head and Spine Trauma** 361
    Judith "Ski" Lower

21 **Hypovolemic Shock, Septic Shock, or Disseminated Intravascular Coagulopathy** 395
    Cathy Bremer

22 **Chest Trauma** 417
    Judy Jo Wells-Mackie

23 **Abdominal Trauma** 435
    P. Howard Cummings
    Sally Pahnke Cummings

24 **Multiple Trauma** 455
    Janet Gren Parker

25 **The Pediatric Patient** 467
    Mitzi M. Lamberth

26 **An Overdose or Poisoning** 491
    Pamela W. Bourg
    Denise A. Gornick

27 **Drug or Alcohol Dependency** 509
    Pamela W. Bourg
    Marilyn K. Bourn

28 A Psychiatric Emergency   529
    Janet Gren Parker

29 Heat Disorders and Cold Disorders   541
    Margaret E. Moser

30 Obstetrical and Gynecological Problems   559
    Mary Ann Brown

PART III EMERGENCY NURSING AND COMMUNITY RESOURCES

31 Disaster Planning   585
    Janet Gren Parker

32 Evolving Trends in Emergency Nursing   595
    June D. Thompson

INDEX   605

AN OVERVIEW OF EMERGENCY NURSING

PART I

1

Introduction to Emergency Department Nursing

Janet Gren Parker

After completing this chapter, the reader will be able to do the following:

1. Discuss the relationship between the emergency department and the hospital.
2. Discuss the relationship between the emergency department and the community.
3. List sociological factors affecting increased public use of the emergency department.
4. Discuss consumer relations and the emergency department.
5. Discuss the past and current roles of the professional nurse within the emergency department.

For nurses who provide emergency health care, life can be demanding as well as dramatic. The medical crises that daily confront the emergency department nurse are only part of the exciting challenge. Vast changes are also taking place within this exciting field. Furthermore, a new awareness is developing that acknowledges the unique contributions made by health care professionals in the emergency department. Emergency nursing, therefore, is a challenging, exciting, and occasionally intimidating, specialty.

Modern medicine has seen an enormous growth in demand for emergency department services. Since World War II, the number of emergency department visits has increased by 600 percent. Nationally, the number of emergency department visits is increasing by 10 percent annually. Moreover, the number of visits by nonacute patients is also increasing (Pisarcik, 1980).

In this chapter, we will discuss a few of the major factors affecting emergency health care. Understanding these influences will help emergency department nurses—whether they are new to the specialty or currently involved in the field—to improve the quality of care that consumers receive in an emergency department.

THE EMERGENCY DEPARTMENT AND THE HOSPITAL

The emergency department formerly was called the emergency room; in fact, most people still call it either the emergency room or the ER. The emergency room itself was primarily located on the basement level, close to the delivery and refuse sites for the hospital. The term "emergency room" was appropriate, because it was indeed a single room, usually staffed with only a clerk, if anyone, and a nurse supervisor on call. Whenever a patient arrived, therefore, the clerk called the nurse, or sometimes the patient himself rang a bell announcing his presence in the emergency room. If the patient had a life-threatening illness or injury, the quality of care delivered was often inadequate.

Today the situation has changed. Most metropolitan emergency departments consist of several rooms, or they may encompass four or five areas, with each area containing several rooms. Nevertheless, inadequate conditions still remain in some rural areas. Seventy percent of all trauma occurs in rural areas, and the mortality rate for trauma victims is four times higher in rural areas than in metropolitan areas. Most emergency departments are now located in highly visible and accessible areas of the hospital. Most departments are staffed with permanent, full-time employees, including nurses and physicians. The quality of care has improved, and the consumer can feel more comfortable about receiving a high level of care in the emergency department.

These improvements did not occur either overnight or automatically. Full-time physician staffing began in the 1960s (Jenkins, 1978). The Department of Transportation established Emergency Medical Service (EMS) guidelines in 1966, as the result of the National Highway Safety Act. In 1968, the American College of Emergency Physicians was organized. The Emergency Department Nurses Association was organized in 1970. Furthermore, the University of Cincinnati established the first residency program in emergency medicine in 1970. In 1972, the Robert Wood Johnson Foundation funded 44 different projects to help establish EMS systems throughout the United States. In 1973, the federal government established a Division of Emergency Medical Services within its organizational structures. In 1979, emergency medicine was recognized as a board-certified specialty by the American Board of Medical Specialists.

Hospital administrators, as well as state and federal organizations, are beginning to recognize the value of the emergency department. Many hospital admissions originate in the emergency department. This financial incentive prompted some administrators to change their conception of the emergency department. Consequently, the emergency department is no longer the stepchild of the hospital; instead, it is one of the hospital's most important links to consumer satisfaction.

THE EMERGENCY DEPARTMENT AND THE COMMUNITY

An emergency was traditionally defined as a threat to life or limb that required immediate attention. Today, however, an *emergency* must be viewed from the consumer's perspective: "An emergency is an illness or injury for which the patient requires or desires the immediate attention of a physician" (Jenkins, 1978, p. 1).

The consumer's definition of an emergency illustrates the role of the emergency department as a *primary* health care facility. Many consumers use the emergency department for all their health care needs, either because they don't have a personal physician or because they prefer the convenience of the emergency department. In fact, only approximately five to ten percent of the visits to an emergency department are made by patients with critical illnesses or injuries. The majority of visits are made by patients with nonacute problems that a clinic or doctor's office could have handled appropriately.

The emergency department also functions in a *secondary* health care role. After the primary health care provider has seen the patient, the patient might be referred to the emergency department for more definitive care. A child, for example, who falls and strikes his head might be taken by his mother to see the pediatrician. The pediatrician, after examining the child, might refer him to the emergency department to be evaluated by the neurosurgeon. Other common referral sources include local clinics and health care centers staffed by nurse practitioners.

Emergency departments function in a *tertiary* health care role whenever they provide care for the critically ill patient or the major trauma victim. Most emergency departments are designed for and equipped to handle this health care role. The tertiary health care role relates to the traditional definition of an emergency.

The primary, secondary, and tertiary roles of the emergency department occasionally create conflicts between the consumer's expectations and the actual events that occur. The patient and the health care provider might establish incongruent priorities, for example, because they use different definitions to describe an emergency. When the emergency department is functioning in the tertiary role, the primary care patient may not realize that treating his sore throat is less urgent than treating the patient experiencing a myocardial infarction. The emergency department health care provider must understand this incongruence and be able and willing to handle it. The community must also be educated concerning the roles the emergency department plays in providing health care.

SOCIOLOGICAL FACTORS AFFECTING EMERGENCY DEPARTMENT USE

Why has the number of visits to the emergency department increased? Why do people use the emergency department as their primary source of health care? Underlying causes may involve sociological factors that have gradually developed within the United States.

Broad and drastic changes have characterized medical technology since World War II. Many consumers, therefore, believe that emergency departments are better informed about the new technology than are doctors or other primary health care providers. According to Hilker (1978), for example, the consumer's nonacute use of the emergency department demonstrates the consumer's preference for using the emergency department's facilities, rather than those of a clinic or doctor's office. Pisarcik (1980) supports this conclusion, identifying consumer attitude as a factor in the use of the emergency department. The consumer perceives a certain competency in the emergency department that is not perceived in the doctor's office or clinic.

Moreover, the consumer today is more mobile. The population migration in the

United States tends to increase the number of nonacute visits to the emergency department. When the consumer is a new resident in a city and he becomes sick, he initially may decide to visit the local emergency department for care. Furthermore, the consumer often tries to locate a primary health care provider after he develops an actual illness or injury, instead of obtaining one before an illness occurs.

Lack of available, personal health care providers eventually increases the number of patients who use the emergency department. According to the U.S. Department of Commerce, Bureau of the Census, the total number of physicians has increased, but the number choosing family practice has declined. (The percentages are illustrated in the following table.)

Year	Percent of Physicians in Family Practice
1970	16.4%
1975	12.6%
1977	11.8%

Even if the consumer tries to locate a primary health care provider difficulties may develop due to the decreasing number of family practitioners available to the consumer.

Third-party reimbursement for health care costs is another factor instrumental in increasing the number of visits to the emergency department. Many insurance policies (private, state, and federal) provide coverage for an emergency department visit, but not for a visit to a clinic or doctor's office. Consequently, the consumer logically uses the facility that is the least expensive, even though this cost eventually will effect an increase in insurance premiums for all consumers.

The major factor increasing emergency department use is consumer and physician convenience. In Hilker's study (1978), 74 percent of the parents of ill children attempted to contact some member of their primary health care group, but they were referred to the emergency department, instead of to the clinic or doctor's office. The medical community itself generates a substantial demand on the emergency department for the provision of nonacute care. Pisarcik (1980) identified the immediacy and the expediency of the emergency department as the primary factors influencing the consumer's use of the emergency department. The consumer felt that faster service was available at all hours of the day, thus making the emergency department more convenient to use than a doctor's office. The frustrated consumer who unsuccessfully tries to reach a primary health care provider quickly learns to use the emergency department during inconvenient hours and for expedient care. The strongest motivation for using the emergency department, of course, is the feeling by the consumer that, indeed, a true emergency exists (Fisher, 1981).

CONSUMER RELATIONS AND THE EMERGENCY DEPARTMENT

Because the emergency department is used as a primary, secondary, and tertiary health care center, traffic in the emergency department is always busy and transient.

The consumer, in fact, may formulate an impression of the entire hospital from the care received only in the emergency department. The emergency department, therefore, frequently is criticized by the consumer. The patient and family in the emergency department are often fearful, anxious, and highly stressed. Waiting time seems to drag, and the family becomes even more anxious. Because patients expect emergency department care to be expedient, they might complain if their care is not appropriate, according to their particular standards.

The staff in the emergency department must alleviate the fear and anxiety exhibited by patients and their families. Establishing an advanced nurse triage system is an excellent way to help improve consumer relations in the emergency department. (This nursing system is discussed in detail in Chapter 4.)

The attitude of the staff in the emergency department plays an important role in consumer relations. The staff, including all health care providers, clerical personnel, financial counselors, and social workers must be sensitive, patient, kind, and efficient. Their gentle caring must be transmitted to patients and their families in both words and actions. A climate of human warmth will help decrease the number of complaints, while it simultaneously enhances a positive image of the emergency department.

THE PROFESSIONAL NURSE IN THE EMERGENCY DEPARTMENT

> Emergency Nursing is a specialty area of professional nursing that involves the integration of practice, research, education, and professionalism. (*Standards of Emergency Nursing Practice*, 1983, p. 3)

This definition of *emergency nursing* was published by the Emergency Department Nurses Association. This definition, however, is being examined and revised to reflect changes in the evolving role of the nursing specialty.

The role of the professional nurse in the emergency department has changed. In the past, the nurse's role included scrubbing floors and walls, maintaining equipment, ordering and stocking supplies, registering patients, assisting the doctor, and, of course, caring for the patient. The role, however, has evolved into that of a specialist whose activities are quite different from those assigned to emergency department nurses in the past:

> The *scope* of emergency nursing practice encompasses nursing activities which are directed toward health problems of various levels of complexity. A rapidly changing physiological and/or psychological status, which may be life-threatening, requires assessment of the severity of the health problem, definitive intervention, ongoing reassessment, and supportive care to significant others. The level of physiological and/or psychological complexity may require life-support measures, appropriate health education, referral, and knowledge of legal implications. (*Standards of Emergency Nursing Practice*, 1983)

Emergency department nursing has evolved gradually into a specialty through the efforts of the Emergency Department Nurses Association. This organization has provided the impetus for change. The association's standards of emergency nursing practice, for example, provide a systematic approach to emergency nursing throughout the country, while concurrently standardizing the role of the professional nurse in the emergency department. Moreover, the association was instrumental in assigning nonnursing tasks to other appropriate hospital departments.

The role of the professional nurse has been expanded to include not only critical, life-saving care, but also preventative care, patient/family health education, and appropriate nursing referrals for continued care. This expanded role has supported the active use of nurse practitioners, clinical specialists, and trauma nurse specialists in emergency departments across the country.

The evolution of a competency-based certificate examination establishes the ability to recognize excellence in emergency nursing practice. This examination was developed by the Emergency Department Nurses Association in close consultation with the American Nurses' Association. After successfully completing the examination, a nurse is called a certified emergency nurse (CEN). This competency-based examination ensures the consumer of the high level of education and skills possessed by the nurse. It also establishes a recognizable baseline for assessing competency within the specialty.

CONCLUSION

Many changes have occurred in the area of emergency health care since World War II. The changes have affected the consumer, the hospital, the community, and the health care professional. The quality of emergency care, which has improved significantly, is continuing to evolve into a unique specialty responsible for monitoring, evaluating, and altering the quality of care the consumer receives.

Emergency nursing as a specialty is characterized by the following: brevity of patient interaction; the stressful climate created by an inability to control the number of patients seeking care; and the limited time frame in which to evaluate the effectiveness of intervention. Emergency nursing includes the care of people of all ages who have perceived physical or emotional alterations that are undiagnosed and may require prompt intervention.

Emergency nurses combine their interests in every subspecialty of nursing into one specialty. The specialty of emergency nursing, therefore, is challenging and frustrating, but also rewarding. The continual, ongoing evolution of this specialty will help to improve the quality of care the consumer receives in the emergency department.

BIBLIOGRAPHY

Fisher, J.: Self-referral to an accident and emergency department. *Nursing Times* 77:196–201 (Jan. 1981).

Friedman, E.: Emergency medical services: What's been done—and what hasn't. *Hospitals* 54:69–73 (1980).

BIBLIOGRAPHY

Hilker, T. L.: Nonemergency visits to a pediatric emergency department. *JACEP* 7:3–8 (1978).

Jenkins, A. L.: *Emergency Department Organization and Management.* American College of Emergency Physicians. St. Louis: Mosby, 1978.

Langhorne, F.: Put out the welcome mat in the emergency department. *Point of View* 16:22 (Oct. 1979).

Pisarcik, G.: Why patients use the emergency department. *Journal of Emergency Nursing* 6:16–21 (1980).

Sadler, A. M.; B. L. Sadler; and S. B. Webb: *Emergency Medical Care: The Neglected Public Service.* Cambridge, MA: Ballinger, 1977.

Simoneau, J. K., and P. McCall: Emergency care update! *Critical Care Update* 6:30–32 (1979).

Standards of Emergency Nursing Practice. St. Louis: Mosby, 1983

Statistical Abstract of the United States. Washington, DC: U.S. Department of Commerce, Bureau of the Census, 1979.

2
Psychological Factors in the Emergency Department

Elizabeth G. Estrada

After completing this chapter, the reader will be able to do the following:

1. Discuss factors that influence the patient's and family's perception of the emergency visit.
2. Discuss actions of the emergency staff that facilitate the emergency visit.
3. Discuss psychological crises in detail.
4. Discuss crisis intervention techniques.
5. List stress factors affecting staff involved in emergency care.

The emergency department, a constantly changing physical and emotional environment, receives the gamut of health conditions—patients of all ages, with diverse medical problems, in various stages of illness, and from different cultural, social, and economic backgrounds. Understanding the effects of psychological factors on the patients, their families, and staff is crucial to ensuring comprehensive delivery of care in the emergency department. Understanding the effects of both psychosocial and emotional forces can provide the key to effective management of a difficult emergency situation.

Whenever a patient appears in an emergency facility for care, anxiety is present. This anxiety, however, cannot always be measured by examining the person's external behavior. The professional providing comprehensive emergency care, therefore, is responsible for developing the assessment and intervention skills required to alleviate the patient's anxiety and stress.

PATIENT'S PERCEPTIONS OF THE EMERGENCY VISIT

Numerous factors can influence the patient's perception of and reaction to an emergency visit: for example, sociological background, physiological condition, economic status, communication skills, educational level, previous emergency facility experience, status of the emergency department environment, personal external stress, and approach of the staff. Any one of these factors will affect the person's response to the health care delivery system.

Sociological Background

Cultural and sociological background may influence the person's perception of health care in general. In some cultures, the hospital is the last place to go, when other cultural remedies are ineffective. These patients may appear in the emergency department only as a last resort, perhaps when death is pending. These patients are usually frightened, when they arrive for care. Patients from other cultural backgrounds, however, might bring their entire families with them to the hospital.

Physiological Condition

The physical condition of the patient upon arrival may cause the person to develop a distorted image of the emergency department. The patient in extreme pain, for instance, may narrowly focus attention on his body, the specific person talking with him, his own stretcher, and his own room. This person may be unaware of anything else that is happening in the emergency department. In addition, this patient's physiological problems might cause problems: for example, the patient may exhibit distorted thought processes, inappropriate behavioral responses, and inadequate coping mechanisms.

Economic Status

Understanding the influence of economic status on the emergency patient is essential. A particular accident or injury that adversely influences the person's ability to maintain job responsibility will be another major source of anxiety. Apprehension concerning additional costs incurred for emergency services, in addition to fear of unemployment and decreased health care benefits, will also increase the patient's anxiety.

Communication Level

Difficulties increase whenever a language barrier exists between the patients and staff. The inability to communicate because of a language barrier can cause numerous misunderstandings. Because the influx of visitors from foreign countries is increasing, a system for facilitating communication is necessary. Using translators could perhaps help to minimize this problem.

Moreover, written and verbal communications often affect the patient's perception. In the case of a deaf and/or dumb person, for example, the communication system will significantly influence the amount of anxiety the person experiences. In addition, misunderstandings often occur whenever patients are subjected to complex jargon.

Educational Level

Educational background may also affect a person's ability to understand the emergency processes and procedures. Explanations given to a patient must be compatible with the person's ability to comprehend the information. Additional knowledge might decrease anxiety in some patients, but increase anxiety in others. A person with a health care background, for instance, may have a higher anxiety level, because the person knows the possible complications that might develop.

Past Emergency Facility Experience

Previous visits to the emergency department will influence the patient's perception of the emergency department. If a previous visit was negative, the individual will experience more anxiety concerning the current visit. If, however, the previous visit was positive, the person will perceive the situation with less anxiety.

Status of the Environment

Number of People
The number of strangers in the environment can also affect a patient's anxiety level. The staff, of course, can offer some comfort. Nevertheless, the number of patients who exhibit various stages of illness and levels of anxiety can affect, and perhaps even escalate, another patient's anxiety.

Amount of Noise
A quiet emergency department may help to calm an anxious individual. Studies in various industrial settings, for example, have demonstrated that excessive noise can increase a person's anxiety level.

Privacy Available
The right to privacy is important to most patients. Revealing internal thoughts and personal history is easier when privacy is available and respected. Physical privacy during examinations is essential, and provisions must be made that are appropriate for the particular emergency department.

Visual Factors

Similar to noise, visual stimuli can influence a person's perception of situations and events. Because the perception of patients under the influence of drugs can be distorted drastically, bright colors may trigger anxiety episodes.

Personal External Stress

Other factors, unrelated to the patient's experiences in the emergency department, may also affect the person's behavior. Personal, family, or work problems, for example, may be additional factors that can affect the person's anxiety level.

Life Changes

Holmes and Rahe (1967) demonstrated that the number of changes (positive as well as negative) in a person's life can increase the possibility that illness and injury will occur. Because change can cause anxiety, a person may be more susceptible to having accidents or to developing altered health conditions.

Table 2.1 contains a sample of the life change scale used for assessment. A person notes how many major events included in the list have occurred in his or her own life in the last 12 months. Each event receives a specific rating. A score between 150 and 199 suggests mild stress, whereas a score higher than 300 indicates high stress. If an individual scores with high stress, the number of changes planned in the future should be reexamined to minimize the potential for incurring illness or injury.

Entering the emergency care system will cause some stress for the patient. In addition, a significant change in health status would produce additional stress.

Approach of the Staff

The approach of the staff can significantly influence the patient's perception of the emergency situation, as well as influence the patient's ability to develop appropriate and adequate coping mechanisms. Competence and professionalism from the staff will help the patient develop confidence in the care delivered.

TYPES OF PSYCHOLOGICAL CRISES

According to Caplan (1964), several factors produce a crisis. First, a precipitating event occurs. Second, the event causes a threat to basic securities. Third, the person is unable to handle the threat with appropriate coping mechanisms.

The types of crises that arise in the emergency department are as follows:

Open anxiety.	Depression.	Acute psychosis.
Verbal aggression.	Grief.	Agitated depression.
Violence.	Panic.	Disaster reactions.

(Many of these crises are discussed in subsequent chapters in this book.)

TABLE 2.1 Life Change Scale

Event Value	Event
100	Death of a spouse
73	Divorce
65	Marital separation
63	Jail term
63	Death of close family member
53	Personal injury or illness
50	Marriage
47	Fired from job
45	Marital reconciliation
45	Retirement
44	Change in health of family member
40	Pregnancy
39	Sex difficulties
39	Gain of new family member
39	Business readjustment
38	Change in financial state
37	Death of close friend
36	Change to different line of work
35	Change in number of arguments with spouse
31	Mortgage over $10,000
30	Foreclosure of mortgage or loan
29	Change in responsibilities at work
29	Son or daughter leaving home
29	Trouble with in-laws
28	Outstanding personal achievement
26	Wife begins or stops work
26	Begin or end school
25	Change in living conditions
24	Revision of personal habits
23	Trouble with boss
20	Change in work hours or conditions
20	Change in residence
20	Change in schools
19	Change in recreation
19	Change in church activities
18	Change in social activities
17	Mortgage or loan less than $10,000
16	Change in sleeping habits
15	Change in number of family get-togethers
15	Change in eating habits
13	Vacation
12	Christmas
11	Minor violations of the law

SOURCE: Holmes and Masuda, 1972.

REACTIONS TO CRISES

James Tyhurst (1957), a social psychiatrist, describes three phases of an individual's reaction to a crisis at the time of a major disaster: impact, recoil, and posttraumatic phases.

The impact phase includes the initial reaction. One person may calmly accept the crisis situation. Another person, however, may be stunned, bewildered, confused, or anxious.

In some instances, the impact phase or shock may last until the person enters the emergency facility. Responses vary, depending on the psychological resources of the individual. The transition from the impact phase to the recoil phase, for instance, may occur in the emergency department. The initial shock may decrease, as the patient gradually returns to selfconsciousness and awareness. In general, the patient must relate his emotions to obtain support. In this phase, the patient is the most receptive to psychological intervention.

In the posttraumatic phase, the patient realizes the major significance of the recent disaster, such as a change in body image, loss of a loved one, continued medical care required, loss of ability to work, and so forth. In this phase, the individual's coping mechanisms may be rigid and more difficult to alter. Depression, for example, may develop. If during the recoil phase, however, the situation was therapeutic, the effects of the posttraumatic phase can be minimized.

CRISIS INTERVENTION

Establishing Priorities

In implementing any approach to a difficult psychological situation, the triage nurse must establish priorities of care. The first priority is protecting the patient, the patient's family, and the staff from physical harm. After ensuring safety, the next priority is establishing rapport between the nurse and the patient. The third priority is assessing psychosocial and emotional symptoms. The fourth priority is implementing an effective intervention.

Ensure Safety

Wickersty (1982) emphasizes the importance of using nonoffensive physical control techniques, not merely self-defensive measures, but actual controlling procedures used to restrain physically aggressive patients. These techniques, as well as the proper use of restraints, should be mastered by health professionals working in an emergency department, because violent reactions to anxiety occur frequently in emergency situations.

Assessment

Assessment of a crisis includes the following: information is obtained from the patient and analyzed; nonverbal data is analyzed; and present interactions are observed. Determining the precipitating factors is also important in the assessment phase. Inappropriate behavior, for example, can be caused by a physiological etiology.

According to Margolin (1980), a Mental Status Examination notes the following characteristics of the patient: general appearance and behavior; stream of speech; mood and affect; mental content; perception; cognitive functioning; and judgment and insight.

Assessment of *general appearance and behavior* would reveal any obvious physical deficits and neurological deficiency, as well as the patient's attitude and general response to the situation. Careful assessment of *speech pattern, mood, and affect* might demonstrate depression, cardiac insufficiency, or neurological deficiencies. Examining a person's *mental content* includes obtaining information about hallucinations, delusions, and suicidal ideology. Assessing a patient's *perception* may reveal intoxication, delirium, or a seizure disorder. Assessing *cognitive functioning* includes examining orientation, attention span, concentration, knowledge, memory, and reasoning. Assessing *judgment and insight* will provide information concerning a person's ability to make decisions and his understanding of his current medical problem.

Paltrow's "Review of Areas" (1980) contains a guideline for making a comprehensive assessment. According to Paltrow, a person expends energy in six possible areas, which include actual, as well as anticipated, events:

1. *Biomedical*—prenatal, birth, family biomedical history; physical, mental, and spiritual illnesses; accidents, operations, hospitalizations; use and abuse of drugs.
2. *Social*—family, friends, marriages; divorces; sexual relationships; children; community and social organizations; religious affiliation; economic status; cultural and national background; travel history; geography of residence.
3. *Vocational*—past, current, and anticipated occupations; industrial hazards, military service; activities of daily living, transportation, and money management.
4. *Recreation*—hobbies, sports, and interests.
5. *Learning*—formal schooling, self-education, and acquisition of skills.
6. *Emotional*—methods for discharging major emotions, such as anger, depression, or anxiety; suicidal or homicidal ideation/attempts; ego defense mechanisms.

The type of detail required for making a psychological assessment depends on the current situation and chief complaint. A complete psychological profile is not necessary in the emergency department. Nevertheless, sufficient data collected from the history and from observing the patient's behavior are required to determine the etiology of the crisis and to select the most effective intervention.

Intervention

Effective intervention involves the following: eliminating communication barriers; using a professional approach; and selecting and implementing an intervention process. One must remain calm and avoid making any snap judgments, while determining the problem or selecting the intervention.

Types of Interventions

To initiate the intervention process, the nurse *assists the individual to accept the existence of a crisis*. If the patient admits feelings of fear and discomfort, for instance, he may relieve some of his tension.

A crisis often contains multiple components: for instance, death of a loved one, injury to self, nobody to care for the children, no health insurance, and so forth. The nurse, therefore, must *assist the patient in confronting the various components one at a time in tolerable doses*.

If misinformation or misperception exists, *clarification and confirmation of facts* might relieve the person's anxiety. Facts about childhood diseases and normal symptoms, for example, might allay the fears of an anxious parent.

If withdrawal or denial prevents the patient from dealing with the problem, helping the patient to *focus on the reality of the present situation* may facilitate appropriate coping mechanisms.

In some situations, the patient might be *directed towards developing adaptive behaviors*. Saying that it is acceptable to cry, when a person struggles desperately not to cry after receiving news of a family member's death, for instance, will direct the patient toward effective coping behavior.

Encouraging a person to talk about his feelings and *listening with a caring attitude* will help a person to release anxiety. In some instances, changing one's volume or rate of speaking may help calm the patient.

Honesty is crucial for establishing an effective intervention. In a crisis, deceptive reassurance and unrealistic promises are inappropriate.

An appropriate *therapeutic touch* often comforts depressed or upset patients. The health professional, however, must slowly enter the borders of a patient's personal space to prevent causing further anxiety through an unexpected intrusion.

If environmental factors are contributing to the patient's stress, the *environment should be manipulated, if possible, to be therapeutic:* for example, dimming bright lights, changing temperature, reducing noise, or changing the patient's room.

If family members are supportive and do not produce additional anxiety for a patient, then *family* members should be included in the crisis intervention. A child or spouse, for example, may remain calmer in the presence of a close relative.

The *appropriate use of humor* can release the tension that a patient feels. Using humor in the form of lighthearted comments or jokes might distract a patient temporarily. Jokes that might belittle the patient's condition or feelings, however, must be avoided.

Chemotherapy may be necessary in crisis intervention. Hazel and Estrada (1980) divide commonly used medications into four categories: antianxiety drugs, antipsychotic drugs, antidepressant drugs, and antimanic drugs. Antianxiety drugs (Librium, Valium, Vistaril, etc.) are fast-acting drugs that cause muscle relaxation and reduction of anxiety. Antipsychotic drugs (Thorazine, Prolixin, Melleril, Stelazine, Haldol, etc.) are used to suppress agitation, rage, hallucinations, and paranoia. These drugs, however, are not immediately effective, since they may take 2 to 21 days to establish a therapeutic level. Antidepressant drugs (Elavil, Tofranil, Nardil, Sinequan, etc.) relieve target symptoms of depression, such as insomnia and anorexia, and they can cause sedation. These drugs reach maximum effect within two to four weeks after therapy is established. Antimanic drugs (Lithium) will take perhaps 10 days to establish a therapeutic level that will prevent exhaustion in a manic individual.

Because many drugs require time to reach a chemotherapeutic level, they are not effective in the emergency care setting. Although antianxiety drugs can be used, drug therapy must not replace psychological intervention. Because the psychological problem may continue after the drug wears off, opportunity to change a person's ineffective coping behavior could be lost.

If the pain or physical condition is a major factor in the patient's anxiety, *relief of the pain or physical problem* can help reduce or even eliminate the crisis situation. Providing comfort, such as a change in position or a pillow, can be effective in decreasing anxiety.

If psychological intervention is not effective, the person's coping abilities may deteriorate, and behavior may escalate into physical aggression. Intervention in this case involves protecting the patient and one's self from harm. (Specific interventions for people experiencing death and grieving, sudden infant death, sexual assault, child and person abuse, and drug abuse will be discussed in subsequent chapters in this book.)

Resolution

Every interaction includes a resolution phase. Necessary referrals should be made before the patient leaves the emergency department. Moreover, the patient might be receptive to suggestions about meeting with a psychologist, social worker, psychiatrist, or crisis worker during the difficult adjustment period after a major incident. Through appropriate intervention and appropriate response to the intervention, however, the patient may develop effective coping mechanisms before leaving the hospital. During the resolution phase, the staff should conduct patient and/or family teaching. Moreover, this time period can be used for additional therapeutic interventions. Careful explanations can allay potential anxiety that occurs whenever patients are not well informed about self-care after discharge. Appropriate resources from the hospital or outside agencies should be made available to the patient.

Carefully documenting not only physical condition, but also significant mental and emotional states is necessary to complete the patient's record.

Evaluation

If a particular patient was upset during an emergency department visit, the staff should call the patient either the next day or soon after. The purpose of the call is to determine whether the patient is coping adequately. The call also demonstrates the hospital staff's concern for the patient. In addition, the staff will receive feedback concerning the effectiveness of their intervention. These calls, therefore, can be effective public relations tools.

Evaluating the effectiveness of staff intervention can be accomplished by scheduling regular "crisis rounds." During a team conference, case studies of patients who have demonstrated extremely anxious behavior and aggressive episodes are discussed. An interdisciplinary perspective permits nurses, physicians, social workers, chaplains, hospital security, and other important personnel to discuss situations that were difficult for them and to propose possible approaches for handling similar situations in the future. These team conferences can be valuable learning experiences for all staff members.

Chart audit should include documentation of psychological interventions. Careful monitoring will reveal continuing education required in the areas of crisis intervention. In addition, the appropriateness of referrals can also be evaluated.

An increase in the number of patients who leave the emergency department against medical advice should alert the staff to investigate possible causes. Waiting time may not be the only factor that causes patients to leave. Some patients may be reacting to perceived inappropriate staff behavior. Perceiving that the staff are under tremendous stress can intensify the patient's already anxious state.

FACTORS AFFECTING STAFF

Stress Factors

Personal Stress
The staff may have personal emotional problems that affect their communication and performance. The staff, therefore, must not allow personal concerns to interfere with their professional duties.

Professional Expectations
Stress also results from anxiety caused by professional expectations. Meeting the expectations of colleagues who expect a specific performance level of practice causes some anxiety. Furthermore, issues of professional ethics occur frequently because members of the health care team must make professional and ethical judgments while they are performing their duties.

Peer Pressure
Role ambiguity and lack of an interdisciplinary philosophy produce inadequate and ineffective communication systems. Personnel who work closely under stressful conditions occasionally create stress for one another, thus, professional energy can be dissipated in peer anxiety.

Stress from Patients and Their Families
Whenever the number of patients and the amount of work increases, the staff will experience additional physical and psychological stress. The number and intensity of difficult psychological reactions from patients and their families can tax the ability of the staff to handle the stress encountered.

Environmental Stress
Working conditions also affect the staff's stress. An area designated exclusively for staff should be used as a place for venting frustration, sharing experiences, and

resting periodically. A well-organized and well-designed unit must consider the influence of environment on the staff. Soothing colors should be chosen. Lounges and rest rooms should be accessible and comfortable. Inadequate, deficient, or outdated equipment and supplies that can cause additional stress should be eliminated from the department.

Effective Use of Stress

A certain amount of stress is considered normal for everyone. Stress creates the impetus to act. Stress, if recognized, controlled, and used appropriately, can assist a person in accomplishing goals.

Each person, however, must develop ways to reduce stress whenever it becomes more frequent, intolerable, or interferes with professional practice. Physical exercise is healthy, and it is also an excellent way to reduce frustration and stress. Health professionals in particular should be concerned with health and fitness. Being physically fit will provide an important resource for patients as well as staff during a crisis.

The ability to relax can be developed through practicing various relaxation techniques, such as deep breathing and imaging or visualization. Through imaging or visualization, a person might relax while visualizing a scene containing a mountain and a stream.

The appropriate use of humor among staff members can be effective in reducing work tensions, although joking should not be done near patients or their families.

Work breaks are important, especially for staff members who are functioning in stressful situations. Unfortunately, breaks frequently are omitted, due to the large number of patients or to the excessive amount of work. Breaks, however, may not only reduce stress, but also increase the staff's efficiency.

Because the number of changes can increase team anxiety, plans for changes in policy, procedures, responsibilities, and so forth should be carefully planned.

Because role ambiguity and conflict can cause professional anxiety and stress among staff members, scheduling conferences to discuss these subjects might assist in reducing the problems. Team agreement on appropriate roles and responsibilities will facilitate staff communication and functioning. Furthermore, agreement will assist the staff in creating a professional climate that produces minimal role anxiety.

CONCLUSION

After ensuring safety, the nurse assesses the situation to determine the etiology of the crisis, then implements appropriate and effective intervention. Skill in crisis intervention includes knowledge of physical and psychological methods to decrease anxiety or to control aggression. Understanding ways to reduce stress can facilitate the staff's ability to handle crisis situations that occur in the emergency department. Distressing behaviors can be less stressful if they are understood and if measures for reducing anxiety are established.

BIBLIOGRAPHY

August, S. C.: Communication in Crisis. In S. A. Budassi and J. M. Barber (eds): *Emergency Nursing: Principles and Practice.* St. Louis: Mosby, 1981, pp. 21–34.

Billings, V.: Providing better emergency care when behaviors bar the way. *Nursing 82* 12:57 (1982).

Cameron, C. T. M.: *Public Relations In The Emergency Department.* Bowie, MD: Bardy, 1980.

Caplan, C.: *Principles of Preventative Psychiatry.* New York: Basic Books, 1964.

Hazel, J. P., and E. G. Estrada: Nursing Process in Crisis Intervention. In *Emergency Department Nursing Association Core Curriculum.* Chicago: EDNA, 1980, pp. 333–356.

Holmes, T., and Rahe, R.: The social readjustment rating scale. *Journal of Psychosomatic Research* 11:213–218 (1967).

Knowles, R. D.: Managing angry feelings. *American Journal of Nursing* 82:299 (1982).

Margolin, C. B.: Assessment of psychiatric patients. *Journal of Emergency Nursing* 6:30–33 (1980).

Murray, R.: What to do with crying, clinging, demanding, seductive, abusive, and withdrawn patients. *Nursing Life* 1:32–39 (1982).

Nichols, N.: Psychiatric interventions in the emergency room. *Journal of the American Medical Women's Association* 33:374–391 (1978).

Paltrow, K.: Review of areas updated. *Postgraduate Medicine* (Jan. 1980).

Pisarcik, G. K.: Psychiatric Emergencies. In S. A. Budassi and J. M. Barber (eds.): *Emergency Nursing: Principles and Practice.* St. Louis: Mosby, 1981, pp. 516–549.

———: Psychiatric Emergencies and Crisis Intervention. In J. L. Spinella (ed.): Symposium on Emergency Nursing. *Nursing Clinics of North America.* Philadelphia: Saunders, 1981, pp. 85–94.

Rada, R.: Violent patient: rapid assessment and management. *Psychosomatics* 22:101–105, 109 (1981).

Speich, P. L.: Taking a psychosocial stress "Pulse." *Journal of Emergency Nursing* 5:43–47 (1979).

Tyhurst, J. S.: The role of transition states—including disasters—in mental illness. In proceedings of the Symposium on Preventative and Social Psychiatry, Washington, DC, 1957, at Walter Reed Army Institute of Research, p. 766.

Wickersty, A.: Controlling aggression in the health care setting (an unpublished workshop manual). Cheverly, MD: Wickersty and Associates, 1982.

3

Legal Issues in the Emergency Department

Nancy Stephens Donatelli

After completing this chapter, the reader will be able to do the following:

1. Understand the hospital's responsibility to provide emergency care.
2. Define malpractice, negligence, statutory law, case law, constitutional law, assault and battery.
3. Identify the four basic elements of negligence that must be alleged and proven for an award to be made.
4. Define two types of consent.
5. Discuss the procedure for obtaining consent for minors.
6. Describe the appropriate procedure to be followed for handling a patient who refuses treatment or leaves against medical advice (AMA).
7. Identify cases that must be reported to the proper authorities.
8. Describe the appropriate procedure to be followed for organ donation.
9. Understand the nurse's role in obtaining blood alcohol levels for legal reasons.
10. Identify the emergency department's responsibility for dead on arrival (DOA) cases.
11. Describe the procedure for dispensing medications from the emergency department.
12. Discuss the procedure for documenting emergency department records.
13. Understand the importance of confidentiality with respect to releasing information and the patient's right to privacy.
14. Identify the requirements necessary for conducting a patient transfer between institutions.
15. Understand the legal implications of giving telephone advice.

16. Identify the important legal aspects of caring for a psychiatric patient.
17. Understand the importance of using available, well-maintained equipment and well-trained staff in the emergency department.

The emergency department nurse must combine skills of quick recall, common sense, and good judgment, while remaining calm within the high pressure environment of the emergency department. In addition, the nurse must also safeguard the patient's welfare and uphold the principle of *primum non nocere* (first, do no harm).

The nurse must understand the legal implications inherent in the care given to patients, in addition to understanding the medical aspects of that care. Health care professionals have become more aware of legal issues in recent years. A chapter relating to legal issues in the emergency department, therefore, is appropriate for a comprehensive book on emergency nursing.

In this chapter we discuss background information necessary for understanding legal considerations affecting the emergency department. Requirements from hospital regulatory agencies, as well as information from legal authorities, are discussed.

THE HOSPITAL'S DUTY TO PROVIDE CARE

To comply with regulations established by agencies that provide third party reimbursement, a hospital must provide emergency care. Furthermore, hospitals maintaining emergency health care facilities may not turn away or refuse patients who ask for emergency health care. Regardless of the patient's definition of an emergent situation, any emergency health care providers refusing to treat a patient could make both the emergency department and themselves vulnerable either to criticism or to legal action. This position has emerged through case law, state laws and regulations, and federal laws, such as the Hill–Burton Act.

According to the Joint Commission on Accreditation of Hospitals (JCAH), "any individual who comes to the hospital for emergency medical evaluation or initial treatment shall be properly assessed by qualified individuals, and appropriate services be rendered within the defined capability of the hospital" (JCAH, 1981, p. 23). This principle must be implemented for the institution to be licensed and thus to be approved for third-party reimbursement. Any hospital that accepts Hill–Burton federal funds is responsible for providing in exchange a certain amount of free medical care to indigent patients.

Case law has played a role in helping to establish the duty of a hospital to provide emergency care, as illustrated in the case of *Wilmington General Hospital* v. *Manlove* (1961):

> In Manlove, the parents of a four-month-old infant with a recent history of fever and diarrhea brought the child to the hospital emergency department. Since the child had been under the care of private pediatricians, no physician or nurse examined or treated the child since the child was, at present, in no acute distress. The child was sent home by the nurse, who explained to the parents that the hospital's policy was to decline emergency treatment to per-

sons already under the care of a private physician. That afternoon the child died of bronchopneumonia. The key issue before the court was whether the hospital had a duty to provide emergency treatment in the face of an unmistakable emergency. The Court held that it did. The hospital's liability was based primarily upon the parents' reliance on the hospital's capacity to render emergency care, and the fact that this was a case that could be held to involve an unmistakable emergency. If a hospital holds itself out to the public as having the capability to render emergency treatment to persons who have reasonably relied on such representations then they may not refuse to give care. Refusal to treat might well worsen the condition of the injured person because of time lost in a useless attempt to obtain medical aid. In the Manlove case this duty outweighed the hospital's internal policies. (George, 1980, p. 20)

Treating anyone who presents for emergency care is the hospital's responsibility. Consequently, implementing such care should be standard policy in the emergency department.

GENERAL LEGAL TERMS

After briefly reviewing several legal terms, we will discuss specific legal issues affecting emergency nursing care.

The term *negligence* is defined by Webster as "failure to exercise the care that the circumstances justly demand." In other words, negligence is a deviation from the accepted standard of care.

Although the terms negligence and malpractice are often used interchangeably, malpractice adds to the definition of negligence the words, "with resultant harm." In *malpractice,* the deviation from the standard of care must invoke harm to the individual.

Four elements of negligence must be alleged and proven in a court of law to sustain a lawsuit for that negligence.

1. *Duty:* Because the health practitioner takes the patient into his care, the law imposes on him a duty to proceed reasonably. In performing this duty, the practitioner must provide the patient with care similar to that given by other health professionals in similar circumstances.
2. *Breach of duty:* The failure to carry out a reasonable standard of care.
3. *Damages:* The person who has filed the complaint must have suffered harm as a result of the incident. Since the purpose of this legal action is to compensate for damages, damage must be apparent.
4. *Proximate cause:* Some reasonable cause and effect relationship between the supposed act of negligence and the damages sustained must exist.

Statutory law, another legal term, is law enacted by a legislative body, such as a state legislature.

Case law, however, is an interpretation by the courts on statutes, administrative rules, and the underlying common law. An example of case law is the ruling made in the Manlove case previously mentioned.

Constitutional law determines the validity of both statutory decisions and case law within the provisions of the fourth, fifth, and fourteenth constitutional amendments.

Assault and battery, terms often associated with criminal action, are two distinct entities. *Assault* is defined as a threat to do harm to another person, without the actual performance of that threatened harm. *Battery* is the actual touching of another person without the person's consent. Obtaining a patient's consent for treatment is thus essential to prevent technically the filing of a charge of battery against the health care provider.

CONSENT TO TREAT

In any emergency department the question concerning consent for treatment frequently arises. This question may pertain to any type of patient, such as a minor, a patient with a psychiatric problem, an intoxicated individual, or a comatose patient. Consent to treat arises out of the law of battery, in essence, the touching of a person without the person's consent.

Two basic types of consent exist. When a patient voluntarily presents for treatment, the consent is *implied*. Implied consent may also exist in cases of mental incompetence due to psychosis, drugs, alcohol, organic disease, or unconsciousness. The patient with any one of these conditions may require treatment to save his life; if that patient could give his consent, he probably would. In the event of a life-threatening situation, therefore, consent is implied, and treatment begins immediately. Failure to treat in this situation could make the health care provider liable for legal redress.

In *informed express consent*, the second type of consent, the patient is informed of any risks, consequences, or alternatives involved in his treatment, before he either verbally or in writing authorizes said treatment. The physician is legally responsible for relaying this information to the patient. It is customarily hospital policy to obtain the patient's express consent in writing. This consent is then dated, timed, and witnessed.

Nevertheless, "the question has been raised as to whether the general express consent to treatment, signed by patients when they register with the emergency department clerk is legally sufficient for subsequent treatment. This initial consent to treatment acknowledges the establishment of a voluntary physician–patient relationship and is satisfactory consent for customary physician–patient procedures (such as physical examination, venipuncture, injections, and x-rays). However, more definitive procedures, such as intravenous pyelograms or lumbar punctures, should be evidenced by a more specific consent form acknowledging these procedures as more than merely routine" (George, 1980, p. 39). The physician performing the procedure must explain to the patient the aforementioned information that relates to the procedure, answer any questions asked by the patient concerning the procedure, and obtain the written consent.

If a patient is physically or mentally unable to give consent and a true emergency situation exists, consent should be obtained from a person whose relationship to the patient authorizes him to act on the patient's behalf. An authorized person may be a relative or court-appointed guardian. "The exact order in which relatives should be contacted may vary from state to state. However, the following order is generally acceptable: spouse, parent, adult child, adult brother or sister, adult aunt or uncle or grandparents" (George, 1980, p. 45).

MINOR'S CONSENT

A minor is any person whose age falls below the legally recognized age of adulthood, or below the age of majority. This age varies from state to state. Some states have lowered the age of majority from 21 years to 18 years. Courts in general have acknowledged that an emancipated minor may consent to treatment. In determining if a minor is emancipated, the practitioner considers the patient's age, maturity, marital status, degree of self-sufficiency, economic independence, and general ability to understand the nature of the proposed treatment. Several states have enacted legislation allowing minors to consent for treatment for specific conditions, such as venereal disease, pregnancy, alcoholism, and drug abuse. The nurse in the emergency department should be aware of specific state laws relating to the treatment of the emancipated minor.

When a nonemancipated minor presents to the emergency department without his parents, consent for treatment must be obtained, unless a life-threatening emergency situation exists. As previously stated, in the event of a life-threatening situation, consent is implied, and treatment begins immediately.

In obtaining consent, one must make every reasonable attempt to contact a parent. After a parent is reached, an informed, express oral consent can be obtained over the telephone and witnessed by another emergency department employee. This consent must be witnessed and documented as such on the emergency department record.

If the parents are legally divorced or separated, consent should be obtained from the parent who has legal custody. When a minor arrives in the department with a form providing signed authorization for treatment in case of an emergency, an attempt to contact the parent to obtain informed, express consent should still be made. Nevertheless, "if the parents cannot be located, it is legally acceptable for the emergency department staff to rely on the signed parental authorization presented by the individual acting in "loco parentis" (in the place of a parent). When in doubt, one should get the informed express written consent of anybody with the minor, as well as the minor himself, if he is sufficiently mature" (George, 1980, p. 48).

If the parent cannot be located, the emergency department nurse "should try to contact a close relative, such as an adult brother or sister, aunt or uncle, or grandparents" (George, 1980, p. 47). Furthermore, "if efforts to locate a close relative are unsuccessful and well documented on the emergency department record, the emergency department staff may reasonably rely on the informed consent given by the person who has custody of the child and who has brought the minor to the emergency department" (George, 1980, p. 48). Obtaining consent often takes a considerable amount of time. The minor, therefore, should be made comfortable, while preliminary first aid is performed.

Good Samaritan laws were enacted to protect citizens from liability for their acts of omissions occurring in attempts to render emergency medical aid to ill or injured persons. Thus, "some states have Good Samaritan laws that cover every person, whereas other states have laws that limit coverage to health care professionals, such as physicians or nurses, or first aid or ambulance squad personnel" (George, 1980, p. 145). Furthermore,

> Generally speaking, any attempts by the emergency physician or nurse to use Good Samaritan immunity for negligent actions that occur in the hospital emergency department are likely to fail in courts. Courts have traditionally been reluctant to extend Good Samaritan immunity beyond emergency care given outside of the hospital.
>
> Thus, it would seem that immunity for prehospital emergency care would exist for EMT-paramedics and emergency physicians and nurses at the scene and enroute to the hospital. It would seem clear that emergency physicians and nurses would not be immune from liability after receiving the patient from the EMTs in the emergency department, unless specific state law granted such immunity. (George, 1980, p. 149)

In view of these facts, it would seem prudent for the emergency department staff to know the Good Samaritan laws governing the state in which they are employed.

REFUSAL OF TREATMENT

Mentally competent adults or emancipated minors, who adequately understand their conditions and the consequences of not being treated, cannot be forced to receive treatment, even during a life-threatening emergency. The key, however, is determining whether the patient is competent to make this decision. Every effort, therefore, should be made to determine why the patient is refusing treatment.

If the patient continues to refuse treatment, the facts surrounding the incident must be thoroughly documented on the record. Moreover, the patient should sign a statement releasing the hospital from any responsibility of liability for nontreatment, since the patient is leaving against medical advice (AMA). If the patient refuses to sign AMA, this refusal must also be documented. If the patient's refusal to receive treatment constitutes a life or death situation, hospital administrators should be informed, and they should become actively involved in pursuing the situation. Administrative action may constitute using a court order to permit life-saving treatment to proceed. The hospital may request the court to appoint a temporary guardian empowered to consent to the appropriate treatment.

REPORTABLE SITUATIONS

Table 3.1 lists typical events that must be reported to the appropriate authorities. Nurses must be aware of special requirements and procedures that are unique to their particular state and/or institution of employment.

In each reportable situation, a detailed history and physical examination is necessary. For reportable communicable diseases, the hospital's infection control nurse

TABLE 3.1 Reportable Events

Event	Detailed History	Physical Exam	Special Consent for Exam	Reportable to	Special Lab Test or Procedure for Legal Reasons	Clothing Kept as Evidence
Motor vehicle accident	×	×		Police	As applicable	
Gunshot or stab wounds	×	×		Police		As advised by police
Hunting accidents	×	×		Police or state game official		As advised by law enforcement officer
Child abuse	×	×	For pelvic exam in some hospitals	Police and child welfare agency		As applicable
Wife abuse	×	×		Police		As applicable
Rape	×	×	×	Police	×	×
Alcohol or drug abuse	×	×	Blood alcohol consent	Police in some cases	×	
Suicide	×	×		Police in some cases		
Reportable communicable diseases	×	×		Health department	×	

should be consulted to determine what cases are reportable, according to the state's specific requirements, since the requirements may vary somewhat from state to state.

RAPE

Rape is usually defined as "unlawful carnal knowledge of a woman by a man, not her husband, forcibly against her will and with penetration, however slight, of the male genitalia into those of the female" (Schwartz et al., 1978, p. 1501).

Treatment of a rape victim includes the following:

Privacy for the patient.
Witnessed consent for the physical examination, specimen collection, photographs (as needed), and release of information to the authorities.
History as it relates to time, person, place, and circumstances surrounding the event.
A complete physical examination.
Collection of all clothing worn at the time of the incident, carefully labeled and held for the police.

Specimens of:
- vaginal vault for mobile sperm and *Neisseria gonorrhoeae,*
- blood for acid phosphatase, VDRL,
- semen for blood group antigens,
- combed and pulled hair from head and pubic area,
- fingernail scrapings, and,
- urine for a pregnancy test.

The specimens should be collected in the presence of a witness, documented in writing, labeled, and then handed directly to the laboratory or police department representative. The person receiving the specimens must sign for them. These procedures must be done carefully to verify the evidence. Failure to protect this important evidence might make the findings inadmissible in court.

Every emergency department should maintain up-to-date policies and procedures for treating rape victims, including the telephone number of the nearest Rape Crisis Center. Furthermore, a specially designed form for rape examination, providing continuity for all phases of the examination, should include the following:

Patient's name, address, telephone number, and age.
Date and time of examination.
Consent for examination, including release of information to authorities.
General observation of the patient's emotional state.
History data.
Physical examination data.
Data from the pelvic examination, with a list of specimens collected.
Treatment plan.
Referral sources.
Signature of the physician and nurse.
Signature of the person to whom the specimens are given.

The sexual assault of one man by another is not technically called rape; instead, this type of assault is called pederasty, buggery, or sodomy, depending on the details of the incident. Nevertheless, the rape examination procedures previously discussed are followed in these cases. Detection of semen on the body and clothing as well as in oral and anal orifices is important. Venereal disease diagnosis and prophylactic treatment should be included in the patient's care. Psychiatric consultation may also be necessary.

CHILD ABUSE

The emergency department nurse must be alert to potential child abuse cases. Child abuse includes not only physical injuries caused by parents or significant others, but also starvation, neglect, and emotional abuse.

The emergency department is one of the primary entry sites into the health care system for battered children. Most states have enacted child abuse laws that make reporting of the abuse mandatory. Failure to report a suspected abuse case can result in legal repercussions.

The nurse must know the reporting procedure required by the state in which he or she is employed. Nursing care includes a thorough history and physical examination, as well as photographs of the child. Furthermore, the nurse documents the interaction between the child and his or her significant other(s).

ORGAN DONATION

The health care provider should realize that a patient may want to donate his organs after his death. In most cases, the prospective donor carries a card indicating his decision. If an apparently healthy individual dies suddenly, usually as a result of an accident, however, the health care provider may decide to discuss the subject of organ donation with the family, if a decision was not previously made by the patient.

The emergency department must have a donor consent form, which, in the absence of a signed request by the patient, the next of kin must sign.

The nurse should know the name of the nearest hospital maintaining a donor team and the procedure for contacting that facility. Once contacted, the donor team will explain the appropriate procedures to be followed by the emergency department. The following organs are being successfully transplanted: bones of the inner ear, heart, liver, kidney, pancreas, cornea, small bowel, bone marrow, and skin.

The brain dead patient who will be an organ donor must be maintained with an adequate cardiovascular system, which maintains a good blood pressure and allows perfusion of the kidneys with adequate urinary output, thus ensuring effective organ procurement.

BLOOD ALCOHOL LEVELS

Intoxicated patients frequently appear in the emergency department. If a patient has been driving while "under the influence" and has been involved in a traffic violation, the staff may be faced with an uncomfortable situation. Police, accompanying this motorist to the emergency department, may request a test to determine the blood alcohol level. Blood alcohol measures the extent to which the body's capacity to eliminate alcohol has been exceeded.

Some states have an implied-consent law: thus, as a condition of accepting a driver's license, the applicant agrees to give a sample of blood or breath, if an officer suspects that the person has been drinking and driving recklessly. The motorist can either undergo one of these tests or accept a six month's suspension of the driver's license.

If a physician requests a blood alcohol level to help in making a differential diagnosis (e.g., head injury versus intoxication), the results may not be admissible in court, if later requested by law officers. The alcohol test in this instance was part of a patient–physician interaction, and therefore, it is considered confidential (*State v Amaniera*, 1975).

If a patient holds out his arm without restraint when informed that a blood alcohol level has been requested by the police officer, he is providing adequate consent. Nevertheless, the patient's action must be documented and witnessed. Written consent is still the preferred method.

An arrest warrant from the police department requiring the patient to enter the emergency department for a blood alcohol test is not considered a consent, if the patient refuses to have the blood drawn. Only a court order can force a patient to have this test done against his will. The police, not the emergency department staff, are responsible for advising the patient regarding the request for a blood specimen to measure either alcohol or drug levels.

Nonetheless, the following procedures should be adhered to in collecting a blood alcohol level for legal purposes:

1. The patient is informed about the test and signs an informed consent for "blood alcohol determination."
2. The skin is cleansed with a nonalcohol preparation, and the record is documented as such.
3. The act of blood drawing is witnessed and documented with site, date, time, and signatures of the person drawing the blood and the witnesses.
4. The blood tube is labeled with the patient's name, hospital record number, date, and time.
5. The signature of the person removing the blood sample from the emergency department is documented on the record.

To avoid confusion and to ensure continuity, these guidelines should be incorporated into one form that can be used for drawing blood alcohol levels for legal purposes. The nurse should research any statutes particular to the state, before developing a policy for a blood alcohol test: for instance, Virginia stipulates that the skin *must* be cleansed with soap and water.

Blood alcohol specimens should not be drawn against the patient's verbal objection or physical resistance. Such force could be interpreted by the courts as assault and battery, and the nurse may not be protected under statutory blood alcohol immunity provisions.

DEAD ON ARRIVAL (DOA)

The physician is responsible for pronouncing the patient dead in cases of DOA. Any tissue or body fluid specimens should be drawn only by the medical examiner. The body should not be disturbed in any way, and handling must be minimal. Good documentation of facts pertaining to the death from relatives or bystanders should be included in the emergency department record. A list of clothing and valuables should be made and signed by the individual who receives the body from the emergency department. A copy of this list should be retained with the hospital record.

DISPENSING OF MEDICATIONS

Dispensing of medications, which includes identifying, counting, packaging, and labeling the drug, must be done by a registered pharmacist, not by a registered nurse. The dispensing of medications for outpatient use is not included in the Nurse Practice Act. Medications can be dispensed by the emergency department only if no pharmacy is open. Any medication that is dispensed should be in a childproof container that was previously labeled by a registered pharmacist.

Generating a list of the most frequently dispensed medications permits the pharmacy to stock the department with appropriate starter dose packages. The pharmacy stocks, and restocks daily, these starter doses in a separate area of the medicine room. All doses are kept in prefilled, childproof, and properly labeled containers. When the starter dose is ordered, the *doctor* completes the patient's name and dosage directions on the label.

THE EMERGENCY DEPARTMENT RECORD

According to JCAH Standards, "a medical record shall be maintained on every patient seeking emergency care and shall be incorporated into the patient's permanent record" (JCAH, 1981, p. 32). JCAH Standards require that the following information be included on the patient's record:

1. Patient identification—name, address, telephone number, age, sex, birth date, race, religion, marital status, occupation, place and address of employment, and name and address of nearest relative or guardian.
2. Date, time, and means of arrival.
3. Pertinent history of the illness or injury and physical findings, including vital signs.
4. Emergency care given to the patient prior to arrival.
5. Diagnostic and therapeutic orders.
6. Clinical observations, including results of treatment.
7. Reports of procedures used and test results.
8. Diagnostic impressions.
9. Conclusions at the termination of evaluation or treatment, including final disposition, the patient's condition on discharge or transfer, and any instructions given to the patient and/or family for follow-up care.
10. Adequate documentation of a patient who leaves against medical advice (AMA).

Who has the ultimate responsibility for the emergency department record? According to JCAH Standards, "the medical record shall be authenticated by the practitioner who is responsible for its clinical accuracy" (JCAH, 1981, p. 32).

In departments with 24-hour physician coverage, the physician is responsible for the record. In departments without 24-hour coverage by a physician, the nurse is responsible for the record. This responsibility shifts back to the physician, if a physician on call enters the emergency department and assumes responsibility for the care of a particular patient.

The nurse is responsible for maintaining accurate and adequate nursing records on all patients. Records should include vital signs of all patients, medications given, treatments performed, and the patient's responses to all measures implemented. Patient teaching by the nurse as well as discharge instructions and provision for follow-up care, must be carefully documented. Furthermore, the physician and nurse must cooperate in resolving any differences of opinion concerning what information should or should not be written on the emergency department record.

The Federal Privacy Act of 1974 gives people the right to inspect federal agency records about themselves, including medical records. This law also gives patients the right to retain a copy of their records. The nurse must be aware of the hospital's procedure for making these records available to the patient.

CONFIDENTIALITY

Photographing a patient for scientific purposes requires consent. Police, if in pursuit of their duty, have the right to photograph a patient. The press, however, may photograph only in public areas, such as in parking lots or in waiting areas, but not inside the treatment area of the department.

Mechanisms should be established to help guide the release of information to the news media by the hospital public relations department or by the shift supervisor. News media calls should not be channeled to a busy emergency department where unauthorized information could easily be released.

Only a court order can release a patient's record without the patient's consent. If the patient requests the release of his records, a consent form must be signed.

The reporting of certain cases is mandated by state law. This reporting mechanism supersedes the patient's right to confidentiality and privacy.

PATIENT TRANSFERS

Emergency departments often confront the question of when to transfer a patient. In general, a patient transfer is appropriate under the following circumstances (George, 1980, p. 242):

1. If the transferring hospital is not clinically staffed to render the necessary care that the patient's condition requires.
2. If the transferring hospital is filled to capacity and, as a result, is physically incapable of accommodating the patient in the type of inpatient setting his condition necessitates.
3. If the patient, after being informed of the consequences of the decision, requests to be transferred to another hospital.

These "transfer rules" should be used only as guidelines, because exceptions always exist.

If the hospital is filled to capacity and a transfer is necessary, but the patient's condition is not stable, then the hospital retains the patient until his condition stabilizes or an inpatient bed can be made available. The first receiving hospital is responsible for this patient, until the person can be safely transferred to another institution.

If a mentally competent patient requests a transfer, but his condition is not adequately stable to effect that move safely, and the emergency department physician has clearly informed the patient of the risks involved, then the patient would be refusing treatment and would have to sign out against medical advice (AMA). (Alternative action, of course, could be pursued through the legal avenues previously discussed.)

TELEPHONE ADVICE

In a busy emergency department where the twentieth telephone advice call has just been received, but the shift is only partially over, the nurse may be tempted to reply as follows: "Take two aspirin and call your doctor in the morning." The nurse must resist this temptation! The information given by the caller may not always be accurate or complete; thus, emergency department staff should never try to diagnose an illness or treat a patient over the telephone.

The patient requesting advice should be told that it is against hospital policy to give advice over the telephone. In addition, if the person calling feels that treatment is required, he should either call his family doctor or be seen in an emergency department. The only exception is the caller with a history of ingestion of a toxic substance; in this case, the following procedures apply:

1. Give the caller the number of the closest Poison Control Center and instruct the person to call that center.
2. Instruct the caller to follow the initial treatment advice given by that center, while waiting for transportation to an emergency department, if required.

THE PSYCHIATRIC PATIENT

The psychiatric patient's mental capacity to give informed consent may be unpredictable. Whenever the patient is in danger of harming either himself or others, or if he is negligent of his own welfare, the nurse must exercise care to protect everyone concerned. Care may include the use of restraints. If a patient is restrained, however, the record should clearly outline the patient's behavior that provoked the need for restraint.

The nurse must know the local proceedings concerning commitment of a patient for psychiatric care or observation. *Commitment* is defined as the proceedings by which mentally ill people are restrained and confined for their own protection and for the general public's safety:

> There are four general categories of involuntary hospitalization or commitment: Emergency, Judicial, Medical, and Observational. *Emergency* hospitalization is a temporary measure for the speedy processing of emergency situations in order to suppress and prevent conduct likely to create a clear and present danger to persons or property. The emergency detention procedure varies from state to state. The procedure generally requires formal application, approval by a magistrate, and certification of the performance of a physical examination. *Judicial* commitment refers to an involuntary hospitalization procedure in which a judge or jury has discretion to determine whether hospitalization is required under the law. This procedure involves formal application, supporting medical evidence, medical examination, and a formal hearing. *Medical* commitment is a procedure whereby one or more physicians may involuntarily hospitalize a patient without his consent for an indefinite period of time. *Observational* commitment is the most practical and efficient commitment tool available to the emergency department staff. This period of observation varies greatly from state to state. The staff should know the exact details of this law for their state. (George, 1980, pp. 225–226)

In involuntary commitment, the patient is examined by the emergency physician and then the patient is admitted for a period of time for observation and psychological examination. "A common law test of insanity, used in many cases to justify involuntary hospitalization, is that the patient is so afflicted as to be likely to harm himself or others or be a menace to the public" (George, 1980, p. 223).

Formal application requesting an examination of a person considered to be mentally ill can be made by anyone observing the patient's irrational behavior. Nevertheless, only a physician or a judge can determine whether this person does indeed require hospitalization.

STAFF AND EQUIPMENT

JCAH Standards II, IV, V, and VI for emergency services require that emergency departments be well-organized, properly directed, and staffed with trained personnel who are guided by written policies and procedures and working in an area that is designed and equipped to facilitate the safe, effective care of patients. At least monthly inservice programs for staff at all levels should be conducted and documented. All staff must have current certification in basic life support. Furthermore, certification in advanced life support is recommended, especially for nurses in emergency departments where 24-hour physician coverage is not available.

All defibrillators, monitors, laryngoscopes, and ventilation equipment must be checked by each shift and documented that they are in good working order. Electrical safety checks should be conducted at least monthly by the department within the hospital responsible for this function.

CONCLUSION

Different legal issues frequently arise in the emergency department. While providing effective and safe patient care, the nurse must be aware of the laws that govern aspects of that care. The staff must remember that statutory law and case law vary from state to state. The nurse, therefore, should be familiar with individual state statutes and should consult the hospital's legal counselors for specific advice and information. Although clear, concise, and accurate records describing patient care and events that occurred during patient treatment may not eliminate legal problems, they will help in recalling and documenting a particular case. Good documentation, therefore, is an invaluable and necessary aid for the emergency department nurse. Most important, the nurse must know the legalities involved in caring for a patient in an emergency department setting.

BIBLIOGRAPHY

George, J. E.: *Law and Emergency Care*. St. Louis: Mosby, 1980.

———.: Law and the emergency department nurse. *Journal of Emergency Nursing* 7:230 (Sept./Oct. 1981).

Joint Commission on Accreditation of Hospitals: *Accreditation Manual for Hospitals*. Emergency Services, 1981, pp. 23–34.

Lanros, N. E.: Legal Implications in Emergency Department Nursing. In *Assessment and Intervention in Emergency Nursing*. Bowie, MD: Brady, 1978, pp. 421–428.

Miller, M.: Law and the emergency department nurse. *Journal of Emergency Nursing* 7:33–34 (Jan./Feb. 1981).

Schwartz, G. R., P. Safer, J. H. Stone, P. B. Storey, and B. K. Wagner: Mediolegal Problems in Emergency Medicine. *Principles and Practice of Emergency Medicine*, Vol. 2. Philadelphia: Saunders, 1978, pp. 1495–1505.

State v. Amaniera, 334A 2D 398 (1975).

Wilmington General Hospital v. Manlove, 184 A 2d 135 (S. Ct., Delaware, 1961).

4

Triage: Concept and Format

Janet Gren Parker

After completing this chapter, the reader will be able to do the following:

1. Define triage.
2. Discuss several different types of triage.
3. Discuss the advantages and disadvantages of the advanced nurse triage system.
4. Discuss the use of the SOAP (subjective data, objective data, assessment, and plan of management) format in triage.
5. List general priorities of care in triage.
6. Discuss nursing documentation in the emergency department.

Triage is a complex and complicated process that presents a constant challenge to the emergency department nurse. Triage has quickly become a necessity in the busy emergency department trying to provide adequate care for all patients who seek treatment. If the general public continues to use emergency departments as primary health care centers, the role of triage will expand, since it can help the emergency department staff to provide the best quality of care.

DEFINITION

The word *triage* is derived from the French *trier,* which means "sorting or choosing." Triage occurs daily in various situations. Parents perform triage when they decide to keep their child home from school due to an illness. Police officials perform triage when they decide to bring someone to the emergency department, instead of taking them to jail. Teachers perform triage when they send a pupil to the school nurse. An employee performs triage when he or she stays home from work and remains in bed due to an illness.

The specific goal of triage in a emergency department, however, is to provide an immediate, brief evaluation of all incoming patients. In addition, triage can help to determine priorities of care for all patients, to define the problems of each patient, and to provide psychological, social, and physical comfort to patients and their families. Most patients are divided into three groups:

1. Emergent.
2. Acute.
3. Nonacute.

Emergent patients have life-threatening conditions that must be treated immediately: for example, cardiac arrest, hypovolemic shock, and blocked airway. *Acute* patients have problems that are not life-threatening, but should be treated by a health care-professional within several hours: for example, lacerations, injured extremities, and transient ischemia attacks. *Nonacute* patients have long-term, chronic conditions, which can wait indefinitely for treatment or can be treated by another clinic: for example, colds, hemorrhoids, and vaginal discharges.

SYSTEMS OF TRIAGE

Within the formal framework of emergency department triage, several systems have been developed (Estrada, 1981):

1. *Nonprofessional*—Receptionist or clerk greets the patient and documents the patient's chief complaint on the emergency department record.
2. *Basic*—Licensed practical nurse or registered nurse greets the patient and assigns the person to the appropriate treatment area.
3. *Advanced*—Registered nurse assesses the patient, identifies the chief complaint, and develops a plan of action, which includes initiating basic first-aid measures as well as ordering x-ray examinations and laboratory studies.
4. *Physician*—Patient is assessed by a physician who may treat and discharge the patient from the triage area.
5. *Team*—A physician and nurse(s) work together in a team approach to triage all incoming patients.

The advanced triage system is the preferred system in most emergency departments. Either the cost effectiveness of a physician triaging or the educational preparedness of a receptionist triaging is debatable. Using emergency medical technicians with developed algorithms (Slay and Riskin, 1976), however, tends to identify triage as a simple, technical skill, rather than the sophisticated, complex, decision-making process that it represents.

Several studies have documented the effectiveness of a formal nurse triage system by measuring the appropriateness of the triage action. Bliss et al. (1971), for example, compared the x-ray studies of distal limbs ordered by both the triage nurse and the physician. This study revealed 100% agreement between the triage nurse and the physician. In a retrospective study (Albin et al., 1977), physicians, using the final, completed chart, agreed with the nurse's triage decision 80% of the time, while identifying 17% of the patients as uptriaged, and only 3% as mistriaged. In another retrospective study (Mills et al., 1976), overall accuracy of nurse triage was 98%, with only 1.9% identified as a mistriage. Willis (1979) documented an accurate triage rate of 87.8%, 3.8% overtriaged, and 4.1% mistriaged. (It is interesting to note that the majority of mistriaged patients presented with the chief complaint of abdominal pain.)

The advanced system of triage is recommended as the preferred choice because of cost effectiveness and accuracy in the decision-making process. Because triage is a sophisticated and complex process, a triage system should reflect its necessity and overall importance in an emergency department.

Advanced Nurse Triage System

In the advanced triage system, the nurse must possess certain characteristics that enable the process to function adequately. The triage nurse must possess adequate knowledge to make decisions. This knowledge is acquired through a formal, inservice education program designed specifically for each emergency department. Moreover, the nurse should acquire experience in emergency nursing, before advancing into the triage position. If this experience is combined with formal, inservice triage education, the nurse will develop a knowledge base adequate for performing nursing triage.

Furthermore, the nurse must also possess adequate communication skills for the process to function smoothly. Attitude is also important because the nurse will deal directly with many different types of people, who have different types of problems. The nurse must have the ability to remain calm in any situation, while continuing to make appropriate decisions during stressful periods. The triage nurse must use common sense, demonstrate leadership abilities, and be capable of solving problems and synthesizing information.

Disadvantages of the advanced nurse triage system, however, do not outweigh the advantages. Although this system costs more to operate than does the receptionist system, it is less expensive than a formal physician triage system. Stress, however, is a major disadvantage. The physical isolation of the triage nurse from the other nurses, in addition to problems resulting from inadequate communication, distressed visitors and patients, the burden of paperwork, and the complexities of the process itself—all contribute to the amount of stress experienced by the triage nurse. Rotating staff between patient care assignments and the expanded role of triage can help to decrease the level of stress. During the nurse's shift of triage, relief should be arranged to allow the nurse the opportunity to relax from the stressful triage activity. Other mechanisms to decrease stress should be identified and incorporated into the emergency department.

The advanced nurse triage system has many advantages. The increase in patient satisfaction is remarkable. The patient and family members are more receptive to waiting, after they have consulted with a nurse who provides simple first aid, reassures them, and initiates the care-giving process. Consequently, public relations in the emergency department improve significantly. Patients appreciate talking immediately with a health care provider, when they arrive in the emergency department. Moreover, the emergency department appears to be more sensitive to the patient's welfare than to the economics of the encounter. Patient care itself is expedited, because the nurse immediately requests an x-ray examination, or draws the blood samples and sends them to the appropriate laboratory. Consequently, delays in patient care, caused by ancillary services, are minimized. Furthermore, the triage nurse also ensures that priorities of care are established according to the acuteness of the patient's condition.

Both congestion and confusion at the entry point of the emergency department decrease. Communication between the patient and the emergency department, however, increases. Explaining the patient's treatment and progress decreases the family's anxiety. Staff nurses' satisfaction increases, because they are functioning in an expanded role, through which their skills and abilities are acknowledged. Furthermore, data from an initial history collected by the triage nurse expedites the physician's work.

Telephone triage is another challenge. Patients who call often expect the nurse to be able to diagnose whether a laceration needs stitches or an ankle needs an x-ray examination. The nurse's most appropriate response is as follows: "We cannot diagnose your problem over the telephone. If you come in, we will be happy to treat you." General health care questions, of course, may be answered over the telephone. In addition to providing an educational service for the public, telephone advice can decrease the number of unnecessary emergency department visits.

TRIAGE FORMAT

Four basic steps in the process of triage include the following:

1. General overview of the patient and a brief history.
2. Brief physical examination dealing primarily with the chief problem area.
3. Analysis of data collected, formulated into problem identification.
4. Plan of management.

These four general steps in the process correlate with the SOAP format of documentation. Because of the close correlation, the SOAP format is recommended for use in the advanced nurse triage system. Using the same organizational system for both the process and the format of triage enables the nurse to make decisions and to document these decisions in a concise, organized manner.

Subjective Data (S)

The subjective data include a general overview of the patient and a brief history as it relates to the patient's chief complaint. All the symptoms that the patient identifies are included in the subjective data. (Subjective data may be incomplete, of course, because the patient is reporting what he feels and thinks is important data.) The pertinent past medical history is documented, in addititon to allergies, current medication, and, if applicable, tetanus toxoid status. Concerns of the family members regarding the patient are included in the subjective data. The triage nurse questions the patient closely regarding the absence of symptoms or signs that might present with each chief complaint. All absent symptoms are called *pertinent negatives*. Age, race, and sex may be included under subjective data, even though they are, in fact, objective data, because they provide a good starting point for most triage nurses. Moreover, the patient's perceptions are documented, and quotation marks are used to indicate the patient's own words:

S: 46 yo Bf with c/o nonradiating midsternal chest pain for 1 hr. before this admission. "Crushing pain" unrelievable, c/o nausea, no SOB, no vomiting. PMH: HTN, NKA, no current medications.

Objective Data (O)

The objective data include a brief physical examination dealing primarily with the chief problem area. Objective data include whatever the triage nurse sees, hears, smells, and touches: in essence, all observable, measurable, and factual data. The amount of distress is noted, and the patient's parameters, such as vital signs, are measured. The patient is described, but unnecessary labels are avoided. As indicated in the following example, the patient is in more distress than can be identified from examining only the subjective data:

O: Obese, diaphoretic, pale, with arm clasped to midsternum, P = 100, regular and strong, skin cool to touch.

The objective data should contain only the vital signs necessary for making an appropriate triage decision: for example, temperature is not necessary in this example, but it would certainly be helpful in a child presenting with a chief complaint of fever.

Assessment (A)

The assessment corresponds to the analysis of the subjective and objective data used to identify and to define the problem. This step in the process is the most difficult, because all of the nurse's knowledge and skills are required to properly identify the problem area. Many experienced emergency department nurses can relate stories of inappropriate assessments. One patient, for example, initially complained of rectal pain, but, thirty minutes later, she gave birth to a child. Patients complaining of chest pain, for example, may be anxious because their neighbor was shot the day before. The triage nurse must consider all the subjective and objective data that have been collected, then compare that data with the nurse's knowledge base to identify and to define the patient's problem. The data occasionally may indicate several problem areas that should be identified and listed under the assessment.

Some people can understand the assessment better, if they equate it with a nursing diagnosis or with the chief complaint. Using the data collected to help support and to define the identified problem correlates with the third step in the triage process. Do not allow labels and words, however, to confuse the issue. The triage nurse must identify the problem to be handled in the emergency department, and the problem identified must be based on the subjective and objective data:

A: Chest pain, possible MI.

Plan of Management (P)

The P in the SOAP format corresponds to the plan of management in the steps of the triage process. The plan of management includes the following: type of health care provider required to see the patient (e.g., medical, surgical, nurse practitioner, psychiatric, etc.), how soon the patient must be seen; and the actions of first aid and other therapeutic tasks that the triage nurse has performed at the triage area. Varying organizational systems in different emergency departments help dictate the documentation required under the particular plan. In some institutions, the option of triage to a clinic is not available. Moreover, the option of requesting different health care providers is not always available. Nevertheless, determining priorities of care is always an integral part of the plan of care developed by the triage nurse.

The plan of management documented in the example would be as follows:

P: Medical evaluation, admit to examination room now.

This documentation may seem complicated and complex, but triage is a complicated, complex activity. As the example illustrates, the triage note may be written after the actual triage process has occurred. With a patient who has chest pain and looks like this patient does, of course, the immediate action of the triage nurse would be to escort the patient to a treatment area. The eventual documentation of the triage nurse's actions, however, is a reliable measure for the department to use in validating their actions whenever questions arise or complaints are filed. (Table 4.1 contains several additional examples of the triage process using the SOAP format.)

Data Collection

Gathering data is sometimes difficult, especially in the emergency department. The triage nurse has the mammoth task of collecting subjective and objective data appropriately and quickly, while not missing an important symptom or piece of history that could drastically alter the assessment and plan of management. The triage nurse must quickly determine whether any life-threatening condition exists, and then provide that patient with the highest priority of care.

A brief overview of each patient as he or she approaches the triage area, therefore, must immediately evaluate the person's respiratory status and circulation. If either function is abnormal, the triage nurse must shift all attention to triaging that patient. If no immediately life-threatening problem is identified in the brief overview, the triage nurse focuses on the history.

Obtaining a history can be a lengthy, complicated task. In the emergency depart-

TRIAGE FORMAT

TABLE 4.1 The Triage Process Using the SOAP Format

S: 32 yo WF with c/o laceration to right hand while doing dishes approximately 20 minutes before admission. Glass broke in her hand. PMH: asthma, NKA, tetanus toxoid UTD.
O: 2 cm superficial lac. on dorsal aspect of right hand, bleeding minimal, ROM nl, sensory nl.
A: Lac. right hand.
P: Surgical evaluation, pressure dressing, elevation, waiting room.

S: 58 yo BM with c/o nosebleed for 2 hrs PTA. PMH: HTN, NKA, Diazide every day.
O: BP 190/130, P 96 strong and regular. Skin warm and dry to touch. Nose brisk bleeding right anterior septum.
A: Epitaxis, related to hypertension.
P: Medical evaluation, HCT sent to lab, admit to examination room as soon as possible, evaluate patient's Diazide compliance.

S: 1 month old WM with c/o vomiting and diarrhea for 24 hr. c/o fever up to 103 Ⓡ, unable to keep anything down, "used 12 diapers last four hours," vomited everything. No other complaints. PMH: none, NKA, no current medications.
O: Fontanel depressed, lethargic child, mucous membranes dry, skin hot to touch, no tears visualized, color pale and grayish, respiration 56 labored.
A: Dehydration with possible sepsis.
P: Pediatric evaluation, admit examination room immediately.

S: 24 yo WM with c/o being involved in motor vehicle accident app. 3 hrs. prior to admission. Transfer patient. Car hit telephone pole and patient thrown from car. PMH: unknown, NKA, unknown tetanus toxoid and current meds.
O: Et tube in place, ventilations assisted, IV of RL infusing at 100 ml/hr, Ⓡ pupil > Ⓛ pupil, responds to painful stimuli, Foley in place, abdomen rigid.
A: Multiple trauma.
P: Surgical evaluation, admit examination room immediately.

ment, a focused interview technique enables the triage nurse to obtain the best history possible in the shortest period of time. The triage nurse explains to both the patient and the family that they are speaking with a nurse. The purpose of the encounter should be explained so that the patient realizes that the nurse is trying to help with the problem. Talking with the patient in private often expedites the conversation: for instance, if the patient has a cyst on his buttock, the nurse might have to ask three or four questions in an open area to obtain that history. In fact, some patients may never tell the triage nurse what is wrong, unless the questioning is done in private. The triage nurse should also remember that the family, if present, can provide additional data.

After the triage nurse asks the patient to identify the problem, the details regarding the onset of the problem are described. Knowing the amount of time between the onset of the problem and the emergency department visit, as well as the patient's current status, can help in determining the acuteness of the patient's illness.

Whenever the problem includes pain of any type, the severity, duration, character (quality), and location of the pain must be identified in the history. Furthermore, associated symptoms, as well as pertinent negatives, are also included in the history.

Interviewing techniques used in the emergency department to obtain data must be open-ended, but directed. Verbal communication is an important factor in obtaining data. The questions, therefore, should be simple and directed. Ask only one question at a time and wait for the answer. Use words that the patient and the family will understand. In addition, remember that nonverbal communication, which often speaks louder than words, can help either clarify or confuse the data collection.

Although the brief physical examination will vary with each patient, it should relate to the chief complaint, and it should be organized to be both rapid and accurate. This examination includes a general overview and specific details relating to the chief complaint.

PRIORITIES OF TRIAGE

Developing a comprehensive, infallible list of priorities of care in the emergency department is impossible. Only general guidelines, rather than comprehensive dissertation on the subject, is possible. General priorities of treatment are as follows:

1. Airway.
2. Circulation.
3. Bleeding and shock.
4. Consciousness.
5. Open wounds.

Assume that everything that could possibly be wrong with the patient is wrong, until the patient has been assessed completely. Do not be misled by the obvious: for instance, do not let the bleeding laceration on the forehead become the first priority, while the patient slowly asphyxiates from a compromised airway. Perhaps the patient lacerated his forehead when he hit the windshield of his car, after he had suffered a massive myocardial infarction, which compromised his airway. Remember the general priorities of care.

Developing priorities in the emergency department requires *caution*. The triage nurse never assumes that the patient has a simple or superficial problem. Always assume that the patient has the worst possible problem, until contrary evidence has been documented. Situations in which caution should be used to determine priorities include the following:

1. Injured alcoholics.
2. Injured comatose patients.

3. A history of loss of consciousness.
4. Chest pain.
5. Abdominal pain.
6. Fever in a child.
7. History of a blow of great force.
8. History of a large amount of bleeding.
9. Abnormal vital signs.
10. Marked pallor.
11. Disorientation (medical versus psychiatric in origin).

Table 4.2 lists several conditions and notes their priorities of care to help provide a few guidelines for the triage nurse.

Another area requiring caution that the triage nurse should remember involves refusing to treat patients. The triage nurse does not have the legal right to refuse treatment to anyone, even though the patient may not require emergency care. Only a physician may refuse treatment to a patient, and even then the treatment cannot be refused in an emergency situation. Thus, do not dismiss a patient, unless the person decides he does not need to see a physician. Some patients, after speaking to the triage nurse, will decide to leave, because they realize that simple first-aid measures performed at home would be adequate treatment. Nevertheless, the physician ultimately defines an emergency. The triage nurse, therefore, must not prevent a patient from seeing a physician. The triage nurse merely determines the priority of care, not whether care should be rendered by a physician.

NURSING DOCUMENTATION

Nursing intervention in the emergency department must be documented. Documentation enables the nurse to care for the patient with a written plan of care, and it establishes a mechanism for auditing the quality of nursing care. Emergency department nurses must acknowledge the care they deliver to the patient by documenting that care.

More often than not the only place for the nurse to document the care given is on the physician's emergency record. This record usually contains both biographical data and medical care data. Additional room rarely exists for the documentation of nursing care. A separate nursing flow sheet, therefore, provides the nurse adequate space to record and document the nursing care delivered to patients in the emergency department.

Each facility will want to tailor its nursing flow record to suit the needs of its particular department. Adequate space should be designed for serial vital signs, serial nursing observations, medication given to the patient, discharge teaching, and nursing referrals to other health care providers. The format of the record should be consistent and should be used for all patients within the department. Consistency enables other health care providers to augment the plan of care initiated by the emergency department.

TABLE 4.2 Priorities of Care

Highest Priority—Treatment Immediately (Emergency Classification)
1. Airway problems of any type, especially with cyanosis, stridor in a child
2. Cardiac and/or respiratory arrest
3. Abnormal vital signs
4. Shock of any type
5. Chest pain
6. Massive hemorrhage
7. Obvious multiple injuries
8. Altered mental state
9. Seizure activity
10. Drug overdose—suicide attempt
11. Major burns
12. Bulging fontanel

Second Priority—Treatment As Soon As Possible (Acute Classification)
1. Severe pain anywhere
2. Continuous vomiting and/or diarrhea
3. Cerebral vascular accident, transient ischemia attack
4. Obvious fractures
5. Major lacerations
6. Acute abdominal pain
7. Sexual assault in last 12 hours
8. Acute headache
9. Patients with an acute problem who also have a significant chronic illness (e.g., cancer, diabetes, kidney disease, congenital heart disease, cystic fibrosis)

Delayed Priority—Treatment Delayed (Nonacute Classification)
1. Minor injuries
2. Nonacute abdominal pain, back pain
3. Chronic conditions
4. Mild anxiety
5. Sore throat, cough

CONCLUSION

Triage is required in every functional emergency department. This sophisticated, complex, decision-making process is best implemented by using the advanced nurse triage system. The SOAP format is recommended as a tool to provide consistent triage documentation. Proper triage action in the emergency department includes the following: assigning correct priorities of care; maintaining patient flow in the emergency department; providing an expanded role for the emergency department nurse, and improving the quality of care that each patient receives from any health care provider in an emergency department.

BIBLIOGRAPHY

Albin, S. L., S. Wassenthial-Smoller, S. Jacobsen, and B. Bell: Evaluation of emergency room triage performed by nurses. *Hospital Topics* 55:45–50 (1977).

Bliss, A., L. Decker, and W. O. Southwick: The emergency room nurse orders x-rays of distal limbs in orthopedic trauma. *Nursing Research* 20:440–443 (1971).

Burney, R. E.: Initial Triage and Diagnosis: A Systems Resource Analysis. In *Emergency Medical Services: Measures to Improve Care.* New York: Macy, 1980, pp. 274–286.

Estrada, E. G.: Triage systems. *Nursing Clinics of North America* 10:13–24 (1981).

George, J. E.: Triage—perils and pitfalls. *Emergency Nurse Legal Bulletin* 5:2–8 (1979).

Mills, J., A. Webster, C. B. Wofsy, P. Harding, and D. D'Acuti: Effectiveness of nurse triage in the emergency department of an urban county hospital. *JACEP* 5:877–882 (1976).

Shanks, L.: Triage, treatment and transfer: scope of duty in the delivery of emergency health care. *Critical Care Update* 7:26–27 (1980).

Slater, R. R.: Triage nurse in the emergency department. *American Journal of Nursing* 70:127–129 (1970).

Slay, L. E., and W. G. Riskin: Algorithm—directed triage in an emergency department. *JACEP.* 5:869–875 (1976).

Willis, D. T.: A study of nursing triage. *Journal of Emergency Nursing* 5:8–11 (1979).

NURSING CARE OF SELECTED EMERGENCIES

PART II

5
Airway Problems

Janet Gren Parker

After completing this chapter, the reader will be able to do the following:

1. Triage a patient with airway problems.
2. Discuss mechanisms of airway maintenance, including the following:
   a. oropharyngeal.
   b. nasopharyngeal.
   c. esophageal obturator airway.
   d. endotracheal intubation.
   e. cricothyrotomy.
   f. transtracheal catheter ventilation.
   g. tracheostomy.
3. Discuss the nursing care of the patient with an obstructed airway.
4. Demonstrate and explain the Heimlich maneuver.
5. Discuss appropriate discharge planning for the patient and family.

Airway maintenance is the most important factor to consider in treating a patient with any imaginable problem. If airway maintenance is neglected, any other treatment will be useless, because, without an adequate supply of oxygen, brain cells start to die within four to six minutes. Airway obstruction or failure is frightening to both the patient and the health care provider. The emergency department nurse, therefore, must calm and reassure the patient, while maintaining the patient's airway as quickly and as efficiently as possible.

TRIAGE

Subjective Data

Quickly obtaining a detailed history from the patient is important, but often difficult, particularly if the patient is either gasping for air or unable to talk because of respiratory difficulty. Nevertheless, it is important to discover the following as soon as possible: What precipitated the attack? How long has it lasted? When did it start? What symptoms has the patient experienced? The triage nurse can acquire information in this situation from family members, friends, or ambulance personnel who brought the patient to the emergency department. Additional questions that should be answered include the following: Did the patient have a fever? Did the patient have any cold symptoms? Did the patient eat recently? Was the patient exposed to any toxic substances? Did the patient have any chest pain or trauma of any type? Has the patient vomited? And if the patient is a juvenile: Was the child playing with small toys? Did the child have a sore throat? All pertinent negatives should be explored to help ascertain a reason for the respiratory distress.

A pertinent past medical history may provide valuable clues to the etiology of the patient's present condition. Does the patient have any heart disease? Does the patient have chronic obstructive pulmonary disease? Does the child have rheumatic heart disease? Is the patient on chronic renal dialysis? Does the child have a history of asthma or cystic fibrosis? Moreover, a thorough history of all current medications, as well as all medications to which the patient might be allergic, should be ascertained to provide data necessary for developing a plan of care.

Objective Data

The triage nurse begins collecting objective data as soon as the patient arrives in the emergency department. These observations will usually reveal whether the patient is acutely or chronically ill. Observations of skin color, use of accessory muscles, ability to talk, facial expressions, or audible respirations will immediately alert the nurse to the seriousness of the situation.

If the patient's status permits, a pertinent, but brief, physical examination should be performed, including assessment of the person's mental, respiratory, and cardiovascular status. As soon as possible, a complete set of vital signs should be taken, including not only the rate of the heart and the respirations, but also the quality and strength of the vital signs. The temperature, an important indicator of the possibility of infection as a causative agent, should be taken rectally or axillary, rather than orally, in a patient with respiratory distress.

Is the patient alert and oriented, or is he confused? Are the breath sounds equal bilaterally, as well as normal in nature, or are rales or rhonchi evident? Does the chest wall move symmetrically? Is the voice hoarse, or is the patient unable to talk at all? Is there cyanosis of the lips, nails, and skin? If circumstances allow, examine the other major body systems and note any abnormal data.

Assessment and Planning

By analyzing the subjective and objective data collected, the triage nurse makes an assessment, or nursing diagnosis, to identify one or more chief complaints, then develops an initial plan of care. The plan of care includes the patient's priority of care, as well as appropriate nursing interventions, such as suctioning, use of oxygen,

AIRWAY MAINTENANCE

TABLE 5.1 Examples of Triage Notes

S: 8 month old WF with c/o cough and runny nose for 2 days. This afternoon awoke from nap with difficulty breathing. No fever, PMH: none, no current meds, NKA.

O: Sitting upright, hunched over in mom's arms, cyanotic around lips and nailbeds, skin pale and dry. RR 56 labored, using accessory muscles.

A: Respiratory difficulty, R/O epiglottitis.

P: Pediatric evaluation, admit to examination area immediately. Keep patient calm and sitting upright. O$_2$ via mask.

S: 24 yo BM with c/o eating steak app. 20 min prior to admission, when had "choking sensation and couldn't talk." Friend at restaurant performed Heimlich maneuver and chunk of meat was dislodged. PMH: asthma, NKA, theophylline, 250 mg BID.

O: Ambulatory, color good, skin warm and dry, alert and oriented, talking normally. RR 12 regular unlabored, breath sounds normal.

A: Foreign body in airway, now dislodged.

P: Medical evaluation, admit examination room as soon as possible, observe closely for possible airway difficulties.

---

positioning, and reassurance. Decreasing the patient's anxiety is important, since anxiety increases the need for oxygen in the patient's body. The family also needs reassurance to decrease their anxiety, and to help them cope with the situation.

Table 5.1 contains two examples of triage notes that might result from a patient presenting with an airway problem. A thorough discussion of airway maintenance, dealing with causes of airway obstructions, as well as airway failure and resultant interventions, follows. Knowledge of this material will aid the nurse in performing triage accurately and appropriately.

AIRWAY MAINTENANCE

Establishing and maintaining the airway is the highest priority in any patient. Without oxygen, brain cells die within four to six minutes. Although the heart may continue to beat and to circulate blood to the body systems, without oxygen added to the blood and carbon dioxide removed from the blood, the patient is surviving on borrowed time. Performing closed cardiac massage without proper airway maintenance is a grave error. The airway is the first priority.

The method used to maintain the airway depends on the condition of the patient, the age of the patient, and the cause of the airway problem. A common error in airway maintenance is establishing the patency of the upper airway, while neglecting the lower part of the airway. The airway, however, is not patent until it is adequately established from the nose to the diaphragm. The airway extends from the nose into the pharynx, then from the hypopharynx, the larynx, the trachea, the bronchi, and the lungs into the thoracic cavity, reaching downward to the diaphragm. Remember that children have smaller airways than do adults; thus, a child's airway can close quicker and become obstructed faster. A bloody nose or congested nasal passage in a child, for example, can cause airway problems. A young child does not realize that he can breathe through his mouth if his nose is blocked. Consequently, the child rarely breathes voluntarily through his mouth.

First Steps

Once breathlessness is established, the first step in maintaining the airway involves opening the mouth of the patient. If the patient is unconscious with a relaxed lower jaw, this procedure is simple; if however, the jaws are clenched shut, they may be difficult to open. Extension of the neck with elevation of the angles of the mandible may open the mouth. Grasping the angles of the jaw and pushing the chin forward may also help unclench the jaws. Before either technique is used, however, the neck must be assessed first to ensure that the cervical spine is not compromised. Using excessive force could injure the cervical spine. The objective is extension of the head at the junction of the neck, rather than hyperextension of the cervical vertebrae. If the cervical spine is injured, the mouth should not be disturbed, though airway maintenance could be attempted through the nasal passage via blind intubation—a technique discussed in detail later in this chapter.

After the mouth is opened, simple extension of the neck may open the airway and reinitiate breathing. This happens because neck extension lifts the tongue, the most common cause of airway obstruction in an unconscious patient, elevating it away from the back of the throat and thus opening the airway. Manually pulling the tongue forward may also stop it from blocking the airway. After the mouth is opened and the tongue is pulled forward use either your finger or a towel to remove any *visible* foreign material. Cautiously remove foreign objects, because a foreign body can easily be pushed even deeper into the airway, thus worsening the situation. Suction apparatus should be available to help remove any secretions from the mouth and nose.

After the airway is opened, rescue breathing is initiated through bag mask, mouth to mask, mouth to mouth, or mouth to nose techniques. The method chosen for the rescue breathing is adequate if the following occur: the chest rises and falls; there is a resistance and compliance of the patient's lungs, while they expand in the rescuer's airway; and, the rescuer hears and feels air escape during expiration.

Oropharyngeal Airway

After the airway is open, and rescue breathing has started, the airway must be maintained in the open position by the insertion of a plastic *oropharyngeal airway*. The insertion can be facilitated by depressing the tongue with a tongue blade. The airway is inserted behind the tongue with the concave side in the upward position, while rotating the airway 180 degrees when it touches the soft palate. If the oropharyngeal airway is too long, its insertion may stimulate the gag reflex in the patient, and aspiration can occur. Suction should be available immediately to help prevent aspiration of any vomitus. Moreover, positioning the patient on his side, if possible, also helps decrease the possibility of aspiration.

Nasopharyngeal Airway

Nasopharyngeal airway is similar to the oropharyngeal airway, except that it is inserted through the nasal passageway. The main objective of the nasopharyngeal airway is to provide air passage into the hypopharynx. Lubricating with a water soluble lubricant is necessary, before insertion is attempted through the nose. Most health care providers feel that the nasopharyngeal airway is inferior to the oral airway, because it decreases the ability to suction the oral cavity adequately.

Special Considerations in Children

More caution is required for children with airway problems, because their airways are smaller and can be obstructed more easily. Using fingers instead of the hand may provide adequate force to extend the neck or lift the chin to open the jaw. After the mouth is open, be careful about sticking any objects, such as tongue blades or fingers, into the airway, because these may cause the complete closure of the airway from epiglottitis, as well as further obstruction from foreign bodies.

Assessing the child who is experiencing respiratory difficulty should include assessment of the child's cry and eating habits. Is the cry normal? Or is it hoarse, muffled, or absent? Has the baby been feeding regularly, or has he had trouble swallowing? Closely assessing these factors can provide the nurse with clues regarding the area of the airway creating the problem. If there is no cry or the voice is hoarse, the problem is in the glottic region; if normal, but weak, the subglottal region is suspect; and, if normal, but muffled, the problem is probably in the supraglottic region. If the child inhales with stridor, the difficulty is probably located at the glottis or above; if the child has stridor during inspiration and expiration, the glottal or subglottal area is suspect; and, if the child is experiencing difficulty in swallowing, the supraglottic area probably contains the problem.

A special conditon that may occur during an infant's first few months of life is a congenital laryngeal stridor. The infant reveals stridor that is worse when the infant is lying on his back and better when the infant is lying on his stomach. The infant rarely experiences serious airway trouble and usually outgrows the condition by the age of two, when the cartilage matures.

TYPES OF AIRWAY MAINTENANCE

After the initial establishment of the airway, if spontaneous respirations do not begin quickly, more extensive airway maintenance techniques must be employed to manage the patient, including using the esophageal obturator airway, endotracheal intubation, cricothyrotomy, transtracheal catheter ventilation, and tracheostomy.

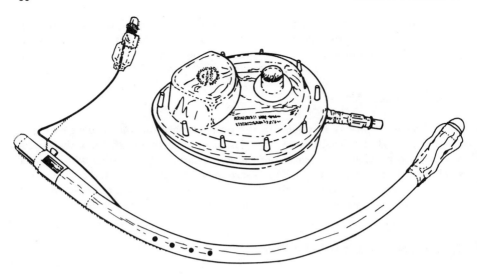

Figure 5.1 An esophageal obturator airway and face mask.

Esophageal Obturator Airway

The *esophageal obturator airway* (EOA) is a cuffed, blind-ended tube with holes located in the upper portion of the tube (see Fig. 5.1). The EOA should be used only in unconscious patients, because it stimulates the gag reflex. If the patient is responsive, he might vomit and tear his esophagus during insertion. The tube is inserted blindly into the esophagus, the cuff filled with approximately 35 cc of air, and the face mask fitted tightly onto the patient. The patient is ventilated, and tube placement is checked by auscultating the lungs and stomach. Air movement should be heard in the lungs, if the holes in the upper part of the EOA are aligned properly in the hypopharynx. The chest wall should rise and fall, and no air should be heard in the stomach. Using the EOA is not recommended for patients with esophageal burns or strictures, or a fractured esophagus, or for anyone under the age of sixteen.

Because the EOA is easy to use, it is ideal for airway maintenance in the prehospital phase. Because it can be inserted blindly with ease, it is particularly useful for treating obese patients. The EOA method delivers and maintains a high oxygen concentration to the patient, while it prevents gastric dilatation and minimizes the possible aspiration of gastric contents. Moreover, an endotracheal tube can be inserted around the EOA. Most important, the EOA must never be removed until another airway mechanism is in place, because of the high incidence of vomiting when the EOA is removed. In removing the EOA, patency of the resulting airway should be ascertained, first, then the patient is placed on his side, the cuff is deflated, the airway is removed, and suction apparatus is used to remove any secretions or material vomited.

Ventilation with the EOA is as effective as ventilation with an endotracheal tube (Meislin, 1980). Arterial blood gas values obtained after EOA insertion, compared with values obtained in the same patient after endotracheal intubation, show no

TYPES OF AIRWAY MAINTENANCE

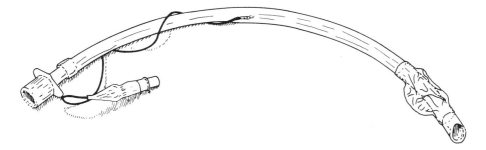

Figure 5.2 A cuffed endotracheal tube.

difference in partial pressure of oxygen (Po_2) or pH. Some data indicate, however, a slightly higher partial pressure of carbon dioxide (Pco_2) when the EOA is in place.

In using the EOA, difficulties may develop: for instance, the mask may leak air; accidental tracheal intubation may occur; the esophagus may accidentally rupture; the ventilation holes may not be in the proper position; and, vomiting and aspiration may still occur.

Endotracheal Intubation

An *endotracheal tube* used in endotracheal intubation is a cuffed, open-ended tube that is inserted into the trachea with the help of a laryngoscope and laryngoscope blade (see Fig. 5.2). After insertion, correct tube placement is checked by noticing bilateral and equal rising and falling of the chest wall, by auscultating bilateral breath sounds, and by examining a chest x-ray film, if time permits. After proper placement is ascertained, the cuff is inflated, and the patient is forcefully ventilated. If the endotracheal tube is inserted too far into the airway, the right bronchus could be blocked completely by the tube itself. If the bronchus is blocked, the tube must be withdrawn until the right bronchus is no longer blocked, which allows both lungs to be ventilated equally. The endotracheal tube should always be taped in place with an oropharyngeal airway to permit suctioning of the oral cavity.

One major advantage of an endotracheal tube is that it can be inserted into the trachea either through the mouth or through the nose. Although the nasal route of insertion is more difficult, because it is a blind intubation attempt, it is useful whenever the patient's jaws are firmly clenched and cannot be opened. Other advantages include actual airway patency and protection, as well as a suction access into the lower parts of the airway.

Endotracheal intubation is difficult to perform. Possible complications that might arise include the following: esophageal intubation; right main stem bronchus intubation resulting in left lung collapse; airway hemorrhage secondary to trauma of insertion; chipping or loosening of teeth; leakage of the tube cuff; and dislocation of the cervical spine. An endotracheal intubation should not be attempted if the health care provider suspects the possibility of a laryngeal foreign body, or laryngeal or tracheal fracture.

For children, the endotracheal tube is not cuffed, because the child's airway cannot accommodate the extra bulk of the cuff. The size of the tube used in a child is usually slightly larger than the diameter of the patient's fifth finger at the terminal joint. The nasal route of insertion in children is usually preferred, because the tube is easier to anchor and less irritating to the child. The tube, inserted orally, can either kink or even come out, if the child moves his head too much.

Cricothyrotomy

A cricothyrotomy provides a rapid access to the airway, particularly to an obstructed airway. In fact, a cricothyrotomy is the preferred choice for treating an obstructed airway whenever esophageal or endotracheal intubation is impossible. After the skin is adequately prepared with an antiseptic solution, a horizontal incision is made over the cricothyroid membrane. The incision can be widened to facilitate passage of a tracheostomy tube through the incision into the trachea, or it can be punctured with a 1 cm vertical stab through the membrane. The cannula used to make the puncture (usually a 14 gauge needle) is left in place, and the patient is ventilated through the cannula. A cricothyrotomy is a temporary measure, used until a tracheostomy is performed or the obstructed airway is cleared.

A cricothyrotomy provides rapid access to the airway and allows the placement of a cuffed tube into the airway to ventilate the patient. Potential complications include too wide a cut through the membrane resulting in a pneumothorax, laceration of the esophagus, a through-and-through laceration of the trachea, false tube passage resulting in subcutaneous and mediastinal emphysema, and the possible creation of a tracheoesophageal fistula.

Transtracheal Catheter Ventilation

Transtracheal catheter ventilation is another method for rapidly accessing the airway. After an antiseptic solution is used to prepare the skin, a large-bore plastic cannula, inserted through the cricothyroid membrane into the trachea is attached to a high-pressure oxygen flow device—a procedure sometimes called needle jet cricothyroidostomy. The high-flow oxygen device is on for one second, then off for four seconds. Since carbon dioxide accumulates quickly with this airway device it should be used for only 30 to 45 minutes.

Possible complications include asphyxia, esophageal perforation, thyroid perforation, possible hemorrhage with exsanguination, and subcutaneous emphysema.

Tracheostomy

Contrary to popular belief, a tracheostomy is neither easily nor quickly performed. In fact, it takes at least 15 to 20 minutes to perform a proper tracheostomy on a child. Tracheostomy, therefore, is not the initial choice for airway maintenance. This technique is usually a long-term mechanism, performed under sterile conditions in a controlled, calm environment, rather than in the heat of the moment in a busy emergency department.

When this technique is used, the patient should have a pillow placed under his shoulders to help place his neck in extension. After the skin is prepared with an antiseptic solution, the tracheostomy is performed, allowing the placement of a cuffed tracheostomy tube. The tube is checked for accurate placement by observing bilateral breath sounds. Then the cuff is inflated, and the incision is dressed, with the tracheostomy tube secured with tracheostomy tape. A ventilator may be attached to the tracheostomy tube. A chest x-ray film should be obtained to verify correct placement of the tube.

Complications of a tracheostomy include hemorrhage, infection, laceration of arteries and nerves, laceration of the thyroid, creation of a tracheoesophageal fistula, perforation of the esophagus, creation of a pneumothorax, and subcutaneous and mediastinal emphysema. Most health care providers feel that a tracheostomy is a surgical procedure that should be done in an operating room, not in the emergency department. The procedure is not recommended for young children, because it makes them prone to long-term tracheal stenosis. An emergency tracheostomy, however, should be performed whenever the patient presents with a fractured larynx or with a pharyngeal foreign body, but only after all other techniques of airway maintenance have been attempted and have failed.

AIRWAY OBSTRUCTION

Foreign body obstruction of the airway accounted for more than 2900 deaths in 1978. Bartlett (1979) stated that 75 percent of all foreign material found obstructing air and food passages occurs in children under five years of age. A large number of people who choke are labeled "café coronaries," because they are in a restaurant eating when they choke on their food. Choking is often mistaken for a coronary occlusion. The nurse must differentiate the patient who has foreign body airway obstruction from the patient who requires cardiopulmonary resuscitation.

Choking is categorized into three types or phases (Nagel, 1980):

1. Choking due to partial airway obstruction by a foreign body with good air exchange.
2. Choking due to partial airway obstruction with inadequate air exchange.
3. Choking due to total airway obstruction resulting in respiratory failure, with the inability to cough, talk, or ventilate.

Management of the patient ranges from simple observation to complicated removal of the foreign body.

Clinical Manifestations

Patients present to the triage nurse with foreign bodies located practically anywhere in the ear, nose, and throat. The nasal foreign body eventually produces a foul-smelling discharge. Little pain is present. A pharyngeal foreign body, commonly found in both adults and children, usually results from a chicken or fish bone. An oversized, poorly chewed piece of meat usually becomes lodged in the laryngeal area. A foreign body in the trachea and/or bronchi produces a cough with a wheeze, decreased breath sounds, and decreased chest expansion. With an esophageal foreign body, the patient usually feels a marked sticking sensation in the throat.

Wherever the foreign body is located, if it obstructs the airway, the patient requires immediate attention. The nurse may observe symptoms and signs including, but not limited to, the following:

Noisy breathing.

Suprasternal and intercostal retractions.

Stridor.

Increased duration of inspiration.

Cyanosis.

Obtundation.

Coma.

In a child, an ineffective cough, high-pitched noises while inhaling, increased respiratory difficulty, and blueness of the lips, nails, and skin may indicate an airway obstruction.

Nursing Care and Related Interventions

Nursing care of the patient with an obstructed airway must be organized and efficient and performed in a calm manner. The nurse must be aware of her or his anxiety and try to remain calm in the situation, while also helping the patient to remain calm. Continued fighting and agitation by the patient may increase obstruction in the patient's airway.

All patients with a suspected foreign body in any location should be placed in a high Fowler's position. Foreign bodies in the nose and pharyngeal area are usually removed with adequate light, suction, and bayonet forceps. An esophageal foreign body, particularly a hard object like a coin or a bead, can be removed by inserting a Foley catheter into the esophagus, past the foreign body, then inflating the balloon and removing the Foley catheter, which pulls the foreign body out of the esophagus. A laryngoscope and endotracheal tube should be accessible in case the airway becomes obstructed. A foreign body in the trachea and bronchi can be easily misdiagnosed as pneumonia or asthma, unless a chest x-ray film (including inspiration and expiration studies) is taken. The film will show trapped air on expiration.

The *Heimlich maneuver,* first developed in 1974, is the preferred action for a patient with a laryngeal foreign body. A foreign body in the larynx is the most common cause of an airway obstruction. The Heimlich maneuver attempts to raise the intrathoracic pressure to a level sufficient to permit expulsion of the foreign body

AIRWAY OBSTRUCTION

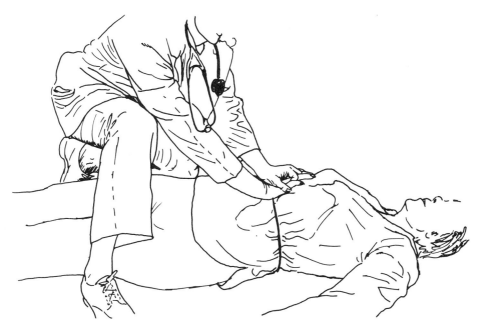

Figure 5.3 The Heimlich maneuver with a supine patient.

from the laryngeal area. If the patient is lying down, he should be rolled onto his side facing the nurse, and four sharp blows should be delivered with the heel of the hand over the spine and between the shoulder blades. The patient should then be rolled onto his back. Then four manual thrusts are delivered to the upper abdomen or lower chest to force air out of the lungs by creating an artificial cough (see Fig. 5.3). The nurse should kneel down beside the patient, with the heel of the hand placed against the patient's abdomen and the nurse's shoulders directly over the patient's abdomen. The chest thrust is necessary in patients with marked obesity, in patients in a state of advanced pregnancy, and in patients with abdominal eviscerations. If the chest thrust is used, the hands should be placed in the middle of the sternum, missing the xiphoid process, and close to the edges of the rib cage. After the back and abdominal (chest) thrusts, the patient should be rolled away from the nurse, and the mouth swept out with the fingers. This maneuver should dislodge the foreign body. The procedure should be repeated until the obstruction is dislodged.

If the patient is sitting or standing (see Fig. 5.4), stand behind the patient, put your arms around the patient's waist, with one hand clenched in a fist and your other hand over it. Place the thumb side of the fist against the patient's abdomen, between the waist and the rib cage. Deliver four quick thrusts. The thrusts should be inward and upward thrusts. No data support whether back or abdominal thrusts should be used first, but combining back and abdominal (chest) thrusts is perhaps the best maneuver to try for opening the airway.

AIRWAY PROBLEMS

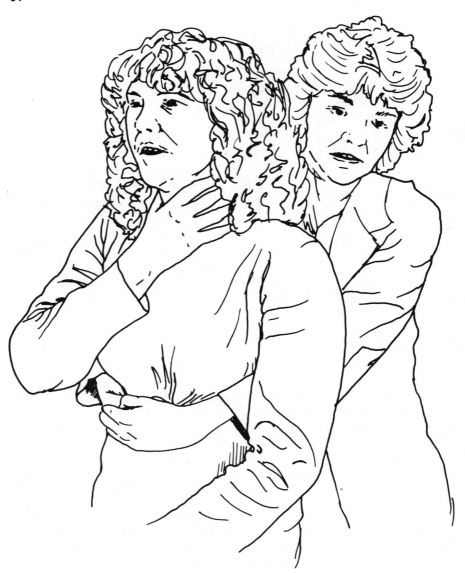

Figure 5.4 The Heimlich maneuver with a standing patient.

Complications
Agia and Hurst (1979) claim that a pneumomediastinum may develop following the Heimlich maneuver. Pain is the most common presenting symptom. A chest x-ray study is required to make a definitive diagnosis. Cases of fractured ribs and ruptured livers and stomachs are other documented complications. Trott (1979) suggests that recurrent airway obstruction is a complication of the Heimlich maneuver. Edema and

subsequent airway obstruction can also occur after the removal of a foreign body from the hypopharynx.

Special Considerations in Children
Abdominal thrusts should not be used in children, due to the possible injury of the abdominal organs, especially the liver. Infants and young children should be lain over the nurse's arm, with the head placed lower than the trunk. Support the child's head with your hand around the child's jaw and chest; be careful to keep your fingers away from the carotid. Four back blows between the child's shoulder blades should be delivered with the heel of the hand. Use less force than is used for an adult. The child should then be turned and placed on the nurse's thigh, and four *chest* thrusts should be done, while continually supporting the child's head and neck.

Older children should be lain across the nurse's thighs, while the nurse kneels on the floor to deliver the back thrusts. The older child should then be placed supine on the floor, and the chest thrusts delivered. The combination of back and chest thrusts should be repeated, until the foreign body has been dislodged, clearing the obstructed airway.

THE USE OF OXYGEN IN AIRWAY MAINTENANCE

Oxygen should be started immediately in any patient with any type of airway problem. Oxygen should not be withheld in order to obtain a set of baseline blood gases. Anyone with airway problems requires the extra oxygen as soon as possible to help decrease anxiety and to improve the oxygen concentration of the blood. Additional oxygen improves the patient's mental state, as well as the status of the person's vital organs.

Oxygen can be delivered via several devices, including nasal cannulas, face masks, reservoir masks, bag-mask devices, and oxygen-powered devices. The nurse should be aware of these devices and be able to select the appropriate device for each patient's specific problem (See Table 5.2). Using oxygen requires the following precautions:

1. Humidify the oxygen whenever possible, except when using a bag-mask or oxygen-powered device.
2. Deliver at least 5 l of oxygen when using a mask device, because expired air can accumulate in the device, resulting in an increase of inspired carbon dioxide and a decrease in inspired oxygen.
3. Gradually reduce the use of oxygen. Do not discontinue its use abruptly.

Discharge Planning

Before the patient is discharged from the emergency department following a relatively minor airway problem, discharge planning is imperative. The planning should include assessment of the patient's and/or family's readiness to learn, teaching, and

TABLE 5.2 Oxygen Delivery Systems

System	Indication for Use	Nursing Considerations
Nasal cannula	Only patient with spontaneous respirations. Patient comfort low-flow system. Does not interfere with the oral cavity, provides continuous positive airway pressure for infants and children.	Flow rate of 2–6 l/min. yields 25–40% oxygen concentration. May cause dry mucous membranes or headache if > 6 l/min. Check for pressure areas under nose and over ears.
Simple face mask	Only patient with spontaneous respirations, who needs higher oxygen concentration than can be achieved with nasal cannula.	Does not dry the mucous membranes of the nose and mouth, cannot deliver > 40% oxygen concentration. Severely dyspneic patients will not tolerate it well. Do not use on patient with COPD. Do not adjust the strap too tightly.
Rebreathing mask (oxygen reservoir mask)	Only patient with spontaneous respirations. Higher oxygen concentration than nasal cannula or simple face mask.	Tight seal necessary to ensure accurate oxygen concentration (90%). Never let the bag totally deflate during inhalation. To fill bag initially, apply the mask as the patient exhales.
Venturi mask	Only patient with spontaneous respirations, who needs a fixed concentration of oxygen.	Connect the mask with correct adapter to deliver the required concentration (24–40%). Observe for signs of oxygen toxicity.
Bag-mask	Patient who either is breathing spontaneously or is apneic. Pediatric size is appropriate for use on a child.	Needs a tight seal around nose and mouth. Use an oropharyngeal or a nasopharyngeal airway with this system. Observe closely for possible emesis. Allows nurse to assess lung compliance.
Oxygen-powered breathing devices	Patient who is apneic and has a mask, EOA, endotracheal tube or transtracheal catheter in place. Only used in children under 12 years of age if a special pediatric adaptor is available.	Observe for gastric distention and overinflation. The time this system can be used is very variable depending on the patient and the operator. Delivers 100% oxygen concentration.

patient/family comprehension and evaluation of the plan. The discharge planning always includes the patient's significant other, such as his family and/or friends.

Before beginning to instruct patient and family, note whether they seem calm enough and ready to absorb the information. The patient who is severely anxious is not ready to learn anything about his care or health maintenance. The family or friends occasionally may be ready to learn before the patient is ready, so they should be taught how to care for the patient's needs. They can then pass that information onto the patient, when the person is ready to comprehend the information.

The discharge teaching should be individualized for each patient situation. Simple mechanisms of opening the airway should be illustrated, such as how to open the mouth and elevate the tongue to remove it from blocking the airway. Parents should be shown the correct procedure for using a bulb syringe to suction their small child. Referrals can be made to the local Red Cross or Heart Association chapter for instruction in more advanced mechanisms of airway maintenance and life support.

To help avoid an obstructed airway, people should be taught to chew slowly and not to talk while chewing their food. They should also be instructed to cut their meat into small pieces and to eat small bites of other foods. Parents should evaluate their child's playthings at home and remove anything that is small enough to become a possible foreign body in their child's airway. Prevention should be stressed. The Heimlich maneuver should be discussed, and the patient referred to a local community agency for provision of definitive instruction and certification. The importance of being certified in basic life support should be stressed to the patient and the family, because no one ever knows when it might be necessary to save another's life. Instruction should also include signs and symptoms that will alert the patient to return, if necessary, to the emergency department. Some symptoms might include difficulty in talking, difficulty in breathing, bluish lips or fingernails, hemoptysis, hematemesis, or noisy respirations in a child. Comprehension should be documented through demonstration by the patient and family or through verbal feedback highlighting the points explained to them.

A thorough understanding of any medication prescribed should be documented, including an understanding of side effects and correct dosage. The patient and family should be given a telephone number where they can reach someone 24 hours a day to ask additional questions or to discuss a change in the patient's condition with a health care provider. A public health nurse referral may be necessary to have someone check on the continuing status of the patient at home. Another mechanism for follow-up is to call the patient at home the next day to check on the person's condition, to reinforce the teaching, and to evaluate the effectiveness of the teaching.

CONCLUSION

The emergency department nurse must be able to care efficiently and effectively for a patient experiencing airway problems. The nurse must understand and be able to manage both the patient's response and the nurse's response to this situation. The first step in caring for all patients involves proper airway maintenance. The emergency department nurse should thoroughly understand all types of airway problems to ensure adequate patient care.

BIBLIOGRAPHY

Agia, G. A., and D. J. Hurst: Pneumomediastinum following the Heimlich maneuver. *JACEP* 8:473–475 (1979).

———: Airway management. *Emergency Medicine* 12:31–42 (1980).

Bartlett, P. C.: Aliens in the ENT. *Emergency Medicine* 11:278–282 (1979).

Budassi, S. A.: Management of cardiopulmonary arrest. *Nursing Clinics of North America* 16:37–57 (1981).

Dailey, R., A. Hyman, J. Redding, and D. H. Rice: Emergency procedures: Update on upper airway management. *Patient Care* 12:233+ (1978).

Meislin, H. W.: The esophageal obturator airway: A study of respiratory effectiveness. *Annals of Emergency Medicine* 9:54–59 (Feb. 1980).

Meislin, H. W.: The esophageal airway: It works, but . . . . *Annals of Emergency Medicine* 9:171 (March 1980).

Nagel, E.: Opening the obstructed airway. *Emergency Medicine* 12:24–30 (1980).

———: Part II—Basic life support in adults. *Emergency Medicine* 12:49–95 (1980).

———: Part III—Basic life support in infants and children. *Emergency Medicine* 12:95–104 (1980).

———: The immature airway. *Emergency Medicine* 10:56–58 (1978).

Trott, A.: Recurrent upper airway obstruction. *JACEP* 8:407–408 (1979).

6
Coma

Janet Gren Parker

After completing this chapter, the reader will be able to do the following:

1. Triage a patient in coma.
2. Explain the Glasgow Coma Scale (GCS).
3. Discuss the pathophysiology of a patient in coma and identify structural, toxic, metabolic, and psychogenic coma types.
4. Recognize the clinical manifestations of a patient in coma.
5. List appropriate diagnostic studies in the management of the patient in coma.
6. Discuss the general nursing care of the patient in coma.
7. Discuss the nursing care of the patient with specific common causes of coma.
8. Discuss the discharge planning for patients with specific causes of coma.

Caring for the patient in coma is challenging for the emergency department nurse, because coma is merely symptomatic of another underlying disease and not, in fact, an actual disease. Identifying the underlying cause of the coma is necessary to ensure providing the appropriate therapy for the patient in coma. A few of the most common causes of coma include alcoholism, trauma, drug overdose, vascular problems, and metabolic disorders.

Coma is derived from the Greek word *koma,* meaning lethargy or deep sleep. Coma is a sleeplike state from which the patient cannot be aroused. Patients in coma are unresponsive to any external stimulation or to internal psychological needs (Spielman, 1981). Coma is the absence of awareness of self and the external environment, even when the patient is externally stimulated (Plum and Posner, 1980). Coma occurs in a broad category of patient types, which can be confusing. To the layperson, as well as to the health care professional, it represents fear of the unknown, brain damage, and death.

The emergency department nurse must be able to do the following: understand all the possible causes of coma; astutely assess the patient in coma; develop and implement a plan of care for the patient in coma, and be attentive to patient discharge planning to help prevent the recurrence of a similar episode.

TRIAGE

The nurse who triages the patient in coma performs an important function. The initial history and assessment form the basis for the care developed and implemented. The triage nurse, therefore, must be as clear and as accurate as possible in collecting data relating to the patient in coma.

Subjective Data

Data collected from the history will facilitate developing a plan of care for the patient in coma. A *chronological* history of the events leading to the patient's present condition is particularly useful. Unfortunately, the patient cannot relate this history. The triage nurse's best sources for obtaining information are the family, friends, or ambulance personnel involved with the patient. Try to reconstruct what happened to the patient that produced the person's condition. Certain complaints the patient expressed earlier, for example, might suggest the cause of the coma. Look for medical alert tags on the arms, legs, and around the neck of the patient. Document how the patient was found, where the patient was found, the presence or absence of odors, pills, or bottles close to the patient, and any behavior by the patient that was unusual. All pertinent negatives or lack of signs and symptoms should also be explored to help ascertain a reason for the coma. If the patient is an infant, ask whether any previous infant deaths have occurred in the family. Ask about the infant's feeding patterns. Has the infant's formula been changed recently? Where was the formula purchased? If the infant is breast-fed, has the mother changed her diet or started taking any new medications? If the infant can walk, did he fall recently? If the patient is a toddler, carefully question the family regarding pill bottles and cleaning equipment. Is the family certain that everything is intact at home? Was the patient recently exposed to illness of any type? With teenagers, question the parents about possible drug abuse. Does a drug problem exist either in the school or on the block at home?

A pertinent past medical history may provide valuable clues regarding the etiology of the patient's present condition. Does the person have chronic renal problems? Is the person a diabetic? Does the child have a seizure disorder? Does the patient have a drug abuse problem? Is hypertension a factor? A thorough history of all current medications, as well as all medications to which the patient might be allergic, should be ascertained to help provide data used to develop a plan of care.

Objective Data

The triage nurse begins a brief, immediate collection of objective data as soon as the patient arrives in the emergency department. Included in the initial assessment is airway, breathing, and circulatory status. If these functions are stable, a more detailed examination is done to help ascertain the possible cause of the coma.

Assessment of the level of consciousness (LOC) is the most important information documented by the triage nurse. Do not label the level of consciousness, but do describe the behavior of the patient. The LOC is best defined when assessed on a

TABLE 6.1 The Glasgow Coma Scale

Category			Response
1. *Eye Opening.* Determine minimal stimulus that evokes opening of at least one eye.	a.	4 points	Eyes open spontaneously.
	b.	3 points	Eyes open in response to speech, either at command or when patient is called by name.
	c.	2 points	Eyes open to painful stimuli.
	d.	1 point	No eye opening in response to painful stimuli.
2. *Verbal.* Determine best response after arousal.	a.	5 points	Patient is oriented to person, place, and time.
	b.	4 points	Patient is confused.
	c.	3 points	Patient uses words or phrases that make little or no sense or uses words inappropriately.
	d.	2 points	Patient responds with incomprehensible sounds.
	e.	1 point	Patient makes no verbal sound, even in response to painful stimuli.
3. *Motor.* Determine the best response with either arm.	a.	6 points	Patient obeys simple commands.
	b.	5 points	Patient purposefully tries to remove painful stimuli.
	c.	4 points	Patient responds to painful stimuli with flexion withdrawal.
	d.	3 points	Patient responds with abnormal flexion (decorticate posture) to painful stimuli.
	e.	2 points	Patient responds with abnormal extension (decerebrate posture) to painful stimuli.
	f.	1 point	Patient has no motor response to painful stimuli.

SOURCE: Jones, 1979.

continuum. The Glasgow Coma Scale (GCS), developed in 1974 at the University of Glasgow in Scotland, is a fast, accurate, and simple tool for evaluating the level of consciousness. (Table 6.1 contains the Glasgow Coma Scale.) The numerical value of each category is added to give the health care provider a sum that objectively measures the LOC. The normal total score is 15; the lowest is 3, signifying brain death; any score below 7 is labeled coma.

The triage nurse should use the sense of smell to discern any odors (such as alcohol) present on the patient's breath. The skin color, integrity, and temperature should be documented. A complete set of vital signs is necessary, as well as a brief examination of the pupils to note size and reactivity. Check for false eyes and contact lenses. The neck should be protected at all times, until trauma has been ruled out as a cause of coma. Assessing the integrity of the skull and scalp, as well as noting any cerebral spinal fluid leakage from the nose or ears, may eliminate trauma as a possible cause of the coma.

Assessment and Planning

By analyzing the subjective and objective data collected, the triage nurse makes an assessment and develops an initial plan of care. This plan of care should include the priority of the patient's care (usually emergent) and appropriate nursing interventions, such as protection of the airway. The family might need reassurance to reduce their anxiety and to help them cope better with the situation. (Table 6.2 contains three examples of triage notes for patients presenting to the emergency department in coma.)

The following sections contain a thorough discussion of the pathophysiology of coma, clinical manifestations, nursing care and related interventions, and specific causes of coma. Knowledge of this material will aid the nurse in performing accurate and appropriate triage.

PATHOPHYSIOLOGY

Coma usually results from a disruptive event affecting cerebral metabolism. Although the brain represents only two percent of the adult body weight, it requires 20 percent of the body's oxygen. Oxygen is not stored in the brain, but is carried to the brain by the vascular system. Coma ensues within 10 seconds after the blood flow to the brain is stopped. The anaerobic metabolic pathway can sustain the brain for only a few seconds. Glucose is the only organic nutrient that is able to cross the blood brain barrier (BBB); thus, it is the only nutrient that supplies the brain with energy. In coma, some disruptive event occurs that alters the normal oxygen and glucose metabolism of the brain.

The disruptive event must affect the cortex and/or the reticular activating system (RAS) to produce coma. Both the cortex and the RAS are usually affected by the development of edema. Brain edema results from an increase in the volume and weight of the organ as a result of an accumulation of fluid. The accumulated fluid in the brain results in a compromise of blood flow or ischemia to the brain. Hyperemia is a form of brain swelling in which there is an increase in cerebral blood flow that exceeds the metabolic needs of the brain. Hyperemia results in cerebral congestion that is due to an increase in blood volume, rather than fluid volume, particularly in pediatric and adult head trauma.

Cerebral edema can be either vasogenic or cytotoxic in nature. If vasogenic, a severe disturbance in the BBB competence causes all of the plasma constituents to leave the vascular confines and to accumulate in the extravascular space—a condition common in neurological conditions. If cytotoxic, the neurons, glia, and endothelial cells of the brain attract fluid and swell, creating a corresponding decrease in the

TABLE 6.2 Examples of Triage Notes for Patients in Coma

S: 10 yo WF with c/o "not feeling well." App. 1 hour prior to admission, patient is on school trip with teacher, teacher relates history of progressive lethargy followed by disorientation, nausea and vomiting. No fever, no h/o trauma. PMH: diabetic, 10 units U100 Reg and 24 units U100 Lente 8 a.m., took insulin this a.m., NKA.

O: Pale, dry skin, ketone smell on breath. RR 52 rapid and labored, GCS 7, makes incomprehensible sounds with appropriate flexion to pain, vomitus on shirt, pupils equal and reactive.

A: Coma 2° to DKA.

P: Pediatric evaluation, admit to examination room immediately, protect airway.

S: 22 yo WF dumped at the entrance from a car, discovered by security lying in the doorway, no other history available. PMH: unknown, allergies unknown, current meds unknown.

O: Pale, disheveled appearance, dirty skin, body odor, GCS 5, responds with flexion to painful stimuli, track marks on arms and legs, malnourished in appearance. RR 4 shallow, pupils pinpoint.

A: Coma. R/O drug overdose/abuse.

P: Medical evaluation, admit examination room immediately, prepare for intubation.

S: 52 yo WM brought by family from funeral for wife. Patient "very emotional," fainted at funeral. Family unable to make patient respond since then, no complaints prior to faint. PMH: HTN, diet controlled, NKA, no current meds.

O: WDWN male, eyelids fluttering slightly, GCS 5, keeps extremity in position where it is placed by nurse, color good. RR 16 normal, P 88 regular, BP 138/90. Skin cool to touch, pupils equal and reactive.

A: Coma, R/O psychogenic cause, anxiety reaction.

P: Medical evaluation, admit examination room now, have family member remain with patient.

---

extracellular fluid space—a condition characteristic of a hypoxic injury that ultimately produces neuronal necrosis.

The result of edema, regardless of the cause, is an increase in the intracranial pressure, which eventually causes a disruption of the cerebral metabolism, thus producing a comatose state. The disruptive events that create the edema are classified into three broad categories (Plum and Posner, 1980): structural disorders; toxic/metabolic disorders; and psychogenic disorders (even though no actual edema is created).

Structural disorders are processes that cause actual physical damage to the brain, such as tumors, strokes, trauma, encephalitis, and intracerebral hemorrhages. Symptoms of structural comas are focal signs, such as hemiparesis and cranial nerve abnormalities. Diseases that either produce endogenous nervous system poisons or delete the nutrients from the brain are *toxic/metabolic disorders*. Coma resulting from the ingestion of toxic substances is also included in this category. Examples of toxic/metabolic disorders include diabetic ketoacidosis, hepatic failure, uremia, heroin overdose, camphor ingestion, and hypoxia. *Psychogenic disorders* are processes of a psychiatric origin that may create a comatose state. Conversion reactions, depression, anxiety reactions, and catatonic stupor are included in this category.

CLINICAL MANIFESTATIONS

The patient must be completely disrobed to enable the nurse to make an appropriate assessment of all the signs and symptoms that may be present. The patient may present with alcohol, fruity, urine, or poison smells on his breath. The patient's skin may be cyanotic, red, jaundiced, or pale, or there may be a rash. The respiratory rate may be elevated, depressed, or normal. The temperature may be elevated or subnormal. The blood pressure may be above or below normal limits. Motor signs may be symmetrical or asymmetrical. Pupillary reactions may be normal or abnormal. In all situations, however, the primary sign will be a decreased LOC. Specific differential characteristics of patients in coma are summarized in Table 6.3. These signs and symptoms will provide the nurse with many clues regarding the possible orgin of the comatose state.

A clinical condition that may be confused with coma is a locked-in state, which occurs when a lesion in the brainstem damages the descending motor tracts to the face and the limbs, but spares the RAS and the innervation to the eyes. The patient is totally awake, but his face and limbs are completely paralyzed.

DIAGNOSTIC STUDIES

Laboratory studies may help to provide a differential diagnosis of the patient in coma. Blood should be drawn for drug and alcohol studies; levels of phosphorus, magnesium, electrolytes, creatinine, calcium, blood urea nitrogen, and glucose; liver function studies, complete blood cell count and differential; and coagulation studies. In addition, thyroid function tests may also be ordered. If a particular cause is suspected due to specific clinical manifestations, some of these studies may be deleted. Arterial blood gas studies should be included whenever cardiorespiratory function is compromised or acidosis is suspected. Patients with serum glucose levels of 70–100 mg/100 ml will present clinically with confusion, and in coma with a 200 mg/100 ml level.

Urine should be obtained for a drug screen, and a urinalysis checked for glucose and acetone levels. If gastric contents are aspirated, they should be analyzed for drug content. An electrocardiogram (ECG) may be ordered if the pulse is irregular, too fast, or too slow. Skull, cervical spine, and chest x-ray studies should be performed to rule out trauma and respiratory problems. A computerized axial tomography (CAT) scan may also be necessary. (See Chapter 20 for a more detailed discussion.)

TABLE 6.3 Differential Characteristics of Patients in Coma

Clinical Manifestation	Possible Cause
Odor	
Alcohol	Alcoholic intoxication
Fruity	Diabetic ketoacidosis
Urine	Uremia
Specific poison	Toxic ingestion
Fecal	Bowel obstruction
Skin	
Cyanotic	Hypoxia, shock
Jaundice	Hepatic failure
Rash, petechial hemorrhage	Meningitis, infection
Needle tracks	Drug abuse
Pale	Hypovolemia, shock, anemia
Red	Heat exposure, alcohol
Red lips	Carbon monoxide poisoning
Vital Signs	
Temperature–elevated	Infection, heat exposure
–subnormal	Dehydration, barbiturate overdose alcohol intoxification, myxedema
Pulse–elevated	Infection, hypoxia
–slow	Overdose
–irregular	Dysrhythmias, anoxia
Respirations–regular, even	Hysteria, postictal state
–slow, regular	Morphine and barbiturate intoxification
–Cheyne-Stokes	Increased intracranial pressure
–Kussmaul	Acidosis (diabetic), uremia, hyperventilation, salicylate poisoning
Blood pressure–hyper	Increased intracranial pressure, CVA
–hypo	Blood loss, overdose, sepsis, myocardial infarction
Pupils	
Constricted, pinpoint	Narcotic overdose
Dilated	Barbiturate overdose
Unequal	Intracranial lesion
Fixed, dilated	Atropine overdose
Small, equal, reactive	Metabolic disorder
Nonreactive	Severe brain damage
Motor Abilities	
Hemiplegia	CVA
Decerebrate	Brainstem involvement
Decorticate	Cerebral cortex involvement
Nuchal rigidity	Subarachnoid, infection
Limb placed in position and remains there	Psychogenic cause
Reflexes	
Dolls-head maneuver absent	Brainstem involvement
Oculovestibular response absent	Pontine centers involved
Babinski present	Pyramidal tract dysfunction
Brudzinski present	Inflammation of meninges
Lid reflex—involuntarily blinks	Psychogenic cause

A lumbar puncture (LP) may be performed as long as no signs of increased intracranial pressure, such as papilledema, exist. Herniation can result if an LP is done inappropriately. The cerebral spinal fluid obtained from the LP should be tested for glucose and protein levels, a cell count performed, and a differential study done. The normal cerebral spinal fluid is clear and colorless. If it is bloody, suspect a subarachnoid hemorrhage; if cloudy, meningitis; and if yellow, an old hemorrhage.

An electroencephalogram (EEG) rarely helps in an emergency situation. Although the EEG might be useful for determining the severity of the situation, it won't reveal the cause of the coma.

NURSING CARE AND RELATED INTERVENTIONS

The primary concern regarding a patient in coma is the patency of the airway. (Chapter 5 discusses this procedure in detail.) Next, a cardiac monitor should be attached to the patient, and a complete set of vital signs should be recorded. Any bleeding present should be stopped with pressure dressings. The patient should be started on oxygen therapy. Blood samples must be obtained before any medications are given or an intravenous (IV) line started. An intravenous line of dextrose 5 percent in water should be started to ensure access to the circulation. Be careful to avoid fluid overload and pulmonary edema. Twenty-five grams of glucose (50 ml of 50 percent solution) should be given intravenously to any comatose patient whose diagnosis is unclear. Although the glucose will prevent brain damage due to hypoglycemia, it will not damage the brain of patients who are not hypoglycemic (Plum and Posner, 1980). Naloxone (0.8 mg) should be given intravenously to rule out narcotic overdosage. If the history of the incident indicates a poisoning or overdose, a nasogastric tube is inserted and gastric lavage performed. A Foley catheter should be inserted to help monitor the circulatory status of the patient and to obtain the necessary urine samples. These steps should be followed whether the patient is an adult or a child.

Special diagnostic tests are then performed to help pinpoint the cause of the coma. During the testing, the nurse continually observes the patient and documents vital signs every 15 minutes. The nurse should observe for seizures, agitation, increased intracranial pressure, dysrhythmias, and any changes in vital signs. The patient will usually be admitted for continuing care.

SPECIFIC CAUSES OF COMA

Hypoglycemia is the most common cause of coma, in addition to diabetic ketoacidosis, hyperglycemic-hyperosmolar nonketotic coma, alcoholic ketosis, uremia, myxedema, trauma, and seizure disorders (Hare and Rossini, 1979). (Coma resulting from trauma is discussed in detail in the trauma chapters.)

The patient with *hypoglycemia* appears diaphoretic and agitated. The patient's LOC decreases gradually, until the person is combative, abusive, and unaware of his actions. The history will usually reveal a diabetic who has increased his insulin dosage, skipped a meal, or increased his activity level. Hypoglycemia is easily corrected with 25 g of glucose given intravenously.

SPECIFIC CAUSES OF COMA

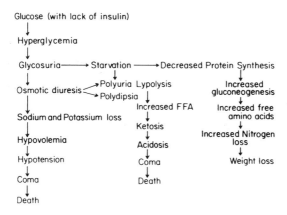

Figure 6.1   The pathophysiology of diabetic ketoacidosis.

Patients with *diabetic ketoacidosis* (DKA) may vary from being fully awake to being in deep coma. (Figure 6.1 illustrates the pathophysiology of DKA.) Common causes of DKA include undiagnosed diabetes, omission of insulin, stress (either positive or negative), and/or an intercurrent disease or infection. The patient may experience polyuria, polydipsia, nausea, vomiting, abdominal pain, dehydration, constipation, Kussmaul respirations, and acetone breath. The patient's urine will be positive for glucose and ketones. Blood results will show a glucose level higher than 250 mg, positive acetone levels, low bicarbonate levels, an acidotic pH level, low sodium levels, and a potassium level that can be high, low, or normal.

The care of the patient in DKA includes fluid replacement with 0.9 percent normal saline. If the blood sodium level rises above 155 mg, switch the fluids to 0.45 percent normal saline. Regular insulin should be given IV as a bolus, and then in continuous infusion with an infusion pump. The amount of insulin depends on the patient's size and glucose levels. Bicarbonate is added to the IV fluid to maintain a serum pH level greater than 7.0. Overtreatment with bicarbonate can create an alkalotic state that can result in dangerous hypokalemia, paradoxical cerebral spinal fluid acidosis, and an impaired oxygen-hemoglobin dissociation. If the serum glucose values are decreased too rapidly, the patient may develop cerebral edema.

Hyperglycemic-hyperosmolar nonketotic coma (HHNC) occurs in elderly patients with undiagnosed diabetes. Patients who present with this condition are usually over age 60 and have either an intercurrent illness or preexisting cerebral, renal, or vascular disease. (Figure 6.2 illustrates the pathophysiology involved.) Patients in HHNC have enough insulin in their circulation to inhibit lipolysis. The patient may experience polyuria, polydipsia, dehydration, bizarre behavior, seizures, and coma. The patient's urine will be positive for glucose, but negative for ketones. The serum glucose level will be extremely high, ranging from 800 mg–2,800 mg. The serum acetone level will be negative; the serum urea nitrogen level elevated; and the pH level normal.

The care of the patient in HHNC is similar to a patient in ketoacidosis. Hydration is the most important step to help prevent or to counteract hypovolemia and hemoconcentration. The fluid used should be 0.9 percent normal saline at two liters

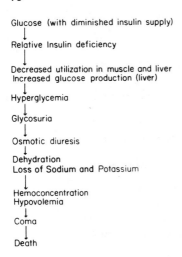

Figure 6.2 The pathophysiology of hyperglycemic-hyperosmolar nonketotic coma.

per hour. After the blood pressure has stabilized, the IV fluid is changed to 0.45 percent normal saline. Insulin may be given to help repair the metabolic derangement along with other electrolytes. The treatment should be cautious and gradual in nature to ensure that more good than harm is done. The mortality rate is 40 to 70 percent, with one-half of the deaths occurring within the first 24 hours. HHNC is frequently confused with cerebral vascular accidents.

Patients who abuse alcohol may present in *alcoholic ketosis*. Alcohol metabolism generates hydrogen ions that form lactic acid. Alcohol also inhibits gluconeogenesis, which leads to hypoglycemia. The nurse should suspect alcoholic ketosis in any patient with a history of alcohol intake, decreased eating habits, and nausea and vomiting with accompanying epigastric pain. Blood studies will indicate metabolic acidosis with a pH level that is frequently below 7.2. The serum glucose level may be high, normal, or low. Treatment involves hydration (IV of 0.9 percent normal saline) and correction of the hypoglycemia, if present. Thiamine 100 mg IV *must* be given before any glucose to prevent precipitating Wernicke's encephalopathy. The thiamine is followed with 25 g of glucose IV. Bicarbonate is given if the pH level is less than 7.1. Recovery is usually prompt, and the mortality is low.

The onset of coma from *uremia* is gradual in nature, with the patient exhibiting neuromuscular and personality changes. In uremia, acid metabolites increase due to the malfunction of the kidneys. The patient may have dry, scaly skin, dehydration, Kussmaul respirations, a uremic frost on the skin, and elevated levels of serum urea nitrogen and creatinine. The patient must be hydrated, and the patient's electrolyte balances must be closely monitored. Treatment depends on the amount of kidney function the patient possesses.

The patient with *myxedema* in crisis usually presents to the emergency department in coma. Myxedema is caused either by the surgical removal of the pituitary gland, which no longer stimulates the thyroid gland or by the hypoactivity of the pituitary gland, which also creates less stimulation of the thyroid. The coma is triggered by hypothermia, hyponatremia, and poor ventilation. Care is directed toward airway maintenance, replacement of sodium, and replacement of thyroxine. Levothyroxine is used intravenously to replace the thyroxine, in addition to some type of steroid replacement. The patient must be placed on the cardiac monitor to observe for signs of cardiac ischemia due to the increased oxygen demands from the thyroxine replacement.

Seizures may be focal or nonfocal in nature, with coma being, in fact, the postictal state. A seizure is a symptom, and the cause of the seizure must be determined. Status epilepticus is a series of grand mal seizures, without an intervening period of consciousness. This condition is serious, because hypoxia can result and cause brain death. The patient may make guttural sounds during the seizure, have urinary incontinence, show an increase in salivation, and cut his mouth, tongue, or lips. The patient usually will not remember the seizure. Moreover, seizures usually are self-limiting, but the patient must be protected so that he does not harm himself or others. Diazepam may be given intravenously to stop status epilepticus. Diazepam should be given slowly (5 mg/minute), and the dosage is variable, depending on the age and weight of the patient. Phenobarbitol may also be used, because it has fewer respiratory depressive side effects than diazepam. Phenytoin (Dilantin) should be given slowly (IV bolus of 50 mg/minute). The dosage is 1–2 mg/kg, and the patient should be on an ECG monitor. This treatment helps with long-term control of the seizures. (Diazepam has a short half-life.) After the seizures have been controlled, attention is directed toward identifying the cause of the seizure disorder.

DISCHARGE PLANNING

Most patients in coma who present to the emergency department will first be stabilized and then admitted to the hospital for further evaluation and monitoring. Diabetics, alcoholics, and patients with seizure disorders may be discharged after treatment in the emergency department. The nurse is responsible for ensuring that discharge planning is done for these patients.

Diabetics should be instructed regarding the importance of a consistent intake, avoidance of concentrated sweets, avoidance of cigarettes and other risk factors, and prevention of hypoglycemia. Ways to prevent hypoglycemia include not skipping meals and snacks, avoiding excessive exertion, and recognizing the symptoms of a pending episode of hypoglycemia. Signs and symptoms include sweating, nervousness, weakness, hunger, headache, and confusion. The patient, as well as significant others, should understand the symptoms. The patient should always carry a simple carbohydrate (such as Life-Savers or hard candy—but not chocolate, because it contains too much fat, making it hard to digest) and a complex carbohydrate (such as milk, half a sandwich with meat, or peanut butter crackers). Stress the importance of wearing a medical alert tag. Explain that commercial preparations of glucagon are available. The patient and family must be referred to appropriate health care professionals for long-term maintenance. The American Diabetes Association sponsors many group activities that may help both the patient and his family.

Instruct the diabetic to take his insulin, even if he is feeling ill. The patient must understand how and when to test his blood and urine for glucose levels. The person should also have a "sick day" diet planned for him by a dietician. The family and the patient must have a good rapport with the primary health care provider and feel comfortable calling for help and advice at any time.

The patient who abuses alcohol should be allowed to talk about his problem. The primary hindrance in helping the alcoholic is the person's refusal to recognize or admit that a problem exists. If the patient realizes he has a problem, adequate nutrition should be stressed and referral made to a local detoxification program, if necessary. The local chapter of Alcoholics Anonymous can provide helpful advice for ways to handle alcoholic patients.

Anyone with a new seizure disorder should be admitted to the hospital for a complete evaluation. People with known seizure disorders, however, are sometimes discharged from the emergency department. The nurse must ensure that someone remains with the patient for 24 hours and drives the patient home from the emergency department. The patient who is receiving seizure medication must understand the dosage, action, and side effects of the medication. Compliance should be stressed. Family and friends should be told what to do if another seizure occurs. They should remain calm, lay the person on a flat surface on his side, loosen tight clothing, insert a soft rag (or handkerchief) between the teeth only if the mouth is open, move objects away from the person so he will not harm himself, and reassure the person after the seizure stops. The physician should be called if the seizures continue, even if the person is on medication. If an outpatient EEG is scheduled, this procedure must be explained to the patient and family members. Appropriate referrals must be made for provision of long-term health care needs.

CONCLUSION

One of the most challenging situations for an emergency department nurse is caring for the patient in coma. All of the nurse's knowledge and skills are used to help plan and implement the care for a patient in coma. Continual evaluation of the care is necessary to meet the changing needs of the patient, as new data are discovered or possible causes of the coma are eliminated from consideration. The quality of patient care is enhanced when the emergency department nurse understands all of the aspects involved in caring for the patient in coma.

BIBLIOGRAPHY

Cavalier, J. P.: Crucial decisions in diabetic emergencies. *RN* 43:32–37 (Nov. 1980).

Finklestein, S., and A. Ropper: The diagnosis of coma: Its pitfalls and limitations. *Heart Lung* 8:1058–1064 (1979).

Hare, G. W., and A. A. Rossini: Diabetic comas: the overlap concept. *Hospital Practice* 14:95–99 (May 1979).

Jarvis, D. A.: . . . And the unconscious child. *Emergency Medicine* 12:45–47 (May 1980).

Jones, C.: Glasgow coma scale. *American Journal of Nursing* 79:1551–1553 (1979).

Miller, M.: Emergency management of the unconscious patient. *Nursing Clinics of North America* 16:59–73 (1981).

———: Never let sleeping drunks lie. *Emergency Medicine* 13:160–161 (1981).

Plum, F., and J. B. Posner: *The Diagnosis of Stupor and Coma.* Philadelphia: Davis, 1980, pp. 1–9, 345–362.

Sneid, D. S.: Hyperosmolar hyperglycemic nonketotic coma. *Critical Care Quarterly* 3:29–43 (Sept. 1980).

Spielman, G.: Coma: a clinical review. *Heart Lung* 10:700–707 (1981).

7
A Respiratory Emergency

Christina A. Ronshausen

After completing this chapter, the reader will be able to do the following:

1. Triage a patient experiencing a respiratory emergency.
2. Differentiate among the respiratory emergencies.
3. Identify the clinical manifestations of specific respiratory emergencies.
4. Recognize the appropriate diagnostic tests to be instituted in each emergency.
5. Implement the nursing care that is appropriate to the specific respiratory emergency identified.
6. Perform discharge planning when indicated for the patient with an acute respiratory problem.

One of the most frightening experiences for anyone is not being able to breathe adequately. A respiratory problem, therefore, can alarm the patient, the patient's family, and the health care provider. In treating the patient with a respiratory problem, the first consideration, of course, is adequate maintenance of the airway, regardless of the cause of the problem. After the airway has been maintained, the cause of the emergency can be identified.

This chapter discusses specific respiratory emergencies in detail. The care of the patient with asthma, inhalation injuries, hyperventilation syndrome, and near drowning will be discussed. The emergency department nurse who understands the principles discussed in this chapter will be able to provide the highest quality of care possible.

TRIAGE

Appropriate triage action can help the nurse to differentiate life-threatening problems from less severe conditions. Most people who present to the emergency department with respiratory distress will be extremely anxious and upset. The triage nurse can reassure patients and decrease their anxiety before the actual registration process occurs. The nurse also makes sure that patients requiring immediate attention receive it.

Subjective Data

The initial subjective history concentrates on the patient's chief complaint. Because respiratory distress may make talking difficult for the patient, the nurse often obtains most of the information from a relative or significant other.

The onset of the respiratory problem must be ascertained, in addition to any precipitating factors, such as where it occurred, when it occurred, duration, prior anxiety or stressful event, exposure to toxins or allergens, exposure to chemical irritants, and whether it is a water-related incident. Any associated conditions should be ascertained, such as neck injuries, respiratory infections, cardiac conditions, any previous incidents, and the presence of any major chronic diseases.

Any medications currently being taken by the patient, any drug allergies, and (particularly important for asthmatic patients) the type and amount of medication taken just prior to admission to the emergency department must be documented.

Objective Data

The severity of respiratory distress must be assessed to determine how quickly the patient must receive care. The rate, quality, and depth of respirations are documented. The skin color, especially around the lips and nailbeds, is generally indicative of the functioning of the respiratory system. The use of accessory muscles in breathing is also noted.

Auscultate the breath sounds and listen for audible wheezes. Does the patient have a productive cough? Does he have a fever? Are there any odors on the patient's breath or clothing? What is the temperature of his skin? Is diaphoresis present?

A brief neurological assessment may help in determining the amount, if any, of anoxia. Is the patient oriented or disoriented? Does the patient have recent and past recall of events? What signs of anxiety is the patient exhibiting?

Assessment and Planning

The nurse uses the subjective and objective data to assess the patient's problem. The plan of care for the patient, which is based on this initial assessment, includes the priorities of care and appropriate nursing interventions. (Table 7.1 contains examples of triage notes for patients experiencing a respiratory emergency.) A thorough discussion of the care of a patient experiencing specific problems follows. Knowledge of this material will aid the nurse in performing accurate and appropriate triage.

ASTHMA

Asthma, which is also called *reactive airway disease,* refers to episodic, reversible reactions of bronchoconstriction and bronchospasm to factors not usually considered

ASTHMA

TABLE 7.1 Examples of Triage Notes for Patients Experiencing Respiratory Distress

S: 19 yo WF with c/o SOB for app. 30 min. PTA. Experienced this at father's funeral. Suddenly started breathing rapidly and couldn't stop. No other complaints. Denies chest pain, fever or cough. PMH: negative, NKA, no current meds.
O: Tears streaming down face, RR 40 rapid and deep, skin color normal, no diaphoresis, equal bilateral breath sounds, no wheezes, can't sit still, constantly moving about on the stretcher, wringing her hands.
A: Hyperventilation syndrome.
P: Medical evaluation, admit examination room, dim lights, provide comfort measures and calmness.
S: 10 yo BF with c/o wheezes since last p.m., wheezes started when it started raining. Slept fitfully through the night. This a.m. no improvement. No fever or cough. PMH: asthma, NKA, currently on Theodur QID.
O: Audible wheezes with RR 40 and labored, sitting forward in chair, diaphoretic with pale lips.
A: Asthma.
P: Pediatric evaluation, admit examination room immediately.

to be irritants. Asthma is characterized by hyperreactive airways. There is edema of the bronchial mucosa, with increased bronchial mucus production. Asthma is also characterized by alternating periods of exacerbations and remissions.

Patients with asthma are classified as either acute or chronic. Patients with acute asthma are symptom-free during some periods. Chronic asthmatics, however, experience symptoms on an almost continual basis for several years.

Several theories regarding the etiology of asthma include the following:

Bacterial infections.
Food allergies.
IgE reaction.
Viral respiratory infections.

IgE reactions and viral respiratory infections are discussed in detail in the following sections.

Pathophysiology

The theory of *IgE reaction* involves circulating antigens that unite with sensitized basophils and mast cells. These basophils and mast cells have a specific antibody immunoglobulin (IgE) on their surfaces. This interaction causes the release of mediators. These mediators then stimulate the development of bronchospasm and increased cellular permeability, which results in edema and inflammation. Mucus production also increases.

The IgE levels in the blood of asthmatics is six times higher than the normal, nonasthmatic level. No correlation exists, however, between the level of IgE and the severity of asthma.

After an *infection,* an inflammatory process with viral colonization results in destruction of epithelial cells. When the epithelial cells regenerate, a wider space or junction exists between them, thus increasing the vulnerability of nerve fibers to stimuli. When the parasympathetic nerve fibers are stimulated, acetylcholine is released, which, in turn, causes bronchoconstriction.

Clinical Manifestations

The most common signs of asthma are dyspnea, wheezing, and a productive cough. The cough may be exaggerated. The patient may appear to be extremely apprehensive and may use accessory neck muscles to assist in breathing. The patient will also be diaphoretic. The patient's expiratory phase may be so prolonged that the expiratory phase becomes greater than the inspiratory phase (the opposite of normal). Breath sounds will be decreased or even absent as a result of mucus plugs and air-trapping. The patient will also be tachycardic.

Diagnostic Studies

A chest x-ray film may indicate atelectasis, infection, and/or air-trapping. Air-trapping is evident by an enlarged overall chest size.

Pulmonary function tests (PFT) sometimes cannot be done during an acute attack, because of the patient's noncompliance. If done, they will be abnormal. In acute asthmatics, the PFTs will probably be normal between attacks.

Arterial blood gas (ABG) studies will reveal hypoxia. In severe cases, respiratory acidosis will be revealed.

White blood cell (WBC) levels may increase either as a result of the inflammatory process or if an infection is present. The eosinophil count will also be elevated.

Sputum for culture and sensitivity may be ordered, if a superimposed infection is suspected. A respiratory infection will frequently trigger an asthmatic attack.

Nursing Care and Related Interventions

The primary intervention includes determining the causative agent, and then removing the patient from that agent if possible. Providing emotional support will alleviate the patient's anxiety. Because asthmatic patients are quite apprehensive, their anxiety tends to exaggerate symptoms. Alleviating the anxiety may help reduce the severity of symptoms. Instructing the patient to concentrate on one thing, such as counting, will distract the patient from his breathing and may reduce the symptoms.

Certain medications will reverse the airway constriction. Epinephrine or terbutaline are given in divided doses subcutaneously. Alupent or isoproterenol via intermittent positive pressure breathing (IPPB) therapy will assist bronchodilation in more severe cases. Aminophylline is often used as a last resort, when other means are ineffective. Giving steroids intravenously (IV), may help in reversing airway constriction through their antiinflammatory action. Continuously monitoring the vital signs is also important, because many drugs used in the treatment of asthma have long-term cardiovascular side effects. Susphrine, a long-acting epinephrine preparation, may be given just prior to discharge, particularly to children.

Fluids given orally or intravenously will help to liquify secretions. This procedure will facilitate removal of secretions by coughing or postural drainage. Postural drainage and percussion may be indicated in patients with significant amounts of secretions and in patients whose cough is ineffective. Attempts to place the patient in positions that facilitate maximum drainage, such as in the Trendelenburg prone position, may be hampered by the patient's dyspnea. The dyspnea may be worsened by placing a patient in these positions, because the diaphragm is forced upward in the chest by the abdominal contents.

After the acute episode subsides, pulmonary function tests may be done to determine the degree of lung dysfunction. This data, in addition to physical assessment and diagnostic tests, are used to determine the appropriate treatment plan for the patient.

Discharge Planning

The patient will require follow-up medical care after discharge from the emergency department. Assistance may be provided to help the patient find suitable medical care.

Patient education will help the patient control asthma. The purpose, action, side effects, and other aspects of medications (such as time of day to take the medicines to prevent side effects) should be explained to the patient.

The patient may be ordered to take the medication via a machine, such as an IPPB machine. The patient must understand how to work the machine: setting it up, instilling the medication, and cleaning the machine afterward. The patient may require assistance in obtaining equipment; for example, names of local distributors, and names of people in the social service department who can assist with purchase or rental of equipment.

Chest physiotherapy, postural drainage, and percussion may help the patient on an ongoing basis. The use of diagrams and booklets will assist the patient to learn and then to replicate the exercises at home. Booklets explaining the procedure for desensitizing the environment to reduce possible causative agents of asthma may also help the patient.

STATUS ASTHMATICUS

A patient with status asthmaticus does not respond to routine therapy. Characteristics of status asthmaticus include airway edema, airway smooth muscle constriction, increased mucus production, and increased air-trapping.

Status asthmaticus evolves in three stages. In the first stage, the patient has nasal flaring and chest retractions, with prolonged expirations. The patient has tachycardia and tachypnea. ABGs reveal metabolic acidosis with respiratory alkalosis. The partial pressure carbon dioxide (P_{CO_2}) is below normal, because the patient is blowing off CO_2.

Nasal flaring and use of accessory neck muscles continue in stage two. The patient also exhibits a decreased ability to cough, and cyanosis is present. A pulsus paradoxus is apparent. The patient is retaining CO_2, which results in a rapid pulse rate and pupillary constriction. The patient feels extremely hot.

Decreased wheezing—a silent chest—occurs in stage three. Due to exhaustion, movement of the chest is minimal, which, in turn, significantly reduces gas exchange. Central nervous system (CNS) changes, such as drowsiness and muscle twitching, become apparent. As the P_{CO_2} level elevates past 70, seizures and coma may occur.

Nursing care and medical management are the same as those used to treat asthma, except applied more rigorously. Artificial ventilation may be instituted.

INHALATION INJURIES

Carbon Monoxide Poisoning

Carbon monoxide (CO) is an odorless, colorless gas that occurs as a byproduct of incomplete combustion. Inhalation of carbon monoxide gas can lead to carbon monoxide poisoning. Depending on the percentage of carbon monoxide in the blood, symptoms of carbon monoxide poisoning can appear due to the hypoxic state that results.

Carbon monoxide can be found in the blood of smokers, industrial workers, and residents of smog-ridden cities. Accidents causing carbon monoxide poisoning can occur at home as a result of faulty furnaces, clogged chimneys, and defective heaters. Inhalation of carbon monoxide can also occur from faulty exhaust systems on cars, and from inhaling gas fumes from cars in enclosed garages and enclosed parking facilities. Carbon monoxide poisoning can also affect campers who use charcoal grills inside their tents.

Pathophysiology
Carbon monoxide poisoning results from combining carbon monoxide (CO) with hemoglobin (Hgb) and the resultant alteration in the transport of oxygen to the tissues. Carbon monoxide has an affinity for hemoglobin that is approximately 200 times greater than oxygen's affinity. Consequently, carbon monoxide-hemoglobin bonding (CO-Hgb) occurs, and fewer hemoglobin bonds are available to combine with oxygen (decreased oxygen saturation—SaO_2). Nevertheless, since the amount of oxygen that can be dissolved in the blood remains the same, the Pa_{O_2} (dissolved portion) remains within normal limits. The Pa_{CO_2} may also be within normal limits. If the patient is hyperventilating, however, the Pa_{CO_2} may be slightly decreased. Furthermore, carbon monoxide has an additional effect on oxygen: in essence, because oxygen that is combined with hemoglobin has a greater affinity for that hemoglobin, less oxygen is given to the tissues.

Depending on the degree of carbon monoxide in the blood, signs and symptoms may indicate hypoxia. In addition, the patient may show evidence of metabolic acidosis. In the presence of hypoxia, the body compensates by initiating anaerobic

INHALATION INJURIES

energy production. Because anaerobic energy production is inefficient, however, excessive lactic acid is produced, which causes metabolic acidosis.

Clinical Manifestations

Because the signs and symptoms of carbon monoxide (CO) poisoning are due to hypoxia (which can also be due to many other causes), obtaining a definitive history of the patient's exposure to carbon monoxide is extremely important. Carbon monoxide poisoning can mimic other disorders, such as a CVA, flu, or intoxication. Because hypoxia exists in CO poisoning, preexisting medical conditions can be aggravated. Death in patients with CO poisoning can be due to other causes, for example, myocardial infarction.

Because CO-Hgb is red, patients may appear to have a cherry-red cast to the skin and lips, and red-striping of the torso and arms. The presence of the cherry-red color is not apparent in all CO poisoning and, therefore, is not a reliable tool for making a diagnosis or for determining the severity of the poisoning. Nevertheless, the absence of cyanosis of the oral mucosa or of the conjunctiva does not eliminate the possibility of hypoxia.

Since the brain and the heart are most sensitive to variations in oxygenation, CO poisoning can precipitate alterations in cognitive ability (decreased memory), personality behaviors (disorientation and agitation), and heart functioning (dysrhythmias, angina, and hypertension). The presence of atherosclerosis can aggravate the clinical picture of the patient. Other signs and symptoms that might exist include nausea, headache, dizziness, bloody diarrhea, lethargy, and tinnitus. Sensory changes can include decreased vision and hearing. In addition, the patient's speech may be abnormal.

Diagnostic Studies

Because the severity of the CO poisoning cannot be determined by observing physical indications or by knowing the duration of exposure, treatment should begin when the patient arrives at the emergency department. Since carbon monoxide dissipates quickly from the blood after administration of 100 percent oxygen, blood samples should be obtained as soon as possible after the patient's arrival.

Blood samples should be obtained for spectrophotometric studies to determine the carbon monoxide content in the blood. This test is the only reliable indicator of the degree of exposure and the severity of the patient's hypoxia. The results of the spectrophotometric studies can be interpreted as follows:

CO Content	*Indication*	*Manifestations*
1–10 percent	Normal	None;
10–20 percent	Mild CO poisoning	Often seen in cigarette smokers; symptoms begin to appear at 20 percent: headache, angina, shortness of breath,
20–40 percent	Moderate poisoning	Headache, tinnitus, nausea, decreased vision, irritability;
40–60 percent	Severe poisoning	Coma.
60–80 percent	Usually fatal	

Electrocardiogram (ECG) monitoring should be initiated as soon as the patient arrives to determine whether hypoxia has affected the heart's functioning. Premature ventricular contractions and tachydysrhythmias are most likely to occur.

Arterial blood samples should be obtained to determine the degree of metabolic acidosis that exists. The state of hypoxia cannot be determined by measuring arterial blood gases, since the Pa_{O_2} (dissolved oxygen) will remain within normal limits, because it is unaffected by the presence of carbon monoxide in the blood. Metabolic acidosis will be evident only by the significantly decreased pH. The Pa_{CO_2} will be normal or slightly below normal limits if the patient is hyperventilating.

Chest x-ray studies may be ordered. The findings, however, will probably be normal. Because the presence of carbon monoxide in the blood may affect coagulation, the presence of pulmonary emboli may be evident on later serial x-ray studies.

Any preexisting medical problems the patient has should be assessed in view of the hypoxic state. The heart and brain are the organs most sensitive to hypoxia. If the oxygen level in venous blood is less than 30 mm Hg, the brain, heart, and other vital organs may be inadequately oxygenated.

Nursing Care and Related Interventions

The goals of therapy are to increase oxygenation, to correct the hypoxia, and to eliminate carbon monoxide. Therapy should be initiated immediately, without waiting for the results from the diagnostic tests.

When the patient arrives at the emergency department, a history of exposure to carbon monoxide should be obtained, if possible. Data should include the length of time of exposure to CO, the time of the incident (relative to the time of arrival at the emergency department), ruling out other possible toxic fumes, and the patient's response to the gas, in essence, respiratory distress and other associated signs and symptoms, as well as the patient's response to therapy, if any, instituted at the scene of the incident.

Therapy should include administration of 100 percent oxygen, starting a peripheral IV line to administer sodium bicarbonate and other emergency drugs, insertion of an arterial line, electrocardiogram (ECG) monitoring, and obtaining blood samples. Administration of 100 percent oxygen through a nonrebreathing face mask for a minimum of four hours will break the CO-Hgb bonds in the shortest amount of time, unless hyperbaric oxygen facilities are available.

The CO-Hgb bonds are most effectively broken by using hyperbaric oxygen therapy (HBO). Placing the patient in an HBO chamber at 2.5 atmospheres for one hour will produce the same beneficial effects as administering 100 percent oxygen (at 1 atmosphere) for four hours. Quickly correcting the hypoxia may possibly avert cerebral damage from hypoxia and/or cerebral edema. HBO should be instituted during the time of the acute episode. Multiple HBO treatments may be required in subsequent hours or days, depending on the patient's condition.

Although cardiopulmonary resuscitation (CPR) may be initiated, it does not effectively maintain oxygenation of the tissues, because high concentrations of oxygen are necessary to break the CO-Hgb bonds so that the Hgb bonds are available for oxygen.

Assessment of the patient with CO poisoning continues even after treatment has been initiated. The patient (and/or the family) should be informed that the patient's

INHALATION INJURIES

admission to the hospital will be necessary to observe, prevent, and treat any complications that might result from the CO poisoning. In subacute poisonings, signs and symptoms may appear slowly. Hospitalization will permit assessment for and treatment of these developments.

Cardiovascular function is continually assessed for the development of hypo- or hypertension or angina (due to the increased workload on the heart to compensate for the hypoxia, which is especially possible in patients with atherosclerosis).

Cerebral edema can occur secondary to the hypoxia. This condition may occur up to three weeks after the initial CO poisoning. Diuretics may be administered to treat or to prevent edema from occurring. The patient's fluid and electrolyte balance must be monitored frequently to avoid side effects of the diuretic therapy. Steroids may also be used to reduce the possibility of cerebral edema occurring.

Central nervous system (CNS) dysfunction may be evident by the appearance of changes in the patient's personality. Aggressive and psychotic behavior, for example, may occur. Changes in the patient's cognitive abilities (e.g., memory) may also indicate CNS dysfunction. The plan of care should include the assessment of and compensation for these changes.

If treatment is not instituted quickly or adequately, complications are more likely to occur. Complications develop primarily as a result of hypoxia. Some complications can also result from cerebral edema. Care, therefore, must be taken to avoid events that will increase the degree of hypoxia or cerebral edema, for example, excitement or chilling. Demyelinization, a dreaded complication, is fatal.

Patients suffering from carbon monoxide poisoning should be admitted to the hospital for observation.

Chlorine Gas Inhalation

Chlorine is a yellow-green gas with a pungent odor that, depending on the amount present, may be either invisible or form a dense cloud. Chlorine is used industrially in the manufacture of plastic and solvents, in water purification, and in hydrochloride production. The risk of industrial exposure and inhalation is minimal. Accidents during transportation and explosions, however, can affect many people simultaneously.

Chlorine inhalation can also occur in and around the home. Chlorine gas in the home is usually produced by the mixing of bleaches containing hydrochlorides with weaker acids, such as ammonia, vinegar, and toilet bowl cleaners. Chlorine gas inhalation can also occur around swimming pools, when chlorine is added to the water.

Because chlorine is extremely corrosive, exposure to the gas can cause complete destruction of the skin and mucous membranes.

Pathophysiology

Chlorine plus water yields hydrochloric acid and other unstable oxidizing agents. The reaction of the oxidizing agents with other compounds actually causes more damage than does the hydrochloric acid.

Twenty parts per million (20 ppm) of chlorine in the air produces pulmonary damage. Chlorine interferes with the mitochondrial and cellular enzyme systems, disrupts protein integrity, and alters intracellular pH, resulting in cell destruction and increased cell permeability. The end result is severe airway and alveolar inflammation. Gas exchange and clearing of foreign material are also impaired.

The extent of injury depends on the length of time of exposure, the concentration of the gas, and the time elapsing between exposure and treatment. Preexisting pulmonary disorders caused, for example, by chronic exposure to gases such as chlorine or to cigarette smoking, set the stage for more serious injury from chlorine inhalation.

Chlorine may affect the endothelium as well as lung surfactant, and it alters the level of surfactant present in the alveoli. As the amount of surfactant decreases, alveoli begin to collapse, and atelectasis follows. Alveolar congestion initially occurs, followed by areas of edema (pulmonary edema). Bronchial and bronchiolar spasm also occur. Gas exchange is thus impaired, resulting in the development of hypoxia and acidosis. The hypoxia affects cell permeability allowing more fluid to enter the alveoli and thus further affect gas exchange.

A granulocyte response may occur several hours after exposure, and the risk of infection significantly increases. The occurrence of hyaline membrane is a later development.

Autopsy findings have revealed sloughing of the alveolar epithelium, the presence of thrombi in the airways, and denuding of the bronchial walls.

Clinical Manifestations
The clinical picture of a victim of chlorine gas inhalation results from direct irritation caused by the gas and from an inflammatory reaction to the injury.

The degree to which signs and symptoms will be apparent depends on the following:

1. The length of time of exposure.
2. The intensity of exposure.
3. The time lapsing between exposure and treatment.
4. Any history of previous exposure.
5. Presence of preexisting medical problems, especially pulmonary or cardiovascular problems.
6. History of cigarette smoking.
7. Type of treatment instituted prior to the patient's arrival at the emergency department.

The patient's condition may deteriorate with time.

The initial signs and symptoms result from irritation of the skin and mucous membranes. Lacrimation, a spastic cough, dyspnea, wheezing, and laryngeal redness are seen first. Glottal spasm with choking also occurs. Cyanosis, secondary to hypoxia and metabolic acidosis, will be apparent. Headache, confusion, dizziness, and vomiting may occur.

Physical examination may reveal moist rales, low blood pressure, and hemoptysis. Signs of neurological depression may be apparent, because chlorine acts as a central nervous system depressant.

Chest x-ray examination reveals infiltrates and, later, pulmonary edema. Arterial blood gas (ABG) studies reveal hypoxia and metabolic acidosis.

Diagnostic Studies

The diagnostic tests will depend on the severity of the patient's condition. Chest x-ray studies and arterial blood gas studies will be done to assess the degree of respiratory involvement. Evidence of infiltrates, pulmonary edema, and atelectasis may be present. An electrocardiogram (ECG) may be ordered to determine the extent of cardiovascular involvement.

Nursing Care and Related Interventions

Therapy involves reversing any irritation and inflammation resulting from the exposure and preventing the development of complications.

After the patient arrives at the emergency department, the patient's clothing should be removed to prevent the patient from breathing any additional chlorine. The body should be washed to eliminate chlorine from the skin. Rinsing out the eyes and mouth is necessary to eliminate irritants. The patient should then be kept warm and placed in a supine position.

Supportive care may involve the insertion of an endotracheal tube, instigation of artificial ventilation using high oxygen concentrations, and perhaps the use of PEEP (positive end expiratory pressure), and the use of bronchodilators. Sodium bicarbonate may be used in the presence of significant acidosis. Antiinflammatory drugs, such as adrenocorticotropic hormone (ACTH), may be used to decrease bronchial edema and thus to increase gas exchange. If congestive heart failure becomes evident, digoxin may be ordered.

Maintaining maximum gas exchange is essential. Postural drainage and percussion will help in removing mucus plugs from the airways. Fluids are limited to prevent fluid from seeping into the lung tissue, thus adding to the patient's breathing problem.

Assessment for the development of complications is an ongoing process. Pulmonary edema, bronchitis with mucus plugs, and bacterial infections may occur. Shock and heart failure may also develop.

The patient may exhibit signs of apprehension and fear. Support and reassurance by the nurse, therefore, are necessary to help alleviate the patient's negative feelings. Depending on the severity of these feelings, increased workload may be placed on the heart and lungs, which may eventually compromise the patient's condition.

Discharge Planning

The patient should be warned of the hazards of being exposed to chlorine gas. Exposure even for brief periods, which may not cause any physical discomfort, can lead to serious injury. The patient should be instructed to avoid mixing any chemicals.

A period of time for convalescence will also be necessary. The duration of convalescence will depend on the severity of exposure and the extent of injury. The patient should know that relapses may occur. Convalescence may take several months to several years, depending on the severity of exposure and the patient's preexisting physical condition. Permanent lung damage may exist.

Parents should be taught how to store dangerous chemicals properly in the home to prevent the possibility of exposure of their children. All of these items should be kept in a locked cabinet in the home.

HYPERVENTILATION SYNDROME

Hyperventilation is a state in which a patient breathes rapidly and/or deeply. Hyperventilation can occur either as a compensatory mechanism in organic dysfunction or in response to acute or chronic attacks of anxiety. Hyperventilation in response to anxiety is termed *hyperventilation syndrome*. Hyperventilation and its associated signs and symptoms are similar in both organic and anxiety-induced states. The etiology of the hyperventilation, therefore, should be determined so that the appropriate intervention can be instituted. Hyperventilation syndrome may be missed as a possible diagnosis. Unfortunately, if no physiologic basis for the symptoms can be found, the patient is frequently incorrectly labeled a neurotic, and then sent home without further intervention.

An estimated 10 percent of all patients have had a hyperventilation attack during their lifetime. The hyperventilation syndrome can occur in patients as young as six years old. It occurs equally in men and women, and it occurs more frequently in younger than in older adults. Moreover, if the syndrome occurs in childhood, it is more likely to continue into adulthood.

Pathophysiology

Regardless of the etiology of the hyperventilatory attack, the effect is the same. Rapid and deep breathing causes the lungs to blow off carbon dioxide (CO_2). The P_{CO_2} may range from 20 to 30 mm Hg (normal: 35–45 mm Hg). This action causes the pH level to rise to 7.55 or higher. Thus, a state of respiratory alkalosis exists. A state of alkalosis causes a drop in the level of the serum calcium, which leads to muscle irritability and tremors. Chest pain can occur in alkalotic states due to coronary vasoconstriction. To compensate for the altered acid-base state, the kidneys will excrete bicarbonate.

The presence of hypocapnia causes cerebral vasoconstriction, and neurological signs and symptoms will be apparent. The presence of a low P_{CO_2} also adversely affects the oxygenation of the tissues. A low P_{CO_2} causes an increased binding between oxygen and hemoglobin. Thus, less oxygen is given to the tissues. This poor oxygenation of the tissues enhances the presence of neurological signs and symptoms.

Involvement of the sympathetic nervous system caused by anxiety also produces cardiovascular abnormalities, such as tachycardia and palpitations.

Clinical Manifestations

Patients experiencing hyperventilation syndrome have been categorized into five types:

Type I: The attacks are frequent and are associated with acute and chronic anxiety. The signs and symptoms of the anxiety are quite apparent.
Type II: Attacks appear to be idiopathic.
Type III: Frequently seen in children with emotional problems or ones who come from problem homes.
Type IV: Attacks occur in response to a specific stress in life.
Type V: Attacks occur after exertion (usually heavy).

Attacks of hyperventilation can last for a few minutes to several hours. Neurological symptoms are the most common symptoms to occur in attacks due to acute anxiety: for example, lightheadedness, dizziness, decreased ability to concentrate, impaired vision, and peripheral paresthesia. Other symptoms may include hyperactivity, dry mouth, fatigue, fidgety movement of the hands, chest pain, breathlessness, a sense of choking, a feeling of impending doom, and confusion. Physical findings may include sweaty palms, tachycardia, tremors, diaphoresis, and urinary frequency. Seizures and loss of consciousness can also occur.

In chronic attacks of hyperventilation, signs and symptoms may include anxiety, depression, headache, irritable bowel, phobias, vomiting, eye blinking, eyelash pulling, and nail biting.

Diagnostic Studies

The extent to which any diagnostic tests will be done depends on the history obtained. If anxiety, acute or chronic, or specific stress incidents cannot be identified, tests must be done to rule out any organic dysfunction. Since the signs and symptoms indicate neurological or cardiovascular dysfunction, tests will focus on these organ systems.

Nursing Care and Related Interventions

Intervention is divided between data collection and treating the hyperventilation. Both occur simultaneously in varying degrees.

Data collection should include assessment of physical signs and symptoms, assessment for a state of fear, and determining the context in which the illness occurred.

A thorough assessment of the signs and symptoms will assist in diagnosing the problem as either organic or anxiety-induced. Because many of the symptoms relate to the neurological and cardiovascular systems, thorough assessment of these systems is important to identify or to rule out an organic cause for the hyperventilation.

A state of fear commonly occurs in hyperventilating patients. The patient may or may not be aware of this fear. The patient may also be afraid to vocalize the fear. Thus, the nurse should ask the patient specifically about being or feeling afraid. The patient may fear dying, being alone, or being insane (due to signs and symptoms of neurological alterations, such as loss of memory and inability to concentrate).

Knowing the context in which the attack occurred is important for diagnosing or ruling out an organic cause. Assessment should include the frequency and duration of attacks and any preceding or precipitating factors, as well as remedies used at home to treat the attack. If the patient has any preexisting medical problems, the possibility that these problems are causing or exaggerating the hyperventilation must be identified.

Therapy for the patient with hyperventilation syndrome may include having the patient breathe into a paper bag, as well as giving emotional support, and reassurance, and instruction. Depending on the data collected, referrals, such as to a psychiatrist, may be included.

Having the patient breathe into a paper bag in order to rebreathe the exhaled air will help to correct the acid/base state, because exhaled air is high in carbon dioxide (CO_2). Rebreathing CO_2, therefore, will cause a reverse in the alkalosis.

Helping the patient to calm down will hasten the person's return to normal breathing. Emotional support and reassurance are vital for helping the patient to recover from this attack. The patient must be reassured that he does not have a disease and that hyperventilating causes no bodily damage.

Discharge Planning

Education of the patient about the hyperventilation attack should begin, while treatment is in progress. Education of the patient and his family should focus on prevention of the attacks. For the educational plan to be effective, the patient must be shown the correlation between his anxiety and the symptoms. Although the patient may not be convinced of the association, initial attempts to convince the patient should be made.

The patient can be introduced to relaxation techniques to use on a routine basis as well as during hyperventilatory attacks. Diaphragmatic breathing exercises will also be helpful.

If the attacks are caused by heavy exertion, the patient again must be shown the correlation between his activities and the attacks, and be given suggestions on how to modify the activities.

The patient's family should be informed of the patient's problem to elicit their support. The family must be aware of the factors that precipitate an attack. If the family is one of the precipitating factors, a referral to an appropriate resource may be necessary. The family should be made aware that they can be supportive of the patient in the person's attempts to prevent attacks, such as avoiding precipitating factors and using relaxation techniques.

The patient may be referred to an outside resource, such as to a psychologist, so that the patient can learn to cope better with stress. This recommendation also applies to hyperventilatory children who have emotional problems or who come from a difficult home situation.

NEAR DROWNING

Submersion for a period of time that does not result in irreversible death of the victim is known as *near drowning*. Whether the person drowns or is a victim of near drowning may be influenced by the person's previous state of health and by the temperature of the water.

In addition to the person's lack of skill in swimming and swimming fatigue, other factors may precipitate a near drowning episode:

Myocardial infarction.
Allergic reaction to the venom of marine life.
Neck injury after diving.
Hyperventilation prior to diving.
Seizures.

Furthermore, struggling to keep one's head above water increases the risk of inhaling water into the lungs. Near drowning can occur in salt water or in fresh water. The victim's pathological process and treatment varies, depending on the type of water inhaled.

Near drowning victims are classified as dry, wet, or secondary. In *dry* near drowning cases, the victim develops a tracheolaryngeal spasm. The victim inhales little or no water. Dry near drowning constitutes approximately 10 to 20 percent of near drowning cases. *Wet* near drowning involves 80 to 90 percent of the near drowning cases, because victims have inhaled a variable amount of water. The influx of water occurs subsequent to a panicky effort to breathe. The classification of *secondary* near drowning refers to the development of complications that occur after successful resuscitation: for example, the development of pulmonary edema.

Pathophysiology

Salt water is a hypertonic solution that draws fluid by osmosis from the vascular bed into the alveoli. A condition of pulmonary edema subsequently develops. An exudative process occurs secondary to the presence of the contaminants in the water. The process also fills the alveoli. The foreign materials may also produce bronchospasm. Consequently, a mismatch of air and blood exists in the lungs. Hypoxia is, therefore, the primary pathological problem. The degree of hypoxia is directly related to the amount of water aspirated.

The osmosis that occurs as a result of the hypertonic solution also produces hypovolemia, which, in turn, causes increased viscosity of the blood, increased osmolarity, and decreased cardiac output. The altered cardiac output will affect perfusion and functioning of vital body organs.

Electrolyte imbalances, especially in serum potassium levels, will occur as a result of hemoconcentration. The hemoglobin level will decrease because of the presence of hemolysis.

Acute renal failure resulting from tubular necrosis will develop secondary to the hypoxia and hypotension.

Fresh water is a hypotonic solution that is drawn by diffusion from the lungs into the vascular bed, which leads to the development of pulmonary edema due to circulatory overload. The pulmonary edema may also be a result of inflammation of the alveoli. With the presence of pulmonary edema, surfactant level decreases, both by direct breakdown of surfactant and by decreased production of surfactant secondary to hypoxia. With the alteration in surfactant levels and the presence of fluid, there is alveolar collapse and a resultant uneven match of ventilation and perfusion. Bronchospasm may also be present, because of the aspiration of the water and its contaminants.

The shift of fluid into the vascular bed has several repercussions. Hemodilution results in a decrease in osmolarity and blood viscosity. Hypervolemia results in circulatory overload. Hemolysis occurs secondary to the influx of water and results in elevated serum hemoglobin levels, but decreased cellular hemoglobin levels. Electrolyte imbalance occurs: decreased sodium and chloride levels due to hypervolemia, and an elevated serum potassium level due to hemolysis and hypoxia. In addition, complications of near drowning include atelectasis, lung abscess, pneumothorax, and empyema.

Clinical Manifestations

The signs and symptoms that will be apparent in near drowning will vary, depending on the following:

1. Length of time of submersion.
2. Temperature of the water.
3. Age of the victim—a child has a large surface area with little padding.
4. General health of the victim.
5. Type of water.
6. Extent of the injury.

Signs that will be apparent in both types of near drowning include tachypnea, progressive dyspnea, wheezing, rales and rhonchi, and a cough producing pink, frothy sputum. Neurological signs include coma, mental confusion, seizures, agitation, and lethargy. Tachycardia will be present. The temperature of the victim will vary, but is usually elevated. Arterial blood gas studies will reveal metabolic acidosis, with overlying respiratory acidosis.

In salt water near drowning, hypotension and tachycardia will be present. Chest x-ray examination will reveal haziness. An elevated CVP exists initially, with a rapid drop and return to normal.

In fresh water near drowning, the blood pressure will be elevated. The CVP will be persistently elevated. Ventricular fibrillation may be present. Chest x-ray examination reveals atelectasis.

Diagnostic Studies

Diagnostic studies will be the same in both types of near drowning. The chest x-ray film will reveal infiltrates of various sizes and density, which may increase during the first 24 hours. Pulmonary hemorrhage, pneumonia, and atelectasis may become apparent.

Electrolyte values may show variations in potassium, sodium, and chloride levels. Complete blood count (CBC) results may indicate hemodilution or hypovolemia. Hemolysis may be apparent with decreasing hemoglobin. The white blood cell (WBC) count may increase in response to the influx of contaminants.

Arterial blood gas studies will reveal metabolic acidosis with an overlying respiratory acidosis. Hypoxia will also be apparent in varying degrees, depending on the severity of the patient's condition.

Nursing Care and Related Interventions

The goals of treatment of near drowning are to promote adequate ventilation and circulation, to prevent complications, and to decrease the victim's anxiety.

Since hypoxia is the primary pathological process of near drowning, the first priority of care is establishing a patent airway and adequate ventilation. Continue CPR as necessary, at least until the patient's core body temperature is normal, if the person is involved in a cold water drowning. An oral airway may be sufficient in conscious patients with adequate blood gases. In other cases, intubation will be necessary, especially if artificial ventilation is indicated. In salt water near drowning, either intermittent positive pressure breathing (IPPB) or positive end expiratory pressure (PEEP) may be necessary to negate the influx of fluid into the alveoli. In fresh water near drowning, periodic hyperventilation will help to combat alveolar collapse due to pulmonary edema. Bronchodilators will be useful in reversing the presence of bronchospasm. Steroids will also increase bronchial diameter, as well as decrease inflammation of the alveoli by their antiinflammatory action. Rigorous postural drainage and percussion will assist to improve gas exchange. All near drowning victims should be hospitalized for two to three days for observation of possible complications.

CONCLUSION

One of the most challenging situations for an emergency department nurse is treating the patient in respiratory distress. All the knowledge and skills the nurse possesses must be used to develop a plan of care for the patient. The care must be continually evaluated to ensure that it meets the changing needs of the patient. The quality of patient care is enhanced when the emergency department nurse understands all of the aspects involved in the care of the patient experiencing respiratory distress.

BIBLIOGRAPHY

Allergies junior grade. *Emergency Medicine* 11:107 (Apr. 15, 1979).

Barber, J. M., and S. A. Budassi: *Mosby's Manual of Emergency Care: Practices and Procedures*. St. Louis: Mosby, 1979.

Beloff, J. S.: Respiratory Distress in Pediatrics. In J. C. Findeiss (ed.): *Emergency Medical Care.* New York: Intercontinental Medical, 1974, pp. 199–208.

Brandenberg, J.: Inhalation injury: carbon monoxide poisoning. *American Journal of Nursing* 80:98 (1980).

A breath of asthma therapy. *Emergency Medicine* 13:63 (Feb. 28, 1981).

A breath of atropine. *Emergency Medicine* 13(13):64 (Feb. 15, 1981).

A breath too frequent. *Emergency Medicine* 13:116 (July 15, 1981).

A breath too many too early. *Emergency Medicine* 13:67 (July 15, 1981).

Burns, D.: Lung Injury Due to Irritant Gases. In R. A. Bordow, E. W. Skool, and K. M. Moser (eds.): *Manual of Clinical Problems in Pulmonary Medicine.* Boston: Little, Brown, 1980, pp. 358–361.

Caudle, J. T.: Emergency nursing of near-drowning victims. *American Journal of Nursing* 76(6):922 (1976).

Chester, E. H., P. J. Kaimal, C. B. Payne, and P. M. Kohn: Pulmonary injury following exposure to chlorine gas. *Chest* 72(2):247 (Aug. 1977).

Clarke, E. B., and E. H. Niggemann: Near-drowning. *Heart and Lung* 1(6):946 (1975).

Conn, A. W.: Cerebral resuscitation for the near-drowned child. *Emergency Medicine* 12(12):16 (June 30, 1980).

Cooper, P.: *Poisoning.* 3rd ed. Chicago: Yearbook Medical, 1974.

Czajka, P. A., and J. P. Duffy: *Poisoning Emergencies: A Guide for Emergency Medical Personnel.* St. Louis: Mosby, 1980.

Decker, W. J., and H. F. Koch: Chlorine poisoning at the swimming pool: an overlooked hazard. *Clinical Toxicology* 13(3):377 (1978).

Deichmann, W. B., and H. W. Gerade: *Toxicology of Drugs and Chemicals.* New York: Academic Press, 1969.

Dewhirst, F.: Voluntary chlorine inhalation. *British Medical Journal* 282:565 (Feb. 14, 1981).

Dreisbach, R. H.: *Handbook of Poisoning: Prevention, Diagnosis and Treatment.* 10th ed. Los Altos, CA.: Lange, 1980.

Ellis, E. F.: The thin line of asthma therapy. *Emergency Medicine* 13:25 (Feb. 15, 1981).

Fint, Jr., T., and H. D. Cain: *Emergency Treatment and Management.* 5th ed., Philadelphia: Saunders, 1975.

Fletcher, M. A.: Intensive Care of Asthma, Cystic Fibrosis, and Other Pediatric Respiratory Diseases. In G. G. Burton, G. N. Gee, J. E. Hodgkin (eds.): *Respiratory Care: A Guide to Clinical Practice.* Philadelphia: Lippincott, pp. 831–871, 1978.

Gaston, S. F., and L. L. Schumann: Inhalation injury: smoke inhalation. *American Journal of Nursing* 80:94 (1980).

Grace, T. W., and F. W. Platt: Subacute carbon monoxide poisoning: another great imitator. *Journal of the American Medical Association* 246(15):1968.

Gracey, D. R.: Carboxyhemoglobinemia and secondary lactic acidosis. *Heart and Lung* 3:817 (Sept./Oct. 1974).

Heeding asthma's warnings. *Emergency Medicine* 11:213 (June 15, 1979).

Henderson, J.: *Emergency Medical Guide.* 4th ed. New York: McGraw-Hill, 1978.

Hollingsworth, C.: Psychiatric Conditions in Pulmonary Medicine. In D. P. Tashkin and S. M. Cassan (eds.): *Guide to Pulmonary Medicine,* New York: Grune & Stratton, 1978, pp. 345–353.

A home guide to asthma. *Emergency Medicine* 12(12):182 (June 15, 1980).

# BIBLIOGRAPHY

Hudgel, D. W., and L. A. Madsen: Acute and chronic asthma: a guide to intervention. *American Journal of Nursing* 80:1791 (1980).

Lawson, J. J.: Chlorine exposure: a challenge to the physician. *American Family Physician* 23:135 (Jan. 1981).

Looking for CO poisoning. *Emergency Medicine* 11:240 (Jan. 1979).

In near-drowning, get the water out. *Emergency Medicine* 11:176 (1979).

For near-drowning x-ray. *Emergency Medicine* 11:43 (May 15, 1979).

McMicken, D. B.: After the emergency. *Emergency Medicine* 11(1):89 (Jan. 15, 1979).

Miller, R. H.: *Textbook of Basic Emergency Medicine.* 2nd ed. St. Louis: Mosby, 1980.

Neuman, T.: Near-Drowning—Diving and Decompression. In R. A. Bordow, E. W. Stool, and K. M. Moser (eds.): *Manual of Clinical Problems in Pulmonary Medicine.* Boston: Little, Brown, 1980, pp. 374–377.

Not so heavy on the steroids. *Emergency Medicine* 12(12):46 (June 30, 1980).

Ochs, M. A.: Poisons. In C. G. Warner (ed.): *Emergency Care: Assessment and Intervention.* 2nd ed. St. Louis: Mosby, 1983, pp. 397–412.

Petersen, W. A.: Pediatric Emergencies. In C. Eckert (ed.): *Emergency-Room Care.* 4th ed. Boston: Little, Brown, 1981, pp. 421–441.

Promisloff, R. A.: Drowning and Near-Drowning. In W. W. Oaks, K. Bharadwaja, and L. Hertz (eds.): *Emergency Care.* New York: Grune & Stratton, 1979.

Rafferty, P.: Voluntary chlorine inhalation: a new form of self-abuse. *British Medical Journal* 281:1178 (1981).

Rebuck, A.: Diagnosis and Treatment of Asthma. In A. Aberman and A. G. Logan (eds.): *Emergency Management of the Critically Ill.* Chicago: Symposia Specialists, 1980, pp. 205–211.

Ronshausen, C. A.: Respiratory Emergencies. In N. M. Halloway (ed.): *Core Curriculum,* 2nd ed. Chicago: Emergency Department Nurses Association, 1980, pp. 241–253.

Schweitzer, M. E.: *Tests Related to Immunology,* edited by P. Beare, V. Rahr, and C. Ronshausen. Philadelphia: Lippincott, 1982.

Simkins, R.: Asthma: reactive airway disease. *American Journal of Nursing* 81:523 (1981).

Summer, W. R., and S. Permutt: Acute Lower Airway Obstruction: Asthma. In E. M. Shibel and K. M. Moser (eds.): *Respiratory Emergencies.* St. Louis: Mosby Company, 1977, pp. 152–169.

Summer, W. R.: Inhalation of Noxious Gases, Fumes, and Vapors. In E. M. Shibel and K. M. Moser (eds.): *Respiratory Emergencies.* St. Louis: Mosby, 1977, pp. 174–181.

Vorosmarti, Jr., J.: Hyperbaric oxygen therapy. *American Family Physician* 23:171 (Jan. 1981).

Wachtel, T. J.: Looking for the origins of hyperventilation. *Emergency Medicine* 14:124 (Feb. 28, 1982).

Watch out for inhalation injury. *Emergency Medicine* 14(1):96 (Jan. 15, 1982).

Westmark, D. O.: Near-Drowning in the Emergency Department. In J. C. Findeiss (ed.): *Emergency Medical Care.* New York: Intercontinental Medical, 1974, pp. 199–208.

What's asthma got to do with psychosis? *Emergency Medicine* 13(7):135 (Apr. 15, 1981).

Wieczorek, R. R., and B. Horner-Rosner: The asthmatic child: preventing and controlling attacks. *American Journal of Nursing* 79:258 (1979).

Winter, P. M., and J. N. Miller: Carbon monoxide poisoning. *JAMA* 236(13):1502 (Sept. 27, 1976).

Zorap, J. S., and P. J. F. Baskett: *Immediate Care.* London: Saunders, 1977.

8

Congestive Heart Failure, Pulmonary Edema, or Pulmonary Embolus

Nancy L. Parrish

After completing this chapter, the reader will be able to do the following:

1. Triage a patient experiencing congestive heart failure, pulmonary edema, or pulmonary embolus.
2. Develop an appropriate nursing plan of care for patients presenting to the emergency department with congestive heart failure, pulmonary edema, or pulmonary embolus.
3. Describe the pathophysiological basis of the clinical manifestations of congestive heart failure, pulmonary edema, and pulmonary embolus.
4. List the major treatment objectives of patients with congestive heart failure, pulmonary edema, and pulmonary embolus.
5. Describe the emergency department nurse's role in meeting the treatment objectives for patients with congestive heart failure, pulmonary edema, and pulmonary embolus.
6. Provide appropriate discharge instructions and patient education relating to congestive heart failure, pulmonary edema, and pulmonary embolus.

Congestive heart failure is an extremely common disorder in the United States. In addition, pulmonary edema and pulmonary embolus, though less common, are often medical emergencies requiring immediate intervention. The emergency department nurse, therefore, must be able to perform a quick, but organized and thorough assessment of, then develop an appropriate plan of care for, patients who present to the emergency department with these disorders.

TRIAGE

Subjective Data

Collection of the initial history from the patient, his family, or the ambulance personnel begins the triage process. Identify what problem or problems caused the patient to come to the emergency department. Patients with congestive heart failure, pulmonary edema, or pulmonary embolus usually complain initially of symptoms relating to cardiovascular or respiratory functions such as difficulty in breathing, cough, fatigue, or chest pain. The nurse's exploration of the patient's chief complaint will depend on the severity of the patient's condition, but it should usually include the following (Morgan and Engel, 1969): (1) Location (Where is it?); (2) Quality (What is it like?); (3) Quantity (How severe is it? How often does it occur? How long does it last?); (4) Chronology (When did it start, and how has it changed until the present time?); (5) Setting (Where was the patient, and what was he doing at the time it started?); (6) Aggravating and Alleviating factors (What seems to make it better or worse?); and, (7) Associated Manifestations (What other signs or symptoms is the patient experiencing, in addition to the chief complaint?).

A pertinent past history may provide valuable clues regarding the patient's current problem. Does he have a history of cardiac, respiratory, peripheral vascular, kidney, or liver disease? Does he have a history of diabetes or cancer? Has he recently experienced any trauma or surgery, or has he been immobilized for a prolonged period of time? What medication is he currently taking, and why? Is he allergic to any substance? Finally, a historical review of systems pertaining to the cardiovascular, respiratory, and peripheral vascular systems may provide pertinent positive, as well as negative, symptoms.

Objective Data

The nurse begins with a general survey to collect objective data from the patient, as soon as the patient enters the emergency department. Simple, close observation will usually reveal whether the patient is acutely or chronically ill. Facial expressions, diaphoresis, and labored or noisy breathing indicate the amount of distress the patient is experiencing, while his skin color, posture, gait, and nutritional status can also be assessed through observation. After the patient is made as comfortable as possible, a complete set of vital signs should be taken.

If the patient's status permits, a pertinent, but brief, physical examination should be performed, including assessment of the person's mental status, cardiovascular, respiratory, and peripheral vascular functions. Is the patient alert and oriented, or is his level of consciousness decreased? Are indications of anxiety, apprehension, or even panic present? Does he show signs of increased respiratory effort, such as the use of accessory muscles? Are his breath sounds vesicular in nature and equal bilaterally? Are any adventitious sounds, such as rales, wheezes, or a friction rub, heard upon auscultation? Is any movement over the precordium detectable? Are any gallops, murmurs, or accentuated heart sounds heard? Are his neck veins distended? If circumstances allow, examine the peripheral vascular system for skin color and temperature, capillary refill time, hair distribution, pulses, edema, and signs of phlebitis.

Assessment and Planning

By integrating both the subjective and objective data collected from the patient and/or his family, the nurse makes an assessment identifying one or more nursing diagnoses, then develops a related plan of care. This plan should include not only the patient's priority of care (for example, should he be placed in an examination room to be seen immediately by a physician, or can he wait for further evaluation?), but also appropriate nursing interventions, such as positioning, reassurance, cardiac monitoring, and oxygen administration. (Table 8.1 contains two examples of triage notes.)

A detailed discussion of congestive heart failure, pulmonary edema, and pulmonary embolus, including their etiology, pathophysiology, clinical manifestations, diagnostic studies, nursing care and related interventions, and discharge instructions

TABLE 8.1 Examples of Triage Notes Related to Pulmonary Edema and Congestive Heart Failure

Pulmonary Edema	*Congestive Heart Failure*
S: 56 yo BF with c/o sudden onset of severe dyspnea while asleep and productive cough for 3 hours. Denies fever, chest pain. PMH: CHF for 5 years, denies COPD, NKA, on digoxin, Lasix.	S: 48 yo WM with c/o SOB with activity ("walking one block"), fatigue for 2 weeks. States "just got over a bad cold." Denies fever, chest pain. PMH: hypertension for 2 years (takes "water pill" q.d.), denies COPD, heart disease. *Allergic* to sulfa drugs, codeine.
O: Restless, anxious, diaphoretic. T 98.6°F, BP 140/90, P 120 weak irregular, RR 30 shallow, with diffuse rales bil., blood-tinged sputum. Skin cool, moist, dusky, distended neck veins, ankle edema bilaterally.	O: T 99.4°F, BP 160/108, P 90 strong regular, RR 24. Skin warm, moist, pink, breath sounds equal bilaterally, without rales/rhonchi, no jugular venous distension, mild ankle edema noted bilaterally.
A: Acute respiratory distress.	A: Mild respiratory dysfunction.
P: Medical evaluation, admit to exam room now, reassurance, high-Fowler's, O$_2$ per mask pending further orders, cardiac monitor.	P: Medical evaluation, admit to exam room ASAP, reassurance, continued observation.

follows. Thorough knowledge of these disorders will aid the emergency nurse in performing appropriate triage action.

CONGESTIVE HEART FAILURE

Congestive heart failure (CHF) is defined as failure of the heart to function as a pump, resulting in inadequate blood flow to the tissues, as well as congestion in the pulmonary and/or systemic circulations. Although CHF can result from any condition that impairs cardiac function, most common causes include the following: (1) arteriosclerotic heart disease; (2) hypertensive heart disease; (3) rheumatic valvular disease; (4) congenital heart disease; and, (5) inflammatory or degenerative diseases of the heart. In many cases of CHF, acute failure is precipitated when an additional burden is placed on the already damaged or overworked heart. The most probable precipitating causes include infection, anemia, thyrotoxicosis, pregnancy, overexertion, emotional crisis, pulmonary embolus, cardiac dysrhythmia, and other acute cardiac disorders, such as myocardial infarction.

Pathophysiology

The basic defect in heart failure is a decrease in the contractile properties of the heart. As the heart begins to fail, the body responds with certain compensatory mechanisms designed to maintain an adequate cardiac output, including an increase in heart rate, ventricular dilation, and myocardial hypertrophy. Dilation of the ventricles, which usually results from the heart's inability to eject its normal volume of blood, results in an increased end-diastolic volume, which augments the stroke volume. An increase in heart rate also helps to restore the cardiac output, while hypertrophy of the myocardium occurs in response to the heart's increased workload.

When these compensatory mechanisms fail, however, the heart is unable to receive its normal flow of blood from the venous system, and it is unable to pump out the required amount of blood through the arterial circulation. Congestion of tissues, therefore, results from increased atrial and venous pressures due to incomplete ventricular emptying. To compound the problem further, as the cardiac output decreases, renal perfusion also decreases, stimulating the release of renin from the kidney which, in turn, stimulates aldosterone secretion; thus, causing sodium and fluid retention and an increase in intravascular volume (Phipps, 1979).

Clinical Manifestations

Since the left and right sides of the heart are two separate pumping systems, either side may fail independently of the other. Since the left ventricle carries the major workload of the heart, left ventricular failure occurs in most patients with CHF. Usually, however, when one side of the heart becomes weakened, the opposite side of the heart also fails. Right-sided failure, for example, often follows left-sided fail-

CONGESTIVE HEART FAILURE 107

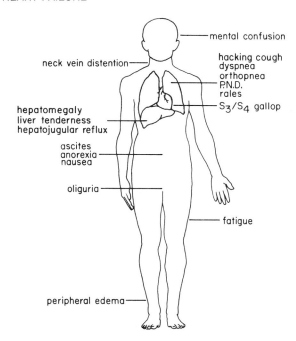

Figure 8.1 Clinical manifestations of left-sided and right-sided congestive heart failure.

ure, because the right side must then pump against the increased resistance in the pulmonary system. The clinical manifestations of either right or left ventricular failure may develop insidiously or acutely, depending on the underlying pathology (see Fig. 8.1)

Left-Sided Heart Failure
Left-sided heart failure results in signs and symptoms that reflect increased pulmonary congestion and pressure, in addition to decreased blood flow to all tissues and organs (Isacson and Schulz, 1978). The earliest symptom is usually *dyspnea* (characterized by rapid, shallow respirations), which, at first, may occur only with physical exertion, but eventually is present even when the patient is at rest. This reaction, which is due to pulmonary congestion that decreases available airspace and increases pressure in the lungs, leads to a decrease in the elasticity and compliance of the lung parenchyma. *Orthopnea* is also a common occurrence, because whenever the patient is lying flat on his back, ventilation decreases and venous return to the heart increases, thereby increasing pulmonary capillary pressure. *Paroxysmal nocturnal dyspnea,* characterized by sudden severe dyspnea and coughing several hours after lying down, is caused by an accumulation of fluid in the lungs, perhaps fluid that has been reabsorbed from edema in dependent sites during recumbency. A persistent *hacking cough* with expectoration of sputum is a frequent symptom of left-sided failure, caused by congestion of the lungs. *Fatigue,* one of the earliest symptoms to

develop, is due to impaired circulation of blood to the tissues and the resulting lack of sufficient oxygen and nutrients for the cells' needs. *Mental confusion* may also occur eventually, as a result of hypoperfusion. An S_3 (ventricular) *gallop* may be auscultated, resulting from increased end-diastolic pressure caused by the weakened left ventricle, while an S_4 (atrial) *gallop,* assumed to be the sound of the atrium contracting against increased ventricular resistance, may also be heard. *Rales,* indicating the presence of fluid in the air passages, may be auscultated as well (Phipps, 1979).

Right-Sided Heart Failure
The major sign of right-sided heart failure is *edema,* because the weakened heart causes blood to dam back into the veins of the systemic circulation. Initially, ankle swelling may be noted only during the day and may disappear overnight, but, as failure continues, the edema becomes more persistent and pronounced. *Ascites,* usually a later development, may occur as the increased pressure within the portal system forces fluid through the blood vessels into the abdominal cavity. *Hepatomegaly* may develop as the liver becomes engorged with blood, at times producing *right upper quadrant tenderness. Distended neck veins* can be seen when the person in right-sided failure is in the sitting position, due to the increased systemic venous pressure. Manual pressure over the liver may cause the neck veins to distend abruptly. This maneuver, known as the *hepatojugular reflux,* indicates marked right-heart distention. *Gastrointestinal disturbances,* such as anorexia, nausea, and vomiting, are also commonly associated with right ventricular failure, due to congestion of the abdominal viscera (Beland, 1981; Phipps, 1979).

Diagnostic Studies

Laboratory studies, although unable to diagnose CHF, are useful in determining the effect of the disorder on other organs and in detecting resultant electrolyte imbalances (e.g., an elevated serum sodium level); therefore, kidney and liver function studies, arterial blood gas analyses, and serum electrolyte studies may be ordered initially. A chest x-ray study not only provides information relating to the size and location of the heart, but also is used to detect early signs of pulmonary congestion. The major purpose of an electrocardiogram (ECG) is to detect myocardial hypertrophy and dysrhythmias associated with heart failure (Beland and Passos, 1981).

Nursing Care and Related Interventions

The major treatment objectives of CHF are as follows: (1) reduce the cardiac workload; (2) enhance myocardial contractility; and, (3) control excessive fluid retention. These procedures do not usually involve emergency measures, although the specific interventions used will depend on the degree and suddenness with which the heart fails.

Reduction of Cardiac Workload
The patient must have both physical and emotional rest to decrease cardiac workload. Rest not only reduces the work of the heart, but also increases the cardiac

reserve, while decreasing blood pressure and oxygen use. In addition, periods of recumbency improve renal perfusion, thereby promoting diuresis (Brunner and Suddarth, 1980). Place the patient in a semi-Fowler's position to facilitate breathing and to reduce the venous return to the heart.

Anxiety is detrimental to the patient with CHF, because it not only increases metabolic activity, which requires additional oxygen, but it also stimulates the sympathetic nervous system, causing vasoconstriction, tachycardia, and cardiac irritability. Promotion of the patient's physical comfort and verbal reassurance may alleviate his apprehension. If not, morphine sulfate (0.2 mg/kg subcutaneously for children, or 4–6 mg intravenously for adults) may be prescribed to allay anxiety and also for its vagal effects. Remember, however, that patients with hepatic congestion are unable to detoxify drugs as rapidly as normal and may react unfavorably to even small dosages.

Oxygen, usually administered by nasal cannula at 2 to 6 l/minute, helps to relieve dyspnea and fatigue, and an antiemetic may be administered when nausea and/or vomiting require control.

Enhancement of Myocardial Contractility

Improving myocardial contractility is achieved primarily through administering cardiac glycosides, such as digitalis, which increase the force of myocardial contraction. Consequently, cardiac output increases, the heart decreases in size, the venous pressure and blood volume decrease, and diuresis is promoted (Brunner and Suddarth, 1980). Digitalis also decreases the heart rate and conduction velocity, which allows time for better filling of the ventricles. For rapid digitalization of adults in emergency situations, deslanoside (Cedilanid-D), 1.6 mg IV, or G-strophanthin (Ouabain), 0.25 to 0.5 mg IV, are usually selected. Digoxin is the most widely used drug for children. (See Table 8.2.) Because a fine line exists between a dosage that is therapeutic and one that is toxic, observe closely for adverse effects of the drug. (See Table 8.3.) Also be aware that several factors predispose an individual to digitalis toxicity, including the following (Meissner and Gever, 1980): (1) electrolyte imbalances, such as hypokalemia, hypercalcemia, and hypomagnesemia; (2) hypothyroidism; (3) liver or kidney diseases; (4) alkalosis; and (5) advanced age.

Control of Excessive Fluid Retention

Control of excessive fluid retention can be achieved by reducing the dietary intake and increasing the urinary excretion of sodium with the aid of diuretics. The amount of sodium restriction actually prescribed, of course, will depend on the severity of

TABLE 8.2 Pediatric Digoxin Doses

Age	Digitalizing Dose (µg/kg)	Maintenance Dose (µg/kg)
Premature	30	10
Term, 0–1 wk	40	10–12
0–2 yr	50–70	15–20
2–5 yr	40–60	12–15
5+ yr	30–50	5–10

TABLE 8.3 Signs and Symptoms of Digitalis Toxicity

Cardiovascular	Neurologic	Gastrointestinal
Ventricular ectopic rhythms	Drowsiness, disorientation	Anorexia
Paroxysmal and nonparoxysmal nodal rhythms	Facial neuralgia	Nausea/vomiting
	Headache	Diarrhea
	Agitation	Abdominal pain
Atrioventricular dissociation	Muscle weakness	
	Apathy	
Paroxysmal atrial tachycardia with block	Mood changes	
	Fatigue	
Bradycardia	Convulsions	
	Green/yellow vision	
	Blurred vision	

the disorder and its resultant signs and symptoms. The patient, however, should be taught how to read labels and to avoid such nonprescription medications as cough syrups, alkalizers, laxatives, and sedatives, because they often contain sodium.

Diuretic therapy also has its complications, including hypokalemia, hyponatremia, hyperuricemia, hyperglycemia, and volume depletion. (See Table 8.4.) Hypokalemia

TABLE 8.4 Signs and Symptoms of Electrolyte Imbalances Related to the Use of Diuretics

Hypokalemia	Hyponatremia
Paresthesias	Weakness
Muscle cramps	Apathy
Muscular weakness progressing to flaccid paralysis	Lassitude
	Muscle weakness
Mental confusion	Fatigue
Anorexia	Headache
Abdominal distention	Hypotension
Paralytic ileus	Vertigo
Irregular cardiac rhythm	Muscle cramps
Heart block	Anorexia
Altered ECG patterns (ST segment depression, flattened or inverted T wave, prolonged Q-T interval)	Nausea/vomiting
	Loss of skin turgor
	Tachycardia
Circulatory failure	Thready peripheral pulse
Hypotension	Collapsed neck veins
Systolic arrest	

is particularly dangerous, because it markedly weakens cardiac contractions and may precipitate digitalis toxicity in individuals receiving digitalis. Consequently, periodic assessment of serum electrolyte values is mandatory, and a potassium supplement or an increase in dietary intake of potassium sources (e.g., orange juice, bananas, dried prunes, raisins, peaches, spinach, and apricots) may be prescribed.

Initial weights, skin turgor checks, and the maintenance of accurate intake and output records will assist in determining the patient's response to diuretic therapy. Moreover, while the patient is in the emergency department, the use of an infusion pump or microdrip IV tubing is recommended to prevent excessive hydration of the patient.

Venous/Arterial Vasodilators
Venous vasodilators, such as isosorbide dinitrate (10-20 mg/po 3-4 times/day), and arterial vasodilators, such as hydralazine (75 mg/po 3-4 times/day), may be used in treating CHF, since they both, by different methods, relieve pulmonary vascular and peripheral vascular congestion, relieve signs and symptoms due to diminished arterial flow, and decrease myocardial oxygen demand. Certain vasodilators, such as nitroprusside and prazosin, have dual actions, resulting in dilation of both veins and arteries (New Concepts, 1981).

Discharge Planning

Unfortunately, many patients continue to return to the hospital for recurrent episodes of CHF. Many recurrences, however, could be prevented through appropriate patient/family education, because they are usually due to the following (Brunner and Suddarth, 1980): (1) failure to follow the drug regimen properly; (2) dietary indiscretions; (3) inadequate medical follow-up; (4) excessive physical activity; and, (5) failure to recognize recurring symptoms.

The nurse should begin teaching by first assessing what the patient knows about his disease and the treatment he has been prescribed. Correct any misconceptions the patient may have; then ask the patient what he wants to know and discuss those areas first. Patients usually signify their readiness to learn by asking questions about their disease or its treatment. During the teaching, try to identify any depression, anxiety, or denial the patient might have, since these feelings can interfere with the patient's ability to learn. Include the family as often as possible in the teaching session to help reassure the patient and to provide him with a support group. The teaching plan should include the signs and symptoms of CHF, the correct usage of medications prescribed, adverse effects of those medications (especially the signs and symptoms of digitalis toxicity), conditions under which the patient should call or return to the emergency department for further evaluation, and the importance of appropriate follow-up care. Reinforce the teaching with written instructions.

Hospital and community resources may be valuable aids in discharge planning. The medical social worker may be able to assist with financial problems, thereby decreasing the patient's anxiety, while a nursing referral to the dietician can aid in appropriate meal planning. Rehabilitation services are available to patients with heart disease through the Office of Vocational Rehabilitation or the American Heart Association (Beland and Passos, 1981). Finally, a public health referral may be necessary to evaluate the effectiveness of the discharge teaching, ensure patient compliance, and prevent recurrences of CHF.

PULMONARY EDEMA

The major complication of CHF is pulmonary edema, the abnormal accumulation of serous or serosanguinous fluid in the lungs, either in the interstitial spaces or in the alveoli. The most common cause of pulmonary edema, of course, is cardiac disease leading to left-ventricular failure. Less commonly, however, pulmonary edema may result from such diverse conditions as inhaled toxins, overinfusion, radiation, renal and hepatic diseases, narcotic overdose, cerebral injury, uremia, anesthesia, near-drowning, disseminated intravascular coagulation, and pulmonary embolus (Jodice, 1978).

Pathophysiology

The development of pulmonary edema usually indicates that cardiac function has become extremely inadequate. When the left ventricle fails and the left ventricular end-diastolic pressure increases, blood backs up into the left atrium, increasing the pressure within this chamber. The increased pressure is then reflected backward into the pulmonary capillary bed, thus increasing capillary permeability and forcing fluids and solutes out of the intravascular compartment into the interstitium of the lungs. The lungs lose their elasticity, and the abnormal accumulation of fluid begins to impair the diffusion of oxygen across the alveolar membrane, resulting in tissue hypoxia. As the interstitium continues to swell with fluids, the lymphatic system can no longer handle the excessive load. Fluid floods into the peripheral alveoli, further aggravating respiratory abnormalities and leading to diminishing lung gas volume, increasing airway resistance, and increasing hypoxemia. In response to the decreasing oxygen supply, the tissues resort to anaerobic metabolism, which results in the accumulation of lactic acid, thus creating metabolic acidosis. The combination of hypoxia and acidosis places the individual in a life-threatening situation (Isacson and Schulz, 1978; Jodice, 1978).

Clinical Manifestations

Although pulmonary edema may have an insidious onset with gradually increasing signs of pulmonary congestion, such as cough, slight hyperventilation, orthopnea, exercise intolerance, and restlessness, it often occurs acutely at night after the individual has been lying down for a few hours. A sudden onset of breathlessness occurs, as well as a frightening sense of suffocation. The person becomes increasingly restless, anxious, and unable to sleep (Brunner and Suddarth, 1980). Sympathetic nervous system discharge produces the following effects: the pulse becomes weak and rapid; the skin becomes cool and moist with a dusky gray appearance; and, the blood pressure rises initially. A persistent cough exists, which, as the condition becomes worse, produces copious amounts of frothy, blood-tinged sputum. Audible rales are present, and some wheezing may occur if bronchospasm is present. The individual may experience chest pain due to stretching of the alveoli in the congested lungs and angina associated with the markedly reduced cardiac output (Beland and Passos, 1981). Signs and symptoms of right-sided heart failure may also be present. An S_3 gallop and decreased heart sounds may be auscultated, and, as the pulmonary edema progresses, the patient's anxiety develops into near panic. The patient's respirations become even more noisy and moist (and can often be heard even without a stethoscope), as the person begins to drown in his own secretions. Cheyne-Stokes respirations frequently enter the clinical picture at this point.

Diagnostic Studies

Because of the dramatic clinical picture usually associated with acute pulmonary edema, studies are performed not to determine a diagnosis, but primarily to provide information relating to the cause and extent of the disorder and to assist health care personnel in determining appropriate treatment. Diagnostic studies that may be ordered include the following (Jodice, 1978):

1. *ECG*—may indicate the basic underlying cardiovascular disease, for example, acute myocardial infarction; may also be used to evaluate the effectiveness of digitalis administration.
2. *Chest x-ray film*—indicates the extent of fluid accumulation in the lungs; may also reveal the presence of a pleural effusion or atelectasis.
3. *Arterial blood gas (ABG) analysis*—provides baseline and continuing data regarding the individual's oxygenation status; early ABG analysis generally reveals a low Po_2 and a low Pco_2.
4. *Digitalis level/serum electrolytes*—provide information about the heart and how it can be expected to respond to digitalis.

Nursing Care and Related Interventions

The major treatment objectives of pulmonary edema include the following: (1) improve ventilation and oxygenation; (2) provide physical and mental relaxation; (3) improve cardiovascular function; and, (4) reduce pulmonary congestion.

Airway Maintenance
The patient's airway must be kept clear. The patient may be able to keep the airway open by coughing. If not, he must be suctioned, or, if necessary, intubated. Continuously assess for airway patency, and note the color, amount, and consistency of the sputum expectorated.

Oxygen Administration
Relatively high concentrations of oxygen are administered either by mask or (for children) by hood or tent to relieve hypoxia and dyspnea. Although infrequently

used, intermittent positive pressure breathing (IPPB), with controlled concentrations of oxygen and humidification, may be ordered. IPPB creates counterpressure on the alveolar capillaries to decrease transudation of fluid from the alveoli; it also helps to retard the venous return by increasing intrathoracic pressure. In addition, IPPB helps to keep the alveoli open, reducing atelectasis and improving respiratory efficiency (Phipps, 1979). If the patient is unable to maintain adequate ventilation on his own, however, (as evidenced by a decreasing Po_2, increasing Pco_2 and decreasing pH), intubation and mechanical ventilation will be necessary. Check ABGs frequently to monitor the patient's oxygenation status.

Positioning
The patient should be placed upright, with the legs in a dependent position whenever possible, because this position decreases the venous return to the heart, decreases the work of breathing, and improves both lung volume and vital capacity. Support the patient with pillows when necessary to prevent fatigue (Brunner and Suddarth, 1980).

Medication Administration
DIURETICS

Either furosemide (40–80 mg IV for adults; 1 mg/kg IV for children) or ethacrynic acid (25–50 mg IV for adults; 1 mg/kg for children) is administered to help eliminate excess fluid and to reduce the circulating blood volume. Furosemide, in addition, causes vasodilation and peripheral vascular pooling, which, in turn, decreases the venous return to the heart. Since electrolytes, as well as water, are excreted in increased quantities, serum electrolyte values must be carefully monitored to detect impending imbalances. A Foley catheter should be inserted, and a careful record of the patient's intake and output maintained. Watch for decreasing blood pressure, increasing heart rate, and decreasing urine output, indicating the total circulation is not tolerating diuresis (Brunner and Suddarth, 1980).

MORPHINE

Morphine, administered IV to the patient in pulmonary edema, alleviates anxiety, reduces the work of breathing, and dilates the periphery with pooling of blood in the veins and reduction in the venous return. Morphine, however, may cause severe respiratory depression even when administered slowly, so give it in increments of only 2 to 4 mg at a time for adults and keep a narcotic antagonist, such as naloxone hydrochloride, as well as intubation equipment, readily available. A dosage of 0.1–0.2 mg/kg subcutaneously is recommended for children. In general, morphine should not be administered to patients with a history of cerebral vascular accident, chronic obstructive pulmonary disease, or to patients in cardiogenic shock (Isacson and Schulz, 1978; Price and Wilson, 1978). Careful monitoring of the respiratory status of the patient with pulmonary edema is obviously essential.

DIGITALIS

Rapid-acting digitalis preparations (see previous section on CHF) may be given intravenously to improve the contractile force of the heart and to increase the left-ventricular output that, in turn, will increase cardiac output. An increased cardiac output will not only enhance diuresis, but will also allow for the reflex withdrawal of increased sympathetic nervous system activity in the peripheral vascular bed leading to systemic arterial and venous dilation. If the patient has been on long-term digitalis therapy or recently has been digitalized, the drug is usually withheld until digitalis intoxication is ruled out (Brunner and Suddarth, 1980; Jodice, 1978).

AMINOPHYLLINE
Aminophylline is primarily administered to relax bronchospasm, when the patient is wheezing significantly. It works secondarily to increase cardiac output by increasing the contractile force of the heart and, in addition, lowers the threshold of the respiratory center to carbon dioxide. Aminophylline, however, must be given slowly to prevent a sudden drop in blood pressure, syncope, or even sudden death (Isacson and Schulz, 1978; Jodice, 1978; Price and Wilson, 1978). Dosages of 250–500 mg IV for adults, and 3.5–5.0 mg/kg IV for children are recommended. Continuous cardiac monitoring should be instituted to detect dysrhythmias, especially premature ventricular contractions.

VASODILATORS
If the patient does not respond to treatment, vasodilators may be used to reduce cardiac preload and afterload by reducing peripheral resistance. With more complete ventricular emptying and increased venous capacity, the left-ventricular filling pressure is reduced, and a decrease in pulmonary congestion is achieved.

Promotion of Physical and Mental Rest
Similar to congestive heart failure reactions, anxiety and fear are harmful to the patient in pulmonary edema, because they increase the work of the heart and the need for oxygen. Reassurance, therefore, is important. Because physical rest decreases the cardiac workload, assisting the patient with his needs will help the person conserve his strength.

Other Treatment Measures
PHLEBOTOMY
Although rarely used as a method of treating pulmonary edema, a phlebotomy, in which 100 to 500 cc of blood is withdrawn from a peripheral vein, may be used to reduce blood volume and thus pulmonary blood flow. Vital signs, of course, should be checked frequently during the procedure. One argument against using this therapy is that hemoglobin and electrolytes are removed, which may further contribute to hypoxemia and electrolyte imbalances (Phipps, 1979). Phlebotomy is contraindicated in patients with anemia.

ROTATING TOURNIQUETS
Although new medications have decreased the use of rotating tourniquets, they may be used in certain circumstances to pool blood in the extremities, thus reducing the venous return to the heart. Whether using automatic or manually applied tourniquets, the nurse's first responsibility is to check and record baseline measurements, including vital signs, mental status, breath sounds, and the quality of peripheral pulses, with special attention given to the warmth and color of each extremity. Mark

the peripheral pulses with a felt-tip marker so that they can be easily located for future monitoring. If available, use blood pressure cuffs, rather than tourniquets, and apply them as high as possible on the three extremities and over a dry washcloth or abdominal pad to prevent maceration of the underlying skin. Do not place a cuff on an arm containing an IV line. Experts disagree on the exact amount of pressure inflation to use, but, in most cases, a pressure of 25 to 45 mm Hg usually retards venous return, without closing off arterial flow. If mottling appears on the arms and legs without their turning blue, if the patient's arterial pulses remain strong, and if his breathing improves and rales decrease, sufficient pressure has been obtained. During the procedure, in which the venous flow of each extremity is retarded for 45 minutes each hour, assess vital signs frequently and keep an eye on the arms and legs to be sure that color, warmth, and pulses are within limits. The process of weaning the patient from rotating tourniquets is also critical; if the venous blood volume is suddenly increased, pulmonary edema will return. Certain contraindications to the use of rotating tourniquets include the following (Frantz and Galdys, 1978): hemorrhagic diathesis, peripheral blood clots, preexistent infection or ischemia, impaired right atrial function, peripheral vascular disease, and shock or impending shock.

Discharge Planning

If the patient will be discharged from the emergency department after treatment of a relatively mild episode of pulmonary edema, patient education is mandatory. Recurrences of pulmonary edema may be attributed to the same factors previously listed that contribute to recurrent episodes of congestive heart failure. The patient's understanding of his prescribed drug therapy, diet, physical activity limitations, and need for appropriate medical follow-up should be assessed. Furthermore, misconceptions should be corrected and additional information with rationale provided as necessary. The patient should be able to recite those signs and symptoms, such as cough, orthopnea, difficulty breathing, increasing exercise intolerance, and restlessness that would necessitate that he immediately contact his physician or return to the hospital emergency department for evaluation and treatment.

PULMONARY EMBOLUS

A pulmonary embolus is an obstruction of one or both branches of the pulmonary artery or its subdivisions (see Fig. 8.2). In the majority of cases, the obstruction is due to a thrombus, dislodged from the deep veins of the legs, that circulates through the blood vessels and the right side of the heart to become lodged in the pulmonary vasculature. Occasionally, the thrombus may originate in other veins, such as in the pelvic or iliac veins, or in the right side of the heart itself. In rare cases, nonthrombotic material, such as fat, air, amniotic fluid, tumor particles, or foreign material, may embolize to the lungs (Beland and Passos, 1981; Dossey and Passons, 1981).

Three major factors that predispose to thrombus formation are as follows: (1) hypercoagulability of the blood; (2) alterations in the integrity of the blood vessel

PULMONARY EMBOLUS

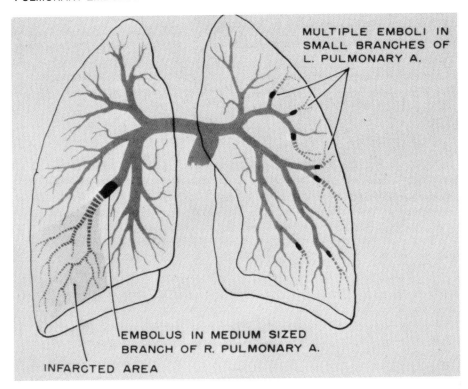

Figure 8.2 Pulmonary embolism and infarction. (Reprinted from *Pathophysiology: Clinical Concepts of Disease Processes* by S. A. Price and L. M. Wilson. Copyright © 1978 by McGraw-Hill, Inc. Used with the permission of McGraw-Hill Book Company.)

walls; and, (3) venous stasis. Anyone with one or more of these factors may be considered at high risk for pulmonary embolus (see Table 8.5).

Pathophysiology

After the embolic obstruction of the pulmonary artery or its branches, alveolar dead space increases, because the area of lung affected, although continuing to be ventilated, receives little or no blood flow. In addition, substances released from the clot (histamine and serotonin) compound the ventilation/perfusion imbalance by promoting bronchoconstriction. The hemodynamic consequences are as follows: (1) increased pulmonary vascular resistance due to reduction in the size of the pulmonary vascular bed; (2) a consequent increase in pulmonary artery pressure; and, in turn, (3) an increase in right ventricular work to maintain pulmonary blood flow. When the

TABLE 8.5 Factors Predisposing to Thrombus Formation

Hypercoagulability	Alterations in Vessel Wall	Venous Stasis
Malignancy	Trauma	Prolonged bedrest/immobilization
Oral contraceptives high in estrogen	Varicose veins	Obesity
	Diabetes mellitus	
Fever	Atherosclerosis	Advanced age
Sickle-cell anemia	Pregnancy	Burns
Pregnancy	Inflammatory processes	Postpartum period
Polycythemia vera		Congestive heart failure
Abrupt discontinuance of anticoagulants		
Myocardial infarction		

work requirements of the right ventricle exceed its capacity, right-ventricular failure occurs. A decrease in cardiac output follows, leading to a drop in systemic blood pressure and the development of shock (Brunner and Suddarth, 1980).

A possible complication of pulmonary embolus is pulmonary infarction, a localized area of ischemic necrosis of the lung parenchyma, usually resulting from embolic occlusion of a medium-sized artery. Pulmonary infarction, however, is an uncommon occurrence (demonstrated in only 10 to 20 percent of cases) due to the lung's dual blood supply, because an increase in blood flow through the bronchial arteries compensates for pulmonary vessel occlusion.

Clinical Manifestations

Pulmonary embolus is difficult to diagnose in the emergency department, because the clinical manifestations are extremely variable, depending not only on the size, location, and number of emboli, but also on the percentage of circulation obstructed and the predisposing factors (Dossey and Passons, 1981). Consequently, the clinical picture may range from no signs at all to sudden and almost immediate death caused by a massive embolus at the bifurcation of the main pulmonary artery. The signs and symptoms of pulmonary embolus are frequently attributed to other cardiopulmonary disorders, such as acute myocardial infarction, dissecting aortic aneurysm, pneumothorax, or pericarditis (Bishop, 1978; Price and Wilson, 1978). Sharp assessment skills and careful evaluation of presenting signs and symptoms are imperative.

The classic syndrome associated with a moderate-sized pulmonary embolus consists of unexplained dyspnea of sudden onset, cough, nonspecific chest or abdominal pain, tachycardia, tachypnea, and anxiety. More than half of the patients will have rales and an accentuated pulmonic component of the second heart sound. Bronchoconstriction may lead to a focal decrease in breath sounds and wheezing. Less frequently, an S_3 gallop, fever, or pleural friction rub will be found, although the latter two are more typical of pulmonary infarction than of a simple embolus. Hemoptysis and pleuritic chest pain may also be present if infarction occurs.

Massive pulmonary embolus, associated with failure of the right ventricle, results in acute cor pulmonale and a sudden, shocklike state with profound dyspnea, tachycardia, hypotension, cyanosis, stupor, or syncope. Death usually follows within minutes. Frequently, however, the symptoms of pulmonary embolus are subtle, such as unexplained fever or worsening of a preexisting cardiac or respiratory condition, such as pneumonia or congestive heart failure (Price and Wilson, 1978).

Diagnostic Studies

Because the differential diagnosis of pulmonary embolus is so broad, some diagnostic studies are primarily used to rule out other conditions, whereas other studies are more definitive for pulmonary embolus.

Laboratory Data
A complete blood cell (CBC) count, an erythrocyte sedimentation rate (ESR), ABG analysis, serum enzyme (SGOT, LDH) and serum bilirubin levels frequently are requested. The ESR and white blood cell count may be elevated if infarction has occurred, although there will be little or no increase in the differential count. The most frequently observed laboratory abnormality is a decreased Po_2 (often below 80 mm Hg), accompanied by a lower than normal Pco_2. Preexisting cardiopulmonary disorders, however, may reduce the usefulness of ABGs in diagnosing pulmonary embolus (Dossey and Passons, 1981; Wyper, 1978). The triad of elevated serum LDH and bilirubin levels and normal SGOT level occurs in less than 15 percent of patients with acute pulmonary embolism and infarction. An elevated LDH level may be demonstrated in as many as 85 percent of patients with pulmonary infarction, but this is not a specific finding.

Chest X-ray Studies
The chest x-ray examination is often useful in ruling out other pulmonary pathology. Most radiographic changes actually associated with pulmonary embolus, if any occur, are subtle and nonspecific. Nevertheless, they may, include the following (Wyper, 1978): (1) elevation of the diaphragm or pleural effusion on the affected side; (2) enlarged pulmonary arteries; or, (3) a triangular shadow indicating necrosis, which may appear with pulmonary infarction.

ECG
Although pulmonary embolus may result in some electrical abnormalities in the heart, the ECG is most useful in ruling out cardiac disease, such as an acute myocardial infarction, because changes associated with pulmonary embolus are often transient in nature and evolve rapidly. A significant embolus, however, may result in a right-bundle branch block with right axis deviation, peaked P waves in the limb leads, and depressed T waves in the right precordial leads.

Lung Scans
Two types of lung scans—perfusion and ventilation—provide valuable data when performed together, because pulmonary embolus, which results in a perfusion defect, does not immediately affect ventilation. With the perfusion scan, radioactive particles are injected intravenously and are carried to the lungs while a scan is performed. Areas of diminished perfusion are revealed by areas of diminished or absent radioactivity. During a ventilation scan, the patient inhales a radioactive-tagged gas as his lungs are scanned to reveal the distribution of radioactivity, which, with pulmonary embolus, should be normal (Dossey and Passons, 1981).

Pulmonary Angiography
Pulmonary angiography is the most definitive procedure for confirming the diagnosis of pulmonary embolus and for estimating the extent of involvement of the pulmonary vasculature. This procedure, however, is invasive, because a contrast media is injected through a catheter in the pulmonary artery, so it should be used only when major embolization is suspected and scanning is not diagnostic. This procedure, however, must be performed before surgical intervention is attempted.

Nursing Care and Related Interventions

The treatment objectives of pulmonary embolus are as follows: (1) to support vital functions; (2) to relieve symptoms resulting from the embolus; and, (3) to prevent further embolization. Measures fulfilling these objectives will vary, of course, depending on the severity of the disorder.

Supportive Measures
The patient is placed on a stretcher, with the head elevated to relieve dyspnea. Oxygen is administered, through nasal cannula or mask, to alleviate respiratory distress and to decrease hypoxemia. Positive pressure or mechanical ventilation may be necessary in severe cases. Analgesics may be administered to relieve pain and apprehension, but, if narcotics are used, they should be carefully monitored in order not to depress the breathing center. An intravenous line is inserted to provide a route for drugs and fluids, and continuous cardiac monitoring is suggested to detect dysrhythmias, which are frequently observed in massive pulmonary embolus. Digitalis may be ordered to aid in managing ventricular failure. Emotional support is also necessary, because fear and anxiety increase the work of both the cardiovascular and pulmonary systems. Frequent monitoring of vital signs and cardiopulmonary function will ensure prompt recognition of impending complications.

Vasopressors
Vasopressors, such as isoproterenol (2 to 4 mg in 1,000 ml of D_5W) or dopamine (200 mg in 500 ml of normal saline) may be used when the patient is experiencing severe circulatory failure. If the patient's hypotension is due to an impediment of blood flow, vasopressors are required to ensure adequate tissue perfusion, and they are titrated by using the urine output as a measure of organ perfusion (Beland and Passos, 1981).

Fibrinolytic Agents
Fibrinolytic agents, such as urokinase and streptokinase, may be used to dissolve both the embolus and the original thrombus. One major side effect of these drugs, however, is bleeding. If given, therefore, these drugs are usually administered before anticoagulant therapy is initiated.

Anticoagulant Therapy
A thrombus is not static, but continuously changing, and it will continue to form at the site of origin and in the lung where it has lodged. Anticoagulants, therefore, are given, to prevent recurrence and extension of the thromboembolism. An initial injection of 5000 to 15,000 units of heparin is quickly administered either by bolus or by constant infusion. Continuous infusion of heparin is preferred, because it causes less bleeding than bolus injections, but it does require close monitoring. Use an intravenous (IV) pump to prevent an inadvertent overdosage by too rapid an administration (Brunner and Suddarth, 1980; Wyper, 1978).

After the loading dose, subsequent dosages of heparin are required to maintain a Lee White clotting time of approximately 2 to 2-½ times that of normal, or a partial thromboplastin time at 1.5 to 2.5 times the control value. Heparin therapy is usually continued for eight to ten days, the estimated time for a clot either to dissolve or to be incorporated into a vein wall (Brunner and Suddarth. 1980; Dossey and Passons, 1981).

Oral anticoagulants, such as warfarin sodium (Coumadin), may be started at the same time as heparin, or they may be delayed for a few days. Coumadin therapy will then be continued for varying lengths of time, from six weeks to indefinitely. Contraindications to the use of anticoagulant therapy include the following (Beland and Passos, 1981; Bishop, 1978): active or recurrent gastrointestinal bleeding; open, fresh wounds; recent surgery; stroke; anemia; and severe hypertension.

Surgical Intervention
Surgical intervention is usually considered only for patients who show the following symptoms (Wyper, 1978): (1) are in profound circulatory failure; (2) cannot be anticoagulated; (3) do not respond to the treatment outlined above; or, (4) have experienced chronic embolism. Two techniques most commonly used are embolectomy and vena caval interruption. An embolectomy involves extraction of the embolus from the pulmonary artery system and requires the use of the cardiopulmonary bypass technique. Vena caval interruption prevents dislodged thrombi from being swept into the lungs and may be used if pulmonary emboli recur despite anticoagulation (Brunner and Suddarth, 1980; Dossey and Passons, 1981).

Discharge Planning

Patients who are diagnosed with pulmonary embolus in the emergency department are usually admitted to the hospital. For those patients who are at risk for pulmonary embolism and who are discharged from the emergency department, however, instruction should be provided, including preventive measures to be taken by the patient, as well as those signs and symptoms that, if they occur, would require the patient to return to the emergency department for further evaluation.

Since pulmonary embolus most frequently results from thrombophlebitis, the patient should be informed of the signs of this disorder—swelling; red, warm, or tender spots; pain in the calf on dorsiflexion—so that he may immediately report them to his physician. Remind the patient not to allow prolonged pressure in one area, sit for long periods of time, sit with his legs crossed or dangling, or wear clothing that restricts circulation to the legs. Demonstrate how to perform dorsiflexion exercises when at rest to enhance venous return from the legs. Patients with conditions predisposing to slow venous return (e.g., varicosities, polycythemia, congestive heart failure) may wear elastic hose to decrease flow to the deep veins of the legs. The hose should be put on before getting out of bed in the morning and taken off before retiring at night (Dossey and Passons, 1981; Moore and Maschak, 1977). A dietary consultation may be necessary to help the obese patient decrease his or her risk of future embolus.

Signs and symptoms that the discharged patient and his family should be instructed to report to his physician include unexplained dyspnea of sudden onset, nonspecific chest or abdominal pain, persistent cough, rapid heart rate, rapid respirations, unexplained anxiety, wheezing, and hemoptysis. Although, as stated previously, these clinical manifestations are not specific for pulmonary embolus, their development warrants prompt evaluation by health care personnel.

CONCLUSION

Recognizing the conditions of congestive heart failure, pulmonary edema, and pulmonary embolus, as well as developing and implementing an appropriate plan of emergency care for individuals with these disorders, ensures a good beginning for the patient's recovery and rehabilitation. When, however, a patient will be transferred to another unit from the emergency department, responsibility for continuity of care must be assumed by the emergency department nurse. Documenting the initial assessment, all therapeutic interventions, and the patient's subsequent response to the interventions will assist all health care personnel in helping patients achieve their health-related goals.

BIBLIOGRAPHY

Beland, I. L., and J. Y. Passos: *Clinical Nursing: Pathophysiological and Psychosocial Approaches*. 4th Ed. New York: Macmillan, 1981, pp. 813–815, 919–934.

Bishop, C. M.: Pulmonary emboli management. *Journal of Emergency Nursing* 4(3):35–39 (1978).

Brunner, L. S., and D. S. Suddarth: *Textbook of Medical–Surgical Nursing*. 4th Ed. Philadelphia: Lippincott, 1980, pp. 490–493, 577–586.

Dossey, B., and J. M. Passons: Pulmonary embolism: Preventing it, treating it. *Nursing 81* 11(3):26–33 (1981).

BIBLIOGRAPHY

Frantz, A., and M. Galdys: Keeping up with automatic rotating tourniquets. *Nursing 78* 8(4):31–35 (1978).

Isacson, L. M., and K. Schulz: Treating pulmonary edema. *Nursing 78* 8(2):42–46 (1978).

Isacson, L. M., and K. Schulz: Congestive Heart Failure: Severe Cardiac Impairment. In *Combatting Cardiovascular Diseases Skillfully*. Horsham, PA: Intermed Communications, 1978, pp. 93–102.

Jodice, J.: Management of acute pulmonary edema. *Journal of Emergency Nursing* 4(2):19–22 (1978).

Miessner, J. E., and L. N. Gever: Digitalis: Reducing the risks of toxicity. *Nursing 80* 10(9):32–38 (1980).

Moore, K., and B. J. Maschak: How patient education can reduce the risks of toxicity. *Nursing 77* 7(9):24–29 (1977).

Morgan, W. L., and G. L. Engel: *The Clinical Approach to the Patient*. Philadelphia: Saunders, 1969.

New concepts in understanding congestive heart failure, part 2: How the therapeutic approaches work. *American Journal of Nursing* 81:357–380 (1981).

Phipps, W. J., et al., eds.: *Medical–Surgical Nursing: Concepts and Clinical Practice*. St. Louis: Mosby, 1979, pp. 1003–1011, 1130.

Price, S. A., and L. M. Wilson: *Pathophysiology: Clinical Concepts of Disease Processes*. New York: McGraw-Hill, 1978, pp. 453–454.

Weldy, N. J.: *Body Fluids and Electrolytes: A Programmed Instruction*. St. Louis: Mosby, 1980, pp. 94–96, 108–112.

Wyper, M. S.: Pulmonary Embolism: Hazard of Immobility. In *Combatting Cardiovascular Disease Skillfully*. Horsham, PA: Intermed Communications, 1978, pp. 133–140.

9

An Upper Respiratory Infection, Croup, or Epiglottitis

Debbie Van Meter

After completing this chapter, the reader will be able to do the following:

1. Triage a patient experiencing an upper respiratory infection, croup, or epiglottis.
2. Name common upper respiratory conditions frequently seen in the emergency department.
3. Identify the upper respiratory infections that are potentially life-threatening.
4. Identify signs and symptoms of common upper respiratory infections, croup, and epiglottitis.
5. Institute appropriate nursing care for patients with an upper respiratory infection, croup, and epiglottitis.
6. Plan appropriate discharge teaching for patients with an upper respiratory infection, croup, and epiglottitis.
7. Identify illnesses associated with the ears and discuss their relationship to upper respiratory conditions.

The respiratory system is composed of the upper respiratory tract and the lower respiratory tract. The upper respiratory tract includes the structures of the nose, paranasal sinuses, pharynx, larynx, trachea, and bronchi. These structures function as open passages leading from the exterior to the lungs. An upper respiratory infection is an infectious process that interferes with the patent airway through numerous anatomical and physiological changes of the upper respiratory tract. A few of the more common upper respiratory infections often treated in the emergency department will be discussed in this chapter. Although these infections are easily treated, mistreatment or the absence of treatment can lead to life-threatening complications.

TRIAGE

Subjective Data

To begin the triage process, the nurse should obtain an initial history of the presenting problem from the patient, his family, ambulance personnel, or significant other. Identifying the motivating factor prompting the patient to enter the emergency department is necessary. The patient usually complains of sore throat, fever, headache, nasal congestion, cough, and perhaps shortness of breath. Depending on the patient's status at the time of his arrival at the emergency department, the triage nurse should conduct a detailed interview with the patient to assess the symptoms exhibited by the person. The length of time the patient has been experiencing the presenting symptoms is also important; data collected from this question often will differentiate a nonacute upper respiratory infection from an emergent one. Furthermore, the triage nurse should consider the patient's contact with other people who have been diagnosed as having an upper respiratory infection, since upper respiratory infections are frequently spread by airborne bacteria and viruses (Hutchinson, 1979).

Objective Data

While entering an emergency department, the patient exhibits many clues to his health status and underlying problem. The triage nurse must capitalize on these clues to obtain the objective data required to assess and plan the patient's care. The patient's color, position, respiratory status, orientation, facial expression, and effort of movement can be observed by the nurse, when the patient enters the emergency department. A complete set of vital signs should be taken, especially an accurate temperature, as soon as the patient is made comfortable. A brief physical assessment of the upper respiratory tract of the patient, which can easily be done by the triage nurse, requires only a few tools. If the patient's condition permits, inspect the patient's face, nares, and oropharynx. If shortness of breath is exhibited, or if labored or noisy, or wet respirations are present, assessment of the lungs and heart is indicated.

Assessment and Planning

After obtaining an initial history, past medical history, and physical assessment, the triage nurse identifies one or more nursing diagnoses and initiates a relevant plan of care for the patient. The plan of care for the patient with an upper respiratory infection considers the emergent nature of the patient's condition. If the patient exhibits respiratory distress, an immediate plan of action is indicated, and physician intervention is required. Nursing measures, such as positioning, monitoring, oxygen administration, and reassurance, are indicated for the patient with an upper respiratory tract emergency. The plan of care for most patients suspected of having an upper respiratory tract infection includes some patient teaching, while the patient waits for physician evaluation. The triage nurse should caution the patient to use a handker-

COMMON UPPER RESPIRATORY CONDITIONS

TABLE 9.1 Examples of Triage Notes for Patients Experiencing an Upper Respiratory Infection

S: 24 yo BF with c/o 3d hx of "runny nose," sneezing, watery eyes, aching all over, headache, possible fever. States "feels hot," denies sore throat, cough, earache, or chills. PMH: occasional cold, NKA, has been taking ASA for aches and fever.

O: Alert, oriented, RR 20, breathing through mouth, clear drainage from nose and eyes. Skin warm and dry, oropharynx pink with no exudates, no tonsils, unable to smell. T 99°F, P 88 regular; BP 110/68.

A: Cold.

P: Medical evaluation, to waiting room with advice to use handkerchief, avoid smoking and close contact with others.

S: 3 yo WM with mother who states child experienced sudden onset of difficulty in swallowing, has become increasingly SOB for 2 hrs. Mother states child has had a 2d hx of irritability, fever up to 102°F, sore throat. PMH: colds and otitis media occasionally, NKA, Tylenol elixir for fever, last dose 2 hrs. PTA.

O: Pale with cyanosis of lips and nail beds, resp. labored, substernal and intercostal retractions with nasal flaring, RR 60, alert. Skin hot and dry, drooling, P 150, BP 90/62, swelling and tenderness in neck area, unable to lie down.

A: Epiglottitis.

P: Pediatric evaluation, admit to examination room immediately, high Fowler's position, O_2 per ped. mask, parent accompany patient, reassurance to child and mother, M.D. notified immediately, continuous monitoring by R.N.

---

chief when coughing or sneezing, to avoid cigarette smoke, and to avoid close contact with others while in the waiting area. Because the patient with the upper respiratory infection often waits long periods of time in a busy emergency department, the triage nurse should emphasize to the patient the necessity of receiving medical care to prevent complications due to an upper respiratory infection. (Table 9.1 contains two examples of triage notes for patients experiencing an upper respiratory tract infection.)

COMMON UPPER RESPIRATORY CONDITIONS

Pathophysiology and Clinical Manifestations

Simple *acute rhinitis,* or the "common cold," is caused by a virus invading the upper respiratory passages. More than a hundred different viruses can cause the common cold. Acute rhinitis is the most prevalent infectious disease among people of all ages (Hutchinson, 1979). The initiation of the inflammatory process by the invading virus interferes with the function of the nose. Thus, temperature and humidity control of the air, particle removal, defensive mechanism, and the sense of smell of the nose is altered. *Allergic rhinitis,* or hay fever, although caused by the allergic response to pollen, dust, and other allergens, also alters the function of the nose.

Allergic rhinitis and simple acute rhinitis have presenting symptoms that are quite similar. The patient with rhinitis complains of sneezing, mild fever, chilliness, malaise, headache, nasal discharge, watery eyes, and muscular aching. Uncomplicated rhinitis is self-limited, and the patient is usually symptom-free after six to seven days. Secondary bacterial infections can complicate the common cold and hay fever. If treatment is not instigated, rhinitis can progress to pneumonia, bronchitis, sinusitis, or otitis media (Luckmann and Sorensen, 1980).

Sinusitis, acute and chronic, is another common upper respiratory infection often seen in the emergency department. Sinusitis is an inflammation of the mucosal lining of the sinuses. This inflammation most often occurs from the spread of a bacterial or viral infection from the nasal passages to the sinuses. The sinuses, as air-filled cavities in the skull, function in lessening the weight of the head. The sinuses, which normally drain secretions from the nose and the nasolacrimal duct, also contain the olfactory sense organs. The inflammation of the mucosal lining, due to acute sinusitis and the thickened mucosal lining of chronic sinusitis, interferes with these functions.

The clinical manifestations of the patient with sinusitis are malaise, lack of appetite, fever, cough, sore throat, headache, pain over affected sinus, puffy face, "heavy" head, nasal discharge, and the inability to smell. Complications of sinusitis that occur with the spread of the infection include orbital cellulitis, septicemia, periorbital abscess, cavernous sinus thrombosis, and brain abscess.

Sore throat is another complaint that is often heard from patients. *Pharyngitis* and acute follicular pharyngitis, or *strep throat,* are common upper respiratory infections frequently seen in emergency departments. Sore throats are most often caused by viruses, with 15 percent of affected throats caused by group A beta hemolytic streptococci. Sore throats due to staphylococcal infections occur occasionally (Luckmann and Sorensen, 1980). The inflammatory process initiated by these invading organisms causes edema, erythema, and pus formation in the lining of the pharynx. If severe enough, the lining of the pharynx can become so edematous that it blocks a patient's airway.

With viral sore throats or pharyngitis, clinical manifestations include a mild fever, mild sore throat, hacking cough, headache, and some difficulty in swallowing. In bacterial throat infections, such as strep throat, symptoms appear abruptly. These symptoms include a high fever, severe sore throat, chills, rash, headache, muscle and joint pain, swollen lymph glands, and malaise. Viral infections usually cause no complications. Streptococcal throat infections, however, can lead to life-threatening complications, such as nephritis and rheumatic heart disease (Luckmann and Sorensen, 1980).

Tonsillitis is the inflammation of a tonsil. The tonsils are two fleshy masses of lymphoid tissue located on either side of the oropharynx. These lymphatic tissues contain numerous lymphocytes that carry antibodies. Since most common infections are airborne, the tonsils act as the first line of defense (Librach, 1979). Tonsillitis can be due to a viral or bacterial infection. Acute tonsillitis is most often due to streptococcal infection (Luckmann and Sorensen, 1980). The inflammatory process, with the characteristic features of edema, redness, and pus formation, occurs with infection of the tonsils. The edema of the tonsils may cause difficulty in swallowing and possible blockage of a patient's airway. Other clinical manifestations associated with tonsillitis include a sore throat, fever, chills, anorexia, muscular pain, headache, and swollen lymph glands.

Peritonsillar abscess, or quinsy, is often a respiratory emergency. An acute streptococcal tonsillitis may cause a peritonsillar abscess to form due to infection of the tissue between the tonsil and the fascia covering the superior constrictor muscle (Luckmann and Sorensen, 1980). The initial history obtained from a patient with peritonsillar abscess involves tonsillitis for several days, before the patient develops pain on one side of the throat and difficulty in swallowing. Other symptoms of peritonsillar abscess include a muffled voice, high fever, and drooling due to the inability to swallow. If the surrounding throat tissue is involved, swelling can progress and cause closure of the upper airway. If closure occurs, the patient presents to the emergency department with signs of respiratory distress (Dupont, 1979).

Laryngitis, an inflammation of the larynx, is caused by an isolated infection involving the vocal cords, or by a general upper respiratory infection, or as a result of vocal abuse. The larynx primarily functions as an airway between the pharynx and trachea. The larynx has important sphincteric functions that help prevent aspiration and increase intrathoracic pressure. The cough reflex is initiated whenever a foreign body touches the highly sensitive laryngeal mucosa. The larynx is also involved in the production of speech by creating sounds as a result of vocal cord vibrations. The edema of the inflammatory process causes alterations in these functions of the larynx and produces hoarseness, the main symptom of laryngitis. Hoarseness may progress to complete voice loss. Other symptoms include a cough, sore throat, fever, chills, and a tickling feeling in the throat. With severe laryngitis, causing massive laryngeal edema, patients may develop respiratory stridor or dyspnea. Complications that can result from laryngitis, in addition to closure of the airway, include septicemia, bronchitis, and pneumonia.

Diagnostic Studies

History and physical examination of the nose, mouth, and oropharynx are the most useful diagnostic tools in determining whether a patient is suffering from an upper respiratory infection. Obtaining an accurate chronological history of the patient's symptoms initiates the process of diagnosing an upper respiratory infection. In examining the nose, note whether the mucosa is a bright, fire red; if it is, the inflammation has been caused by acute rhinitis. In allergic rhinitis, on the contrary, the mucosa appears normally pink to grayish in color and glistens. Any exudate found in the nasal cavity should be noted for color, consistency, amount, and smell. Pus in the nasal cavity suggests sinusitis. If sinusitis is suspected, symmetry of the face and puffiness over the affected sinus is often diagnostic. Other diagnostic tests of sinusitis include pain in the face when bending over and pain on palpation of the sinuses. Sinus x-ray studies that show transillumination (presence of pus) are diagnostic for sinusitis. A nasal pharyngeal culture is done to determine the exact organism causing the sinusitis. Testing for the sense of smell also helps diagnose rhinitis and sinusitis.

History differentiates acute from chronic sinusitis. In examining the nose of an infant, remember that infants are obligatory nose breathers and develop their sense of smell late.

In diagnosing an upper respiratory infection of the oropharynx, one can use throat cultures and examination of the oropharynx. Throat cultures should be done on all patients suspected of pharyngitis or tonsillitis to screen for streptococcal infection. In examining the oropharynx and tonsils, one notes the color of the mucosa and assumes that evidence of swelling, exudate, symmetry, and ulcerations are diagnostic clues indicating an upper respiratory infection. In viral pharyngitis, the posterior pharyngeal wall appears red and infected on examination. In streptococcal pharyngitis, however, yellow or white pus in the cryptae of the tonsils (if present) or on the posterior wall of the pharynx, along with redness and swelling, is present. Lymph nodes of the neck are often enlarged with streptococcal pharyngitis. Another diagnostic tool that may differentiate viral pharyngitis from streptococcal pharyngitis is a white blood cell count (WBC). In viral pharyngitis, the white blood cell (WBC) is often less than 10,000/cu mm, but in streptococcal pharyngitis, the WBC is elevated (Luckmann and Sorensen, 1980).

Peritonsillar abscess is diagnosed from the patient's presenting symptoms as well as from a history of acute streptococcal or staphylococcal tonsillitis for the past few days. On examining the tonsils, the nurse may notice a red bulge on one tonsil and severe swelling of the surrounding tissues that occludes the airway (Luckmann and Sorensen, 1980).

Laryngitis is also diagnosed by throat culture, oropharynx examination, white blood cell count, and history. The differentiating factor is hoarseness or aphonia.

Nursing Care and Related Interventions

General nursing care of the patient with any of the upper respiratory infections discussed includes rest, fluids, observation for complications, placing the patient in high Fowler's position, obtaining the temperature, and administering cooling measures if fever is present. Rest decreases the metabolic need of the patient, and thus decreases the body's needs for oxygen, an especially important factor in the patient with a compromised airway. Fluids keep a patient hydrated in the presence of a fever and help loosen secretions. Intravenous fluids may be necessary if a patient is severely dehydrated, such as in infants, the aged, and debilitated patients. The nurse should observe for signs of dehydration and begin hydration measures as soon as possible if dehydration is present.

Observation of life-threatening complications, such as closure of the airway, is an important nursing function, while the patient is in the emergency department. Placing the patient in a high Fowler's position facilitates breathing. With an infant, parents should be instructed to hold the infant upright or prop him against pillows, making sure to avoid hyperextension of the neck, to ensure adequate respiration.

Measuring the patient's temperature and administering appropriate antipyretics are other important nursing measures for the patient with a suspected upper respiratory infection. If fever is present to an extreme degree (103°F or above), other measures such as sponge baths and ice bags may be necessary, especially for infants, because they lack temperature control mechanisms.

Providing humidity for patients with sinusitis facilitates drainage of the sinuses. For the person with laryngitis, asking yes and no questions allows the patient's voice to rest and encourages healing of the larynx.

A patient with a peritonsillar abscess may require suctioning if spontaneous rupture of the abscess occurs. Maintenance of an open airway is an important nursing measure for these patients. Often an ice collar can help alleviate the swelling of a compromised airway.

An actual cure for the common cold still eludes the medical profession. Because colds are viral in origin, antibiotics are not necessary. Decongestants, antihistamines, and cough suppressants are sometimes prescribed to relieve the patient's cold symptoms. Nose drops are usually not recommended because of their rebound engorgement of the nasal mucosa (Hutchinson, 1979). Treatment of allergic rhinitis consists of desensitizing the patient to known allergens.

Sinusitis, if bacterial in origin, is treated with appropriate antibiotics. Pain medications are given to relieve the discomfort of sinusitis. Irrigation of the sinuses may be necessary in severe cases of sinusitis to promote drainage of the sinuses and to remove purulent matter. Antihistamines may be given to the patient with sinusitis, but these medications thicken nasal secretions and may prevent adequate sinus drainage. Treatment of chronic sinusitis is aimed at alleviating the underlying cause, such as obstruction due to polyps or to a deviated nasal septum (Luckmann and Sorensen, 1980).

Antibiotic therapy is necessary for the patient with streptococcal pharyngitis or tonsillitis to prevent possibly serious complications from developing. Antibiotics are prescribed only after a positive throat culture has been obtained. Antibiotics are not prescribed for patients with viral pharyngitis. Penicillin is the preferred drug for treating patients with a streptococcal infection. If the patient is allergic to penicillin, treatment with erythromycin or tetracycline can be prescribed. Pain medication may be required for the patient with a severe sore throat, and an antitussive may relieve a persistent cough in the patient with pharyngitis or tonsillitis. If a patient's airway is compromised, or if the patient is unable to swallow due to severe swelling of the pharynx, hospitalization, and the administration of intravenous antibiotics may be necessary (Luckmann and Sorensen, 1980).

Therapy for the patient with a peritonsillar abscess includes incision and drainage of the abscess. Hospitalization with intravenous hydration and antibiotics is necessary for the patient with a peritonsillar abscess, due to the possibility of an occluded airway.

Discharge Planning

Discharge teaching by the emergency department nurse is important in the care and treatment of the patient with an upper respiratory infection. If detailed and understandable teaching and planning are done, the incidence of return visits to the emergency department is significantly reduced. When planning discharge, the nurse considers the patient's educational level and cultural and environmental background, as well as the person's financial status and adjusts the discharge teaching appropriately.

General education of the patient with an upper respiratory infection includes the importance of rest, increased fluid intake, humidity to loosen secretions, warm saline gargles for sore throats, a good general diet to increase host resistance, mouth care to prevent secondary infections, local heat to the face for patients with sinusitis, avoidance of smoking, the use of antipyretics and their potential side effects, and the observation of temperature. Parents should be taught how to take their child's rectal temperature and how to read a thermometer.

Discharge teaching also explains that, because upper respiratory infections are contagious, measures to prevent cross contamination should be taken. These measures include not eating or drinking from the same utensils as an affected person, avoiding kissing others, and covering the mouth and nose when coughing and sneezing.

Patients should be taught to avoid blowing the nose forcefully, because this irritates the nasal mucosa and further aggravates the swelling. In addition, epistaxis may occur with the increased pressure due to nose blowing. Infants, since they are obligatory nose breathers, should have their nares frequently bulb-suctioned to remove secretions. Parents should be taught how this is done and explained that care must be taken to prevent traumatization of the infant's nose.

The importance of obtaining a positive throat culture before using antibiotic therapy should be explained to the patient. The patient should receive instructions on how to inquire about culture results and how follow-up care should be arranged.

Other important discharge teaching measures concern the prescription of drugs for the treatment of an upper respiratory infection. Stress that the patient must continue to take all antibiotics as prescribed, even if symptoms are relieved, to avoid a recurrence of the upper respiratory infection. Antibiotic action, administration, and side effects should be explained. In addition, explanation of the lack of antibiotic therapy for patients with viral upper respiratory infections is necessary. Explain the side effects of drowsiness and lethargy from using antihistamines and analgesic medications, and also stress the need to avoid driving and dangerous activities that require alertness.

For patients with peritonsillar abscess, the importance of sleeping with the head of the bed elevated and observing for complications, such as respiratory distress, should be explained in discharge teaching. The possibility of a future tonsillectomy should also be mentioned. Patients with laryngitis are advised to rest their voices and to use throat lozenges for their soothing effects.

Another long-term discharge procedure includes maintaining a record of the frequency of upper respiratory infections an individual experiences. Underlying disease processes may be discovered by analyzing these records.

ACUTE AND CHRONIC BRONCHITIS

Pathophysiology

Bronchitis, defined as the inflammation of the bronchi, can be either acute or chronic. Bronchitis can be viral or bacterial in origin, or it can be caused by irritants, such as smoke. Bronchitis frequently is caused by an extension of a general acute upper respiratory infection. Invasion of the bronchi by a bacteria or virus impairs the cleaning mechanism performed by the cilia lining the bronchi. Thus, exudate and cellular wastes accumulate and initiate the most common symptom of bronchitis—a productive cough (Luckmann and Sorensen, 1980).

Chronic bronchitis is characterized by a recurrent productive cough. Chronic bronchitis is due to recurrent upper respiratory infections involving the bronchi, and it is almost always associated with heavy cigarette smoking. The onset of chronic bronchitis is insidious, progressing throughout a period of years and leading to potentially debilitating respiratory disorders. Degenerative changes that occur in the bronchi include hypersecretion of bronchial mucus and hypertrophy, as well as hyperplasia of the bronchial mucosal glands. Cilia are absent, and the bronchi appear to be dry and inelastic, thus requiring greater effort to cleanse the upper respiratory tract. In addition, due to the impairment of the cleansing function of the bronchi, the bronchi provide a media for repeated respiratory infection.

Clinical Manifestations

The clinical presentation of a patient with acute bronchitis includes a general malaise, irritating dry cough progressing to sputum production, anorexia, fever, chills, chest tightness, dyspnea, and sore throat. In a patient with chronic bronchitis, a cough with clear sputum production on waking and then continuous throughout the day is the major symptom. The patient with chronic bronchitis presents to the emergency department with signs and symptoms of acute exacerbation of an upper respiratory infection. Some patients with progressed chronic bronchitis exhibit shortness of breath and signs of hypoxia during these periods of acute exacerbation.

Diagnostic Studies

Both acute and chronic bronchitis are diagnosed by history and clinical presentation. Chest x-ray studies are done to determine if any underlying disease or complication, such as pneumonia, is present. Sputum cultures are obtained to rule out bacterial origin. Chest auscultation occasionally reveals rhonchi and wheezes in the patient with acute bronchitis (Iveson, 1981). In chronic bronchitis, ventilatory function tests and arterial blood gases are performed to determine the severity of the patient's condition (Luckmann and Sorensen, 1980).

Nursing Care and Related Interventions

The nursing care for the patient with acute or chronic bronchitis is essentially the same as for patients with any other general upper respiratory infection. Rest, fluids, humidity, and good general health care are recommended. In the emergency department, oxygen therapy and intravenous fluids may be necessary for the patient with severe bronchitis, especially for infants, the aged, and debilitated patients. Treatment for acute bronchitis includes antibiotics, if the cause of the infection is bacterial, and bronchodilators, if bronchospasm is present. Cough depressants are not usually prescribed, since the lungs should be cleared of accumulated secretions.

For the patient with chronic bronchitis, nursing care focuses on reducing symptoms. Improving ventilation and respiration by positioning and oxygen therapy prevents hypoxia and possible respiratory failure. Relief of bronchospasm includes removal of irritants, such as cigarette smoking, antibiotics to destroy infectious bacteria, and the administration of bronchodilators. The nurse administering bronchodilators in the emergency department must observe the patient's vital signs and be aware of the side effects of these drugs (Luckmann and Sorensen, 1980).

Discharge Planning

Discharge teaching and planning for patients with bronchitis are similar to the teaching for patients with an acute upper respiratory infection. The emergency department nurse should emphasize the avoidance of cigarette smoking. Other discharge instructions include an explanation of drug therapy (side effects, actions, and administration) of antibiotics and bronchodilators and follow-up care, especially for the patient with chronic bronchitis.

ILLNESSES ASSOCIATED WITH THE EARS

Otitis Media

Pathophysiology
Because of the proximity and connection via the eustachian tube of the ear to the upper respiratory tract, upper respiratory infections are commonly associated with infections of the ear. *Otitis media,* or infection of the middle ear, is more common in children than in adults due to the narrower eustachian tube that can be occluded easily. The eustachian tube functions by opening and closing to equalize pressure between the middle ear and barometric pressure. When this function fails, an effusion may develop within the middle ear and cause an infection to develop. Otitis media can be either viral or bacterial in origin and is described as serous, secretory, or suppurative otitis media (Sataloff and Colton, 1981).

Clinical Manifestations
The child who presents to the emergency department with otitis media exhibits symptoms of hearing loss, earache, pulling at the ears, drainage from the ears, fever, malaise, "fussiness," irritability, and feeding problems. In an adult, severe ear pain and hearing loss with fever and malaise are the common symptoms of otitis media.

Diagnostic Studies
Diagnosis of otitis media is done by history and by clinical presentation. Other diagnostic measures include otoscopic examination, which may reveal a bulging of the tympanic membrane, presence of pus, obscured bony landmarks, and erythema of the tympanic membrane. A pneumatic otoscopic examination and testing for hearing identifies impairment of the tympanic membrane. If otitis media is not treated diligently, serious complications can develop, such as intracranial abscess, meningi-

tis, neck abscess, jugular thrombosis, mastoiditis, and permanent hearing loss (Kasonof, 1980).

Nursing Care and Related Interventions
Nursing care for the patient with otitis media includes rest, checking the temperature and administering appropriate cooling measures, observing for dehydration, especially in children and the aged, and initiating fluid replacement if necessary. Unless severe dehydration or secondary complications are present, otitis media can be treated effectively in the home. Decongestants and antibiotics are routinely prescribed. Pain medication for severe ear pain occasionally is prescribed.

Discharge Planning
Discharge teaching of the patient and family is important to prevent serious complications. Side effects, and administration of antibiotics, decongestants, and pain medications should be explained. Stress to patients and parents of children experiencing otitis media that they should observe for fever and dehydration and should increase fluid intake. Also important is the feeding technique parents use for their infants. Otitis media often develops because the infant's head is held too low during feeding so that milk and other food particles enter the eustachian tube and provide a media for the development of infection. Parents and babysitters should keep the infant's head elevated as much as possible during feeding. Instructions for follow-up care are necessary for patients with otitis media to evaluate antibiotic treatment and to prevent complications. In addition, if otitis media is a recurrent problem in an individual, underlying causes, such as adenoid hypertrophy, should be evaluated.

External Otitis

Pathophysiology
Another common ear infection seen in the emergency department is swimmer's ear, or *external otitis*. This condition is a painful inflammation of the skin of the outer ear canal, usually caused by an accumulation of water in the ear.

Clinical Manifestations
The clinical manifestations of external otitis include severe pain in the affected ear and possibly pain radiating over the entire affected side of the head. The patient often complains of fullness in the ear and impaired hearing.

Nursing Care and Related Interventions
Treatment for external otitis includes the insertion of an ear wick to prevent total closure of the ear canal due to edema. The ear wick remains in place for 48 hours. Antibiotic ear drops are prescribed to apply to the wick, while it remains in place.

Discharge Planning
Discharge instructions for the patient with external otitis should include an explanation of the ear wick and the use of the antibiotic drops. To prevent further complications, the patient should be instructed to keep his ear out of water, while the wick is

in place. A cotton ball moistened with petroleum jelly should be placed in the patient's outer ear to keep the ear dry, while the person is washing his hair or taking a shower. The patient should avoid using cotton swabs or other foreign objects to clean the ear. If pain is severe, a pain medication may be prescribed (Dupont, 1979).

Infected Adenoids

An underlying cause of chronic ear infections is infected and hypertrophied adenoids. Adenoids are a collection of lymphoid tissue that grows from the roof and posterior wall of the nasopharynx. Adenoids are rarely present in adults, since they atrophy during puberty. Children, therefore, are the most common sufferers of infected adenoids. Repeated adenoid infection causes hypertrophy of this lymphoid tissue, eventually leading to obstruction of the eustachian tube and a change in the ears, which leads to chronic infections and hearing loss. Hypertrophy of the adenoids indicates the need for surgical removal (Luckmann and Sorensen, 1980). In treating children seen in the emergency department with repeated ear infections, the nurse should discuss with the family the possibility of adenoids as an underlying cause and emphasize the need for follow-up care.

DIPHTHERIA

Diphtheria, a severe disease involving the pharynx and other structures of the throat, most often affects children and is caused by the bacillus *Corynebacterium diphtheriae*. Immunization during the last 50 years has significantly decreased the evidence of diphtheria. Because of the recent lack of emphasis on immunizing children, however, diphtheria infections have occasionally been seen during the last few years. Diphtheria produces a white or gray membrane in the throat that advances rapidly to cover all structures of the throat and extends into the trachea. Acute inflammation develops on the mucosal surfaces of the throat in response to the diphtheria exotoxin. Necrosis and desquamation develop with large amounts of exudates (Luckmann and Sorensen, 1980).

The patient with diphtheria is severely ill and presents with a severe sore throat, fever, and possibly airway obstruction and respiratory difficulty. Treatment must be given immediately to prevent serious complications. Admitting the patient to the hospital and placing him in strict isolation is necessary. The administration of antitoxin and antibiotics should begin immediately (Luckmann and Sorensen, 1980).

WHOOPING COUGH OR PERTUSSIS

Another upper respiratory infection, whose incidence is increasing due to lack of immunization for children, is whooping cough or pertussis. This acute, highly contagious bacterial disease, caused by *Bordetella pertussis,* is characterized by a paroxysmal or spasmodic cough that ends in a prolonged, high-pitched, crowing inspiration or whoop. The bacteria causing pertussis invades the mucosa of the upper respiratory tract and produces symptoms due to the inflammatory process: for example, anorexia, nasal congestion, and cough. Pertussis has a high mortality rate in young children, but is rarely serious in older children or in adults. Treatment involves alleviating symptoms and supporting the respiratory system. Antibiotics are not usually prescribed.

SUBGLOTTIC CROUP OR ACUTE LARYNGOTRACHEOBRONCHITIS

Pathophysiology

Croup, a common childhood disease, usually occurs during the winter months, is more prevalent in males, and occurs between the ages of three months and three years (Simkins, 1981). Croup is, in fact, a symptom that refers to the harsh, barky cough typical of laryngotracheobronchitis. Laryngotracheobronchitis is an inflammation of the larynx, trachea, and bronchi due to viral or bacterial infections. Croup is primarily viral in origin, and parainfluenza viruses are the most common causative agents. Other viruses, such as respiratory syncytial virus, adenovirus, or influenza virus, may also cause croup (Page, 1981). The harsh, noisy cough arising in the larynx is due to the narrowing of the larynx caused by edema and is an important sign of potential airway obstruction.

Clinical Manifestations

Laryngotracheobronchitis or croup is usually preceded either by a cold or by another upper respiratory tract infection producing cough, low-grade fever, and nasal congestion. After a few days, the child develops the harsh, barky cough typical of croup and stridorous respirations that become worse at night. Most croup is not serious, and treatment at home can alleviate symptoms. If a child's breathing becomes labored, with restlessness or cyanosis, emergency care is indicated. Adults may also experience croup. Presenting symptoms include hoarseness, sore throat, and cough. Complications of croup, if not treated adequately at home or in the emergency department, include airway obstruction with respiratory failure, epiglottitis, bronchitis, pneumonia, and septicemia (Page, 1981).

Diagnostic Studies

Diagnosis of croup is primarily done by examining the patient's history and clinical presentation. The harsh, barky cough associated with croup is often diagnostic of this disorder. Further studies are done to eliminate the possibility of epiglottitis. An x-ray film depicting the lateral view of the neck is recommended. In the patient with croup, the x-ray study shows a normal epiglottis with constriction of the subglottic area. Examination of the larynx is also done to exclude the diagnosis of epiglottitis (Simkins, 1981). A throat culture is done to establish a viral or bacterial cause for the croup. If a white blood cell count is indicated, for instance with high fever, the count is usually normal in the patient with croup (Page, 1981).

Nursing Care and Related Interventions

The nursing care for the adult or child experiencing croup involves providing a patent airway. The nurse must continuously monitor the patient's respiratory status, while the patient is in the emergency department. Changes in vital signs, the patient's mental state, color, and respiratory effort can provide clues regarding impending respiratory distress. The patient should be placed in a high Fowler's position to facilitate breathing. Supplemental oxygen administered with humidity often prevents hypoxia due to respiratory insufficiency. Suction should be available at all times for the patient with croup. An endotracheal tube and the necessary equipment for intubation should also be made available. Reassurance and explanation of procedures decrease the anxiety of the patient and prevent an increase in oxygen requirements of the body.

Antibiotics are usually not necessary for the patient with croup, since most croup is viral in origin. Nevertheless, some physicians occasionally prescribe antibiotics to prevent secondary bacterial infections.

Nebulized racemic epinephrine administered by intermittent positive pressure breathing (IPPB) has been advocated by several pediatric centers for the effective treatment of the acute symptoms of croup (Simkins, 1981). Epinephrine acts as a local vasoconstrictor and decreases laryngeal swelling. Administration of racemic epinephrine remains controversial due to studies demonstrating that a rebound effect with rapid recurrence of obstructive symptoms may occur (Luckmann and Sorensen, 1980). The nurse administering racemic epinephrine in the emergency department must closely observe the patient and monitor vital signs to recognize possible rebound effects.

Steroids, such as Decadron and Solu-Medrol, have also been advocated for the treatment of croup, because of their anti-inflammatory actions. These drugs, however, are controversial due to their numerous side effects (Simkins, 1981).

Hospitalization may be necessary for the patient with croup to continue monitoring the person's respiratory status and to administer oxygen therapy. Sedatives are contraindicated for patients with croup, due to their respiratory depressive actions (Simkins, 1981).

Discharge Planning

Frequently, the exposure of the patient to moist cool air outside the home, while enroute to the emergency department, eliminates the symptoms of respiratory distress associated with croup. The nurse in the emergency department should explain this phenomenon to the patient and to the patient's family and instruct them to use humidification in the home. If a humidifier is not available, showers can be used to acquire the desired humidity.

The patient and his family should be taught to observe for signs and symptoms of respiratory distress and cautioned to return to the emergency department immediately if these symptoms reappear. Rest and decreasing the activity of the patient will decrease the patient's oxygen needs. Fluids should be encouraged to prevent dehydration and to loosen secretions. Furthermore, sleeping with two pillows aids in respiratory function. If medications are prescribed, such as antibiotics or steroids, their side effects, administration, and actions should be explained. Follow-up care instructions concerning throat cultures and further medical care should be given to the patient and his family on discharge from the emergency department.

EPIGLOTTITIS OR SUPRAGLOTTIC CROUP

Pathophysiology

Epiglottitis is an extremely rare and emergent disease. It most often occurs in children (especially in boys) between the ages of one to seven, but it can also occur in adults. Epiglottitis is an extremely acute inflammation and swelling of the epiglottis that tends to obstruct the glottic opening and leads rapidly to respiratory obstruction. The inflammatory process also involves the aryepiglottic folds and supraglottic areas, thus significantly diminishing the opening of the airway. (Figure 9.1 depicts the normal anatomy of the oropharynx.) Epiglottitis is usually bacterial in origin, and it most often is caused by the *Hemophilus influenzae* type B organism (Fried, 1980).

Clinical Manifestations

Epiglottitis differs from the common viral croup infection, because it immediately develops into an acute medical emergency. (Table 9.2 describes the differences between croup and epiglottitis.) The patient with epiglottitis has a history of sudden

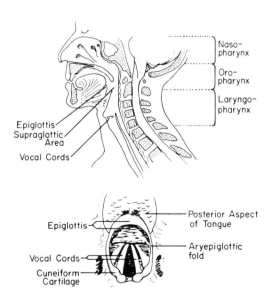

Figure 9.1 The anatomy of the oropharynx.

TABLE 9.2 Differences Between Croup and Epiglottitis

Criteria	Croup	Epiglottitis
Age	3 months to 3 yrs	1 yr to 7 yrs
Sex	Male	Male
Occurrence	Winter	All seasons
Cause	Viral	Bacterial
Clinical symptoms	Cough (harsh, barky)	No cough
	Sore throat	Severe sore throat
	Low-grade fever	High fever
	Onset over period of days	Onset within 2–4 hrs
	Normal white blood cell count	High white blood cell count
Diagnostic findings	Normal-sized epiglottis	Enlarged cherry-red epiglottis

onset of discomfort in the throat and fever, progressing rapidly over a two-to-four-hour period to inspiratory stridor and to extreme difficulty in breathing. The patient may show signs of hypoxia, such as cyanosis, lethargy, or disorientation. Other clinical manifestations of epiglottitis include muffled voice sounds, drooling due to the inability to swallow, sore throat, inability to lie down, high fever, malaise, and usually no coughing. If the clinical manifestations of epiglottitis are not recognized immediately by medical personnel, death of the patient can result within a few hours (Fried, 1980).

Diagnostic Studies

Diagnosis of epiglottitis is made by history, clinical presentation, and direct visualization of the epiglottis and aryepiglottic folds. A throat culture should not be done due to the possibility of creating a spasm and complete airway obstruction. Lateral neck views on the x-ray film exhibit an enlarged epiglottis and a narrowing of the supraglottic area. Visualization of the epiglottis should be done extremely cautiously. Equipment for intubation must be available before the examination. On direct visualization, the patient with epiglottitis will have an edematous and cherry-red epiglottis. A white blood cell count in the patient with acute epiglottitis will be markedly high due to the bacterial origin of the disease. Arterial blood gas values may be indicated to ascertain the degree of respiratory insufficiency.

Nursing Care and Related Interventions

Nursing care of the patient with epiglottitis is similar to treatment discussed for croup. The main nursing objective is to provide a patent airway. In addition to the nursing care recommended for the patient with croup, the patient with epiglottitis must never be left alone by health care professionals. Airway obstruction and death can occur suddenly and at any time. Intubation equipment must be on hand at the patient's bedside at all times. Hospitalization is mandatory for the patient with epiglottitis to prevent respiratory failure and death. Intravenous antibiotics, steroids, and racemic epinephrine are often prescribed for the patient with epiglottitis (Page, 1981).

Because of the development of extremely soft, flexible, and fine plastic endotracheal tubes that are nontraumatic to the patient, tracheotomies are rarely done in the emergency department. If a tracheotomy is necessary, it is done under general anesthesia, using aseptic surgical techniques (Page, 1981). Even though epiglottitis is a potentially life-threatening disease, it is treatable and curable in the hospital setting.

CONCLUSION

Because upper respiratory infections are usually nonacute disorders, nurses in the emergency department often forget the possibility that life-threatening complications may occur with these disorders. The emergency department nurse, therefore, must make an accurate and thorough assessment of the patient presenting to the emergency department with symptoms of an upper respiratory infection to avoid mistriaging a possibly emergent situation. The emergency department nurse, who understands acute and nonacute upper respiratory disorders and who develops expertise in assessing, treating, and teaching patients with an upper respiratory infection, can provide quality nursing care to patients and can prevent life-threatening complications from developing.

BIBLIOGRAPHY

Dupont, J.: EENT emergencies. *Nursing 79* 9:65–70 (Nov. 1979).

Fried, E.: Acute epiglottitis. *Issues in Comprehensive Pediatric Nursing* 4:29–36 (Sept./Dec. 1980).

Hutchinson, R.: The common cold primer. *Nursing 79* 9:57–61 (Mar. 1979).

Iveson-Iveson, J.: Acute bronchitis. *Nursing Mirror* 152:24 (May 1981).

Kasanof, D. M., ed.: Current care for otitis media. *Patient Care* 14:31–48 (Dec. 1980).

Librach, I.: Layman's guide to common complaints. *Nursing Mirror* 149:18–19 (Sept. 1979).

Luckmann, J., and K. Sorensen: *Medical-Surgical Nursing: A Psychophysiologic Approach.* Philadelphia: Saunders, 1980.

Page, H. S.: Croup and epiglottitis: Sudden trouble for young children. *American Lung Association Bulletin* 67:9–11 (Mar. 1981).

Sataloff, R. T., and C. M. Colton: Otitis media: a common childhood infection. *American Journal of Nursing* 81:1480–1483 (Aug. 1981).

Simkins, R.: Croup and epiglottitis. *American Journal of Nursing* 81:519–520 (Mar. 1981).

10

Angina, Myocardial Infarction, or Cardiogenic Shock

Molly P. Bronaugh

After completing this chapter, the reader will be able to do the following:

1. Obtain the appropriate triage data from patients with angina, unstable angina, and myocardial infarction.
2. Explain the pathophysiology of angina and myocardial infarction as it relates to atherosclerosis, ischemia, and myocardial cellular death.
3. List and correlate symptoms or signs associated with cardiac chest pain to their pathophysiological basis.
4. Describe the nursing responsibilities involved in the care of patients with angina or myocardial infarction.
5. List the anticipated early complications of unstable angina and myocardial infarction.
6. Explain the pathological sequence of events leading to cardiogenic shock.
7. Pinpoint the clinical manifestations of cardiogenic shock.
8. Describe current nursing management techniques used to reverse the shock state.

Each year approximately 1.3 million people in the United States suffer from acute myocardial infarction (MI), resulting in 15 to 20 percent of all natural deaths (Alpert and Braunwald, 1980; Lown, 1980). The two major causes of death following myocardial infarction are lethal dysrhythmias and severe heart failure. Approximately half of the deaths occur in the prehospital setting within two hours after the onset of symptoms, and ventricular fibrillation is the primary cause of death in a majority of these patients (McIntyre and Parker, 1980).

With the extensive development of coronary care units during the past 20 years, in-hospital mortality from lethal dysrhythmias has markedly declined; thus, the most severe form of heart failure, cardiogenic shock, is now the leading cause of in-hospital death after MI (Dracup et al., 1981.) More than 80 percent of patients developing cardiogenic shock die, despite aggressive management (Foster and Canty, 1980).

The emergency department, a vital link between the prehospital and coronary care units, mandates adequate nursing knowledge for the care of patients suffering from angina, myocardial infarction, or cardiogenic shock.

TRIAGE

Subjective Data

Because myocardial infarction is a potentially life-threatening condition, patients complaining of cardiac chest pain must be triaged quickly, often with initial stabilization already in progress. The subjective history includes data pertaining to the pain onset, duration, quality, site, relief, and associated symptoms.

The onset of cardiac chest pain is sudden, and it is associated with angina if related to activity. Onset at rest is correlated with myocardial infarction, because in the majority of these patients no precipitating factor can be found (Alpert, 1980). Stable anginal attacks last 30 seconds to 30 minutes (Helfant and Banka, 1978); if the patient reports pain of longer duration, the triage nurse should be concerned about the possibility of unstable angina or myocardial infarction. Unstable angina may last for 45 minutes, and chest pain of longer duration is usually associated with infarction (Cohn and Braunwald, 1980).

The quality of cardiac chest pain will vary with the individual and according to severity. It is classically characterized as tight, squeezing, heavy pain, although some patients may complain only of mild chest discomfort. The patient may report burning pain, describe it as something heavy sitting upon the chest, or portray the pain with complaints that mimic indigestion. The site of the pain is typically midchest or substernal and can radiate from the chest to the arms, jaw, neck, or subscapular area.

When the initial event is relieved by rest and nitroglycerin, the pain is considered angina. If the patient's pain is not relieved by those actions, the possibility of myocardial infarction increases. A notation of associated symptoms completes the initial subjective history. Both angina and infarction can be accompanied by the complaint of shortness of breath. The triage nurse should further question the patient about nausea, which is more commonly related to myocardial infarction.

Using the "PQRST" mnemonic may help the triage nurse obtain the subjective history. The mnemonic is derived from the complexes seen on normal ECG. Table 10.1 explains what each letter represents when used to obtain the subjective cardiac chest pain history.

In addition to obtaining standard past medical history data, the triage nurse must identify "risk factors" strongly associated with cardiac chest pain. Risk factors are either biologic characteristics of the patient or chronic problems. If obtained in the past medical history, risk factors increase the chances that chest pain complaints are cardiac in origin. Among the risk factors presented by Levy and Feinleib (1980) are

TABLE 10.1 Useful Mnemonic in Obtaining Subjective Data

P—Provokes	"What brought on the pain?"
Q—Quality	"What does the pain feel like?"
R—Relief	"Have you done anything to relieve the pain?"
S—Site	"Point to where it hurts."
T—Time	"How long have you had this pain?"

the unalterable biologic characteristics of age, sex, and race. Chronic problems that increase risk include hypertension, diabetes, cigarette smoking, obesity, and stress. Although they do not comprise the entire spectrum of risk factors, they are the risks most readily assessed by the triage nurse.

The significance of the risk factors is determined by the manner in which they are interpreted by the triage nurse. If a patient is 44, male, black, and has a past medical history of hypertension, for example, his complaints are more likely to be cardiac in origin, compared to a 24-year-old white female with chest pain complaints.

Information regarding the patient's current drug therapy and allergies completes the past medical history notation. Medications reflect the nature of chronic underlying problems that might not otherwise be reported by the patient. Drugs taken that directly relate to a previous history of angina pectoris include Isordil, Inderal, Nitro-Bid paste, and nitroglycerin.

The triage nurse is frequently able to determine whether the patient's subjective complaints are cardiac in nature or due to some other cause. Several other urgent and nonurgent conditions produce chest pain. Table 10.2 compares chest pain with various causes and explains the differences in signs and symptoms.

Objective Data

Objective data noted during triage is obtained from a rapid assessment of presenting signs; thus, the nurse briefly examines the patient's respiratory, cardiovascular, integumentary, and neurologic body systems.

Respiratory Assessment
In patients with cardiac chest pain, the respiratory rate increases, and depth may be shallow. Auscultation for rales should be performed if the patient appears dyspneic.

Cardiovascular Assessment
Unstable angina and myocardial infarction may be accompanied by a variety of pulse and blood pressure findings. The patient may have a pulse rate that is extremely slow or fast or that is weak or irregular, and can be hypertensive or hypotensive. Alterations in pulse and blood pressure are not uncommon, although the patient may have a normal pulse and blood pressure (Kapoor and Dang, 1978). The pulse and blood pressure values obtained, as well as their characteristics, depend on the degrees of myocardial irritability, the extent of injury, and the patient's physiologic response to the stressful event.

TABLE 10.2 Chest Pain Differentiation

Origins	Characteristics
Chest Wall Pain	
1. Muscular strain (myalgia)	1. Pain is associated with movement, muscle tenderness to palpation
2. Trauma to bony thorax	2. Sharp, well-localized pain directly over traumatized area, respiration splinted
3. Thoracic spine pain	3. Stabbing pain, accentuated with movement. Pain referred to lateral and anterior chest wall. Patient has history of back pain
Pain From the Respiratory System	
1. Pleuritic pain	1. Localized, stabbing pain, increased by coughing and breathing
2. Spontaneous pneumothorax	2. Severe pain, dyspnea, decreased breath sounds on affected side
3. Hyperventilation	3. Sharp, anterior chest pain accompanied by very rapid breathing. Patient may complain of numbness and tingling in extremities
Cardiovascular Pain Sources	
1. Pulmonary embolism	1. Pleuritic chest pain, dyspnea, cough, friction rub on auscultation. Severe events produce hypotension, cyanosis, and tachycardia
2. Dissecting aortic aneurysm	2. Severe, intense, tearing pain, located substernally and radiating to back. Pain is deep and constant
Gastrointestinal and Related Abdominal Organ Pain	
Conditions producing epigastric and low anterior chest pain:	
1. Esophagitis	1. "Heart burn," gnawing pain, relief obtained with antacids
2. Peptic ulcer, gastric ulcer	2. Gnawing or burning pain, relief obtained by eating or ingestion of antacids
3. Cholecystitis	3. Onset gradual or sudden, initial lower substernal pain localizes to RUQ, associated complaints: fever, chills

While severe derangements in pulse and blood pressure will always require immediate emergency attention, the patient with stable vital signs must also be treated just as seriously due to the high incidence of lethal dysrhythmias that can occur during the period immediately after acute cardiac events.

Integumentary Assessment
The skin, which is assessed for color, temperature, moisture, and perfusion, may be pale, cool and clammy, or diaphoretic. Capillary refill should be examined at the nailbeds; a nailbed that remains blanched for more than three to five seconds suggests poor peripheral perfusion.

Neurologic Assessment
The level of consciousness and behavior are the important components of the neurologic system to be noted by the triage nurse. While many patients are alert and oriented, a decrease in the level of consciousness suggests poor cerebral perfusion due to a dysrhythmia or severe mechanical impairment of the left ventricle from extensive injury. Patients suffering from angina will exhibit anxious behavior and the need to rest, while patients with more severe pain due to infarction will feel doomed and exhibit restless behavior.

With the exception of the blood pressure and auscultation, initial objective data may be obtained rapidly. By placing two fingers on the ventral aspect of the wrist, the triage nurse can note the temperature, color, and moisture of the skin, as well as the rate, strength, and regularity of the pulse, while simultaneously observing the chest for the character and rate of respiration. Conclusions regarding level of consciousness and patient behavior are made when the patient reports his complaints.

Assessment and Planning

Initial assessment is based on the subjective and objective data. Cardiac chest pain is classified as stable angina, unstable angina, or myocardial infarction.

Stable angina pectoris is ischemic chest pain that is relieved completely by rest or nitroglycerin. The chest pain is the same in duration and precipitated by activity similar to activity that produced chest pain on previous occasions.

According to Hurst (1982), *unstable angina* is a group of syndromes intermediate between stable angina pectoris and myocardial infarction. Previously termed "preinfarction syndrome," unstable angina describes angina that either has occurred for the first time, has increased in frequency, occurs at rest, is provoked more easily, or is prolonged. Variant, or Prinzmetal's angina, and acute coronary insufficiency are other syndromes classified as unstable angina. Unstable angina is taken seriously, because it often signifies impending myocardial infarction and electrical instability.

Myocardial infarction, the most serious event represented by cardiac chest pain, occurs when some heart muscle cells are so severely deprived of blood flow (oxygen and nutrients) that cellular death occurs, leaving a localized area of permanently nonfunctional myocardial cells.

Differentiating among the more serious classifications of cardiac chest pain is difficult during initial emergency care. Patients may exhibit some, all, or none of the

TABLE 10.3 Example of Triage Notes for Patients Experiencing Chest Pain

S: 44 yo BM c/o heavy, constant substernal chest pain radiating to LA for 35". Pain unrelated to activity, unrelieved by rest or NTG, c/o SOB, nausea. PMH: HTN for 5 years, NKA, meds Aldomet, Inderal, Lasix.

O: AAO × 3, skin cool and moist, P 68 slightly irregular, BP 106/72, RR 24 shallow, anxious behavior, cap. refill good

A: Chest pain, R/O MI.

P: Admit to exam room now, medical evaluation.

S: 52 yo WM per ambulance stretcher semiconscious, in respiratory distress. Family says no recent trauma or bleeding problems. Patient c/o progressive chest pain with lethargy for 45 minutes prior to admission. PMH: HTN, hx CAB × 2 in 1978, NKA.

O: Responds by moaning to verbal stimuli. Skin diaphoretic, lips cyanotic, RR 28, noisy, access. resp. muscle use noted. P 120, BP 80 palp. IV D_5W in place per paramedic, O_2 per face mask at 6 l/min

A: Possible MI, severe hypotension, shock.

P: Admit to exam room now, medical evaluation.

symptoms and signs indicating their problem. Definitive diagnosis, based on clinical and laboratory findings, often is not completed until after the patient is admitted to the intensive care unit. Patients with severe cardiac chest pain may develop sudden and unforeseen lethal dysrhythmias, particularly within the first hour of the event (Sobel and Braunwald, 1980). Thus, immediate intervention to stabilize the patient is mandatory and must be documented with phrases, such as "admit to exam room now." Furthermore, the triage nurse must also summon the emergency staff responsible for cardiac patients. Table 10.3 contains two examples of triage notes in which the assessment is chest pain.

PATHOPHYSIOLOGY

The most common cause of angina and myocardial infarction is atherosclerosis. The term *coronary atherosclerotic heart disease* (CAHD) indicates that the disease exists in the coronary arteries. Atherosclerosis is a vascular disease causing the development of fatty plaque within the walls of blood vessels. The plaque is composed of cholesterol-containing fat (lipid) deposits, fibrous tissue, assorted cellular debris, and calcifications. The plaque protrudes into the lumen of the vessel and, in severe cases, limits blood flow to tissues supplied by the vessel. The rough endothelial surface creates an environment that encourages thrombus formation.

The precise mechanisms by which atherosclerosis develops into plaque remain controversial. Evidence points to a number of mechanisms that combine to produce mature, obstructive plaque. These mechanisms include endothelial injury, high blood lipid levels, hemodynamic stress at arterial bifurcations or curvatures, and the risk factors that seem to accelerate the process.

According to one theory, hemodynamic shearing forces, together with risk factors such as hypertension, high fat diet, and stress, cause damage to inner vessel walls, making them permeable to the influx of fats and other substances found in the blood (Wissler, 1980). Contact between the inside of the damaged vessel wall and blood platelets causes platelet adherence. Substances released from the platelets, along with certain types of lipids, cause proliferation of the vessel wall's smooth muscle cells, resulting in formation of plaque (Ross, 1982). Theorists assert that plaque develops more extensively in the coronary arteries, rather than in other arteries, due to the hemodynamics of flow in the tortuous coronary vessels (Wissler, 1980).

Hypertension may accelerate the plaque formation process, because it creates chronic excessive pressure against the arterial walls, increasing endothelial injury. Diabetes mellitus may generate the atherosclerotic process due to the body's inability to metabolize fats, thus creating an environment for the acceleration of fat deposition within arterial walls. The precise mechanism, however, is still controversial (Levy and Feinleib, 1980).

Ischemia is a state of reversible oxygen lack to tissue cells secondary to reduced perfusion. Ischemia occurs in the myocardium when the narrow and stiff atherosclerotic coronary arteries are unable to dilate, preventing delivery of sufficient blood flow to meet myocardial oxygen demands.

The myocardial cells respond to insufficient oxygen by reverting to inefficient anaerobic metabolism for the production of energy. The end result is lactic acid production, as well as cellular release of histamine, bradykinin, and enzymes. Because blood flow is inadequate, the removal of these substances is impaired (Sobel and Braunwald, 1980). Chest pain results from irritation of local visceral sensory pain fibers (Guyton, 1981). This pain, produced by myocardial ischemia, creates *angina pectoris* in the adult. Angina pectoris in infants and children is rare.

An oxygen supply and demand imbalance is inherent in myocardial ischemia. The imbalance relates to patient activity and physiological factors. Activities that increase myocardial work and may thus precipitate angina in patients with CAHD include excessive physical exertion, emotional stress, environmental temperature changes, sexual activity, smoking, and eating. These activities physiologically precipitate ischemia by increasing preload, afterload, heart rate, and contractility, thereby increasing myocardial demand for oxygen—a demand that cannot be met due to the diseased coronary vessels. When the heart's workload is reduced, blood supply can match myocardial oxygen demands, and the pain of angina pectoris resolves.

Unstable angina describes a set of syndromes in which atherosclerotic disease progresses more rapidly than the development of collateral circulation (Hurst, 1982). The condition thus indicates more than oxygen supply and demand imbalance because severe ischemia and even cellular injury may have developed, yet no clinical evidence exists indicating actual infarction at the time the patient presents to the emergency department. Because unstable angina may progress to infarction, in the initial stages of care it must be treated as seriously as though infarction had already occurred.

Myocardial infarction denotes obstruction of a coronary artery that is so severe that some of the myocardial cells supplied by that vessel die from lack of oxygen and nutrients. Most myocardial infarctions involve the thicker left ventricular wall. Infarctions of the right ventricle comprise less than three percent of all infarcts (Alpert and Braunwald, 1980). Discussion, therefore, of pathophysiology will be limited to the left ventricular myocardium.

Infarction is caused either by ulceration of mature atherosclerotic plaque creating a clot, or by severe narrowing of the affected coronary artery (Wissler, 1980; Ridolfi and Hutchins, 1978). Other causes include accumulation of platelets around the atheromatous protrusion and emboli. Another possible cause now being studied is vasospasm. Regardless of the cause, the affected coronary artery is occluded, precipitating cellular death.

After acute deprivation of blood flow, affected muscle cells begin to die, irreversibly affecting the most severely involved cells within 20 to 40 minutes (Allison et al., 1977). The patient's complaints of chest pain are indexed by time, because the longer the pain-producing, noxious stimuli are secreted from injured cells, the greater the possibility that infarction either is impending or has already occurred.

Surrounding the central zone of dead cells is a precarious zone of severely ischemic cells that receive a small supply of blood from vessel branches other than from the obstructed one. Here the balance of oxygen supply and demand can be tipped in either direction causing addition of this zone to the infarcted tissue if oxygen demands are not maintained at an absolute minimum (Opie, 1980).

The outer edges of the damaged tissue usually receive blood flow from healthier arteries, since this area is farthest from the obstructed vessel. Consequently, this region has the best chance of returning to normal function post MI. Figure 10.1 illustrates a myocardial infarction with the zones of injury.

Loss of normal cellular electrical or mechanical function and sympathetic nervous system compensation result from the death of or severe injury to myocardial cells. These events provide the pathophysiologic basis for symptoms and signs seen in patients with cardiac chest pain.

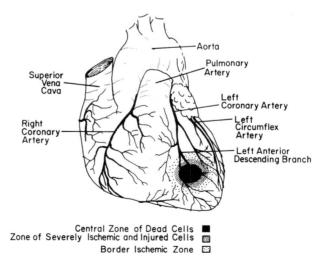

Figure 10.1 Myocardial infarction of the left anterior ventricular wall due to the occlusion of the left anterior descending coronary artery.

Mechanical Cell Involvement

Mechanically, the infarcted tissue is akinetic; in other words, the dead area no longer contracts with the rest of the ventricle, while the ischemic area's contractile activity is usually weak, creating a paradoxical bulge as the healthy areas of the ventricle contract more vigorously to compensate for the loss (Hillis, 1977). This akinesis creates abnormal wall motion and increases heart workload, since most force must be generated by healthy tissue in the struggle to empty the ventricle during systole.

The areas of reduced and absent wall motion can decrease left ventricular systolic contractile efficiency, thus reducing stroke volume and cardiac output (Alpert and Braunwald, 1980). Both infarction and ischemia also impair ventricular diastolic relaxation (compliance). The combination of decreased stroke volume and impaired ventricular relaxation increases left ventricular end-diastolic volume and pressure (Hillis, 1977). The effect of increased left heart pressure is increased pressure in the pulmonary vascular beds, producing the transient shortness of breath seen in both infarction and angina patients (Sobel and Braunwald, 1980). Large left ventricular infarctions can cause progressive pulmonary congestion producing the same clinical picture that accompanies acute left congestive heart failure.

Electrical Cell Involvement

Severe ischemia creates an irritable and electrically unstable environment within the myocardium. Furthermore, occlusion of certain coronary artery branches will produce conduction defects. The result is dysrhythmias—the earliest and most common complication of unstable angina and myocardial infarction, as well as one of the major nursing care concerns. Additional factors also increase the possibility of dysrhythmias with myocardial injury. These include sympathetic activity, vagal influence, lactic acid production, hypoxia, and hemodynamic problems (Price and Wilson, 1978).

The types of dysrhythmias depend on the coronary artery occluded, as well as the location and function of the myocardial tissue that the artery supplied. Infarction of the inferior portion of the left ventricle, for example, is associated with sinus bradycardia, due to an increase in vagal stimulation. All degrees of heart block may be involved, because inferior infarctions usually result from right coronary artery obstruction, whose branches supply portions of the conduction system. Ventricular premature beats as well as life-threatening ventricular tachycardia and fibrillation, accompany unstable angina and infarction regardless of the damage location, primarily due to ischemia and early sympathetic stimulation (Sobel and Braunwald, 1980).

Sympathetic Nervous System Involvement

Three mechanisms cause a compensatory sympathetic nervous system response in the patient with severe unstable angina or myocardial infarction. First of all, baroreceptors in the aortic arch and carotid bifurcations, which sense the reduction in stroke volume and cardiac output, send messages to the medulla to stimulate sympathetic activity. Secondly, the persistent noxious stimuli to pain receptors significantly increase the sympathetic activity (Bonica, 1979). Finally, the extreme anxiety associated with severe cardiac chest pain elicits a physiologic stress response that compounds sympathetic outpouring.

Two catecholamines produce the sympathetic response: norepinephrine at the autonomic nerve endings, as well as both epinephrine and norepinephrine from the adrenal gland. Norepinephrine vasoconstricts the blood vessels supplying the skin and stimulates sweat secretion, producing the frequently observed pale, cool, clammy skin. Sympathetic vasoconstriction increases peripheral arterial resistance causing the initial blood pressure increase in some patients.

Epinephrine, which stimulates the heart by increasing the force of contraction and heart rate, helps to compensate for any fall in cardiac output. Unfortunately, the increase in preload, afterload, force of contraction, and heart rate raises myocardial oxygen demands. Since oxygen supply to the ischemic areas surrounding the infarct is limited, sustained sympathetic activity will extend the infarct. A substantial portion of the emergency nursing care of the patient, therefore, involves resolving pain and reducing anxiety in an effort to decrease stimuli for sympathetic activity.

NURSING CARE AND RELATED INTERVENTIONS FOR STABLE ANGINA

The nursing care of patients with stable angina includes the knowledge of clinical manifestations, diagnostic studies, and the objectives required to care for the patient. The clinical manifestations of stable angina are summarized in Table 10.4. Nursing objectives for patient management include reduction of myocardial oxygen demands, patient teaching, and discharge planning.

Diagnostic Studies

The physician may request a 12-lead ECG to determine any electrocardiographic changes accompanying the event, and a chest x-ray study to determine the presence of left ventricular enlargement. If the patient has been followed in the hospital, old records should be obtained for comparative study. Specific leads may show ST segment depression and T wave inversion during the anginal attack. The changes electrically reflect the effect of ischemia upon ventricular repolarization (Horan and Flowers, 1980).

Nursing Care and Related Interventions

The myocardial oxygen supply and demand imbalance causing stable angina pectoris is modified through reduction of demand by placing the patient at rest and administering nitroglycerin. Nitroglycerin primarily reduces preload, although it also reduces afterload as well. Nitroglycerin relieves angina by manipulating the loads against which the myocardium is pumping, thereby reducing O_2 demands. While nitroglycerin may dilate healthy coronary arteries, it does not affect diseased coronary arteries and, therefore, does not increase blood supply to the ischemic area supplied by atherosclerotic vessels (Rice et al. 1981).

TABLE 10.4 Summary of Clinical Manifestations of Patients with Cardiac Chest Pain

Symptoms	Stable Angina	Unstable Angina	Myocardial Infarction
Onset	Sudden	Sudden	Sudden
Precipitating factors	Activity: eating, smoking, stress, temperature change, physical exertion	Altered: pain has increase in frequency, duration, is provoked easily, occurs at rest, or occurred for the first time	Usually none
Duration	30 sec to 30 min	Up to 45 min	Longer than 30–45 min
Site	Substernal, may radiate to arms, jaw, neck, subscapular area	Same as angina; may radiate to new site	Same as stable or unstable angina
Quality	Tightness, discomfort, aching, burning, or squeezing pain	Pain may be more severe	Severe, crushing squeezing pain
Relief	Rest and NTG gives complete relief	Relief obtained by rest and NTG incomplete	Morphine
Associated symptoms	Shortness of breath	Shortness of breath, nausea	Shortness of breath, nausea, vomiting
Signs			
Respiratory	No sustained alteration	↑ respiratory rate and depth	↑ respiratory rate, may use accessory muscles
Cardiovascular	No sustained alteration	BP may be stable, ↑ or ↓, pulse may be ↑ or ↓, weak or strong, regular or irregular, dysrhythmia may be present	Same as unstable angina
Neurologic	Alert, feels need to rest	Usually alert, anxious	Usually alert, restless, feels doomed
Integumentary	May be pale and moist until pain is relieved	Pale, moist, cool, may be diaphoretic	Same as unstable angina

Nitroglycerin reduces preload by dilating systemic veins, thereby reducing venous return, ventricular end-diastolic volume, and, as a result, decreasing the contractile force needed for systolic emptying (Lewis and Gotsman, 1980; Weber and Janicki, 1979). Arterial vasodilation is a secondary effect that reduces peripheral arterial resistance, thus decreasing afterload. The nitroglycerin tablet, which comes in 1/100 grain, 1/150 grain, and 1/200 grain strength, should be given sublingually every five minutes until complete pain relief is obtained, or up to three tablets, whichever occurs first.

The systemic vasodilation produced by nitroglycerin causes headaches in many patients, and the reduction in afterload may produce hypotension and reflex tachycardia. Vital signs, therefore, are checked and documented every five minutes after nitroglycerin is administered. Immediate measures to correct a hypotensive episode include the following: (1) raising the patient's legs; and, (2) holding the next tablet. The tablets are light sensitive and are stored in a dark container. Nitroglycerin should be replaced every six months; if the tablets do not produce a burning sensation under the patient's tongue, they are inactive.

Medications that act similarly to nitroglycerin, but produce a more sustained effect, include Isordil and Nitro-Bid paste. Isordil is a long-acting nitrate and is given orally or sublingually to prevent episodes of chest pain from occurring. Similarly, Nitro-Bid paste is applied topically every three to four hours for continuous absorption, thus producing a more long-term effect. Inderal, another drug that may be administered orally to patients with angina, acts to block sympathetic effects upon the heart, and thus decreases myocardial oxygen demands by decreasing heart rate, force of contraction, and blood pressure.

Discharge Planning

Patients with stable angina may be admitted for further study, but are usually discharged from the emergency department. If the patient is discharged, follow-up is required, and the emergency nurse is responsible for discharge planning.

Cardiac patient education in the emergency setting is challenging. Unfortunately, other responsibilities often take precedence. In addition, anginal attacks are disturbing emotional stressors to the patient, and they will interfere with the patient's capacity to absorb large quantities of information (Hast, 1981). Although education can decrease the patient's and family's anxieties, the patient's underlying psychologic state will significantly affect readiness to learn (Miller, 1981). Factors that will influence the outcome of the patient teaching include the degree of psychological distress, culture, motivation, personal strengths, socioeconomic factors, and past experiences with members of the health care system. Because the emergency department nurse may be the first professional contact for the patient, the educational foundation established is important.

Appropriate emergency department education for the patient with chronic stable angina includes instruction in modification of risk factors, exercise, medication teaching, and careful instructions regarding actions to be taken in the event of a future anginal attack.

1. *Risk factors:* The emergency nurse identifies the risk factors by referring to the triage note and questioning the patient. Diet teaching is required if obesity, diabetes, hypertension, or hyperlipidemia have been identified. Written instructions regarding ADA, low cholesterol, low sodium, or low caloric diets should be provided for the patient's specific needs in postdischarge reference material. Specific measures that alter the habits of a tobacco smoker include incremental diminution of the number of cigarettes smoked per day, a switch in cigarette brands, and an effort to smoke less of each cigarette, since nicotine is most heavily concentrated near the filter. Written information pertaining to diabetes and hypertension should be given and explained to patients with those risk factors.
2. *Exercise:* Precautions include instructions not to smoke before or during exercise, the avoidance of exercise during periods of emotional stress, and to delay exercise for two hours after eating (Comoss et al., 1979). The family should know where the patient is during exercise. The patient may be advised to schedule two or three periods of uninterrupted rest during times of fatigue or stress. Unless otherwise advised by the physician, the patient can continue sexual activity, but may need to take nitroglycerin or a similar drug if angina occurs during intercourse.
3. *Medications and future chest pain episodes:* Patients must be taught the action, dose, route, and side effects of any prescribed medications and be provided with written information regarding the drugs. Patients are instructed to carry nitroglycerin with them at all times. For further episodes of chest pain, the patient is advised to do the following:
   a. Stop activity and sit or lie down.
   b. Take one nitroglycerin tablet every five minutes for a maximum of three tablets in ten minutes.
   c. If chest pain continues unrelieved or is only partially relieved by three tablets and rest, call for an ambulance or go to the nearest emergency department immediately.

   Family members should map the quickest route to the nearest emergency department and may be referred to the local American Heart Association chapter for further information regarding the patient's condition, risk factors, and Basic Life Support courses.
4. *Follow-up health care:* Because the emergency department may be the patient's only entry into the health care system, physician follow-up arrangements must be made and confirmed prior to discharge. Although basic instruction is provided in part by the emergency nurse, further diagnostic study, physician evaluation, and individualized education are required.

NURSING CARE AND RELATED INTERVENTIONS FOR UNSTABLE ANGINA AND MYOCARDIAL INFARCTION

The syndromes classified as unstable angina and myocardial infarction are managed similarly in terms of diagnostic studies and nursing care. The clinical manifestations of both unstable angina and myocardial infarction are summarized in Table 10.4.

Diagnostic Studies

The studies needed for definitive diagnosis of infarction are cardiac enzymes (CPK, LDH, SGOT) and a 12-lead ECG. Other baseline studies obtained in anticipation of the patient's hospital course include arterial blood gases, admission venous blood samples (SMA-6, SMA-18, CBC, PT/PTT), urine sample for analysis, and a chest x-ray film.

Although cardiac enzymes are drawn, they probably will not assist the emergency team in determining whether the patient is in the throes of a preinfarction angina syndrome or has already infarcted. The duration of ischemia determines the amount of cellular injury. It is not until cell membrane integrity is impaired that enzymes will move into local interstitial spaces, then into the blood stream. The onset of elevation occurs in 2 to 24 hours, depending on the enzyme (Roberts, 1981).

The 12-lead ECG is obtained to determine electrocardiographic evidence of injury, infarct, and conduction impairment. Each lead reflects depolarization and repolarization of the myocardium from a different angle, making it possible to pinpoint the location of damage. While this is often possible, the ECG, however, may not be helpful because damage is not always electrically evident in early stages.

Myocardial damage is reflected in the QRS complex and ST segment of leads that view the injured myocardium. During the acute phase, changes include ST segment elevation (signifying cellular injury from prolonged ischemia) and, on occasion, significant Q waves (denoting cellular death). The changes are an electrical "current of injury," due to some combination of the injured tissue's failure to depolarize and inadequate repolarization of the ischemic region during diastole (Hillis, 1977). Conduction problems from bundle-branch blockage may also be detected by studying other characteristics of the ECG.

Nursing Care and Related Interventions

The nursing goal in the management of the patient with prolonged chest pain suggesting unstable angina or myocardial infarction is to prevent further myocardial damage.

Initial Stabilization and Further Assessment

Initial interventions and evaluation of the patient's status require coordinated teamwork. Life-threatening dysrhythmias may develop, even if the patient's vital signs are stable (Lown, 1980). In anticipating this possibility, a portable cardiac monitor with a defibrillator unit attached is connected by lead placement to the patient, and an intravenous (IV) drug line is established as quickly as possible. The patient is usually connected to lead II with the positive electrode on the left chest wall near the nipple, and the negative electrode under the right clavicle. The heart's electrical activity is assessed frequently for changes.

The IV solution of choice is 250 to 500 cc of 5 percent dextrose in water (D_5W), infused via microdrip tubing at a keep open rate. This solution is used because it is hypotonic to extracellular body fluids. As D_5W infuses, portions of it move osmotically out of the vascular space and into the interstitial space, thus preventing an increase in venous return and preload to the damaged heart. The smaller amount of fluid, tubing size, and infusion rate serve to prevent accidental fluid overload. The IV serves as a drug line and provides immediate access to venous circulation if it becomes necessary to administer antidysrhythmic or other emergency drugs.

The nurse caring for the patient must reassess the patient's neurologic, respiratory, cardiovascular, and integumentary status continually, while observing for any departure from the way the patient initially presented in the emergency department. Referring to the triage note, listening to the physician's interview of the patient, and questioning the patient for changes in symptoms as therapy progresses will ensure prompt and appropriate intervention.

Reduction of Sympathetic Stimulation

Reducing sympathetic stimulation is critical to prevent further myocardial damage. The objective is attained through actions that reduce pain and relieve anxiety because these mechanisms cause excessive sympathetic activity.

The pain of unstable angina may be relieved through administrating nitroglycerin, occasionally combined with propranolol (Inderal) or morphine, if necessary (Cohn and Braunwald, 1980). Care must be taken to prevent the occurrence of hypotension and reflex tachycardia that can result from nitroglycerin therapy—two side effects that create the danger of extending injury by decreasing coronary artery perfusion and increasing myocardial oxygen demands.

The preferred drug for pain relief in the infarction patient is morphine sulfate. From 4 to 8 mg are given intravenously in 2-mg increments every 5 to 15 minutes, until pain relief is obtained. Morphine acts as a powerful analgesic, reducing sympathetic activity and relaxing peripheral vasculature, thus decreasing myocardial workload. Side effects can include respiratory depression and hypotension. Respiratory depression is reversed by administering Narcan. Hypotension accompanied by the vagal response of bradycardia is corrected by administering atropine and elevating the patient's legs (Sobel and Braunwald, 1980). Sustained tachycardia in infarction resulting from sympathetic activity may be treated with intravenous Inderal, which blocks sympathetic activity and, therefore, decreases myocardial oxygen demands. The initial intravenous dose is 1.0 mg during a five minute period, followed by 0.5 mg per minute to a maximum dose of 0.1 mg per kilogram of body weight (Rice, 1981). Because of the side effects of hypotension, heart failure, and AV block, the nurse must monitor the patient's blood pressure and rhythm while administering the drug.

Oxygen therapy is started at 2 to 4 l per minute by nasal cannula to correct hypoxemia and to reduce anxiety. Hypoxemia is associated with unstable angina and myocardial infarction due to the transient pulmonary congestion often affecting these patients.

Specific actions related to reassurance must be taken to reduce sympathetic stimulation resulting from anxiety. The major concerns in these patients include fear of sudden death and fear of further chest pain (Miller, 1981), as well as anxiety and concern regarding an unfamiliar environment. Measures that reduce anxiety include the following:

1. The nurse's introduction by name and assurance of his or her constant availability as long as the patient remains in the emergency department.
2. Assurance that pain will be relieved through medications.

3. Simple explanations of the monitor, IV, and nasal cannula.
4. Explanation of procedures as they are carried out.
5. Support by attentive listening if the patient expresses concerns.
6. Allowing the patient to see family members or significant others, if possible, and if such interaction is deemed helpful to the patient.

Recognition and Treatment of Dysrhythmias
Serious dysrhythmias will manifest symptoms and signs of decreased perfusion in the patient. Sinus bradycardia, sinus block, atrial rhythms with slow ventricular response, slow junctional rhythms, and heart blocks require treatment when they create heart rates below 40 to 50 beats per minute. At these rates, cardiac output falls and coronary artery perfusion becomes worse, thus increasing the risk of infarct or injury extension. Clinically, the patient exhibits signs of decreased perfusion, such as low blood pressure, poor skin color, decreased level of consciousness, and reduction in the speed of capillary refill.

Rapid dysrhythmias, such as atrial and junctional tachycardia, create similar problems when the rates exceed 150 to 160 beats per minute. At these rates, cardiac output is compromised due to shortened diastolic filling time, and the patient again exhibits symptoms and signs of decreased perfusion (McCarty, 1981).

Irritable dysrhythmias, such as atrial, junctional, and ventricular premature beats, may alter stroke volume. More importantly, ventricular premature beats often herald ventricular tachycardia and ventricular fibrillation. Recognition and treatment of ventricular premature beats can prevent the occurrence of these life-threatening dysrhythmias. Dysrhythmias and indications for treatment, as well as suggested therapy, are discussed in detail in Chapter 12.

Reduction of Preload and Afterload
The fourth nursing objective is attained, in part, by limited intravenous fluid administration and the decrease in sympathetic activity through reducing pain and anxiety. In addition, inability of the damaged myocardium to handle the physiologic loads will manifest in clinical signs of left heart failure. The diuretic furosemide (Lasix) is administered if the patient exhibits respiratory signs of left heart failure. Administered intravenously, 40 mg will decrease preload by reducing venous return through an increase in urinary output. Furosemide decreases preload, which in turn, decreases pulmonary congestion prior to the onset of diuresis by dilating systemic veins (Sobel, 1980). These actions allow the damaged left ventricle to empty its contents more efficiently helping to resolve respiratory difficulty by decreasing pulmonary congestion.

Nitroglycerin may be used as a vasodilator in patients experiencing infarction with evidence of left ventricular failure. The medical literature supports the use of an intravenous route, rather than sublingual doses, because the former can be more carefully controlled, thus preventing dangerous episodes of hypotension and reflex tachycardia (Sobel and Braunwald, 1980). Parenteral nitroglycerin is given in increments of 10 µg per minute every five minutes, while vital signs are carefully monitored.

Infarction patients with seriously progressive signs of heart failure require more aggressive therapy to maintain cardiac output, often involving the administration of multiple vasoactive drugs. (Discussion of more complex treatment modalities and related nursing care follows in the section on cardiogenic shock.)

Safe Transport to the Intensive Care Unit
Transport requires the knowledge that complications may occur in transit. The patient must be accompanied by the monitor and defibrillator unit, portable oxygen, ambu bag, and lidocaine for treatment of irritable ventricular dysrhythmias should they occur. The family should be informed of events and given directions regarding the location of the patient in the hospital.

CARDIOGENIC SHOCK

Cardiogenic shock occurs when the heart as a pump fails to meet the oxygen and nutritive demands of body tissue. While definite signs of congestive heart failure are seen with infarctions involving 20 percent of the left ventricular myocardium, infarctions of more than 40 percent of the left ventricular wall will produce cardiogenic shock (Rackley et al., 1979).

Cardiogenic shock affects 10 to 15 percent of the patients admitted to intensive care units (Price and Wilson, 1978) and often develops in the first 24 hours after infarction (Goldberger, 1977). The treatment of cardiogenic shock remains controversial, and it is unsuccessful in the vast majority of patients. The profound myocardial damage often makes shock irreversible after it has developed (Kuhn, 1978). Every effort must be made to recognize shock due to myocardial infarction in its earliest compensatory stages so that aggressive therapy may reverse the process.

Pathophysiology

Shock is defined as a decrease in tissue perfusion so severe that oxygen and nutrients fail to reach tissue cells, while cellular waste products are not removed, resulting in cellular damage and eventually cellular death (Abboud, 1982). Cardiogenic shock satisfies the definition most often by failure of the left ventricle, because it confronts more pressure loads than does the right ventricle and because it is the usual location of infarct (Sobel, 1980). Shock develops when the infarcted akinetic area of the myocardium produces contractile failure of the left ventricle, resulting in decreased stroke volume and cardiac output that is 30 percent to 50 percent below normal (Weil and Henning, 1979).

The decrease in cardiac output produces a sequel of compensatory and degenerative events that terminate in a vicious downward cycle that is difficult to reverse. Reducing stroke volume and cardiac output lowers the arterial blood pressure which stimulates neuro and hormonal sympathetic activity, causing initial arterial vasoconstriction and an increase in total peripheral resistance. This may raise the blood pressure slightly, but, unfortunately, it also creates an increase in afterload. Because the failing left ventricle cannot efficiently empty against the increased afterload, left ventricular end-diastolic pressure becomes higher. Further increase in sympathetic activity increases the heart rate and the force of contractions in remaining healthy tissue, adding more oxygen demand and workload to the heart, which already is confronting hypotension and coronary artery obstruction (Goldberger, 1977; Weil and Henning, 1979).

Although sympathetic activity may compensate for the decrease in cardiac output at first, the resulting increase in myocardial workload cannot be handled due to the large, preexisting infarction. Thus, hypotension progresses. The combination of hypotension (low arterial blood pressure) and increased myocardial oxygen demands produces a downward spiral of pathologic events. Because of their atherosclerotic disease, the coronary arteries cannot dilate to satisfy increased myocardial oxygen demand and depend on adequate diastolic arterial blood pressure for sufficient flow (Foster and Canty, 1980). Because the hypotension reduces the pressure required for perfusion of the stiff coronary arteries, oxygen demands are not satisfied, and the area of myocardial ischemia enlarges (Gutowitz et al., 1978).

The extension of myocardial ischemia results in further decrease of contractile tissue, causing a decrease in left ventricular function. The reduction of left ventricular function progressively decreases cardiac output and arterial blood pressure, which further lowers coronary artery perfusion (Alpert and Braunwald, 1980). The reduction in coronary artery perfusion accentuates ischemia and reinitiates the vicious cycle. The shock becomes progressively more severe, as the pathologic events spiral downward.

Decreased perfusion to the body tissues eventually initiates anaerobic metabolism, an increase in lactic acid production, metabolic acidosis, and a subsequent decrease in the function of vital organs and secondary body systems (Weil and Henning, 1979).

Reduced pulmonary blood flow and subsequent hypoxia of the lung tissue reduce alveolar gas exchange, decreasing the amount of oxygen in the arterial blood (hypoxemia) (Goldberger, 1977). In addition, because the blood is no longer being effectively pumped out, the volume and pressure within the left ventricle rises (increased left ventricular end-diastolic pressure and volume). This "back-side" pressure can increase left atrial pressure and then increase pulmonary pressure, possibly resulting in transudation of fluid out of the vascular bed and into the lungs, creating the pulmonary edema that occasionally accompanies cardiogenic shock. Some patients confront the terrible combination of circulatory and respiratory failure.

Clinical Manifestations

The patient in cardiogenic shock presents with the signs and symptoms produced by intense sympathetic activity, decreased perfusion to vital bodily systems, extending myocardial ischemia and, in some cases, pulmonary edema. Similar to all types of shock, the worse the condition, the more severe the signs.

The increase in left heart pressures and/or inadequate perfusion of the alveoli produces the clinical condition of respiratory distress with moderate to severe signs and symptoms. The patient may be dyspneic, using accessory respiratory muscles, and have rapid, shallow respirations. Signs of pulmonary edema may be evident, including rales on auscultation and even copious pulmonary secretions with subsequent airway compromise. A severe decrease in perfusion can result in central ner-

CARDIOGENIC SHOCK

vous system dysfunction, producing a Cheyne-Stokes respiratory pattern in the patient (Sobel, 1980).

Assessment of the cardiovascular system reveals a systolic pressure of less than 80 to 90 mm Hg and a narrow pulse pressure with a diastolic value of less than 50 mm Hg. A drop of more than 50 mm Hg pressure in the previously hypertensive patient signifies similar underlying problems. An ultrasound device should be used to obtain the systolic pressure until the intra-arterial pressure can be monitored. The heart rate exceeds 100 beats per minute, and peripheral pulses are weak and thready. Dysrhythmias commonly associated with cardiogenic shock include sinus tachycardia, premature complexes, sinus bradycardia, atrioventricular (AV) block, and complex dissociative rhythms (Sobel, 1980). The appearance of premature ventricular beats and fatal ventricular dysrhythmias reflects critically low coronary artery perfusion due to low blood pressure (Weil and Henning, 1979). Conscious patients will often complain of persistent cardiac chest pain (Manescalco and Whipple, 1978).

Due to the decrease in perfusion, the patient will exhibit initial hypoxic signs of restlessness and agitation. As the pathologic process progresses and brain cells are further deprived of oxygen, the patient will become confused, listless, or stuporous, and finally comatose.

Assessment of the skin and nailbeds often reveals dramatic alterations, because of increased sympathetic activity, poor peripheral perfusion, and inadequate tissue oxygenation. The skin is cool and clammy, or diaphoretic, and extremities may acquire a mottled appearance (Goldberger, 1977). Skin color may be pale, ashen, or cyanotic, and capillary refill is poor.

The urinary output is less than 20 to 30 cc per hour, initially due to compensatory vasoconstriction of renal vascular beds. As the shock progresses, the oliguria becomes a sign of renal failure.

Diagnostic Studies

Extensive laboratory studies and related tests are obtained due to the severe cellular, metabolic, and vital organ derangements associated with cardiogenic shock. Table 10.5 lists several studies and relevant information.

Nursing Care and Related Interventions

The patient in cardiogenic shock requires rapid intervention based on the presenting priority problems. As previously mentioned, the management of cardiogenic shock is both complex and controversial.

Establish Airway and Maintain Ventilation

1. Clear the airway of any excessive pulmonary secretions using appropriate suctioning technique.
2. In patients with depressed neurologic status, insert an oral airway to displace the tongue from the pharynx.

TABLE 10.5 Diagnostic Studies in Cardiogenic Shock

Diagnostic Studies	Rationale
12-lead ECG	To reflect location and extent of infarction. Q waves are present. May also have ST segment elevation. Serves as baseline.
Chest x-ray	To detect presence and extent of pulmonary edema. Baseline study.
SMA 18, CBC with differential, PT/PTT, platelet count, serum enzymes (CPK, LDH, SGOT)	To obtain baseline and for the detection of electrolyte, renal, clotting, blood count, and hepatic derangements associated with shock.
Arterial blood gases	To determine presence and degree of metabolic imbalance reflected in the pH and Pco_2, to monitor the Po_2 as basis for oxygen therapy. Serves as baseline.
Arterial lactic acid	Concentrations above 1.8 mmol/l confirm perfusion failure (Weil and Henning, 1979). Serves as baseline.
Urine analysis	Helps to determine baseline renal function.

3. Patient positioning is preferably supine; in instances of severe respiratory compromise, elevate the head of the stretcher 15 to 30 degrees.
4. If the patient is breathing spontaneously and adequately, administer humidified oxygen per face mask at flow rates of 8 to 15 liters per minute to maintain an arterial Po_2 of 70 mm Hg or higher.
5. Assist ventilations and prepare for endotracheal intubation under the following circumstances:
   a. unconscious patient with struggling or agonal respirations.
   b. unconscious patient who may risk aspiration (in essence, is unable to handle secretions).
   c. the patient with an arterial Po_2 less than 70 mm Hg.

Relative advantages of endotracheal intubation include a decrease in the work of breathing and a subsequent decrease in myocardial oxygen consumption, reduction of pulmonary edema via positive pressure to decrease preload, and airway control in the event of respiratory arrest (Foster and Canty, 1980).

Furosemide (Lasix) or ethacrynic acid (Edecrin) are indicated when the patient is in pulmonary edema with ventricular filling pressure substantially higher than 20 mm Hg (Sobel, 1980). Although the drugs have other actions, reduction of pulmonary congestion and edema will improve ventilation of the alveoli, thus enhancing oxygen-

CARDIOGENIC SHOCK

ation of arterial blood. Aminophylline may be used in the event of bronchospasm to dilate the airways; however, this drug must be used with extreme caution in the patient with cardiogenic shock, due to its excitatory effects upon the heart.

Assist in Establishing Assessment Parameters
Establishing assessment parameters may be superseded by life-threatening conditions in the patient. The speed at which all of the objective's components are satisfied depends on the number of people available to manage the patient and the needs of each individual patient.

1. Attach a monitor to the patient and obtain a 12-lead ECG.
2. Start an IV of D_5W with microdrip tubing and obtain venous samples for laboratory study.
3. Obtain arterial blood gas sample.
4. Insert a urinary catheter with attachment for precise monitoring of urinary output.
5. Assist the physician in the placement of hemodynamic monitoring devices, if the equipment is available. Arterial lines and Swan Ganz catheters may be inserted in the emergency department or in the coronary care unit.

Improve Vital Organ Perfusion
Vital organ perfusion can be improved by reversing the reductions in arterial blood pressure and coronary artery perfusion. In patients with severe pump failure and profound hypotension, the use of *vasopressor drugs,* such as norepinephrine (Levophed), metaraminol (Aramine), or dopamine (Intropin), may be used initially in an effort to save the patient's life (Kuhn, 1978). At systolic pressures of less than 80 mm Hg, insufficient force exists behind the blood flow to maintain perfusion of the pressure-dependent coronary arteries, and the patient will develop premature ventricular beats, as well as fatal ventricular dysrhythmias, if action is not taken (Weil and Henning, 1979).

Norepinephrine and metaraminol have direct peripheral vasoconstrictor effects that raise blood pressure, potentially establishing sufficient coronary artery perfusion to sustain the patient long enough for further therapy. The problem with these drugs is an accompanying increase in afterload that increases myocardial oxygen demand. They are thus used for the shortest time possible only as initial emergency measures to elevate the arterial blood pressure.

Some sources state that the two drugs best tolerated in the setting of cardiogenic shock are dopamine and dobutamine because they deal more satisfactorily with underlying abnormalities. Table 10.6 summarizes information about the drugs and nursing actions that accompany their administration.

Bradycardias and tachycardias are extremely undesirable in the setting of cardiogenic shock. They can cause reduction in cardiac output and a subsequent fall in blood pressure, thus compromising coronary artery perfusion. In cardiogenic shock, the antidysrhythmic drugs are given more cautiously, because the mass of ischemic myocardium is often more sensitive to the adverse effects of antidysrhythmic drugs, occasionally increasing left ventricular failure (Cohn, 1982).

TABLE 10.6 Drugs Commonly Utilized in the Management of Cardiogenic Shock

Drug	Actions	Indications	Dose	Nursing Considerations
Vasopressors				
Norepinephrine (Levophed)	Immediate Vasoconstriction of blood vessels in the skin, gut, and kidney to ↑ BP	To raise arterial blood pressure quickly when coronary artery perfusion must be improved to sustain patient's life	2 mg in 500 ml infused at 2–4 µg/min, titrated to ↑ BP to 100 mm Hg systolic	1. All vasopressors can increase myocardial oxygen demands through excessive vasoconstriction and afterload; titrate to maintain 90–100 mm Hg systolic pressure so that coronary artery perfusion is assured with minimal increase in myocardial damage.
Metaraminol (Aramine)	Action similar to norepinephrine	Indications are the same as for norepinephrine	Mix 200 mg in 500 ml D$_5$W titrated to ↑ BP to 100 mm Hg systolic	2. The vasopressors can cause tachycardic dysrhythmias, including ventricular dysrhythmias. Monitor ECG closely and document the strips during administration. (The exception to this rule is norepinephrine, which is more likely to cause reflex bradycardia.)
Dopamine (Intropin)	*Low dose:* vasodilation of renal vascular beds	To raise arterial blood pressure and thus improve coronary artery perfusion or to improve myocardial contractility and/or improve renal perfusion (may be used in combination with Nipride)	*Low dose:* 2–5 µg/kg/min	3. If allowed to infiltrate, vasopressors will damage local tissue and even cause tissue sloughing. Check IV site frequently for signs of accidental infiltration.
	Moderate dose: increased myocardial contractility which improves cerebral blood flow by ↑ CO		*Moderate dose:* 5–20 µg/kg/min	4. Hemodynamic monitoring is strongly recommended for safe administration of these drugs.
	High dose: vasoconstriction of all vasculature with subsequent ↑ BP.		*High dose:* > 20 µg/kg/min	

Drug	Action	Indication	Dosage	Nursing Implications
Dobutamine (Dobutrex)	↑ myocardial contractility, ↑ CO, minimal effect upon blood vessels	To improve myocardial contractility without the vasoconstriction associated with dopamine	Mix 250 mg in 500 ml D$_5$W. Infuse 2.5–10 µg/kg/min.	
Vasodilators				
Nitroprusside (Nipride)	Dilates arterial vessels, reducing afterload. Dilates veins, decreasing preload. Result is decrease in left ventricular filling pressure and oxygen demands.	Indicated for ↑ left ventricular filling pressure with low CO as long as systolic BP is 90 mm Hg or greater	Dilute 50 mg in 2–3 ml D$_5$W and add to 250–500 ml D$_5$W. Infuse at rates which administer 0.5–10 µg/kg/min.	1. Use only D$_5$W 2. Cover bottle with foil; solution is light sensitive. Give only with infusion pump. 3. Assess patient for desired signs of improved CO and peripheral perfusion 4. Monitor systolic blood pressure every 2–5 minutes; drug effects are adverse if BP falls below 80–90 mm Hg.
Diuretics				
Furosemide (Lasix)	Both diuretics alter Na$^+$ transport mechanisms in the loop of Henle to ↑ urinary output. Lasix also produces venous dilation, which decreases preload.	Clinical evidence of pulmonary edema in addition to cardiogenic shock	Lasix: 40 mg IV bolus over 1–2 min.	1. Diuretics will decrease pulmonary congestion prior to reabsorption of alveolar and pulmonary edema. Observe for decrease in signs of respiratory distress. 2. Foley catheter must be in place at onset of diuresis.
Ethacrynic acid (Edecrine)			Edecrine: 50 mg IV bolus	

Although it seems paradoxical to risk overload of a left ventricle that apparently cannot handle preexisting loads, *fluid challenge* may be instituted under certain circumstances (Rackley et al., 1979). Because the injured ventricle has a large, stiff, akinetic area, the ventricle is not as distendible, resulting in left ventricular end-diastolic pressures that are higher than the pressure the left ventricular end-diastolic volume would normally create. Thus, preload may be less than required to maintain effective cardiac output, particularly if the patient has become hypovolemic due to diaphoresis or vomiting. Volume expanders in these instances are administered to increase cardiac output via the Starling's law phenomenon (Sobel, 1980; Manescalco and Whipple, 1978).

Fluid challenge involves the administration of albumin, plasma protein, or dextran in 50 ml boluses (Cohn, 1980). Left ventricular filling pressures are monitored via the Swan Ganz catheter, if available, while assessing for clinical evidence of increased cardiac output, including assessment for improvement in the level of consciousness, skin, urinary output, and vital signs. Increase of left ventricular filling pressure to upper limits of normal (18 to 20 mm Hg) signifies optimal diastolic fiber length and improvement of cardiac output (Sobel, 1980; Foster and Canty, 1980). The fluid challenge is halted if clinical signs of improvement are not manifested.

If vasopressor drugs and/or fluid challenge do not improve the patient's status, the use of nitroprusside (Nipride) may be instituted either alone or in combination with dopamine, although combined drug therapy remains controversial. (See Table 10.6).

Nitroprusside (Nipride) acts to produce *systemic vasodilation,* reducing preload and afterload. This reduction may seem paradoxical because decreased afterload would appear to lower blood pressure when every effort has been made to raise blood pressure. Nevertheless, because Nipride reduces afterload, the heart workload is decreased, occasionally permitting the drug to promote a sufficient increase in stroke volume and cardiac output to counteract any decrease in blood pressure, thus maintaining coronary artery perfusion while improving blood flow to vital organs and peripheral tissues (Foster and Canty, 1980; Cohn, 1982). Nipride is obviously administered extremely carefully to prevent the blood pressure from falling dangerously low.

Both Nipride and dopamine may be used simultaneously in the treatment of cardiogenic shock. Combined, the two drugs optimally reduce preload and afterload, while increasing myocardial contractility. Consequently, oxygen supply and demand ratios improve with increased myocardial performance (Dracup et al., 1981). When titrated to meet the requirements of the individual patient, the two drugs "check and balance" each other, allowing the desired drug effects to enhance myocardial performance.

Morphine may be utilized for complaints of persistent chest pain, to reduce preload, and for *reducing anxiety and sympathetic activity*.

Decreased perfusion in shock results in *metabolic acidosis* that requires treatment, because it depresses myocardial function, among other effects. Sodium bicarbonate is administered carefully to prevent overdosage and subsequent metabolic alkalosis. Alkalosis can increase the incidence of ventricular dysrhythmias, and it can create a metabolic environment that makes those fatal dysrhythmias relatively irreversible. Consequently, sodium bicarbonate should be administered only when the arterial pH level is below 7.25 in doses of 1 mEq/kg (Weil and Henning, 1979).

CONCLUSION

This chapter has covered the triage, pathophysiology, clinical manifestations, diagnostic studies, and nursing interventions of patients experiencing angina, myocardial infarction, and cardiogenic shock. Understanding the mechanisms underlying these clinical syndromes will assist the nurse in caring for patients, and it will contribute to further decreasing the mortality statistics associated with coronary atherosclerotic heart disease.

BIBLIOGRAPHY

Abboud, F. M.: Pathophysiology of hypotension and shock. In J. W. Hurst (ed.): *The Heart, Arteries and Veins* . . . . New York: McGraw-Hill, 1982.

Allison, T. B., C. A. Ramey, and J. W. Holsinger: Transmural gradients of left ventricular tissue metabolites after circumflex artery ligation in dogs. *Journal of Molecular Cell Cardiology* 9:837–852 (1977).

Alpert, J. S., and E. Braunwald: Pathological and clinical manifestations of acute myocardial infarction. In E. Braunwald (ed.): *Heart Disease: A Textbook of Cardiovascular Medicine.* Philadelphia: Saunders, 1980.

Bonica, J.: Important clinical aspects of acute and chronic pain. In R. F. Beers and E. G. Bassett (eds.): *Mechanisms of Pain and Analgesic Compounds.* New York: Raven, 1979.

Braunwald, B., F. H. Sonnenblick, and J. Ross: Contraction of the normal heart. In E. Braunwald (ed.): *Heart Disease: A Textbook of Cardiovascular Medicine.* Philadelphia: Saunders, 1980.

Clements, S. D.: Emergency evaluation and treatment of disorders resulting from coronary atherosclerotic heart disease. In Schwartz, et al. (eds.): *Principles and Practice of Emergency Medicine.* Philadelphia: Saunders, 1978.

Cohn, J. N.: Recognition and management of shock and acute pump failure. In J. W. Hurst (ed.): *The Heart, Arteries, and Veins.* New York: McGraw-Hill, 1982.

Cohn, P. F., and E. Braunwald: Chronic coronary artery disease. In E. Braunwald (ed.): *Heart Disease: A Textbook of Cardiovascular Medicine.* Philadelphia: Saunders, 1980.

Comoss, O. M., E. A. S. Burke, and S. H. Swails: *Cardiac Rehabilitation: A Comprehensive Nursing Approach.* New York: Lippincott, 1979.

Dracup, K. A., C. S. Breu, and J. H. Tillisch: The physiologic basis for combined nitroprusside-dopamine therapy in post-myocardial infarction heart failure. *Heart and Lung* 10(1):114–119 (1981).

Foster, S. B., and K. A. Canty: Pump failure following myocardial infarction. *Heart and Lung* 9:293–297 (1980).

Goldberger, E.: *Treatment of Cardiac Emergencies.* St. Louis: Mosby, 1977.

Gutowitz, A. L., B. E. Sobel, and R. Roberts: Progressive nature of myocardial injury in selected patients with cardiogenic shock. *American Journal of Cardiology* 41:469–475 (1978).

Guyton, A. C.: *Textbook of Medical Physiology.* Philadelphia: Saunders, 1981.

Hast, A. S.: Anxiety in the coronary care unit: Assessment and intervention. *Critical Care Quarterly* 4(3):75–82 (1981).

Helfant, R. H., and V. S. Banka: *A Clinical and Angiographic Approach to Coronary Artery Disease.* Philadelphia: Davis, 1978.

Hillis, L. D., and E. Braunwald: Myocardial ischemia. *New England Journal of Medicine* 296(17):971–978 (1977).

Horan, L. G., and N. C. Flowers: Electrocardiography and Ventrocardiography. In E. Braunwald (ed.): *Heart Disease: A Textbook of Cardiovascular Medicine*. Philadelphia: Saunders, 1980.

Hurst, J. W., et al.: Atherosclerotic heart disease, angina pectoris, myocardial infarction, and other manifestations of myocardial ischemia. In J. W. Hurst (ed.): *The Heart, Arteries, and Veins*. New York: McGraw-Hill, 1982.

Kapoor, A. S., and N. S. Dang: Reliance on physical signs in acute myocardial infarction and its complications. *Heart and Lung* 7(6):1020–1021 (1978).

Kuhn, L. A.: Management of shock following AMI. *American Heart Journal* 95(4):529–533 (1978).

Levy, R. I., and M. Feinleib: Risk factors for coronary artery disease and their management. In E. Braunwald (ed.): *Heart Disease: A Textbook of Cardiovascular Medicine*. Philadelphia: Saunders, 1980.

Lewis, B. S., and M. G. Gotsman: Current concepts of left ventricular relaxation and compliance. *American Heart Journal* 99(1):101–112 (1980).

Lown, B.: Cardiovascular collapse and sudden death. In E. Braunwald (ed.): *Heart Disease: A Textbook of Cardiovascular Medicine*. Philadelphia: Saunders, 1980.

Manescalco, B. S., and R. L. Whipple: Cardiogenic Shock. In G. R. Schwartz et al. (eds.): *Principles and Practice of Emergency Medicine*. Philadelphia: Saunders, 1978.

McCarty, E.: Hemodynamic effects and clinical assessment of dysrhythmias. *Critical Care Quarterly* 4(1):10 (1981).

McIntyre, K., and M. R. Parker: Standards for cardiopulmonary resuscitation and emergency cardiac care: 1979 National Conference. *JAMA* 244(5):453–509 (1980).

Miller, L. S.: Covert anxiety in the acute MI patient. *Critical Care Update:* 21–23 (Nov. 1981).

Opie, L. H.: Myocardial infarct size: Basic considerations. *American Heart Journal* 100(3):355–372 (1980).

Price, S. A., and L. H. Wilson, eds.: *Pathophysiology: Clinical Concepts of Disease Processes.* New York: McGraw-Hill, 1978.

Rackley, C. E., et al.: Cardiogenic shock. *Medical Times:* 33–38 (Sept. 1979).

Rice, V. S., P. Vaughan, and N. J. Shepard: *Critical Care Syllabus*. Knoxville, TN: Institute for Public Service, The University of Tennessee, 1981.

Ridolfi, R. L., and G. M. Hutchins: The relationship between coronary artery lesions and myocardial infarcts: Ulceration of atherosclerotic plaques precipitating coronary thrombus. *American Heart Journal* 93:468 (1978).

Roberts, R.: Diagnostic assessment of myocardial infarction based on lactate dehydrogenase and creatine kinase isoenzymes. *Heart and Lung* 10(3):487 (1981).

Ross, R.: Factors influencing atherogenesis. In J. W. Hurst (ed.): *The Heart, Arteries, and Veins*. New York: McGraw-Hill, 1982.

Ryan, J. L.: Dobutamine vs. Dopamine. *Critical Care Nurse:* 18–19, 63, 66 (Nov./Dec. 1980).

Schlant, R. C., et al.: Normal physiology of the cardiovascular system. In Hurst, J. W. (ed.): *The Heart, Arteries, and Veins*. St. Louis: Mosby, 1982.

Sobel, B. E.: Cardiac and noncardiac forms of acute circulatory collapse (shock). In E. Braunwald (ed.): *Heart Disease: A Textbook of Cardiovascular Medicine*. Philadelphia: Saunders, 1980.

BIBLIOGRAPHY

Sobel, B. E., and E. Braunwald: Coronary blood flow and myocardial ischemia. In E. Braunwald (ed.): *Heart Disease: A Textbook of Cardiovascular Medicine*. Philadelphia: Saunders, 1980.

Steingart, R. H., and Scheuer, J.: Assessment of myocardial ischemia and infarction. In J. W. Hurst (ed.): *The Heart, Arteries, and Veins*. St. Louis: Mosby, 1982.

Weber, K. T., and J. S. Janicki: The metabolic demand and oxygen supply of the heart: Physiologic and clinical considerations. *American Journal of Cardiology* 44:722–729 (1979).

Weil, M. H., and R. J. Henning: Shock complicating myocardial infarction. In *The Handbook of Critical Care Medicine*. New York: EM Books, 1979.

Wissler, R. W.: Principles of the pathogenesis of atherosclerosis. In E. Braunwald (ed.): *Heart Disease: A Textbook of Cardiovascular Medicine*. Philadelphia: Saunders, 1980.

11
Cardiopulmonary Arrest

Judy Stoner Halpern

After completing this chapter, the reader will be able to do the following:

1. Triage a patient experiencing cardiopulmonary arrest.
2. State objective signs of cardiopulmonary arrest.
3. List the initial emergency care measures used to resuscitate a person in cardiopulmonary arrest.
4. Recall possible etiologies for cardiac or respiratory arrest.
5. Discuss advanced therapy for a person in cardiopulmonary arrest.
6. Identify approaches that may assist a person to handle the grieving process.

The emergency department is one area within a medical facility dedicated to providing immediate care for the critically ill or injured. Few situations tax a department's staff or resources more than a patient experiencing a cardiopulmonary arrest. A patient who has lost the ability to oxygenate his tissues or to produce an effective cardiac output will die unless medical intervention is instituted within minutes. Often referred to as "the five-minute emergency," cardiopulmonary arrest creates a situation that is incompatible with life. A rescuer must recognize this emergency and be able to intervene immediately. The emergency department must be prepared to handle this situation on a moment's notice. For effective care of a patient with this problem, the nurse should anticipate patients who are most in jeopardy, be able to identify a cardiopulmonary arrest, and be able to begin immediate intervention to the maximum level of preparation and liability coverage.

In addition to providing direct patient care, the nurse may also be requested to provide emotional support to others who are affected by the crisis. Family, friends, or fellow staff members may require emotional support from a person who is available to help with this important aspect of personalized care.

Patients in Jeopardy of Cardiopulmonary Arrest

People at high risk for cardiopulmonary arrest are those with heart disease. In the United States, more than 1,000 people die each day from sudden cardiac death (American Heart Association, 1980). More than one-half of the deaths occur outside of the hospital, with nearly 50 percent dying without premonitory signs of heart disease. The medical profession, therefore, must identify potential victims who are at risk of dying, but who do not exhibit clinical signs or symptoms.

Heart disease can be predicted in some individuals by identifying factors that may be associated with cardiac pathology. Men, for example, are affected by the disease more often than women; most victims are over the age of 35; and, in general, a positive family history of cardiac disease usually exists (Andreoli et al., 1979). The presence of other metabolic disorders may increase the probability of disease, such as diabetes mellitus, hypertension, hyperlipidemia, obesity, increased catecholamine levels, hypothyroidism, and hyperuricemia. Individuals engaged in high-stress, sedentary occupations, and those who smoke tobacco are also at greater risk.

Heart disease is not the only etiology for cardiopulmonary arrest. Trauma is the leading cause of death in people under the age of 40. The physiologic stress created by hypoxia, hypovolemia, or central nervous system depression may precipitate myocardial compromise and fatal cardiac dysrhythmias.

Toxic emergencies, such as drug overdose, accidental ingestion, or inhalation, may cause cardiac arrest. The emergency department nurse who is alert for abnormal signs and responses to therapy, or notes an unusual history may actually discover the medical cause for arrest and can direct efforts for more appropriate treatment.

Infants without congenital defects are not often considered to be potential victims of sudden cardiac arrest. Some situations, however, create demands that exceed a baby's ability to cope with or respond to therapy. Infants may arrest from hypothermia, respiratory distress, electrolyte imbalance (hypoglycemia), poisoning, near drowning, or trauma (Gray, 1980). Newborn infants are obligatory nose breathers and may have a respiratory arrest if the nares are occluded.

TRIAGE

A patient in cardiopulmonary arrest has immediate priorities of care, but an assessment is still necessary. Triage is an approach that helps the nurse to recognize life-threatening conditions, as well as to collect data that provide a framework for the planning and delivery of care.

Subjective Data

Because the patient is unresponsive and unable to give information, the collection of subjective data begins with family members or ambulance personnel. Obtaining a chronological sequence of events to determine the length of time involved and the possible etiology is important.

All symptoms that the patient complained of prior to the arrest should be docu-

TRIAGE

mented to help determine probable cause. Actions of bystanders or rescuers should be recorded. Past medical history, if obtainable, is important and should include all present and past medical conditions, medications, and allergies.

Objective Data

The nurse must immediately assess the airway. The nurse inspects for breathing efforts and auscultates the chest for breath sounds, if no exchange of air can be felt coming from the nose or mouth. In cardiopulmonary arrest, the patient is not breathing.

Cardiac function is assessed by palpating for arterial pulses (preferably carotid or femoral on adults, but brachial on infants) or by auscultating the apical pulse on adults. All pulses will be absent in a cardiac arrest. The skin may provide further clues to a loss of perfusion by being cool to touch or by appearing pale, mottled, or cyanotic. Cerebral signs of loss of perfusion include a loss of consciousness with no response to any stimuli, in addition to dilated, unresponsive pupils.

By observing the total patient, the triage nurse notes external signs that may provide clues regarding the possible etiology of arrest. Nitroglycerine paste, old thoracotomy or cardiac catheterization scars, clubbing of fingertips, or a barrel chest may be associated with cardiopulmonary disorders. Medication bottles, medical alert bracelets, or soft tissue injuries associated with trauma may also be helpful.

Assessment and Planning

By comparing the subjective and objective data, the nurse can assess the patient's needs and develop a plan of care. Of highest priority with this type of patient are life-saving measures, including basic life support (see Table 11.1) and preparation for

TABLE 11.1 Guide to Providing Artificial Ventilation and Circulation According to Age

Age	Rate of Ventilation	Rate of Compression	Compression/Ventilation Ratio
Less than 1 yr	1 every 3 sec (20 times/min)	100/min	5:1
1–8 yrs	1 every 4 sec (15 times/min)	80/min	5:1 (Single rescuer)
8 yrs–adult	Single rescuer: 2 every 15 sec (12 times/min)	15/10 sec (60/min)	15:2
	Two rescuers: 1 every 5 sec (12 times/min)	1 every sec (60/min)	5:1

SOURCE: American Heart Association, 1980.

TABLE 11.2 Examples of Triage Notes for a Patient in Cardiopulmonary Arrest

S: 47 yo M found slumped over steering wheel. Pt. initially awake, c/o of "sharp" chest pains, SOB, and nausea. App. 1 min. later patient unconscious with dilated pupils, apneic, #7 Et tube placed with bilateral breath sounds. Monitor v fib. Defib. × 1 without change. PMH: unknown, cigarettes in coat pocket, Med-Alert bracelet "allergic to PCN."

O: No respirations, lips dusky, skin pale, cool, diaphoretic. No palpable pulses, no apical pulse. CPR in progress.

A: CPR.

P: Admit cardiac bed. Continue BLS. Have IV, lab, x-ray available. Crash cart at bedside. Social worker notified and with family.

S: 68 yo WM found in bed app. 20 minutes prior to admission. Unresponsive to wife. Initiated CPR and called ambulance. Patient was napping for 30 min. PMH: HTN, diazide 250 mg BID, NKA.

O: No respiratory effort, no palpable pulses, skin cool and clammy, lips and nails cyanotic. Basic CPR being done. Pupils fixed and dilated.

A: CPR.

P: Medical evaluation, admit examination room immediately, continue basic CPR, prepare for advanced CPR. Chaplain called to be with wife.

advanced life support when it is available. Appropriate resources should also be identified for the family, such as a social worker or clergy. (Table 11.2 contains examples of triage notes written for a patient in cardiopulmonary arrest.)

PATHOPHYSIOLOGY

Cardiopulmonary arrest is a nonviable condition if not corrected immediately. All tissues require oxygen and glucose for energy production and cellular function. Without ventilation, carbon dioxide cannot be exchanged for oxygen. A circulatory arrest causes a loss of perfusion to the tissues, resulting in an acute loss of oxygen and glucose to the cells and allowing an accumulation of carbon dioxide. Loss of ventilatory and circulatory functions starts a number of processes that cause further metabolic deterioration.

Excess carbon dioxide in the tissues produces an increased amount of carbonic acid. Without oxygen, cells convert to anaerobic metabolism, which produces lactic acid as a byproduct. Consequently, the multiple acids lower the serum and tissue pH levels and create metabolic acidosis. Bicarbonate is normally produced in the kidney and provides a major buffering system for metabolic acids. Without adequate renal perfusion, sufficient amounts of bicarbonate cannot be made, and the amount on hand is quickly consumed by the rapidly increasing amounts of acids. Acid-base imbalance alters many body functions and affects the distribution of electrolytes. An acidotic environment interferes with the catecholamine's ability to function, making it more difficult for the heart to respond to stress.

PATHOPHYSIOLOGY

Different tissues have various responses to the loss of oxygen, but the central nervous system appears to be the most sensitive. After approximately four to five minutes of ischemia time, except in special circumstances (e.g., hypothermia), the brain does not recover to a prearrest functional level (Southwick and Dalglish, 1980).

The exact mechanism responsible for cardiac arrest in heart disease is not completely understood. Clinical studies have revealed three possible etiologies: myocardial muscle disease, myocardial conduction disturbances, and autonomic nervous system abnormalities.

Myocardial Muscle Disease

As stressed previously, normal tissue function requires adequate circulation. One typical finding in patients who suffer from cardiac disease is an altered coronary blood flow, which produces ischemic muscle areas (Olivia, 1980). The coronary arteries may have occlusive atherosclerotic plaques that reduce the diameter of the vessel and, thus, the flow. Emboli, platelet aggregations, or a thrombosis may produce the same effect. Spasms of a coronary artery produce a functional occlusion (Gorlin, 1982). Loss of arterial perfusion, with a resultant ischemia, subjects the tissue to electrical instability and the possibility of life-threatening dysrhythmias.

Myocardial Conduction Disturbances

Some patients, however, suffer a sudden cardiac death without muscle infarct or vascular occlusion (Cowan, 1979). Histologic studies of myocardial tissue from these individuals reveal a selective myocardial cell necrosis, despite the presence of free-flowing arterial blood supply. The necrotic cells appear in a random patchy distribution. The cause of this unusual pathology is still unknown, but it has been reproduced in animal myocardial cells by injecting isoproterenol subcutaneously. It has also been identified in autopsies of patients who have had open-heart surgery, subarachnoid hemorrhage, and pheochromocytoma.

The cardiac conduction system exerts electrical dominance over muscle cells by controlling the rate and direction of depolarization. Myocardial cells are normally triggered from a pacemaker within the conduction system. A synchronized impulse is generated, and muscular contraction is produced in this manner. If the dominant cells, or foci, originate *outside* the normal conduction system, an abnormal pattern of depolarization can occur. Synchronized contraction and electrical stability may be lost. Rapid rates and/or ineffective contractions create a hypoperfusion state that further aggravates the myocardial oxygen requirements and creates the potential for ventricular fibrillation (Zeluff et al., 1979).

Autonomic Nervous System Abnormalities

The effect of the autonomic nervous system on the heart as a cause of arrest is being researched. Because many patients who experience sudden cardiac death do not have structural changes, some clinicians believe that neural abnormalities cause electrical instability (Lown, 1980).

Stress is another factor associated with sudden death. Life events, such as the loss of a spouse, divorce, change of a job, or altered social patterns require the individual to make a significant adjustment. Illness and injury frequently are associated with such events. Unfortunately, a major source of stress for a patient is hospitalization. Patients in coronary care and other intensive care units often have detrimental cardiac changes when stressful events occur within their environment, such as suctioning, disturbing conversations, or observing other patients in distress (Lynch, 1977).

As previously noted, a change in the autonomic stimulation occurs early in a myocardial infarction—usually within the first 30 minutes after onset. Increased sympathetic or parasympathetic activity may be seen. Exaggerated catecholamine levels have been measured with physical and psychological stress. Epinephrine and norepinephrine can produce ST segment and T wave alterations on the electrocardiogram, as well as an increase in the frequency of premature ventricular contractions (Lown, 1980). Arteriolar constriction due to sympathetic stimulation may participate with platelet aggregation to further reduce blood flow and cause anoxic changes in the heart (Rossi and Gaetano, 1981). Parasympathetic stimulation may cause excessive vagal tone resulting in heart block, bradycardia, and asystole.

CLINICAL MANIFESTATIONS

Because cardiopulmonary arrest can be produced by many causes, prevention is extremely difficult. The early recognition of contributing factors and the monitoring of susceptible individuals will help to provide timely treatment.

Approximately 75 percent of people who experience sudden cardiopulmonary arrest do have a known myocardial disease (Southwick and Dalglish, 1980). Careful assessment and treatment, of course, can be instituted for patients who are most susceptible to cardiac disease.

Myocardial Infarction
A serious consequence of heart disease is actual muscle injury. Early symptoms of injury include pain (in the precordial area, jaw, down the left arm, and radiating to the back), precordial pressure, feelings of indigestion, weakness, dyspnea, nausea, fatigue, and palpitations. Patients with these complaints should be evaluated medically for further evidence of infarct and be admitted for careful observation and treatment (see Chapter 10).

Conduction System Instability
Premature contractions may first be noted by the patient as "skipped beats" or palpitations. Individuals may complain of associated symptoms of "shortness of breath" or "light-headedness." Not all premature ventricular contractions (PVCs) require treatment, but those associated with myocardial disease should be evaluated carefully for treatment.

Conduction abnormalities cause a greater risk of sudden cardiac death. Accessory pathways set up the myocardium for early stimulation during the vulnerable period of repolarization, while a prolonged QT interval effectively increases the period of vulnerability (Zeluff et al., 1979), both of which may produce ventricular fibrillation.

An accessory conduction pathway usually does not present a risk of cardiac death, but sudden death has been reported with Wolff-Parkinson-White syndrome. The rapid tachydysrhythmia, resulting from the aberrant conduction, creates a high metabolic demand on an already compromised ventricle. Coronary artery flow that occurs during diastole may be reduced significantly with a rapid rate. Ventricular fibrillation due to hypoxia and ischemia can quickly follow.

Bradydysrhythmias present a potential for asystole. Failure to generate an adequate cardiac output results in a decreased ability to perfuse the heart, central nervous system, and renal tissue.

Previous History of Ventricular Fibrillation
A patient who has once suffered ventricular fibrillation is at higher risk of having it reappear. Most cases of recurrence tend to be at 20 weeks after resuscitation from a previous infarct (Zeluff et al., 1979).

DIAGNOSTIC STUDIES

The diagnosis of cardiopulmonary arrest is based on an absence of respirations and cardiac output. Further studies may be done to verify the diagnosis, to determine probable cause, and to direct therapy.

The electrocardiogram (ECG), which documents electrical activity of the heart, can show patterns of injury, ischemia, or infarct. The reliability of the ECG must be tempered with the acceptance that it will be used as a tool along with physical assessment to diagnose cardiac patterns. The patient must *always* be checked for a loose lead, interference, or equipment failure before aggressive therapy is instituted, because dangerous "lookalike" patterns can mimic life-threatening patterns. (See Table 11.3 for patterns associated with cardiopulmonary arrest.)

Arterial blood gas studies will vary with therapy and can be used as a guide. One can expect the carbon dioxide concentration in the blood (Pa_{CO_2}) to rise, while the oxygen concentration (Pa_{O_2}), bicarbonate (HCO_3) levels, and pH levels would decrease in an untreated or poorly managed cardiac arrest patient.

Serum electrolyte levels depend on many variables, but they could indicate the cause of cardiac arrest. The heart is extremely sensitive to potassium, sodium, calcium, and magnesium levels.

A chest x-ray study will not document the presence or absence of cardiopulmonary arrest, because it is a static film. It may be helpful, however, in identifying the cause of arrest or complications of therapy.

NURSING CARE AND RELATED INTERVENTIONS

Depending on a nurse's level of skill, training, and the authority under which she or he works, the nurse will respond to a cardiac arrest with either basic life support or

TABLE 11.3 Electrocardiographic Rhythms Associated with Cardiopulmonary Arrest

Potential for Arrest
1. Premature ventricular contractions
   Significant if they –occur in patients with organic heart disease.
   –occur close to the T wave.
   –are frequent (over 6 per min).
   –appear in groups (coupling as in bigeminal and trigeminal rhythms or appear in groups of 2 or 3 before another normal complex occurs).
   –are multifocal in nature.
2. Ventricular tachycardia
   Significant because the rapid ventricular rate does not allow for adequate cardiac output and coronary artery perfusion. The failure to perfuse the heart makes the possibility of ventricular fibrillation more likely. Loss of cerebral perfusion may produce loss of consciousness and respiratory depression.
3. Third degree (complete) heart block
   Complete heart block produces a bradycardia, which cannot sustain an adequate cardiac output. Either ventricular fibrillation due to hypoxia or asystole will result.

Definitive Arrest
1. Ventricular fibrillation
2. Asystole
3. Electromechanical dissociation
4. Idioventricular rhythm

---

more advanced interventions. Immediate care is essential to provide the maximum chances for recovery.

Priorities should be followed. The *"ABC" rule* (airway, breathing, circulation) describes the priority of actions. *Airway* and *breathing* are started with the simplest, yet most effective, method available. Mouth-to-mouth breathing can be implemented, while other equipment and personnel are being summoned. (Table 11.4 outlines options available for rescue breathing, and Chapter 5 discusses these options in greater detail.) Supplemental oxygen should be started as soon as possible.

Artificial *circulation* can be managed effectively with external chest massage, except in unusual situations, such as in cardiac arrest associated with hypovolemia, in massive chest wall defects, or in penetrating chest or upper abdominal trauma, which may require internal cardiac massage. Chest compressions may be associated with undesirable complications, such as fractured ribs, lacerated vessels, or punctured organs. Recognizing potential complications and the additional care that may be required to remedy the complications are critical. The development of a tension pneumothorax, for example, would require a needle thoracostomy to correct. Assistive devices can be used to aid circulatory efforts. Mechanical compressors, designed to depress the sternum to a predetermined depth via power supplied by pressurized

NURSING CARE AND RELATED INTERVENTIONS

TABLE 11.4 Airway Adjuncts Used With Artificial Ventilation

Supplemental oxygen
Oropharyngeal airway
Nasopharyngeal airway
Pocket mask
Bag-valve mask
Esophageal obturator airway
Endotracheal airway
Cricothyrotomy tube
Mechanical ventilators, preferably manually triggered or volume sensitive

---

gas, require placing the patient, positioning and adjusting the chest plate, and supplying a continuous gas source. Disadvantages with a mechanical compressor include the following: the compressor plate may slip from over the sternum; and, the force of the compressions cannot be varied. MAST (military antishock trouser) garments are being used to treat patients in cardiac arrest. The garment effectively reduces the size of the vascular bed by externally occluding the blood vessels in the lower torso. A major disadvantage to the MAST is the loss of circulation to a part of the body, which can precipitate anaerobic metabolism. Patients who have had the MAST in place for several hours may suffer a drop in serum pH levels, when the trousers are deflated. Nonperfused tissues tend to accumulate lactic acid that will reenter the circulation once the circulation is restored to these tissues. Using the MAST eliminates emergency venous access in the lower extremities.

After satisfying basic priorities, the professional nurse must consider more definitive methods of care. An intravenous infusion should be started as soon as possible for administration of cardiotonic drugs. Peripheral arm veins are generally preferred, because they can be entered easily, especially during cardiopulmonary resuscitation (CPR). If a central vein access is desired or necessary, the femoral, external jugular, or internal jugular vein is used, rather than a subclavian, which requires the interruption of CPR to perform. Five percent dextrose in water is the solution of choice.

Drug therapy is directed towards correcting life-threatening dysrhythmias and correcting acid-base, electrolyte or volume disorders. Table 11.5 lists medications used in cardiopulmonary arrest. The sequence in which the drugs will be used depends on the cause of arrest, how long the patient has been without an effective cardiac output or ventilation, and the response to other therapies. (The triage nurse should review more extensive resources for the rationale for using various drug combinations.)

Continuous monitoring of the electrical activity of the heart documents the dysrhythmia and the effectiveness of therapy. A cardiac monitor, or 12-lead ECG machine, should be attached to the patient for a continuous documentation of care. Caution must be used when using "quick-look" paddles. Several monitoring systems have a monitoring mode available in the defibrillation paddles. The patient's cardiac pattern, however, is obtained only when the paddles are *on the chest*. With the paddles removed, the monitor screen may show a wavy line not unlike ventricular

TABLE 11.5 Medications Used for Treatment of Acute Cardiopulmonary Arrest*

Medication	Desired Response	Method of Administration*	Adult Dose	Pediatric Dose	Nursing Considerations
Atropine	Increase heart rate in bradycardia	Given IV push	0.5 mg IV every 5 min until 2 mg are given or patient has responded	0.01–0.03 mg/kg	A rapid increase in the heart rate may also increase myocardial oxygen consumption. Observe patient for possible extension of infarct area
Bretylium (Bretylol)	Suppress ventricular fibrillation or tachycardia	Undiluted: Given *rapid* IV push Diluted: dilute 10 ml (500 mg) to 50 ml Infusion: mix 500 mg in 250 ml NS or D_5W (= 2 mg/ml)	Initial: 5 mg/kg; if second dose needed after one unsuccessful defibrillation, give 10 mg/kg at 15–30 min interval Inject 5–10 mg/kg over 8–10 min Infuse 2 mg/min	Safety in children has not been established	Hypotensive side effects are best treated with IV fluids and modified Trendelenburg position. Some may become nauseated with this drug
Calcium chloride	Increase force of contractions in electromechanical dissociation or asystole	Given *slow* IV push	5–6 mg/kg (2.5–5 ml of 10% solution) every 10 min	0.10–0.30 mg/kg in 10% solution	May precipitate digitalis toxicity if given to patient who has been digitalized. This drug will precipitate in sodium bicarbonate solutions

Dopamine	Increase heart rate, force of contractions, and BP	Infusion: mix 200 mg in 250 ml D$_5$W (= 800 µg/ml)	*Dose dictated by desired action* *2–10 µg/kg/min:* increased rate and force of contractions *10–20 µg/kg/min:* increased vascular resistance *> 20 µg/kg/min:* renal and mesenteric vascular constriction	2–10 µg/kg/min	1. Dose must be calculated on the basis of patient weight and desired action. Infusion pumps can be a useful adjunct for providing more accurate dosages 2. Dosage is titrated until a desired response is obtained (increase in BP, urine output, and tissue perfusion)
Epinephrine	Increase heart rate, force of contractions, and BP in asystole; also convert fine ventricular fibrillation to course ventricular fibrillation in preparation for cardioversion	Given IV push	0.5–1 mg IV (5–10 ml of 1:10,000 solution) every 5 min	0.10 mg/kg in 1:10,000 solution	Catecholamines do not function well in extremes of pH. Correction of respiratory acidosis must be done to allow epinephrine to function. Sodium bicarbonate infusions are very alkaline and can also inactivate this drug. Be sure to flush the intravenous tubing of any bicarbonate before giving epinephrine

TABLE 11.5 (continued)

Medication	Desired Response	Method of Administration*	Adult Dose	Pediatric Dose	Nursing Considerations
Isoproterenol (Isuprel)	Increase heart rate and force of contractions with severe bradycardia or asystole	Infusion: mix 1 mg in 250 ml D$_5$W (= 4 µg/ml)	2–20 µg/min, titrated to desired response	Start at 0.10 µg/kg/min and titrate to desired response	Careful attention must be paid to infusion. Rapid administration may cause an excessive heart rate, hypertension, and tachydysrhythmias. Infusion pumps are helpful aids to prevent overdose
Lidocaine	Suppress ventricular dysrhythmias	Given IV push, and as infusion—mix 1 g in 250 ml D$_5$W (= 4 mg/ml)	Initially give 1 mg/kg bolus followed by a 1–4 mg/min infusion to maintain serum levels	IV push: 1 mg/kg per dose Infusion: 30 µg/kg/min	1. Myocardial and central nervous depression may occur with excessive doses of lidocaine. Observe the ECG for signs of conduction delay. If the patient complains of muscle twitching or has a grand mal seizure, stop infusion until cause of disturbances can be determined

			2. Patients with poor hepatic function or CHF may become lidocaine-toxic due to decreased metabolism of the drug. Smaller doses should be given to these individuals
Oxygen	Correct respiratory acidosis		100% concentration	100% concentration
Sodium bicarbonate	Correct metabolic acidosis	Given IV push	1 mEq/kg initially, then half the original dose every 10–15 min or as blood gases indicate	1–2 mEq/kg/dose in a *diluted* form (or 0.3 × kg × base deficit)	Most drugs will become inactive or precipitate in the alkaline solution of sodium bicarbonate. Flush all lines before and after giving this medication

SOURCE: Sharer, 1979; White, 1981.

*The sequence in which the medications will be given depends upon the etiology of arrest, whether the arrest was witnessed by a rescuer, and the length of time before drug therapy was started after the arrest.

TABLE 11.6 Emergency Use of Cardioversion or Defibrillation with Cardiopulmonary Resuscitation

Emergency Cardioversion

Indication: For the use of terminating tachydysrhythmias that cause hypotension, loss of consciousness, or other indications of hemodynamic instability.

Special considerations: Used with extreme caution in patients who are being treated with digitalis. Discharge of current will be in synchrony with QRS complex. Emergency procedure starts with a dose of 200 joules of delivered energy.

Emergency Defibrillation

Indication: Ventricular fibrillation

Special considerations: Used with extreme caution in patients who are being treated with digitalis. Dose is related to attempts: Initial, 200–300 joules of delivered energy. If first attempt unsuccessful, repeat at same setting for second defibrillation. If second is unsuccessful, continue basic and advanced life support until medications can be circulated, then attempt a third defibrillation at 360 joules of delivered energy (400 joule setting on defibrillator).

Indication: Internal defibrillation

Special considerations: Requires sterile internal paddles. Dose begins low (5 joules) and is gradually increased up to 40 joules.

Indication: Pediatric defibrillation

Special considerations: Most children will respond to basic life support without electrical intervention. Use paddles appropriate to child's size. Dose is related to attempts: Initial, 2 joules/kg. If first attempt is unsuccessful, double the next dose. If second unsuccessful, reassess basic and advanced life support before attempting higher doses.

---

fibrillation, agonal rhythm, or asystole. Remember to check both the patient and the monitor before administering electrical countershock, because it may be an artifact and not an actual dysrhythmia. Table 11.6 lists indications and special considerations for electrical therapy in cardiac arrest. Nurses should familiarize themselves with the equipment to learn how to attach pediatric or internal paddles, as well as how to adjust energy for defibrillation versus cardioversion.

Heart block or certain lethal ventricular dysrhythmias may terminate when the myocardial conduction system is electrically dominated and paced with an external pacemaker. Emergency pacing via catheters, placed through a central vein or chest wall, may be used to "overdrive" the myocardium, thus interrupting lethal rhythms and enabling a more viable one to recover. Emergency insertion of a pacemaker is an invasive procedure, which may be associated with various complications, such as pacer-induced dysrhythmias and electrical hazards.

The unconscious arrest victim should receive additional therapeutic and diagnostic interventions. A nasogastric tube that empties the stomach of air and gastric contents serves two purposes: to decompress the stomach to permit maximum lung expansion; and to decrease the risk of aspiration. A uretheral catheter should be inserted to empty the bladder and to gauge renal perfusion via urinary output.

After patients have been successfully resuscitated and stabilized, they should be transferred to a critical care unit for further monitoring and care. Furthermore, family or friends who are present will also need consideration and support from hospital personnel. Many people tend to gauge the quality of care delivered to their loved one by the amount of interest and concern given to them. Emotional support, consisting of communication and consideration, is important in the care of a critically ill patient.

THE UNSUCCESSFUL RESUSCITATION

Many patients die, despite the aggressive efforts of the emergency department staff. This phenomenon presents a paradox to many professionals: How does one switch from an emotionally charged resuscitative effort to one of calm, reassuring support? By recalling a few basic principles, the staff can provide effective and individualized emotional support. An awareness of how the grieving person may respond, and what interactions are appropriate, can help the nurse to be more effective in handling emotional aspects of care.

The process of grieving occurs in various stages, such as shock, denial, anger, and resolution. Individuals will vary in their response, and their behavior will be affected by their social mores, previous experience, and culture (Schultz, 1980). The nurse should be prepared to encounter any type of behavior and to accept the person who exhibits it, regardless of the way that person ventilates feelings. Acceptance is difficult if the survivor begins to attack the hospital, the staff, or the individual nurse. Although it is very difficult not to become defensive, trying to reason with a distraught person is not always successful. The person often forgets this initial outburst of anger, because his feelings were based on a sense of loss, rather than on an actual problem with the staff (Schultz, 1980). The family should be given an opportunity to grieve in private.

Whenever children are involved, either as the patient or as the survivor, special considerations exist. If the deceased is a child, parents and siblings often experience guilt (Gaffney, 1976; Cordell and Apolito, 1981). By carefully phrasing questions, the nurse will not sound accusatory or critical. Strong emotions surround the death of a child and place difficult strains on a marriage. Divorce frequently occurs after a child has been lost.

All survivors, including children, are touched by the loss of a significant other (Schultz, 1980). A child comprehends death and grieves according to his age and psychosocial adjustment. Except for the new infant, everyone will exhibit some form of emotional reaction to the death. The child should be included in the traditional mourning or burial activities. To remove or shield the child from these activities in the attempt to protect him may only make him feel left out or rejected. Children often fantasize to explain the circumstances and may develop an excessive fear of death, which may persist into adult life.

Because preschoolers do not comprehend the meaning of permanent change, they may ask about the deceased, or they will want to know when they will see the deceased again. Four- and five-year-olds may develop fears and associate death with monsters or demons. Schoolage children have difficulty separating themselves from death. They may fear that others will die, while they are at school, or they may fear personal death if they enter the environment in which someone else died. Because they may associate death with the hospital, they may have significant fears about returning to the hospital in the future.

Because adolescents are dealing with a changing body and mental image, they often need to escape from their feelings of vulnerability. They may respond to the news of a death by running outside or by engaging in physical activities to forget.

Many hospitals provide professionals, such as counselors, specialists, clergy, social workers, or volunteer advocate groups, who can assist the grieving individual. Nurses in particular may be contacted for support.

A few simple guidelines exist to help one deal with a crisis. During the resuscitation, the family should be prepared for the severity of the situation (Sharer, 1979). Providing false hope or misleading statements, however, may create feelings of distrust in family members. Instead, the nurse either reports, "We are doing our best to help," or gives short facts, such as, "We are breathing for him." Because no set answers will be appropriate for every situation, discretion should be the guide. Several types of statements, however, are inappropriate, including argumentative statements, clichés (such as, "His reward is in Heaven"; or, "You are strong and can have another child"), or admonishments to "pull yourself together."

After resuscitation efforts are stopped, the physician should speak with the family. The survivors recognize the physician as the one in charge, and they deserve the courtesy of having an authority figure who personally relays the news and offers condolences. If possible, the nurse should accompany the physician, because the family members frequently ask the nurse for further clarification, after the physician leaves.

The nurse should also permit the grieving friends or family to see the body. Parents, for example, may need to hold, caress, or bathe their child—one last thing they can do for the person. Adults who want to see, touch, or kiss a dead person should not be discouraged. Nurses can make the environment less traumatic by removing offensive sights or drainage. A badly injured body can be partially exposed to enable the survivor to recognize a ring, tattoo, or mark. Seeing and touching the dead will help the grieving person to accept the reality of death, thereby aiding the process of grieving.

Professional or volunteer groups can be quite valuable in helping the family overcome the long-term effects of grieving. Parents who share a common bond, such as death due to sudden infant death syndrome, are usually willing to become immediately involved. A list of support groups should be kept in the emergency department for appropriate referral of family members.

Religious affiliations can provide significant support, even if the patient is not an active member of a particular church. A nurse might even offer to call a member of the clergy for the patient. Many faiths and cultures have special rites that are performed at or near the time of death of a member.

Patients who have had a chronic illness may be affiliated with an organization that will provide different types of aid to family members after a death. Hospice groups, for example, are not necessarily limited in their ability to provide care for a specific person. The nurse should ask the family "*Whom* may I call for you?", rather than, "*Can* I call someone for you?" Because the first question requires a reply, not just consent, it is more likely to receive a positive response.

Caring for the emotional needs of the grieving family and friends is more than just an act of kindness. It may also offer the nurse a chance to confront or deal with personal feelings experienced with the loss of a patient and the pain observed in others.

CONCLUSION

Cardiopulmonary arrest represents a clinical situation in which a patient will inevitably die, if not treated immediately. The professional nurse is responsible for knowing how to intervene, even if it is possible to provide only basic life support. Cardiopulmonary resuscitation is a skill requiring abilities, as well as knowledge, and nurses should be responsible for maintaining both.

Although this chapter should familiarize the reader with various aspects of cardiopulmonary arrest, it is not intended to be a definitive resource. Priorities of care, adjuncts of diagnosis or therapy, and special considerations for grieving family and friends are the salient principles of nursing care.

BIBLIOGRAPHY

American Heart Association: Standards and guidelines for cardiopulmonary resuscitation (CPR) and emergency cardiac care (ECC). *JAMA* 244:453–509 (1980).

Andreoli, K., V. Fowkes, D. Zipes, and A. Wallace: *Comprehensive Cardiac Care*. 4th ed. St. Louis: Mosby, 1979.

Bjork, R., B. Snyder, B. Campion, and R. Loewenson: Medical complications of cardiopulmonary arrest. *Archives of Internal Medicine*. 142:500–503 (Mar. 1982).

Cordell, A., and R. Apolito: Family support in infant death. *JOGN Nursing* 10:281–285 (1981).

Cowan, M.: Sudden cardiac death and selective myocardial cell necrosis. *Heart and Lung* 8:568–574 (1979).

Gaffney, K.: Helping grieving parents. *Journal of Emergency Nursing* 2:42–43 (1976).

Gorlin, R.: Role of coronary vasospasm in the pathogenesis of myocardial ischemia and angina pectoris. *American Heart Journal* 103(4, part 2):598–603 (1982).

Gray, M.: Neonatal resuscitation. *Journal of Emergency Nursing* 6:29–32 (1980).

Gurley, H., T. McAsian, E. Nagel, and M. Weisfeldt: Cardiopulmonary resuscitation. In G. Zuidema, R. Rutheford, and W. Ballinger (eds.): *The Management of Trauma*. 3rd ed. Philadelphia: Saunders, 1979.

Holland, L., and L. Rogich: Dealing with grief in the emergency room. *Health & Social Work* 5:12–17 (1980).

Lown, B.: Cardiovascular collapse and sudden cardiac death. In E. Braunwald (ed.): *Heart Disease: A Textbook of Cardiovascular Medicine*. Philadelphia: Saunders, 1980.

Lynch, J.: *The Broken Heart: The Medical Consequences of Loneliness*. New York: Basic Books, 1977.

McIntyre, K.: Cardiovascular pharmacology: Part II. In K. McIntyre and A. Lewis (eds.): *Textbook of Advanced Cardiac Life Support*. American Heart Association, 1981.

Olivia, P.: Sudden coronary death: predictors and prevention. *Medical Times* 108:57–65 (1980).

Rossi, L., and T. Gaetano: Recent advances in clinicohistopathologic correlates of sudden cardiac death. *American Heart Journal* 102:478–484 (1981).

Schultz, C.: Sudden death crisis: pre-hospital and in the emergency department. *Journal of Emergency Nursing* 6:46–50 (1980).

Sharer, P.: Helping survivors cope with the shock of sudden death. *Nursing '79* 9:20–23 (1979).

Southwick, F.; and P. Dalglish: Recovery after prolonged asystolic cardiac arrest in profound hypothermia. *JAMA* 243:1250–1253 (1980).

White, R.: Cardiovascular pharmacology: Part I. In K. McIntyre, and A. Lewis (eds.): *Textbook of Advanced Cardiac Life Support*. American Heart Association, 1981.

Zeluff, G., G. Pratt, and D. Jackson: Sudden death—how can we prevent it? *Heart and Lung* 8:568–574 (1979).

12

Cardiac Dysrhythmias

Susan K. MacArthur

After completing this chapter, the reader will be able to do the following:

1. Triage a patient experiencing cardiac dysrhythmias.
2. Define the major pathophysiological disturbances that can cause a dysrhythmia.
3. Recognize by single channel rhythm strip the following groups of dysrhythmias: sinus dysrhythmias, atrial dysrhythmias, atrioventricular junctional dysrhythmias, ventricular dysrhythmias, and heart blocks.
4. List major clinical manifestations for each dysrhythmia.
5. State the appropriate nursing interventions and medical therapy for each dysrhythmia.

Cardiac dysrhythmias occur in all age groups and types of patients in the emergency department. A dysrhythmia is defined as an abnormal heart beat. Dysrhythmias are produced when one of three conditions exist (Wolf, 1977): (1) the heart rate is too slow or too fast; (2) the site of the heart's impulse formation is abnormal; or, (3) the conduction of cardiac impulses is abnormal.

A cardiac dysrhythmia can be the primary problem or a symptom of an underlying diagnosis. Nevertheless, the effect of the dysrhythmia on the patient's cardiac output is the focus of the nursing and medical intervention.

TRIAGE

Subjective Data

The subjective data for a patient experiencing a dysrhythmia are the signs and symptoms of an inadequate cardiac output. The patient usually is unaware of the change in his heart rhythm, but recognizes the changes that have occurred in other body systems. The patient should be questioned to discern if he has a history of heart disease. What are the symptoms he has experienced in the past, and what is the present complaint? Specific to a dysrhythmia, the patient may be experiencing angina, dyspnea, palpitations, dizziness with or without syncope, constant cough, dependent edema, and weakness. Prescribed and over-the-counter medications may have a dysrhythmogenic effect. Their use, therefore, should be documented. Allergies must be listed, since a recent exposure may have precipitated the present visit to the emergency department. Carefully listening to and documenting the patient's complaints are the first steps in gathering the triage data.

Objective Data

The actual electrocardiogram (ECG) monitoring of the patient provides the base for the objective data. A 12-lead ECG should be taken as soon as possible to identify the dysrhythmia and to determine if any myocardial damage has occurred. After the 12-lead ECG is taken, the patient should be placed on a standard 3-lead monitor, until a decision is made regarding his condition.

A physical assessment of the patient will substantiate the effect of the dysrhythmia on the cardiac output. Careful attention to the cardiovascular system is necessary. The apical pulse should be taken for one full minute, listening for rate and regularity. Continued auscultation will identify any extra heart sounds. An apical-radial pulse should be taken to identify a pulse deficit. Blood pressure in both arms, noting all sounds heard, must be documented. An auscultatory gap or paradoxical pulse may be heard in the symptomatic patient. Respiratory rate and pattern are noted. Auscultate the lungs for the presence of adventitious sounds. Check for skin color, temperature, and capillary refill. The presence, volume, and quality of the peripheral pulses are checked. Examine the neck veins, palpate for liver enlargement, and check for dependent edema to assess the competency of the venous circulation. Document all information that is obtained upon initial assessment. The same dysrhythmia can produce various symptoms in different patients, depending on the underlying status of the patient's cardiovascular system (Andreoli et al., 1979).

Assessment and Planning

Information the nurse derives from the objective and subjective data will determine the remaining triage action. The patient, not the dysrhythmia, is being treated. The plan must include the priority of care for the patient, as well as the immediate placement of the patient on a standard 3-lead monitor. (Table 12.1 contains examples of triage notes for patients experiencing dysrhythmias.)

PATHOPHYSIOLOGY

The major causes of cardiac dysrhythmias can be divided into the following categories, with accompanying etiologies (Holloway, 1979):

PATHOPHYSIOLOGY

TABLE 12.1 Examples of Triage Notes for Patients Experiencing Dysrhythmias

S: 62 yo WM with c/o "dizziness, pounding in the chest at times and being short of breath after walking." PMH: gallbladder removed 10 years ago, NKA, no prescribed meds, takes ASA for arthritic pains.
O: Oriented × 3; BP 110/80/60, P 74–120 weak and irregular, RR 28, rales both bases; skin pink and warm, JVD at 45°, +1 ankle edema.
A: Irregular heart beat with congestive heart failure.
P: Admit to exam room, place on cardiac monitor, perform 12-lead ECG, Fowler's position, O$_2$ per nasal cannula 2–3 l/min, medical evaluation.

S: 40 yo BF with c/o "palpitations, feel pounding of my heart every now and then, I get dizzy and feel like I may faint." PMH: negative, *allergic* to Demerol.
O: Anxious and upset; oriented × 3; BP 150/90, P 85–60, apical-radial pulse deficit noted, RR 30, lungs clear, skin cool and moist.
A: Irregular heart beat.
P: Admit to exam room, place on cardiac monitor, perform 12-lead ECG, keep room quiet, nurse to stay with patient to keep her calm, Fowler's position; O$_2$ 2–3 l/min, medical evaluation.

1. *Myocardial hypoxia*—coronary artery insufficiency, myocardial infarction, shock, and anemia.
2. *Electrolyte imbalance*—hypokalemia, hyperkalemia, hypocalcemia, hypercalcemia, and hypermagnesemia.
3. *Catecholamine stimulation*—endocrine disorders, hypotension, hypertension, emotional excitement, exercise, sympathomimetic drugs, and organic stimulants (caffeine, nicotine).
4. *Vagal stimulation*—vagal maneuvers (tracheal suctioning, vomiting, straining with a bowel movement) and digitalis intoxication.
5. *Interruption of the conductive system*—cardiac surgery, congenital heart defects, myocarditis, and ventricular dilatation (and hypertrophy).

Electrophysiology

The unique properties of automaticity, conductivity, rhythmicity, and excitability of the heart's conduction system create the propagation of the normal cardiac impulse. The normal conduction system of the heart begins with the sinoatrial (SA) node, the heart's pacemaker. The SA node's inherent rate is 60–100 beats per minute (bpm). This rate is faster than rates in any of the other parts of the normal conduction system. From the SA node, the impulse is transmitted by the internodal tracts and Bachmann's bundle through the atria to the atrioventricular (AV) node. Evidence of this electrical activity is the P wave on the ECG. (See Fig. 12.1). A delay, repre-

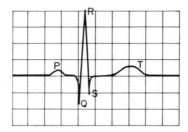

P wave
Atrial depolarization

PR interval
Beginning of atrial depolarization to the beginning of ventricular depolarization
Length: 0.12-0.20 sec.

QRS complex
Ventricular depolarization
Length: 0.06-0.10 sec.

QT interval
Beginning of ventricular conduction to the end of the T wave
Length: Variable with heart rate; 1/2 the preceding R-R interval for normal heart rates

Figure 12.1 The normal cardiac complex with ECG intervals.

sented by the PR interval, occurs to allow the ventricles to fill completely before systole, and it also protects the ventricles from high atrial rates. The impulse is then conducted in the ventricles by the bundle of His, right and left bundle branches, and ends in the Purkinje fibers. Electrocardiographically, this activity is seen as the QRS complex.

Automaticity, the ability to generate a spontaneous impulse, is a property inherent in the heart's conduction system. The SA node, which discharges at the fastest rate (60-100 bpm), serves as the heart's pacemaker. If the SA node discharges too slowly or if its normal impulse transmission is blocked, an escape pacemaker will begin to control the heart's rhythm. In descending order, lower areas of the conduction system have the following inherent rates: the AV node, 40-60 bpm; and, Purkinje system, 40 bpm (Andreoli et al., 1979).

The property of *conductivity* permits the transmission of impulses throughout the myocardium via the conduction system. *Rhythmicity* refers to the regular cyclic response of the cardiac cells in response to an electrical impulse. Cardiac cells also possess *excitability,* the ability to be depolarized by a stimulus. Many factors influence cardiac excitability, such as drugs and ischemia. Evidence of excitability exist as premature beats on the ECG.

Cardiac Monitoring

Before placing the patient on a cardiac monitor, the nurse explains to the patient and to the family the purpose of the monitor. It is an upsetting experience for the patient

PATHOPHYSIOLOGY

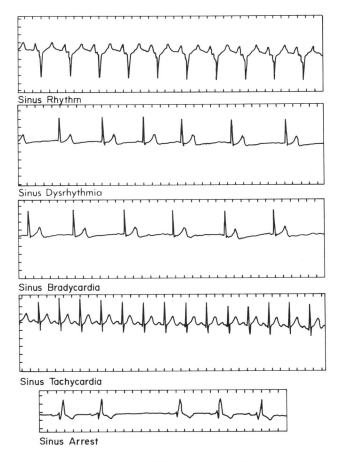

Figure 12.2 Sinus dysrhythmias.

with an illness in the emergency department. If, without forewarning the patient, strange monitors are placed on the patient to watch his heart, then deleterious psychological effects can be produced. Reassuring and supporting the patient and family are important, because they are in a strange and, at times, uncontrollable environment.

For electrode placement, lead II is commonly selected. The negative electrode is placed below the right clavicle, the positive electrode on the left lower chest, and the ground somewhere on the right lower chest. In lead II one can see a complex of good amplitude, and all deflections are upright (check normal sinus rhythm strip, Fig. 12.2). Factors to consider when placing electrodes include avoiding large muscle masses because they produce interference, not placing electrodes on the chest where they could interfere with defibrillation paddles, and preparing the underlying skin for good electrode contact by shaving excess hair or rubbing the skin with alcohol, applying benzoin, or rubbing electrode paste into the skin.

TYPES OF DYSRHYTHMIAS

Deviations from the normal cardiac complex will determine the ECG requirements of the dysrhythmia. (See Figure 12.1 for the normal PQRST complex and intervals.)

Normal sinus rhythm (NSR) personifies the normal cardiac complex. All ECG requirements fall in normal limits. A slight variation may be 0.04 sec. in the PR interval. Ventricular and atrial rates are 60–100 bpm and equal in rhythm. As the name indicates, the normal sequence of conduction is followed with the impulse originating in the SA node. A variation is sinus dysrhythmia, in which a cyclic increase with inspiration and a decrease with expiration of the sinus rate is evident. Sinus dysrhythmia commonly occurs in children and young adults. (See Fig. 12.2 for examples of all sinus dysrhythmias.)

SINUS DYSRHYTHMIAS

Sinus Bradycardia

In sinus bradycardia, the sinus rate is less than 60 bpm. All other parameters remain within normal limits. An accompanying sinus dysrhythmia is commonly seen.

In most instances, this dysrhythmia is benign, and it often appears in athletes and in elderly people. Pathologically, sinus bradycardia can occur in the early periods of myocardial infarction. Any form of vagal stimulation (sleeping, vomiting, carotid massage, administration of excessive digitalis or morphine sulfate), as well as increased intracranial pressure, can cause sinus bradycardia.

Clinical Manifestations
Normally the patient is asymptomatic. If the patient is symptomatic, signs of a decreased cardiac output will be evident. These symptoms include hypotension, weakness, syncope, pallor, dyspnea, and associated signs of heart failure. The patient may complain of angina, indicative of a myocardial infarction. In a head trauma victim, bradycardia is a late sign of increasing intracranial pressure.

Nursing Care and Related Interventions
The patient should be placed in a semi-Fowler's position to maximize cardiac output. If vagal stimulation is the cause of the bradycardia, an attempt should be made to alleviate it: in essence, relieve vomiting. All patients who are symptomatic with a dysrhythmia should have an intravenous (IV) fluid line established. Most of the time, a keep-open line of 5 percent dextrose in water (D_5W) is used. The nurse must be cautious of the vagal response when inserting an IV, because it can produce further reduction in the heart rate.

If the hemodynamic status of the patient is in jeopardy, 0.5 mg of atropine can be given IV every five minutes, up to a total of 2 mg. Isoproterenol 1.0–2.0 µg/minute IV drip is also effective. If these measures fail, then electrical pacing may be required (Andreoli et al., 1979).

Sinus Tachycardia

In sinus tachycardia, the sinus rate is higher than 100 bpm, but does not usually exceed 180 bpm. All other parameters remain within normal limits. According to Wenger (1980), with increases in the heart rate up to 200 bpm, the P wave may merge into the preceding T wave and may appear as atrial flutter or atrial tachycardia. To differentiate between sinus tachycardia and atrial flutter, examine the regularity of the heart rate. In sinus tachycardia, the rate will vary slightly from minute to minute, whereas the rate is consistent in atrial flutter and atrial tachycardia.

Numerous factors can cause sinus tachycardia. It occurs in the normal heart as a normal response to exercise, excitement, and anxiety. Organic stimulants like coffee, tea, and nicotine can also induce tachycardia.

Pathological causes of sinus tachycardia include fever, anemia, pulmonary emboli, pericarditis, hyperthyroidism, shock, hypovolemia, congestive heart failure, and myocardial ischemia. Sinus tachycardia is deleterious in patients with preexisting ischemic heart disease, because the heart's increased oxygen requirements are due to the fast heart rate. In these patients, a tachycardia can induce further ischemia and heart failure.

Clinical Manifestations
If the heart rate is near 160 bpm, the patient may state that his heart is "racing", and the person may be dyspneic and anxious. Signs of a reduced cardiac output, angina, and heart failure will be evident in patients in which sinus tachycardia complicates existing ischemic heart disease.

In children, sinus tachycardia is the norm. Normal resting heart rates for an infant average about 140 bpm; for a one-year-old child, 110 bpm; and, for a two-year-old, 100 bpm (Reece, 1978).

Nursing Care and Related Interventions
Care is best directed at correcting the cause of the tachycardia, because it is only a manifestation of the clinical problem. The patient should be placed in a semi-Fowler's position in a quiet room, then he is connected to a cardiac monitor. Oxygen at 2 to 3 l/minute by nasal prongs can be started if the patient has no history of chronic pulmonary disease. Reassuring the anxious patient is accomplished by the nurse's presence and verbal support. Question the patient regarding the use of organic stimulants. If the patient is experiencing angina, the angina should be relieved to avoid contributing to the tachycardia. A 12-lead ECG must be done, and the patient observed for signs of cardiac decompensation.

Vagal stimulation (Andreoli, et al., 1979) via carotid massage may provide immediate relief by temporarily slowing the tachycardia during the time when pressure is applied. Atrial tachycardias will respond to carotid massage with a sudden reduction in ventricular rate or normal sinus rhythm (Wenger et al., 1980). A Valsalva maneuver will temporarily slow the heart rate. Sedation can be given to the anxious patient, if a pathological cause for the tachycardia has been ruled out. Digitalis is reserved for the patient in whom tachycardia is due to heart failure. For a maintenance drug, propranolol 10–60 mg, given orally four times a day, may be used (Andreoli et al., 1979).

Sinus Arrest

Sinus arrest is the complete absence of the normal cardiac complex on the ECG, creating asystole. The SA node fails to discharge, which is seen as the absence of the normal ECG complex. The period of asystole is not a multiple of the underlying sinus cycle. The rhythm, therefore, is irregular (Holloway, 1979). This condition can occur with infarction of the sinus node, increased vagal stimulation, fibrosis of the conduction system, and, most commonly, with digitalis toxicity.

Clinical Manifestations
Depending on the length of asystole, the patient may experience dizziness or syncope. Escape rhythms from lower pacemakers may arise. If the heart rate is adequate, the patient will be asymptomatic.

In patients with a brady-tachy syndrome, periods of sinus arrest or bradycardia alternate with a supraventricular tachycardia. The patient may complain of dizziness, then feel his heart "racing away."

Nursing Care and Related Interventions
The patient must be in a safe environment to prevent injury if syncope occurs. For patients on digitalis, the possibility of an overdose of digitalis should be addressed.

Initially, atropine 0.5 mg IV can be given and repeated if necessary. If unsuccessful, isoproterenol 1.0–2.0 µg/minute IV should be tried to speed the SA node. A temporary pacemaker can be inserted, if drug treatment fails. If the patient has prolonged asystole and arrests, CPR must be initiated. Long-term therapy for patients with a brady-tachy syndrome uses a combination of medications and electrical pacing (Andreoli et al., 1979).

Discharge Planing for Patients with Sinus Dysrhythmias

If the patient is either symptomatic or has questionable ECG changes, admission to a special care unit for further monitoring is indicated. In transferring the patient from the emergency department to another unit, the nurse must document the specific interventions used to treat the patient in the emergency department, as well as the patient's clinical and electrographic responses. All rhythm strips and a 12-lead ECG must be sent with the patient for inclusion in the record.

For patients released from the emergency department, nursing care includes patient teaching. Patients with sinus tachycardia due to an organic stimulant must be educated regarding the effect stimulants have on the heart. Drug information on new prescriptions must be reviewed with the patient before release. A handout with all pertinent medication information listed should be given to the patient to review at

ATRIAL DYSRHYTHMIAS

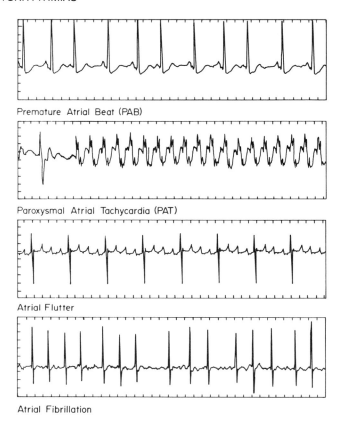

Figure 12.3 Atrial dysrhythmias.

home. The patient should be instructed that, if symptoms return, he should report back to the emergency department.

ATRIAL DYSRHYTHMIAS

Premature Atrial Beat (PAB)

The cardiac rhythm becomes irregular due to the premature atrial beat. The P wave of the PAB is early and similar in morphology to the normal sinus P wave (see Fig. 12.3). The P wave may be buried in the preceding T wave. The PR interval of the PAB may be either normal or prolonged. The QRS complex is usually normal, but may be aberrantly conducted. If the PAB is blocked because the ventricles are in a refractory period, then only the premature P wave will be evident on lead II; it will not be followed by a QRS.

Noncompensatory pauses follow the PABs. In other words, the premature atrial beat resets the sinus mechanism so that the interval between the PQRS complex preceding the PAB and the interval of the PQRS complex after the PAB is less than twice the normal PQRS interval.

An ectopic foci in the atria gives rise to the premature beat. In normal people, the PABs can be produced by a variety of stimulants, such as alcohol or anxiety. Premature atrial beats are frequently seen in elderly people with ischemic heart disease. Infectious states can also produce PABs. In some cases, frequent PABs precede a run of supraventricular tachycardia.

Clinical Manifestations
Most patients are asymptomatic. If the PABs are frequent, the patient may feel palpitations. If the patient is asymptomatic, the PABs must be observed on the monitor to note their frequency and to see if they progress to a supraventricular tachycardia.

Nursing Care and Related Interventions
If symptomatic, the patient should be placed in a quiet environment to reduce extraneous stimuli. Question the patient carefully regarding the use of organic stimulants and reassure the anxious patient. Sedation may be used for some patients. Digitalis with procainamide or quinidine can be used to control the PABs in warranted cases (Andreoli et al., 1979).

Paroxysmal Atrial Tachycardia (PAT)

Paroxysmal atrial tachycardia is a rapid, regular tachycardia with sudden onset and termination at rates between 150–250 bpm. In children, the rate may increase to 250 bpm. This rhythm is also known as paroxysmal supraventricular tachycardia (PSVT) or paroxysmal junctional tachycardia (PJT) (Andreoli et al., 1979). The P wave has a different contour than the normal sinus beats. It may be superimposed on the preceding T wave, occur during the QRS complex, or even occur after the QRS. If the PR interval can be measured, it will be consistent. The QRS complex is normal or aberrantly conducted.

Paroxysmal atrial tachycardia can occur at any age, with or without ischemic heart disease. It is associated frequently with thyrotoxicosis. Heavy use of organic stimulants or emotional stresses can trigger an occurrence of PAT.

Clinical Manifestations
Because of the rapid heart rate, the patient will be nervous, anxious and, complain of a "racing heart." Angina, shock with decreased blood pressure, syncope, and heart failure can occur with prolonged PAT.

Nursing Care and Related Interventions
A quiet room and reassurance for the anxious, symptomatic patient is critical. The nurse should question the patient regarding the frequency of use of organic stimulants. All episodes of PAT should be documented by a rhythm strip. A 12-lead ECG should be obtained initially and, if possible, during a PAT episode. For patients in

ATRIAL DYSRHYTHMIAS

TABLE 12.2 Digitalis Dosage for Paroxysmal Atrial Tachycardia

Type of Digitalis	Dose (Andreoli, 1979)	Total Dose Not to be Exceeded in 24 Hours
Ouabain	0.25–0.50 mg IV followed by 0.1 mg every 30 to 60 min	1.0 mg per 24 hrs
Digoxin (Lanoxin)	0.5–1.0 mg IV followed by 0.25 mg every 2 to 4 hrs	Less than 1.5 mg per 24 hrs
	Children* (Wieczorek, 1981) IV digitalizing dose is 0.04–0.05 mg/kg. One half is given immediately, one quarter in 6 hrs, and the last quarter in 6 hrs or more	Maximum of 0.8 mg/kg
Deslanoslide	0.8 mg IV followed by 0.4 mg every 2–4 hrs	Less than 2.0 mg per 24 hrs

*Digitoxin should be used to convert the child who is not in acute distress.

failure or shock, appropriate nursing measures outlined in Chapters 8 and 10 should be followed.

The giving of medication is determined by how well the patient is tolerating the tachycardia. Sedation may be given to the anxious patient. Vagal stimulation via carotid massage usually will terminate PAT. Intravenous digitalis can also be given. (Table 12.2 contains the dosages of digitalis.) Synchronized cardioversion at low settings (joules 50–100) will terminate PAT. The patient should be given intravenous Valium prior to the cardioversion to induce sedation and amnesia. Propranolol IV 0.5–1.0 mg/minute, up to a total of 3.0 mg, may be tried (Andreoli et al., 1979). Propranolol is contraindicated in patients with heart failure and chronic lung disease. A calcium antagonist, verapamil, can be used at doses of 5–10 mg IV bolus, or in a constant infusion of one mg/minute, up to a maximum of 20 mg (White, 1981). Verapamil is also indicated for supraventricular dysrhythmias and atrial flutter or for atrial fibrillation with a rapid ventricular response.

Atrial Flutter

When the atria begin beating at a rate of 250–350 bpm, producing P waves that are regular with a saw-toothed appearance (flutter waves), the patient is experiencing atrial flutter. The ventricular rate is frequently one-half of the atrial rate due to the protective blocking of the AV node. The ventricles will respond at a slower rate when the patient is treated with drugs for atrial flutter or has altered AV conduction. In children and patients with hyperthyroidism, a one to one conduction ratio may exist through the AV node. The presence of atrial flutter usually indicates underlying ischemic heart disease. Pulmonary emboli and mitral valve disease can also cause atrial flutter.

Clinical Manifestations
The clinical picture depends on the resultant ventricular rate. If the patient is symptomatic, he or she will have the signs and symptoms of paroxysmal atrial tachycardia.

Nursing Care and Related Interventions
Nursing care is the same for this type of patient as for the one with PAT. Synchronized cardioversion is the preferred medical treatment in a patient with a deteriorated clinical picture. Digitalis may be used in the nonacute setting. The dose will vary, and it occasionally may be in the toxic range to adequately control the atrial flutter.

Atrial Fibrillation (A-fib)

In atrial fibrillation, a total disorganization of the atria occurs, since they beat at 350–600 bpm. This phenomenon is seen in a fibrillatory, undulating baseline representing the ineffectual atrial contractions. The PR interval is not measurable. The ventricular response is irregular at a rate of 120–180 bpm, if untreated, and 100–160 bpm, if treated with digitalis.

Chronic atrial fibrillation is seen in patients with ischemic heart disease. It is also seen in patients with rheumatic mitral valve disease, thyrotoxicosis, hypertension, cardiomyopathy, and pericarditis.

Clinical Manifestations
The clinical picture depends on the ventricular response. Signs of a decreased cardiac output may be seen due to the loss of effective atrial contraction. According to Andreoli et al. (1979), systemic and pulmonary emboli are seen as a complication in about 30 percent of the patients with atrial fibrillation.

Nursing Care and Related Interventions
Because the patient has a reduced cardiac output, therapeutic measures should be used to minimize the work on the heart. These measures include placing the patient in a semi-Fowler's position, total bedrest for the patient, and giving the patient supplemental oxygen.

Treatment is directed at slowing the ventricular rate and restoring effective atrial contraction. Synchronized cardioversion at low watt settings (up to 100 joules) is the preferred treatment for the patient in distress (Andreoli et al., 1979). Digitalis (see Table 12.2) is given in nonacute settings. Oral quinidine, combined with digitalis, is most successful in converting atrial fibrillation to a sinus rhythm for long-term maintenance.

Discharge Planning for Patients with Atrial Dysrhythmias

For patients with PABs and PAT due to organic stimulants, education is necessary. Patients should be warned to avoid or reduce their intake of the offending agent. Family members and significant others should be included in teaching. Patients with symptomatic PAT or atrial flutter or fibrillation must be admitted to the hospital for further cardiac monitoring. Patients with chronic atrial fibrillation combined with an adequate ventricular response must be given information on the impending signs of emboli. These signs include discoloration of an extremity with coolness, an absent or diminished pulse, paresthesia, dizziness, syncope, as well as difficulty in moving an extremity or slurred speech.

ATRIOVENTRICULAR JUNCTIONAL DYSRHYTHMIAS

(Figure 12.4 illustrates the atrioventricular junctional rhythms.)

Premature Junctional Beat (PJB)

Similar to a premature atrial beat, a premature junctional beat (PJB) is an early, premature beat, but the site of impulse formation is in the AV node or bundle of His. The site at which the premature beat arises plus the speed of its conduction deter-

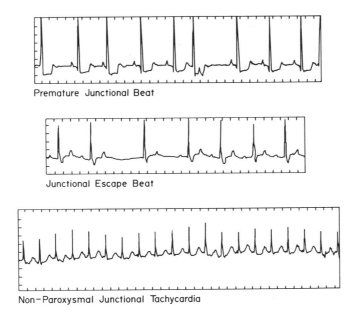

Figure 12.4 Atrioventricular junctional dysrhythmias.

mine the placement of the P wave. The P wave can appear prematurely before, buried in, or after the QRS complex. A compensatory pause normally follows the PJB. Premature junctional beats are seen in people with normal hearts and in patients with ischemic heart disease.

The patient with a PJB has clinical manifestations identical to the patient with premature atrial beats. The nursing care is also identical for the patient with a PAB.

Junctional Escape Beats

The discharge rate for the junctional escape beat is between 40–60 bpm, which is the pacemaker rate of the AV node. The requirements for the P wave are the same as those discussed in the PJB section. Usually the QRS is normal, but it may be aberrantly conducted. A series of junctional escape beats is called a junctional rhythm.

Escape beats are a protective mechanism of the heart to prevent ventricular asystole. If the SA node fails to pace the heart or if its impulse is blocked, then following the normal order of the heart's hierarchy of conduction, the AV node will assume the role of pacemaker of the heart.

Junctional escape beats can occur in the normal heart in response to increased vagal tone. An escape rhythm may arise during periods of pathological heart block, for example, in a patient with an acute inferior myocardial infarction.

Clinical Manifestations
Most patients are asymptomatic with junctional escape beats. The patient's clinical status is determined by the frequency and underlying cause of the dysrhythmia.

Nursing Care and Related Interventions
The symptomatic patient must be observed for signs of inadequate cardiac output due to a slow heart rate. If heart block is coexistent, the rhythm must be closely monitored for further progression of the block. A 12-lead ECG should be performed. Judicious use of sublingual nitroglycerine and/or IV morphine is warranted, in order to prevent the complication of hypotension. Oxygen at 2 to 3 l/minute by nasal cannula can be used if no chronic obstructive pulmonary disease (COPD) is present. In patients with COPD, judicious use of oxygen at 1 to 2 l/minute via pediatric flow meter should be used to give supplemental oxygen. Intravenous atropine or isoproterenol (the same dosage listed for sinus arrest) can be used to increase the rate of discharge of higher pacemakers.

NonParoxysmal Junctional Tachycardia (NPJT)

The ECG will show a pattern of gradual onset and termination of nonparoxysmal junctional tachycardia. This pattern differs from the rapid onset and rapid termination of paroxysmal junctional tachycardia (PJT) discussed earlier. The rhythm is set at a rate of 60–140 bpm (Wenger, 1980). This rate is considered to be a tachycardia for the AV junction; therefore, it is called nonparoxysmal junctional tachycardia (NPJT) (Andreoli et al., 1979). The P wave and QRS complex follow the same criterion discussed for junctional escape beats.

VENTRICULAR DYSRHYTHMIAS

Digitalis toxicity is the most common cause of NPJT. Other causes include myocardial infarction, rheumatic myocarditis, and as a complication in the postoperative phase of the open-heart surgery patient.

Clinical Manifestations
The patient's response to the dysrhythmia is determined by its frequency and underlying cause. Similar to abnormalities of the rhythm of the heart, the patient should be observed for low cardiac output syndrome. If the patient has had an acute myocardial infarction, the nurse must institute the care required for a patient experiencing a myocardial infarction.

Nursing Care and Related Interventions
Patients on digitalis must be carefully questioned regarding their use of the drug. The first, common signs of digitalis toxicity are the gastrointestinal (GI) disturbances of anorexia, nausea, and vomiting, with possible accompanying abdominal pain. The patient may experience disturbances in vision, seeing yellow-green halos around objects, blurred vision, or diplopia. Central nervous system symptoms can range from headache to coma. Any change in behavior or patterns of living should be questioned. Digitalis toxicity commonly produces conduction disturbances, supraventricular dysrhythmias, and premature ventricular beats. A digoxin blood level above 2.5 mg/ml is considered toxic (Nursing '79 Books, 1979). If digitalis toxicity is determined to be the cause, the management is to withhold the drug, to monitor the patient for other dysrhythmias, and to replace slowly any potassium deficit by giving orally 30–45 mEq initially or 0.5 mEq potassium chloride per minute in 5 percent dextrose and water for a total of 30–60 mEq (Andreoli et al., 1979). Constant ECG monitoring is mandatory, because the potassium may have an additional blocking effect on the AV node. If digitalis toxicity is ruled out, and the patient is exhibiting signs of failure or compromised cardiac output, then IV digitalis (see Table 12.2) is given. Low joule synchronized cardioversion can be used when IV digitalis is unsuccessful (Andreoli et al. 1979).

Discharge Planning for Patients with Atrioventricular Junctional Rhythms

For asymptomatic patients with premature junctional beats, the discharge planning is the same as for patients with premature atrial beats. Symptomatic patients with junctional escape beats and nonparoxysmal junctional tachycardia will usually be admitted for continued cardiac monitoring and evaluation.

VENTRICULAR DYSRHYTHMIAS

Premature Ventricular Beat (PVB)

The first visual clue to a premature ventricular beat (PVB) is a premature, wide (greater than 0.11 seconds), bizarre QRS, which usually has a larger T wave reflected in the opposite direction of the QRS (see Fig. 12.5). The P wave is absent, or it may

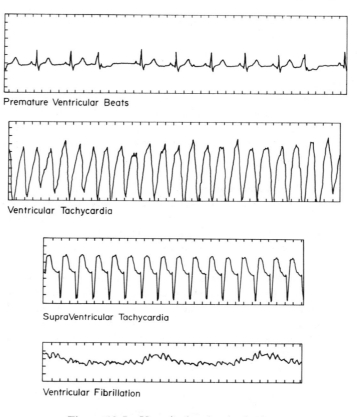

Figure 12.5 Ventricular dysrhythmias.

follow the QRS. The sinus node is not reset. A compensatory pause, therefore, follows the PVB.

Different names are given to PVBs, depending on their timing, configuration, and frequency. *Unifocal* PVBs derive from one ectopic focus. Each time the ectopic focus fires, the same configuration of a PVB is seen. *Multifocal* PVBs arise from several ectopic foci, all having different configurations. *Bigeminy* is the term used to denote timing of a PVB every second beat. *Trigeminy* denotes a PVB every third beat. A *fusion* beat is an intermingling of a normally conducted QRS and PVB, so that the PVB has characteristics of both beats. If the PVB is sandwiched between two normal beats without a compensatory pause, it is termed an *interpolated PVB*.

If the normal sinus pacemaker fails and the next highest pacemaker does not begin conducting, then a ventricular escape rhythm will arise. This rhythm may be multifocal in nature, occurring at a rate of 20–40 bpm.

"R on T" PVBs can occur during the vulnerable period (at the apex of the T wave) in the cardiac cycle. At this point, the myocardium has the potential to respond to an extra induced stimulus. The response at this time could be as chaotic as ventricular fibrillation.

Premature ventricular beats occur at all ages in patients with normal and abnormal hearts. Conditions predisposing to PVBs include ischemic heart disease, myocardial infarction, hypokalemia, digitalis toxicity, and as a complication in the postoperative phase of the open-heart surgery patient.

Clinical Manifestations
If the patient is having frequent PVBs, he may complain of palpitations. Patients with a history of heart disease may have angina and become hypotensive with frequent PVBs. The radial pulse will be irregular, or there may be a bigeminal pulse, or there may be a pulse that varies in volume. An apical-radial pulse deficit can be counted.

Nursing Care and Related Interventions
For the anxious, hemodynamically stable patient, reassurance is the best intervention. In symptomatic patients with angina, an IV of D_5W should be started immediately. Oxygen should also be started. If the dysrhythmia is not a ventricular escape rhythm, a bolus of lidocaine IV (1 mg/kg body weight) should be administered. A lidocaine drip is then started at a rate of two to four mg/minute. A second and third lidocaine bolus can be given at approximately 10 to 20 minute intervals at a dose of one-half the first bolus. To prevent lidocaine toxicity, the total dose should not exceed 300 mg/hour. The signs and symptoms of lidocaine toxicity center on central nervous system disturbances. These symptoms include confusion, slurred speech, light-headedness, paresthesia, muscle twitches, tinnitus, blurred or double vision, hypotension, and coma.

Procainamide is used when lidocaine is ineffective. Intravenous boluses of 50 to 100 mg every one to three minutes, up to a total of 750 to 1000 mg is given. A drip of 2 mg to 6 mg per minute can be started (Andreoli et al., 1979). The blood pressure must be carefully monitored because of the complication of profound hypotension from procainamide administration.

Ventricular Tachycardia (V-T)

Ventricular tachycardia is defined as three or more PVBs occurring in a row at a rate of 110–250 bpm. The rhythm is usually regular with P waves seen at various points in the rhythm.

A supraventricular dysrhythmia with aberrant conduction can mimic ventricular tachycardia. The two can be differentiated if any one of the following symptoms is demonstrated (Andreoli et al, 1979): (1) an ectopic P wave initiates supraventricular tachycardia; (2) capture and fusion beats are seen with V-T and not with supraventricular tachycardia; (3) complete heart block rarely occurs with supraventricular tachycardia but usually with V-T; (4) Carotid massage slows supraventricular tachycardia, but does not slow V-T; or (5) IV lidocaine terminates V-T, but it may only slow a supraventricular tachycardia so that the P waves can be recorded. Until it can be discerned whether the dysrhythmia is either V-T or a supraventricular tachycardia with aberrant conduction, the patient should be treated as though the dysrhythmia is V-T.

All conditions discussed for the PVBs can account for ventricular tachycardia. The patient will most likely have some sign of cardiac disease. An occurrence of V-T is common in the first one to three hours after an acute myocardial infarction.

Clinical Manifestations
Ventricular tachycardia is an acute emergency. The patient may or may not be conscious. If conscious, the patient may complain of palpitations, dizziness, dyspnea, and chest pain. The blood pressure will be low. Depending on the cardiac status and the length of V-T, heart failure may be present. The patient may quickly become unconscious and need to be treated with life support measures.

Nursing Care and Related Interventions
The protocol listed under PVBs is followed for the conscious patient in V-T. In the unconscious patient, emergency cardioversion at 200 joules should be given immediately (Creed, 1981). Vital signs must be taken every two to three minutes. The patient's cardiac rhythm must be closely watched for any progression to ventricular fibrillation. The patient should be prepared for transfer to an acute care unit.

Ventricular Fibrillation

Ventricular fibrillation is represented by large, irregular, ineffective, and undulating ventricular contractions at a rate of 150–300 bpm. Atrial activity may be present, independent of the ventricles.

Ventricular fibrillation occurs in situations similar to ventricular tachycardia and PVBs. Most commonly, the event is associated with an acute myocardial infarction or an episode of severe hypoxia. Drug toxicity (digitalis, procainamide, quinidine) can also precipitate ventricular fibrillation.

Clinical Manifestations
The patient is in profound shock and is pulseless, with no spontaneous respirations. A seizure may precede the event. Death will ensue in three to six minutes, unless life support measures are immediately instituted.

Nursing Care and Related Interventions
Without delay, defibrillation at 200 to 300 joules must be delivered (Creed, 1981). Cardiac monitoring is imperative to assess any change in the patient's rhythm. Emergency life support measures should be initiated.

The hypoxia induced by ventricular fibrillation produces metabolic acidosis. This condition is corrected with proper ventilation, intravenous sodium bicarbonate, and serial blood gas analysis. Lidocaine may be given, using the same guidelines discussed in the management of PVBs. Intravenous epinephrine may be used to change a fine ventricular fibrillation to a coarse ventricular fibrillation, which is easier to convert to a normal rhythm.

If ventricular fibrillation persists after a series of cardioversions, IV lidocaine, and management of hypoxia, then IV bretylium is given. The initial dose of bretylium is 5 to 10 mg per kilogram body weight, which is repeated up to a maximum dose of 30 mg/kg. For intravenous maintenance with bretylium, a 1 to 2 mg/minute drip rate is administered (White, 1981).

Discharge Planning for Patients with Ventricular Dysrhythmias
Because of the lethal nature of ventricular dysrhythmias, these patients will be admitted to an acute care monitoring unit. Stabilization of the patient in the emergency department before transport is essential. A physician and nurse, who accompany the patient to the unit, should be prepared to administer life support measures, if required.

HEART BLOCKS

First Degree Heart Block—First Degree AV Block

In first degree heart block, a delay in conduction occurs at the AV node, creating a PR interval that is greater than 0.20 seconds. All other ECG parameters are normal (see Fig. 12.6).

The dysrhythmia occurs in all age groups and in people with normal and diseased hearts. Antidysrhythmic drugs (digitalis, procainamide, quinidine, and propranolol) can prolong the PR interval.

No clinical signs or symptoms of first degree AV Block exist. No treatment for the dysrhythmia is required. For patients taking an antidysrhythmic drug, measurement of the drug level should be obtained. This measurement will indicate whether the patient is in a therapeutic or toxic range.

Second Degree Heart Block—Mobitz I or Wenckebach Block

In Mobitz Type I, an impairment exists in conduction through the AV node. This condition is seen as the PR interval progressively lengthens with each beat, until a QRS complex is dropped. A cyclic fashion of atrial impulses to ventricular responses occurs, and it can present in a ratio of 5:4, 4:3, and so forth.

In an acute inferior myocardial infarction or digitalis toxicity, Wenckebach rhythm is a common phenomenon (Wolf, 1982). The block is transient and does not usually progress to a higher degree of block.

No clinical manifestations of Wenckebach usually exist, unless there are frequently dropped beats that significantly alter the patient's hemodynamic status. An irregular pulse will be present due to the dropped beats.

The patient should be placed on a cardiac monitor, and an IV of D5W started. If the patient is experiencing any symptoms of an acute myocardial infarction, further evaluation will be required. Patients taking digitalis must have drug levels drawn.

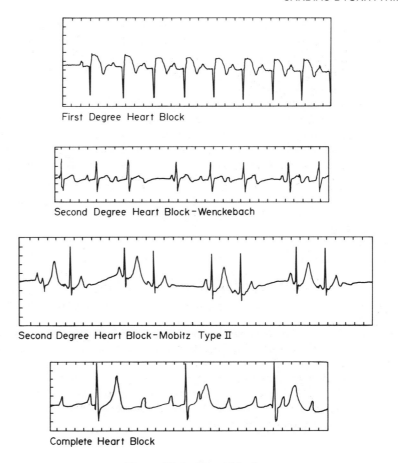

Figure 12.6 Heart blocks.

Second Degree Heart Block—Mobitz II

In Mobitz Type II, the block in conduction exists beyond the AV node and is located in the bundle of His and bundle branches. P waves are blocked. The PR interval for conducted beats may be either prolonged or normal, but it remains constant. "The ventricular rate is a fraction (1:2, 1:3, 1:4, and so forth) of the atrial rate" (Wolf, 1982, p. 132). The QRS complexes are wide. A Mobitz Type II exists when there is a severe impairment in the AV conduction, such as in a patient with an acute anterior myocardial infarction.

Similar to Mobitz Type I, the patient is asymptomatic. If the ventricular rate is extremely slow, signs of a decreased cardiac output will be seen.

Mobitz Type II can progress to complete heart block, requiring the patient to have continuous cardiac monitoring and a patent IV line. If complete block occurs, isoproterenol 1.0–2.0 μg/minute by intravenous drip can be given to increase the ventricular rate. Atropine is not recommended, because it will increase only the atrial and not the ventricular rate (Andreoli et al., 1979). The nurse should be prepared to help in the insertion of a temporary pacemaker.

Third Degree Heart Block—Complete Heart Block (CHB)

In third degree heart block, a complete block exists in the conduction between the atria and ventricles. No P waves are conducted to the ventricles. The atrial activity is controlled by an independent focus, usually a sinus mechanism beating at 60–100 bpm. Ventricular activity is controlled by a separate focus at a rate less than 40 bpm. The PR interval bears no relation to the succeeding QRS. The QRS is prolonged (greater than 0.11 seconds), because it originates within the ventricles.

Numerous factors cause CHB. In children, it can be either a congenital problem or a complication from open-heart surgery. In adults, possible causes include degeneration of the conduction system, acute myocardial infarction, digitalis toxicity, myocarditis, and open-heart surgery.

If the ventricular rate is adequate, the patient may be asymptomatic. More commonly, the patient will show signs of a decreased cardiac output, manifested by the signs and symptoms of heart failure or Stokes-Adams attacks. Stokes-Adams attacks refer to cardiac standstill and syncope from CHB.

Similar to the patient with Mobitz Type II, the patient with CHB may require IV isoproterenol and a temporary pacemaker. The patient must be closely monitored for cardiac asystole.

Discharge Planning for Patients with Heart Block

In all cases of heart block, the discharge instructions given to the patient will depend on the underlying cause of and treatment of the block. When the block is due to drug toxicity, the patient may require a review of pertinent drug information and/or a readjustment in medication dosage. For patients who have a history of cardiac disease and have changes on their 12-lead ECG consistent with an acute myocardial infarction, preparation for transport and admittance to an acute care unit is necessary.

CONCLUSION

Care of the patient experiencing a dysrhythmia always centers on the entire person, not just on the patient's ECG changes. The emergency department nurse is responsible for appropriate triage of the patient so that the person's condition can be stabilized and plans made for future care. The nurse must be able to recognize the basic dysrhythmias and develop the plan of care for the patient. Adequate discharge instructions must be included in the plan for the patient discharged from the emergency department. More often, however, the patient's care will continue in an acute care unit. The emergency department nurse helps provide the appropriate initial care for the patient experiencing a dysrhythmia.

BIBLIOGRAPHY

Andreoli, K. G., et al.: *Comprehensive Cardiac Care.* 4th ed. St. Louis: Mosby, 1979.

Braun, H., and G. Diettert: *Coronary Care Unit Nursing.* Reston, VA: Reston, 1980.

Conover, M., and E. Zalis: *Understanding Electrocardiograpy.* St. Louis: Mosby, 1976.

Chernoff, H. L., and M. B. Kriedberg: Arrhythmias, Cardiac. In R. N. Reece (ed.): *Manual of Emergency Pediatrics.* Philadelphia: Saunders, 1978, pp. 15–23.

Creed, T. D., et al.: Defibrillation and Synchronized Cardioversion. In D. M. McIntyre, and A. J. Lewis, (eds.): *Textbook of Advanced Cardiac Life Support.* Dallas: American Heart Association, 1981, Chapter 7.

Daly, B.: *Intensive Care Nursing.* New York: Medical Examination, 1980.

Garson, A.: Supraventricular Tachycardia. In P. C. Gillette, and A. Garson (eds.): *Pediatric Cardiac Dysrhythmias.* New York: Grune & Stratton, 1981, pp. 177–253.

Goldberger, E.: *Treatment of Cardiac Emergencies.* St. Louis: Mosby, 1977.

Holloway, N. M.: Arrhythmias and Conduction Defects. In N. M. Holloway, (ed.): *Nursing the Critically Ill Adult.* Menlo Park, CA: Addison-Wesley, 1979, pp. 77–145.

Knoll Pharmaceutical Company: *Isoptin* Print #1063. Whippany, NH, 1981.

Margolis, et al.: Episodic drug treatment in the management of paroxysmal arrhythmias. *American Journal of Cardiology* 45:621–626 (1980).

Marriott, H.: *Practical Electrocardiography.* 6th ed. Baltimore, MD: Williams & Wilkins, 1977.

Nursing '79 Books: *Nurse's Guide to Drugs.* Horsham, PA: Intermed Communications, 1979.

Opie, L. H.: Antiarrhythmic Agents. *Lancet* 1(8173): 861–867 (Apr. 19, 1980).

Sokolow, M. and M. McIlroy: *Clinical Cardiology.* Los Altos, CA: Lange, 1977.

Stanford, et al.: Antiarrhythmic Drug Therapy. *American Journal of Nursing* 80:1288–95 (July 1980).

Wenger, N. K., et al.: *Cardiology for Nurses.* New York: McGraw-Hill, 1980.

Wieczorek, R. N., and J. N. Natapoff: *A Conceptual Approach to the Nursing of Children.* Philadelphia: Lippincott, 1981, pp. 377–401.

White, R. N.: Cardiovascular Pharmacology: Part I. In D. M. McIntyre, and Lewis, A. J. (eds.): *Textbook in Advanced Cardiac Life Support.* Dallas: American Heart Association, 1981, Chapter 8.

Wolf, P. S.: Assessment Skills for the Nurse: Cardiovascular System Arrhythmias and Conduction Disturbances. In C. N. Hudak, T. Lohr, and B. M. Gallo (eds.): *Critical Care Nursing.* 3rd ed. Philadelphia: Lippincott, 1982, pp. 119–138.

13

Thrombus, Embolus, Hypertensive Crisis, or Cerebrovascular Accident

Carol Beth Pulliam

After completing this chapter, the reader will be able to do the following:

1. Triage a patient experiencing thrombus, embolus, hypertensive crisis, or cerebrovascular accident.
2. Explain three mechanisms in the pathophysiology of thrombosis.
3. Recognize the various heart conditions that are often the primary sources of emboli.
4. Discuss educational needs for patients receiving anticoagulant therapy.
5. Identify and select the most appropriate antihypertensive for each crisis situation.
6. Discuss and identify eight situations in which rapid blood pressure reduction is required.
7. Explain the etiology of hypertensive emergencies.
8. Discuss the clinical manifestations of and treatment of the various etiologies of hypertensive crisis.
9. Identify and discuss factors that increase the possibility that stroke will occur.
10. Discuss the three causes of cerebrovascular occlusive disease and the clinical manifestations of each cause.
11. Discuss the acute and long-term nursing interventions required for treating patients with cerebrovascular disease.

Lower extremity thrombosis occurs in about 2.5 million people annually. Frequently, patients present with this condition as the result of complications due to another illness. The urgency of treatment is evident by virtue of possible clot detachment and its migration to the pulmonary vasculature. Hypertensive crises, though occurring less frequently since 1975, continue to be a challenge for emergency department nurses. Severe hypertension, venous thrombus, and arterial embolus have the potential to cause a disruption in cerebral blood flow and result in a stroke or cerebrovascular accident. Any one of these interrelated conditions may be seen in an emergency department, and each requires immediate attention and intervention.

This chapter deals with the initial evaluation of and management of patients presenting to the emergency department with a thrombus, embolus, hypertensive crisis, or cerebrovascular accident. The nurse's understanding of these conditions will facilitate the triage process.

TRIAGE

Subjective Data

Subjective data are collected by interviewing the patient, his family, or ambulance personnel. The primary concern is the nature of the complaint, or precisely what prompted the patient to visit the emergency department. Patients, for example, with thrombus or embolus usually complain of symptoms related to ischemia, while those with hypertensive encephalopathy or cerebrovascular accident may present with neurological deficits. Further questioning of the patient with possible thrombosis should elicit information regarding the presence of pain, the location of pain, and its quality or severity. An immediate past medical history of any operation or illness requiring bed rest can be significant in establishing the diagnosis.

Patients with hypertensive encephalopathy or cerebrovascular accident often initially complain of a headache, followed by a change in neurological status. The emergency department nurse must question the patient or family about the onset of the headache and the sequence of events that followed. This information is important in differentiating hypertensive encephalopathy from a cerebrovascular accident. The nurse must also ascertain whether the patient has any focal or lateralizing neurological signs, such as hemiplegia. In addition, the nurse should determine if the patient is experiencing ataxia, dysphagia, or visual disturbances.

The patient's past medical history, current medication regimen, if any, as well as allergies should be determined.

The decision to delve further into the chief complaint depends on the seriousness of the patient's condition. If the patient is unable to provide the necessary information, the emergency department nurse may question family members or ambulance personnel.

Objective Data

The triage nurse collects objective data primarily through direct observation of the patient, as soon as the patient enters the emergency department. Facial expressions, such as grimacing or wincing, may indicate pain. Observation of an extremity for color and warmth as well as palpation of pulses provides information regarding the quality of peripheral blood flow. Measurement of vital signs, particularly the blood pressure and pulse, are essential in diagnosing a hypertensive emergency. In addition, fundoscopic examination provides valuable information about the severity of the hypertensive vascular disease. Assessment of neurological status requires the triage nurse to observe the patient for any motor or sensory deficit, as well as for disorientation or confusion.

Assessment and Planning

Once the nurse has collected both subjective and objective findings, a determination regarding the cause of the complaint and the appropriate intervention(s) can be made. The initial nursing intervention(s) will depend on the priority of care the patient's condition demands. (Examples of triage notes for a patient with lower extremity thrombosis and for a patient with malignant hypertension are included in Table 13.1.)

THROMBUS—VENOUS AND ARTERIAL

The occlusion of an artery or a vein by a blood clot is called a *thrombus*. Thrombus formation, accompanied by inflammation of a vein, is called *thrombophlebitis*.

Thrombus formation occurs more frequently in the venous system than in the arterial system and may involve both the superficial and deep veins. *Superficial*

TABLE 13.1 Examples of Triage Notes for Patients With Venous Thrombosis and Malignant Hypertension

S:	52 yo WM with c/o gradual onset of pain in right calf for 2 days PTA. PMH: recent MI requiring inactivity, NKA, no regular meds.
O:	Right lower extremity swollen, reddened, nonpalpable cord, pedal pulses present and normal. T 99.6°F, P 96, BP 136/90.
A:	Deep venous thrombosis 2° to immobility from recent MI.
P:	Admit to treatment room as soon as possible. Elevate affected extremity, apply hot compresses, medical evaluation.
S:	42 yo BF with c/o onset severe headache accompanied by blurred vision approximately 1 hour prior to admission. PMH: HTN 4 years, NKA, Inderal, Lasix, Minoxidil, has not taken for 1 week before admission.
O:	Oriented × 4, BP 240/140, P 90. Fundoscopic exam: grade IV hypertensive retinopathy. Apprehensive.
A:	Malignant hypertension 2° to noncompliance.
P:	Admit to treatment room immediately, medical evaluation, begin IV D_5W TKO, obtain BP's q 10–15 minutes, observe for any alterations in mental status.

venous thrombosis occurs most commonly in the long and short saphenous veins, while *deep venous thrombosis* occurs most frequently (88 percent) in the veins of the posterior and anterior tibial compartment and in the soleus and gastrocnemius.

Less commonly, deep vein thrombi may also originate in the pelvic, iliac, common femoral, deep femoral, or popliteal veins, and they are more serious. Deep vein thrombosis requires immediate intervention to alter the risks of pulmonary embolism and venous insufficiency (Bloom, 1981).

Pathophysiology

The development of thrombosis may be attributed to one of the following factors: (1) inflammation or trauma to the vascular wall occurring with mechanical injury, heat, or ischemia; (2) alterations in the blood flow, such as venous stasis occurring with immobility; or, (3) hypercoagulable properties of the blood seen in patients with malignancy, blood dyscrasias, or in patients taking oral contraceptives. One or more of these factors can promote intravascular coagulation, which becomes the basis for thrombus formation (Sharnoff, 1980).

A thrombosis may occur in any portion of the circulatory system. The formation is initiated when clusters of platelets attach or adhere themselves to an injured vascular wall, to an atheromatous plaque, or in an area of sluggish blood flow. Platelet adherence produces fibrin deposition and red blood cell aggregation on the vascular wall. Repeated layers of these components increase the size of the thrombus, until occlusion of the vessel occurs (Price, 1982).

The majority of *venous thrombi* can be attributed to venous stasis, secondary to immobility after a surgical procedure. Absence of calf muscle contraction with immobility prevents propulsion of the blood forward. This condition, which causes pooling of the blood in the lower extremities, is conducive to thrombus formation. Other medical conditions that may predispose a person to thrombosis are malignancy, cardiac disease, pregnancy, and obesity.

An *arterial thrombosis* may result from damage to arterial endothelium after a vascular operation, but, in most instances, it develops on an atheromatous plaque. Arterial thrombi have the same composition and structure as venous thrombi. The location for deposition varies, but most arterial thrombi have the propensity to develop near bifurcations of the aorta, particularly near the iliac-aorta junction (Maschak, 1981).

Clinical Manifestations

A superficial vein thrombosis is easily assessed, since it can be seen and palpated. The acute phase is manifested by warmth, pain, and redness along the pathway of the thrombosed vein. Fever may occur in some patients. Deep vein thrombosis is more difficult to recognize and is asymptomatic 50 percent of the time. Nevertheless, patients presenting with symptoms have swelling, pain, and tenderness in the affected extremity. The skin is warm to the touch and has a reddish hue. Some patients may develop fever and tachycardia (Douglas, 1978).

Because of the acute symptoms accompanying ischemia in an arterial occlusion, arterial thrombi are more readily assessed than are venous thrombi. Most patients with arterial thrombi present with the chief complaint of sudden onset of numbness and pain in an extremity that appears pale in color and cold to the touch. Peripheral pulses distal to the point of obstruction are not palpable.

Diagnostic Studies

Venography with a 90 percent accuracy rate is the most widely accepted tool for establishing the diagnosis of venous thrombosis. The test involves injection of contrast material through the common femoral vein or through a dorsal foot vein, after which x-ray studies are taken to determine the location of the occlusion.

The ^{125}I *fibrinogen test* involves the injection of radioactive fibrinogen. Once in the body, radioactive fibrinogen is converted to fibrin by local thrombin, and it then becomes a part of the forming thrombus. A scintillation counter is used to scan the affected extremity and to detect the location of the thrombus in the area with increased radioactivity. This test, however, is not extremely accurate in detecting thrombosis that originates in the proximal thigh veins (Bloom, 1981).

The *Doppler ultrasound* flow study is a noninvasive test often used to diagnose a deep venous or arterial occlusion. A Doppler probe is used to determine audible signals from a reflected ultrasound beam that is sent through an acoustical gel on the skin. The audible signals are compared to the corresponding extremity. The signals differentiate between normal and obstructed blood flow (Fischbach, 1980).

Impedance plethysmography is a study based on the principle that electrical impedance occurs in an extremity with occlusion. Occlusion of the extremity is accomplished by placing a pneumatic cuff on the patient's thigh and inflating it, thus occluding the venous return. Deflation of the cuff results in changes in impedance (resistance) that are determined by calf electrodes and recorded on an ECG strip. This test is accurate in detecting thrombosis in the popliteal, femoral, or iliac veins (Sharnoff, 1980).

Prothrombin time (PT) and partial thromboplastin time (PTT) are blood tests used to measure the ability of the blood to coagulate. These tests are necessary for patients receiving warfarin and heparin to determine that adequate anticoagulation has been achieved.

Complete blood count (CBC) is a blood test that helps determine the presence of an infection and is used as a baseline for assessment of bleeding as a complication of anticoagulation.

Nursing Care and Related Interventions

The major management objectives include the following: (1) to restore blood supply to the ischemic extremity; (2) to prevent the thrombus from detaching and traveling to the pulmonary vasculature; and, (3) to provide relief from pain and discomfort.

The nursing care of patients with superficial vein thrombosis or thrombophlebitis includes application of heat, elevation of the affected extremity to promote venous return, and administration of antiinflammatory agents. Antiinflammatory agents frequently used are phenylbutazone (Butazoladin) in a dose of 100 mg three to four times a day with meals or indomethacin (Indocin) in a dose of 25 to 50 mg four times a day with meals. Neither of these agents should be administered routinely in children under 14 years of age. Patients who do not have a fever or infection may be discharged from the emergency department and managed on an outpatient basis.

On the other hand, patients with deep vein thrombosis usually require hospitalization and bedrest to reduce the risk of pulmonary embolism. Hot compresses can be applied to the extremity to alleviate pain, in addition to administration of analgesics such as propoxyphene (Darvon) or acetaminophen (Tylenol). Elevation of the extremity is necessary to reduce edema and to decrease venous stasis by enhancing venous return. The administration of anticoagulants should be initiated immediately to arrest the growth of the clot. For adult patients, a bolus injection of 5,000 to 10,000 units of heparin intravenously is frequently ordered to ensure immediate anticoagulation. This loading dose is followed by a continuous intravenous infusion of 1,000 units/hour using an infusion pump. For children, the loading dose is 50 to 100 units per kilogram of body weight. This dose is followed by a continuous infusion of 25 units per kilogram per hour. Patients receiving heparin must have their partial thromboplastin time (PTT) measured to ensure adequate anticoagulation.

The PTT should be maintained at 1.5 to 2.5 that of the normal control. Anticoagulation therapy is required for several months after a thrombotic episode (Maschak, 1981). The major complication that can occur with anticoagulation is massive bleeding. Should massive bleeding on heparin occur, it is treated immediately by the intravenous administration of the heparin antagonist, protamine sulfate. A dose of 1 mg of protamine per 100 units of heparin in the circulating blood is necessary to reverse the anticoagulant effect of heparin.

The management of patients with arterial thrombosis depends on the threat to the viability of the involved extremity. Since irreversible tissue damage and necrosis can occur, immediate hospitalization and surgical intervention is necessary. Long-term anticoagulation with warfarin (Coumadin), an oral anticoagulant, occasionally is indicated.

EMBOLUS

An *embolus* is a clot composed of blood, fat, tissue, or bacteria that detaches from its place of origin, migrates within the arterial system, and causes obstruction to blood flow. Similar to an arterial thrombus, the embolic occlusion causes ischemia in the tissue distal to the obstruction, and necrosis will result unless intervention is implemented immediately.

Pathophysiology

An acute arterial embolism frequently originates in the heart and causes obstruction in a healthy artery. Embolic occlusion occurring in a cerebral, mesenteric, or peripheral artery may be due to one of several cardiac conditions. Mural thrombi developing in the left ventricle after a myocardial infarction can become detached and lodge in a major artery. Left atrial myxoma (primary tumor of the heart) is often a source of arterial embolism, if some of the tumor tissue detaches and travels through the systemic arterial circulation causing obstruction at some point. The stagnation of blood, sometimes occurring as a result of inadequate atrial emptying during atrial fibrillation and mitral stenosis, is a predisposition for thrombus and, hence, embolism. In bacterial endocarditis, fibrin and platelets that can adhere to the infected myocardium may become detached and embolize to any blood vessel. In addition to cardiac conditions, an atherosclerotic aneurysm of the abdominal aorta may cause embolic obstruction if a clot or cholesterol plaque breaks off and occludes a vessel (Isselbacher, 1980).

Clinical Manifestations

Signs and symptoms vary, depending on the location of the embolism and the severity of obstruction. Symptoms may not be manifested until the embolic mass completely obstructs blood flow. If the embolus occludes the cerebral artery, severe neurological deficits ensue. (This particular type of occlusion will be discussed later in the chapter.)

Peripheral embolism is characterized by an acute onset of pain with coldness and numbness (paresthesia) of the affected extremity. The extremity takes on a pale appearance and lacks palpable pulses. The absence of pulses is an important physical finding. The tissue may become gangrenous due to ischemia, unless intervention is implemented immediately.

Diagnostic Studies

Careful physical assessment is the key to identifying not only the site of embolization, but also the source. An arteriogram, however, is usually required to determine the location of an embolus. An electrocardiogram (ECG) is required to ensure that no related cardiac condition exists that might be the underlying cause of the embolus.

Nursing Care and Related Interventions

The goal of intervention is to restore the circulation as quickly as possible. Nursing measures include maintaining the extremity in a position of slight dependency and protecting it from trauma. Most patients are maintained on bed rest in the emergency department. Immediate anticoagulant therapy with intravenous (IV) heparin is initiated, and analgesics are given to relieve pain. The anticoagulant dosage for treatment of an embolus is the same as treatment for a thrombus.

Most acute arterial occlusions require embolectomy. An embolectomy involves insertion of a balloon (Fogarty) catheter into the involved artery. The catheter is passed beyond the embolus, and then the balloon is inflated. Withdrawal of the inflated balloon catheter removes the embolus and restores circulation to that area.

Once the acute episode has been treated, a thorough investigation regarding the primary source of embolism should be made (Armstrong, 1979).

Discharge Planning

Many patients may return to the emergency department with thromboembolic recurrence. These patients, therefore, must recognize the symptoms, such as warmth, pain, swelling, and discoloration of an extremity, that may indicate a recurrence and require medical attention.

Patients also must be informed of prophylactic measures to prevent recurrences. They should be instructed to elevate the extremity when sitting and to never dangle their legs. They should be cautioned against riding in cars or sitting with their legs in a dependent position for long periods of time. Elastic stockings should be worn and active exercises of the lower extremities performed if the patient is confined to bed for several days. Instruct patients not to wear girdles, garters, or socks with elasticized bands, because these constrict the circulation and encourage thrombosis (Rose, 1979; Tikoff and Prescott, 1979).

The nurse should instruct the patient to complete the entire course of anticoagulation therapy. Cooperation from the patient can be facilitated by his understanding of the necessity for taking the drug. Patients must know that bleeding is the most common complication of anticoagulant therapy, and, therefore, a periodic blood sample is required to monitor the patient's prothrombin time. Patients at high risk for bleeding include the elderly patient, the hypertensive patient, the ulcer patient, and obese people over 65 years old. All patients, but particularly patients at high risk, should be instructed to avoid the following activities: participating in sports, since injury from body contact or falls can traumatize skin tissue; taking aspirin, since it inhibits platelet function and increases the risk of bleeding; receiving intravenous fluids, injections, or arterial puncture; using straight razors; using toothbrushes with hard bristles; and going barefoot. Patients must be aware of other side effects from anticoagulation requiring medical attention, such as red/brown urine, red or black stools, excessive menstrual flow and bruises that enlarge. The complication of bleeding can often be avoided, however, through adequate patient education and conscientious maintenance of the prothrombin time (Maschak, 1981).

HYPERTENSIVE CRISIS

Hypertensive crisis occurs when blood pressure elevation poses an immediate risk to life or health. The settings in which a hypertensive crisis can occur include accelerated and malignant hypertension, hypertensive encephalopathy, pheochromocytoma, hypertension complicated by acute dissecting aortic aneurysm, hypertension associated with heart failure, pregnancy-induced hypertension, primary renal disease with rapidly deteriorating renal function, stroke, and myocardial infarction. Elevated diastolic blood pressures in the 120–140 range, however, are not necessarily congruous with a hypertensive crisis. Nevertheless, severely elevated arterial

HYPERTENSIVE CRISIS

pressure in the presence of life-threatening conditions constitutes a hypertensive emergency.

Accelerated and Malignant Hypertension

Accelerated hypertension commonly occurs as a result of uncontrolled essential hypertension in the patient who has diastolic pressures greater than 120 mm Hg and Grade III hypertensive retinopathy, characterized by hemorrhages and exudates on fundoscopic examination. If untreated, accelerated hypertension can progress to the malignant phase. *Malignant hypertension* exists when a patient demonstrates diastolic blood pressures in the 120–140 mm Hg range and has Grade IV retinopathy with hemorrhage, exudates, and papilledema in the eyegrounds. Grade I–IV hypertensive retinopathy is illustrated in Figure 13.1.

Pathophysiology
In malignant hypertension, the severely elevated arterial pressure causes damage to the endothelium of the arteries. This damage contributes to the adherence of platelets and deposition of fibrin on the endothelial surface. The subsequent lesion, known as *fibrinoid necrosis,* may involve all body organs, but is most often seen in the renal arterioles. When necrosis affects the kidneys, constriction of the renal arterioles occurs and causes renin to be released. Renin, in turn, causes increased formation of angiotension II, which raises the aldosterone level and causes severe vasoconstriction, further elevating the blood pressure (Moore, 1980).

Hemorrhage and exudates in the eyegrounds occur in response to severe arteriolar spasm in the ocular fundus.

Clinical Manifestations
Symptoms of malignant hypertension occur as a result of damage to the major body organs, that is, brain, eyes, heart, and kidneys. Diastolic blood pressure greater than 130–140 mm Hg is a common finding. Damage to cerebral arteries can cause severe vasospasm resulting in a headache and dizziness. Damage to the eyes results in visual impairment, in addition to hemorrhages, exudates, and papilledema in the eyegrounds. Cardiac involvement may be demonstrated by the onset of chest pain or palpitations. In addition, many patients have left ventricular failure and cardiomegaly complicating the malignant phase.

Diagnostic Studies
Fundoscopic findings of hemorrhages, exudates, and papilledema with the clinical picture of severely elevated blood pressure confirm the diagnosis of malignant hypertension. Laboratory tests, therefore, are done to determine target organ damage. Blood samples are routinely drawn to determine electrolytes, creatinine, urea nitrogen and uric acid levels. Patients with malignant hypertension will most probably have elevated blood urea nitrogen and creatinine levels reflecting damage to their kidneys. Urinalysis is necessary to test for protein (albumin), sedimentation, and electrolytes in the urine. In addition, the urinalysis often reveals red blood cells. A

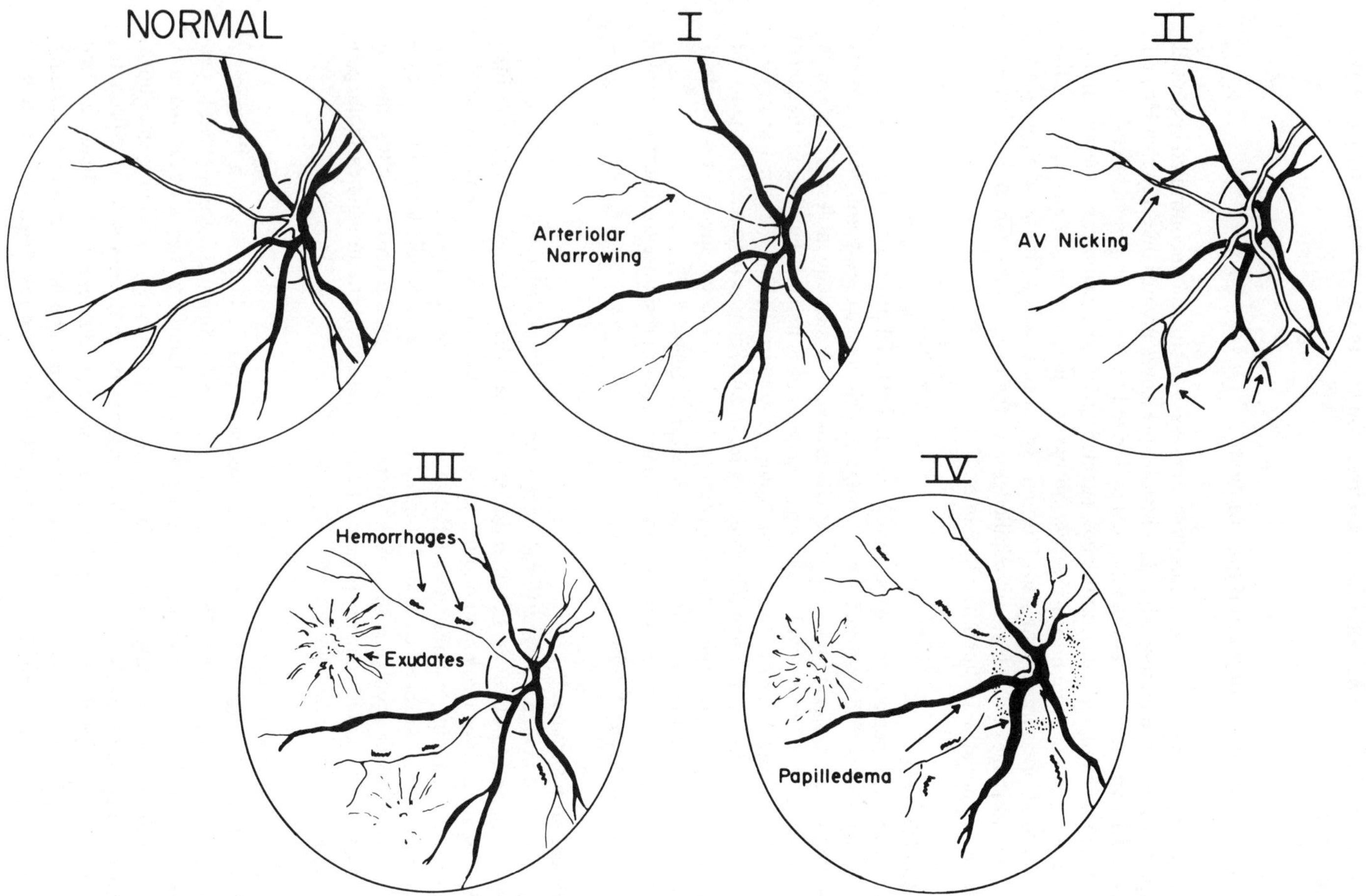

Figure 13.1 The grades of hypertensive retinopathy.

chest x-ray study provides information about the heart size. An ECG is ordered to determine whether cardiac abnormalities, specifically left-ventricular hypertrophy, exist.

Once the blood pressure has been controlled, and the malignant phase has subsided, further diagnostic studies may be performed to determine any underlying etiologies.

Nursing Care and Related Interventions

Malignant hypertension mandates prompt reduction of the blood pressure to reverse the malignant phase. These patients are considered medical emergencies and require hospitalization, bedrest, and intravenous medication to reduce their blood pressure. The two most reliable antihypertensive agents used to lower blood pressure are sodium nitroprusside (Nipride) and diazoxide (Hyperstat). Both of these intravenous vasodilators are capable of achieving an immediate blood pressure response. Diazoxide may be preferred in the emergency department, since it can be given as an intravenous bolus injection. Nitroprusside requires continuous intravenous infusion, using an infusion pump. This drug also deteriorates in light; therefore, the bottle must be wrapped in an opaque material such as aluminum foil. (For specific information about drugs, see Table 13.2.)

Patients presenting to the emergency department with severely elevated blood pressure readings without evidence of vascular damage may not require hospitalization. They are often treated with antihypertensive agents and then observed for several hours. The oral antihypertensive currently used in the emergency situation is clonidine (Catapres). The starting dose is 0.2 mg, followed by 0.1 mg every hour, until a blood pressure response is observed. The dosage should not exceed 0.6 mg. If the patient's blood pressure quickly responds to treatment, the person can be sent home with a prescription for oral antihypertensives and an appointment with his physician in a few days for follow-up care (Pascual, 1981; Finnerty, 1981).

Discharge Planning

Patients with hypertension who are discharged from the emergency department must be instructed regarding the importance of blood pressure control. They must realize that the absence of physical symptoms does not mean they are cured or even under adequate blood pressure control. They must understand that uncontrolled hypertension may progress to malignant hypertension with resultant damage to the brain, eyes, heart, or kidneys. The emergency department nurse must ascertain the patient's understanding of the medications and stress the importance of establishing and adhering to a daily schedule. Since most patients with hypertension are discharged on a diuretic, symptoms of hypokalemia should be explained to the patient. Potassium depletion is often manifested by muscular weakness, tingling, muscle spasm, and dizziness when standing. These symptoms suggest that the person's potassium level is low and that they should notify their physician for a potassium supplement, as well as begin eating foods rich in potassium, for example, bananas, peanuts, dried peas, or beans. The necessity of a sodium-restricted diet should be discussed, as well as the identification of high sodium foods, such as table salt, salt cured pork, celery, preprocessed meats, canned vegetables, soups, and dill

TABLE 13.2 Antihypertensive Medications Commonly Used in Hypertensive Emergencies

Drug & Action	Dosage	Advantages	Disadvantages	Indications for Use	Relative Contraindications
Diazoxide (Hyperstat). Directly relaxes the arteriolar smooth muscle, decreasing arteriolar resistance and BP. The lower arterial pressure activates the baroreceptor reflex, resulting in cardiac stimulation with increased heart rate and cardiac output.	Initially, 75 mg bolus IV in 10–15 sec. If no response, repeat the 75 mg bolus at 5–10 min intervals. The initial dose in children is 5 mg/kg of body weight infused over a 10-min period.	1. Rapid onset of action usually 3–5 min. Duration of action 2–24 hrs. 2. Does not require continuous monitoring or careful titration. 3. Lack of sedative side effects allows assessment of mental status.	1. Excessive hypotension can occur but is unlikely with this dosage regimen. 2. Causes fluid retention and may require addition of a potent diuretic such as furosemide. 3. Transient hyperglycemia. 4. In pregnancy can cause cessation of labor. 5. Associated with increased cardiac work (tachycardia and increased stroke volume).	1. Malignant hypertension 2. Hypertensive encephalopathy 3. Eclampsia 4. Severe HTN associated with acute glomerulonephritis 5. Renovascular hypertension	1. Dissecting aortic aneurysm 2. Patients with coronary insufficiency 3. Acute myocardial infarction 4. Diabetes

Drug	Dose	Comments	Indications	Contraindications
Nitroprusside (Nipride). Directly relaxes the smooth muscle of both arteries and veins resulting in a decrease in peripheral resistance and venous return.	0.1–10 µg/kg/min. Average dose is 3 µg/kg/min. This drug is packaged in a 50-mg vial that must be dissolved in 2–3 ml of D_5W and then placed in 250–500 ml of D_5W. 50 mg in 500 ml D_5W (= 100 µg/ml) 50 mg in 250 ml D_5W (= 200 µg/ml)	1. Onset of action is immediate. 2. Not associated with tachycardia. 3. Excessive hypotension can be reversed by slowing or stopping the infusion.	1. Requires continuous IV infusion and expert supervision. 2. Nitroprusside metabolizes to thiocyanate. Thiocyanate toxicity can occur. This requires (a) monitoring of thiocyanate concentrations (should not exceed 10 mg/ml); (b) monitoring patient for symptoms of toxicity—tinnitus, delirium, blurred vision, seizures, coma. 3. Deteriorates in light. Bottle must be wrapped in an opaque material and changed every 24 hours.	1. Malignant hypertension 2. Hypertensive encephalopathy 3. Acute pulmonary edema 4. Congestive heart failure 5. Acute hypertension associated with acute glomerulonephritis 6. Renovascular hypertension	1. Hepatic insufficiency 2. Eclampsia

TABLE 13.2 *(continued)*

Drug & Action	Dosage	Advantages	Disadvantages	Indications for Use	Relative Contraindications
Trimethaphan (Arfonad). Ganglionic blocking agent that blocks sympathetic impulses to arterioles, veins, and heart. Cardiac output is decreased directly and indirectly by decreased venous return and afterload.	Dose is titrated until BP control is achieved. The drug is prepared by mixing 500 mg in 1000 ml D_5W and infused slowly at 0.25–0.5 mg/min. An infusion rate as high as 6 mg/min may be necessary to achieve BP control.	1. Potent drug with onset of action in 3–4 min. 2. Hypotensive effect is reversed by stopping the infusion and placing the patient in Trendelenburg position. 3. Free of cardiac stimulation.	1. Requires careful monitoring of the infusion. 2. Short duration of action. 3. The effect is primarily orthostatic and therefore large doses are required to decrease BP in the supine position.	1. Malignant hypertension 2. Congestive heart failure 3. Dissecting aortic aneurysm 4. Hypertensive encephalopathy	Eclampsia
Phentolamine (Regitine). Alpha adrenergic blocking agent that blocks sympathetic impulse at alpha adrenergic receptor sites, resulting in vasodilatation and decreased BP.	0.5–1 mg intravenously by bolus injection every 5 min until BP control is achieved.		Has a short half-life and requires reinjection at 5–10 min intervals.	Pheochromocytoma	1. Angina 2. Coronary insufficiency

Drug	Dose	Comments	Indications	Side Effects/Cautions
Furosemide (Lasix). Potent diuretic that acts by enhancing renal excretion of fluid, thereby reducing blood volume and electrolytes.	Initially 20–40 mg intravenously.	1. May cause deafness in patients with impaired renal function. 2. May require incremental doses to achieve effect. 3. May cause hyperglycemia.	All hypertensive emergencies where fluid overload is a factor	1. Hypokalemia 2. Thiazide sensitivity
Hydralazine (Apresoline). Direct arteriolar vasodilator that reflexively increases heart rate and cardiac output.	20–40 mg IV or IM. Onset of action is 30 min after intramuscular injection and 10 min after intravenous injection.	1. Hypotension is rare. 2. Absence of sedation and somnolence.	Should not be used in patients with coronary insufficiency.	1. Accelerated hypertension 2. Eclampsia 3. Malignant hypertension 4. Hypertension associated with acute glomerulonephritis
				1. Dissecting aneurysm 2. Heart failure 3. Coronary insufficiency

pickles. Weight reduction, cessation of smoking and avoidance of stress should be emphasized.

These patients would probably benefit from a public health referral. The public health nurse can enhance and reinforce the emergency department nurse's teaching efforts, as well as evaluate the home situation, verify compliance, and determine factors that could precipitate blood pressure elevations.

Hypertensive Encephalopathy

Hypertensive encephalopathy is a syndrome characterized by abrupt, severe elevation of arterial pressure in the presence of neurological symptoms. This type of hypertensive crisis does not occur with any one particular type of hypertension and can potentially complicate any form of severe hypertension.

Pathophysiology
The primary pathologic findings in hypertensive encephalopathy are severe arterial spasm and cerebral edema. One theory postulates that the increased arterial pressure perhaps produces arterial spasm that, in turn, increases capillary permeability. Thus, fluid leaks from the capillaries into the tissues, and cerebral edema occurs. Another theory proposes that a disturbance in cerebral autoregulation causes increased cerebral vasoconstriction, with a decrease in cerebral blood flow (Pascual, 1981).

Clinical Manifestations
Clinical characteristics of patients with hypertensive encephalopathy include a diastolic blood pressure reading higher than 140 mm Hg with Grade IV retinopathy (hemorrhages, exudates, and papilledema), severe headache, and blurring of vision. Patients may also complain of nausea and vomiting. Some patients experience transient neurological deficits, such as hemiparesis or aphasia. Disorientation and confusion are present and may progress to a coma. Convulsions are likely to occur in children with encephalopathy.

Diagnostic Studies
A rapid response of blood pressure to antihypertensive treatment suggests encephalopathy. *Brain computerized tomography scan* (CT) may be ordered, and it is useful in differentiating encephalopathy from cerebral infarction or hemorrhage. A *lumbar puncture* may also be done to ascertain cerebral involvement. Cerebrospinal fluid is clear in patients with encephalopathy and bloody in patients with cerebral hemorrhage. Most diagnostic tests are deferred until the blood pressure is controlled. A detailed evaluation of underlying causes, of course, is necessary.

Nursing Care and Related Interventions
The goal of intervention is the immediate reduction in blood pressure to ameliorate the symptoms and to arrest damage to body organs. This intervention is accomplished through hospitalization of the patient in an intensive care unit and through administration of parenteral vasodilators, such as diazoxide or nitroprusside. (For more specific information, see Table 13.2.) A potent diuretic, such as furosemide

(Lasix), can be given in conjunction with these agents, because they have sodium and water retaining properties.

The primary problem with aggressive therapy of patients with encephalopathy is underperfusion of the cerebral vessels, thus increasing the risk of thrombosis. These patients, therefore, require meticulous monitoring of their blood pressure to prevent severe hypotension. The goal diastolic blood pressure should be 90–100 mm Hg in all patients, except in pregnant women and in children whose diastolic blood pressure should be maintained in the 60–70 mm Hg range. Since these patients have alterations in their mental status, neurological checks should be made to determine improvement or regression of symptoms.

Pheochromocytoma

A pheochromocytoma is a tumor usually located in the adrenal medulla, but it may be found anywhere along the sympathetic nerve chain. This tumor releases excessive amounts of catecholamines, resulting in episodic hypertension that reaches life-threatening levels.

Pathophysiology
The elevated arterial pressure in the presence of a pheochromocytoma results from excessive release of epinephrine and norepinephrine. These hormones stimulate the alpha adrenergic receptors in the arterioles, resulting in constriction and increased vascular resistance. These hormones also stimulate the beta adrenergic receptors in the myocardium and cause tachydysrhythmias.

Clinical Manifestations
Because the catecholamine hypersecretion can be intermittent, the symptoms can occur episodically. Characteristically the patient presents with the sudden onset of hypertension accompanied by complaints of headache, palpitations (tachycardia), excessive perspiration, and cold, clammy skin.

Diagnostic Studies
Twenty-four-hour urine collections for vanilmandelic acid (VMA), catecholamines, and metanephrines are necessary in establishing the diagnosis. If the patient, however, voids in the emergency department, the urine should be saved. In addition, a computerized tomography (CT) scan of the abdomen may help to localize the tumor(s). After the blood pressure has been controlled, more invasive tests, such as adrenal vein sampling, may be done.

Nursing Care and Related Interventions
Patients should be hospitalized to control the hypertension and paroxysmal symptoms and to reduce the risk of possible complications. Immediate blood pressure reduction can be achieved through using an alpha adrenergic blocking drug, such as phentolamine (Regitine) or phenoxybenzamine (Dibenzyline). Phentolamine is given at a dose of 0.5–1 mg intravenous bolus. Phenoxybenzamine is an oral alpha blocker given most often at a dose of 10–120 mg daily in two to four divided doses. Beta

adrenergic blockers may be used concomitantly to control dysrhythmias, but are used after alpha adrenergic blockers are given to prevent increasing the blood pressure when the beta blocker is used alone. The beta blocker propranolol (Inderal) often is used in the dose range of 40–320 mg daily in two to four divided doses.

Patients presenting to the emergency department with the probable diagnosis of a pheochromocytoma should be admitted to the hospital for a thorough evaluation.

Hypertension Complicated by Acute Dissecting Aortic Aneurysm

Long-standing, severe hypertension and atherosclerosis can weaken the arterial muscle wall and further stretch and thin the elastic tissues of the arteries, producing dilatation—a condition known as an *aneurysm*. With each heart beat, blood is pumped not only through the artery, but also through the dilated portion, decreasing the ability of the arteries to contract. An aneurysm that threatens to rupture or dissect produces an emergency situation (Pascual, 1981).

Severe elevated arterial pressure can cause progression of the dissection, rupture, and death. Immediately reducing the blood pressure, therefore, is necessary. Trimethaphan (Arfonad) is the preferred drug, because it reduces the force of blood across the aorta. Moreover, the combination of propranolol and nitroprusside has also been used successfully. (See Table 13.2 for information regarding dosage.) (Clinical manifestations of acute dissecting aortic aneurysm and appropriate interventions are discussed in detail in Chapter 14.)

Hypertension Associated with Heart Failure

Patients with acute severe hypertension may develop hypertrophy of the left ventricle. When hypertrophy occurs, the pumping ability of the left ventricle is reduced, subsequently resulting in left-ventricular failure and pulmonary edema. Prompt reduction of the blood pressure is necessary to reverse the symptoms of pulmonary edema. Potent diuretics, such as furosemide (Lasix) or metolazone (Zaroxlyn), are given to reduce the total blood volume. In addition, antihypertensive agents, such as trimethaphan and nitroprusside, also are indicated, because they decrease the venous return, but do not increase the cardiac workload. Associated left-ventricular failure often results from inadequately controlled blood pressure. It can be prevented, therefore, if patients adhere to their therapeutic regimens (Finnerty, 1981). (See Chapter 8 for a further discussion of heart failure.)

Pregnancy–Induced Hypertension

Preeclampsia occurs during the last trimester of pregnancy and is manifested by severe arterial pressure, edema, and proteinuria. If untreated, the process may progress to eclampsia, which occurs when the patient develops a convulsion. Neurological signs in eclampsia are similar to those occurring with hypertensive encephalopathy. The pathophysiology of eclampsia is unclear. Management of these patients is aimed at reducing blood pressure, prevention of convulsions, and termination of pregnancy (Finnerty, 1981). (This condition is discussed in detail in Chapter 30.)

Hypertension Associated with Primary Renal Disease with Rapidly Deteriorating Renal Function

Most patients with renal insufficiency eventually develop hypertension. Hypertension probably results from the retention of sodium and water that expands extracellular fluid volume. Secretion of renin in primary renal disease can also result in sustained hypertension at crisis levels.

The goal of intervention is reduction of blood pressure, without further compromise of the kidney function. Intervention is often difficult, because reducing blood pressure also reduces kidney perfusion pressure and may cause kidney failure. Methyldopa (Aldomet), propranolol, and hydralazine (Apresoline) can be used to reduce the blood pressure gradually in these patients. The dosage prescribed for these antihypertensives varies, but should fall within the following ranges: methyldopa–250 to 2000 mg per day; propranolol–20 to 320 mg per day; and hydralazine–10 to 200 mg per day. Patients who have hypertensive retinopathy with deteriorating renal function require a more rapid reduction in blood pressure and, hence, larger dosages of these medications (Moore, 1980).

Strokes

A cerebrovascular accident can precipitate a hypertensive emergency, but, most often, hypertension occurring in association with a stroke results from chronic, essential, uncontrolled hypertension. In this condition the blood pressure must be lowered slowly to prevent ischemia of brain tissue and further progression of the stroke.

Myocardial Infarction

Elevated diastolic blood pressure in patients suffering from an acute myocardial infarction can cause extension of the infarction. Reduction of the blood pressure must occur promptly. (Chapter 10 discusses the nursing care and related interventions for a patient experiencing a myocardial infarction.)

CEREBROVASCULAR ACCIDENT

An impairment in the cerebral blood supply, whether from an embolus, thrombus, or hemorrhage, causes a cerebrovascular accident or stroke and initiates an emergency situation. Cerebrovascular disease is currently the third leading cause of death in the United States. Each year more than a half a million Americans are victims of a cerebrovascular accident. Early recognition of certain factors known to increase the occurrence of stroke and their prompt reduction could significantly reduce the incidence of stroke. These risk factors include hypertension (the greatest risk factor), cardiac abnormalities, and dysrhythmias or existing cerebral occlusive disease evident by transient ischemic attacks. The more risk factors a person has, the greater the possibility that cerebrovascular disease and stroke will occur (O'Brien and Pallett, 1980).

Each condition leading to cerebrovascular accidents will be discussed in detail. Although the pathophysiology of each condition is different, the clinical manifestations, with the exception of onset, are similar. Because the development of neurological deficits varies, information regarding time of onset, progression of symptoms, and premonitory symptoms is useful for establishing whether a stroke is evolving or has been completed, as well as for selecting the appropriate interventions to initiate.

Transient Ischemic Attacks

Pathophysiology
Prior to the development of the cerebrovascular accident, 50 percent of the victims will experience a *transient ischemic attack* (TIA). These attacks are temporary, focal symptoms that often preface a more severe neurological deficit and require immediate evaluation and treatment to prevent progression to a completed stroke.

Transient ischemic attacks occur when cholesterol/platelet emboli, originating from an atherosclerotic plaque, produce symptoms of inadequate cerebral circulation. Symptoms include weakness or paralysis, parethesias, speech disturbances, and partial or complete loss of vision in one or both eyes. The onset of a TIA is rapid, and the duration rarely exceeds 30 minutes, with full recovery within 24 hours (O'Brien and Pallett, 1980; Byer and Caston, 1980).

Nursing Care and Related Interventions
Intervention is directed toward halting the occurrence of attacks and toward preventing progression to cerebral infarction. These goals can be accomplished by anticoagulation therapy, antiplatelet therapy, or by surgical endarterectomy.

Since stroke prevention is a primary concern, nursing care should include adequate education for the patient and his family prior to leaving the emergency department. The patient must understand that anticoagulant therapy, antiplatelet therapy, antihypertensive therapy, dietary cholesterol restriction, cessation of smoking, and carotid endarterectomy can reduce transient ischemic attacks and prevent strokes. Furthermore, the patient should also be informed that symptoms, such as visual, auditory, or sensory disturbances, headaches, or seizures, may indicate that a TIA is recurring and will require medical attention. The emergency department nurse must procure a follow-up appointment for the patient with the patient's primary care physician, prior to the patient's discharge from the emergency department. The importance of keeping the appointment, as well as the need for monitoring one's blood pressure and prothrombin time, should be stressed (O'Brien and Pallett, 1980).

Cerebral Thrombosis

Pathophysiology
Thrombosis, the primary cause of cerebral occlusion, is often associated with atherosclerotic disease. A thrombosis may develop in one of the cerebral hemispheres causing ischemia, which produces neurological deficits in the opposite side of the body, because the right cerebral hemisphere governs the left side of the body, and vice versa. Thrombus formation most frequently occurs in either the right or left internal carotid artery. Other common sites of origin include the middle cerebral artery near the corpus collosum, as well as in the vertebral and basilar arteries (O'Brien and Pallett, 1980).

The clinical picture may vary depending on the location of the thrombus and on the amount of tissue involved. Symptoms may develop slowly during a period of several days. The slow onset is attributed to the gradual ischemia occurring with the thrombus formation. This type of stroke is preceded by transient ischemic attacks, and the primary symptoms resemble a TIA—for instance, transient aphasia, hemiplegia, or paresthesia to half of the body, which may progress to paralysis. Strokes from cerebral thrombosis often occur during sleep or soon after awakening.

Cerebral Embolus

Pathophysiology
Embolism, the second most common cause of cerebrovascular accidents, is primarily related to heart disease. When embolic material, usually from a thrombus within the heart, detaches and lodges in a cerebral blood vessel, ischemia and stroke will occur. Heart conditions that can lead to cerebral embolism include atrial fibrillation, bacterial endocarditis, myocardial infarction, mural thrombus, rheumatic endocarditis, and congenital heart disease (O'Brien and Pallett, 1980).

The onset of symptoms in a cerebral embolic stroke is sudden, with no warning signals. Clinical manifestations frequently include weakness, hemiplegia, aphasia, and visual impairment in a person who is awake and active. The exact neurological deficits, however, will depend on the area of brain affected by the embolic occlusion. Brainstem involvement, for instance, causes changes in the level of consciousness, and left hemisphere involvement results in aphasia. Patients with cerebral embolism can often be differentiated from patients with thrombosis by the sudden onset of symptoms and by the previous history of cardiovascular disease.

Cerebral Hemorrhage

Pathophysiology
The third cause of a stroke, cerebral hemorrhage, accounts for about 10 percent of all strokes. This type of stroke occurs most often in hypertensive patients who are either untreated or inadequately treated. The rupture of a cerebral blood vessel in the presence of existing hypertension causes a cerebral hemorrhage. Bleeding into the tissue occurs and results in compression and displacement of brain tissue. If vital

centers are compressed, coma, and eventually death, will occur. The most common site of origin for cerebral hemorrhage is the putamen. Hemorrhage, however, also can occur in the thalamus, cerebellum, and brainstem (O'Brien and Pallett, 1980).

Clinical manifestations will depend on the location and on the severity of the hemorrhage. Most patients suddenly develop headaches and nuchal rigidity, accompanied by vomiting, vertigo, and ataxia. Changes in the patient's level of consciousness will occur as the hemorrhage becomes worse.

Diagnostic Studies

Diagnostic tests are performed in stroke patients to determine the underlying etiology. The following diagnostic studies are commonly performed.

Computerized tomography (CT) scan, a noninvasive test, is useful in confirming the size and location of a cerebral infarction or hemorrhage. The procedure for the test involves placing the patient's head in the scanning unit, and then scanning the head and making several pictures of the brain tissue. Cerebral infarctions may not be identified for several days, while hemorrhages are identified immediately (Fischbach, 1980).

Four-vessel arteriogram, a radiographic study of the cerebral vessels, is useful in confirming an obstruction in either one or both of the internal carotid arteries.

Electroencephalogram measures and records electrical impulses in the brain. Although an electroencephalogram is sometimes used in diagnosing cerebral infarcts and hemorrhages, its findings are not always valuable. Alterations in the brain wave pattern occur in patients with large superficial lesions, but may not occur in patients with small, deep, vascular lesions.

An electrocardiogram is often ordered and is used to determine cardiac rhythm disturbance or recent myocardial infarction. These findings suggest that the cerebral infarction may be embolic in origin.

Lumbar puncture for the purpose of examining cerebrospinal fluid may be done. This test is particularly indicated whenever a question of subarachnoid hemorrhage exists, or if the diagnosis is uncertain. Extreme caution should be used in lumbar puncture to prevent brain herniation.

Nursing Care and Related Interventions

The acute care of a stroke patient presenting to the emergency department will be the same, regardless of etiology. In an unconscious or semiconscious stroke patient, the first priority is establishing a patent airway. The nursing care then can be directed toward providing the following supportive measures: (1) maintenance of an adequate airway; (2) prevention of aspiration by positioning the patient in a semiprone position; (3) administration of oxygen therapy in cyanotic patients; (4) placement of electrodes for cardiac monitoring; and, (5) insertion of catheters to administer intravenous fluids. The nurse must also perform neurological checks to assess changes in the level of consciousness, ability to move, pupillary response, and vital signs (Luckmann and Sorensen, 1980).

An increase in the intracranial pressure may occur after a cerebrovascular accident; therefore, the nurse must also observe and monitor the patient for signs of increased intracranial pressure. Early signs are lethargy or change in the level of responsiveness, accompanied by headache, nausea, and projectile vomiting. As the cerebral pressure increases, later signs include bradycardia, decreased respirations, papilledema, hyperthermia, and an elevation in the systolic blood pressure.

The blood pressure of stroke patients should be maintained at slightly higher than normal levels to ensure adequate cerebral perfusion. The systolic blood pressure should be between 150 and 180 mm Hg, and the diastolic between 95 and 110 mm Hg.

The two goals of intervention in stroke patients are to decrease the size of the infarcted tissue area and to increase the oxygen supply to the infarcted tissue. The medications often used to treat stroke patients include cerebral vasodilators that improve cerebral blood flow, barbiturates to reduce cerebral metabolic demands, and steroids and osmotic diuretics to reduce cerebral edema (Neubaur, 1980).

Anticoagulants may be used to treat stroke patients, only after the diagnosis of a cerebral hemorrhage has been eliminated.

The cerebral vascular accident and resulting neurological deficits often require approximately three weeks to stabilize. Most patients are hospitalized during this period, and treatment includes preventing complications of immobility and providing rehabilitative measures to assist the patient's recovery.

CONCLUSION

All the cardiovascular conditions previously discussed may constitute emergencies that could probably be prevented. Early recognition of and intervention into risk factors that predispose a patient to thrombus, embolus, hypertensive crisis, or cerebrovascular accident may reduce the probability of occurrence. Assessment and intervention in the immediate emergency situation begins with the triage nurse. Appropriate and effective nursing assessment and care must continue throughout the patient's stay in the emergency department and during the convalescent period to prevent complications and disabilities and to provide the patient with the highest quality of care possible.

BIBLIOGRAPHY

Armstrong, M. D., et al., eds.: *McGraw-Hill Handbook of Clinical Nursing*. New York: McGraw-Hill, 1979, pp. 812–823.

Becker, C. E., and N. L. Benowitz: Hypertensive emergencies. *Medical Clinicians of North America* 63:127–138 (1979).

Bloom, A. L., and D. P. Thomas eds.: *Haemostasis and Thrombosis*, New York: Churchill Livingstone, 1981.

Byer, J. A., and J. D. Caston: Therapy of ischemic cerebrovascular disease. *Annals of Internal Medicine* 93:742–756 (1980).

Douglas, A.: Venous thrombosis: a disease of hospitals. *Nursing Mirror* 147:44–46 (1978).

Finnerty, F.: Treatment of hypertensive emergencies. *Heart and Lung* 10:275–283 (1981).

Fischbach, F.: *A Manual of Laboratory Diagnostic Tests*. Philadelphia: Lippincott, 1980.

Hartshorn, J. C.: Hypertensive crisis. *Nursing 80*: 37–45 (1980).

Isselbacher, K. J., et al., eds.: *Harrison's Principles of Internal Medicine*. New York: McGraw-Hill, 1980.

Joist, J. H., and L. A. Sherman eds.: *Venous and Arterial Thrombosis: Pathogenesis, Diagnosis, Prevention and Therapy*. New York: Grune & Stratton, 1978.

Luckman, J., and K. Sorensen: *Medical Surgical Nursing*. Philadelphia: Saunders, 1980.

Maschak, C. B., and K. Moore: Anticoagulation therapy. *Critical Care Update* 8:5–13 (1981).

Mendlowitz, M.: Management of hypertensive emergencies. *Hospital Medicine* 15:63–71 (1979).

Moore, M.: Hypertensive emergencies. *American Family Physician* 21:141–146 (1980).

Neubaur, R. E.: Hyperbaric oxygenation as an adjunct therapy in strokes due to thrombosis. *Stroke* 11:297 (1980).

O'Brien, M. T., and P. J. Pallett: *Total Care of the Stroke Patient*. Boston: Little, Brown, 1980.

Pascual, A. V.: Hypertensive crisis: diagnosis and strategies in treatment. *Hospital Medicine* 11:43–59 (1981).

Price, S. A., and L. M. Wilson: *Pathophysiology–Clinical Concepts of Disease Processes*. New York: McGraw-Hill, 1982.

Rose, S. D.: Prophylaxis of thromboembolic disease. *Medical Clinicians of North America* 63:1205–1219 (1979).

Sharnoff, J. G.: *Prevention of Venous Thrombosis and Pulmonary Embolism*. Boston: Hall, 1980.

Tikoff, G., and S. M. Prescott: Axioms on thrombophlebitis and phlebothrombosis. *Hospital Medicine* 15:36–59 (1979).

14

Abdominal Pain

Barbara Knezevich

After completing this chapter, the reader will be able to do the following:

1. Triage a patient experiencing abdominal pain.
2. Discuss common causes of abdominal pain.
3. Discuss clinical manifestations, diagnostic studies, and nursing care of patients experiencing abdominal pain.
4. Identify appropriate discharge planning activities for the patient experiencing abdominal pain.

Abdominal pain is associated with a variety of illnesses. Causes observed most frequently in the pediatric patient include the following:

Lead poisoning.
Sickle-cell disease.

Causes more frequently observed in the adult patient include the following:

Inferior wall myocardial infarction.
Narcotic withdrawal.
Peritonitis.
Lobar pneumonia.
Renal colic.
Diabetic ketoacidosis.

The problem may be as simple as constipation or as complex and serious as an aneurysm. (See Chapter 25 for more detailed information regarding pediatric abdominal pain.)

TRIAGE

Subjective Data

Subjective information should be obtained from the patient and from family members. Since abdominal pain frequently is mistriaged, the nurse must collect all available information carefully. The patient should be asked to describe the following:

Onset of pain—whether gradual or sudden.
Intensity of pain—does it come and go; is it crampy; does it exist all of the time?
Severity of pain.
The movement of the pain, if any.
Conditions that aggravate or intensify the pain, such as walking, eating, or lying down.
What seems to relieve the pain, if anything.
Any changes in eating habits.
Time of last meal.
Any previous abdominal problems.
History of fever.
Epigastric discomfort, if any.
Loss of appetite.
Foods that cause abdominal pain.
Change in bowel habits.
Abnormal menstrual cycle.
Cervical discharge.
Past medical history.
Any allergies to food, medication, and so forth.

(Table 14.1 identifies areas of pain and possible related illnesses.)

Objective Data

Examination of the abdomen should begin with inspection, followed by auscultation, percussion, and palpation. The examiner should take a few moments to inspect the abdomen for the following:

Contour.
Scars.
Visible masses.
Engorged veins.
Visible peristalsis.

TABLE 14.1 Areas of Pain and Related Illnesses

Right Costal Margin—Five cm Right of the Sternum	Four cm Above The Umbilicus
Acute cholecystitis	Appendicitis (early)
Acute pyelonephritis	Acute pancreatitis
	Acute intestinal obstruction
Right Hypogastric Region	Acute gastritis
Appendicitis	Coronary occlusion
Duodenal ulcer	**Four cm Below The Umbilicus**
Pyelonephritis	Obstruction/transverse colon
Acute pancreatitis	
Meckel's diverticulitis	**Left Costal Margin**
Acute cholecystitis	Splenic rupture
Left Hypogastric Region	
Diverticulitis of colon	
Cancer of colon	

Old scars will appear silvery, while recent scars are pink or blue. Striae or stretching occurs most commonly in the abdomen. In normal skin, stretching causes rupture of the elastic fibers in the reticular layer of the cutis. Bluish purple scars are usually seen with a distention of the abdomen in pregnancy, obesity, and ascites.

A pulsating abdomen may be due to an aneurysm. Distention of the lower abdomen could be due to an ovarian tumor or to a distended urinary bladder. The skin should be observed, and its color noted. Both jaundice and icterus color the skin yellow. The patient should be asked to describe whether the following symptoms exist:

Inability to void.

Blood in the urine.

Flank pain.

Flank tenderness.

A change in the color of urine.

A change in the odor of urine.

A history of urinary tract infections.

Auscultation is the next step in assessing abdominal pain. An abdominal aneurysm is indicated by turbulent blood flow, such as the murmur heard in an aortic aneurysm. The abdomen should be auscultated for peristaltic sounds. The diaphragm of the stethoscope is placed on the abdomen below the umbilicus. If bowel sounds are not heard immediately, it is advisable to listen for five minutes. When listening for bowel sounds, start at the right of the umbilicus and listen carefully for two to five minutes in each of the four quadrants.

Normal bowel sounds are high-pitched, gurgling noises. Bowel sounds vary in frequency, depending on the presence or absence of food in the gastrointestinal tract.

It is significant when there are no sounds or extremely loud sounds. Decreased bowel sounds indicate inhibition of mobility, and increased bowel sounds may result from gastroenteritis or from a laxative.

The examiner should next percuss the abdomen to detect the following:

Masses.
Fluid.
Gaseous distention.
Solid structures.

Solid organs or masses will sound dull, whereas tympany will be heard over the bowel. Percussion of the liver, spleen, and stomach will give the examiner vital data that may indicate any abnormality.

Light abdominal palpation helps to evaluate major organs in the abdominal cavity. Light palpation will also identify areas of tenderness and areas of increased resistance or guarding. By identifying areas of tenderness, the examiner can perhaps avoid producing pain that would result in voluntary rigidity of abdominal muscles that could interfere with further investigation.

All four quadrants of the abdomen should be examined. Rebound tenderness (Blumberg's sign) is elicited when the examiner gently presses the fingers into the abdomen in an area away from the tenderness, and then suddenly withdraws the fingers. The transmission of pain is a reverse response to stimulus palpation. Rebound tenderness may be a sign of peritoneal inflammation.

Pain, its location, duration, and quality is commonly a diagnostic key. Pain may travel or change location, such as in appendicitis in which pain is felt first in the epigastrium and later in the right lower quadrant. Acute abdomen, a term used to describe a variety of disorders, is usually not associated with chronic diseases. The sudden onset of pain, however, may be due to an acute phase of a chronic illness.

Assessment and Planning

After both the subjective and objective data have been collected and analyzed, a nursing diagnosis identifying all patient problems is made, and a plan for care is established and prioritized. Most patients with abdominal pain are triaged to the surgical service and allowed to wait in the waiting room. Exceptions include patients with signs of shock or patients exhibiting signs of unbearable pain. (Table 14.2 includes two examples of triage notes for patients experiencing abdominal pain.)

SPECIFIC DISEASES CAUSING ABDOMINAL PAIN

Urinary Tract Infections

The urinary tract system is responsible for maintaining and regulating both the fluid volume and the electrolyte composition and for excreting metabolic wastes. Compo-

SPECIFIC DISEASES CAUSING ABDOMINAL PAIN

TABLE 14.2 Examples of Triage Notes for Patients Experiencing Abdominal Pain

S: 10 yo BF with c/o leg pain, lower midabdominal pain and back pain for approximately 1 hour prior to admission. "I've had this pain one other time, but not this bad." PMH: negative, NKA, no urinary complaints, normal bowel habits, c/o fever of 100°F.

O: Pale, diaphoretic, appears to be in extreme pain. T 104°F, knees curled up in fetal position.

A: Acute abdominal pain, R/O sickle-cell disease.

P: Pediatric evaluation, admit to examination room immediately.

S: 43 yo WF with c/o lower abdominal pain for 24 hours with burning on urination. Bowel habits and menstrual cycle normal. Pain is increased during urination and sexual intercourse. No cervical discharge. c/o low-grade fever 99–100°F, no blood in urine, c/o strong odor to urine.

O: Skin warm to touch, T 101°F, skin color slightly flushed, bowel sounds normal, c/o moderate pain during palpation of lower abdomen.

A: Abdominal pain, R/O UTI.

P: Medical evaluation, admit to examination room as soon as possible.

---

sition of body fluid, waste, and electrolytes is controlled by the kidneys. Furthermore, the kidney is also responsible for maintaining acid-base balance within the body. Collectively, the ureters, bladder, and urethra serve to filter, secrete, and eliminate waste products.

Pathophysiology

Dysuria, or painful urination, is usually a sign of a *urinary tract infection*. The patient frequently will complain of burning on urination. Frequency and urgency to void often accompany dysuria. Low-grade fever (100°F) and fatigue may be present. Examination of the urine may reveal clear, cloudy, or purulent urine.

Changes in micturition, such as hematuria (red blood cells in urine), are serious symptoms. The color of the bloody urine is determined by the pH. Acidic urine is dark and smoky, while alkaline urine is red. Moreover, hematuria can also be caused by a systemic blood dyscrasia, anticoagulent therapy, or neoplasm.

The examining emergency department nurse must obtain the most complete history that is possible. The symptom of pain does not always indicate a severe form of urinary tract disease. Pain in the flank and lower abdomen, radiating to the testis or labium, may be kidney stones. Painless hematuria, however, may indicate neoplasm in the urinary tract.

Proteinuria, also called albuminuria, is an excess of serum proteins in the urine. Urine normally does not contain protein in any significant amount. Proteinuria is characteristically seen more frequently in glomerulonephritis, rather than in pyelonephritis. Because albumin and globulin are released through the damaged glomerular capillaries in huge amounts, they cannot be reabsorbed in the tubules. Mild proteinuria may be seen in urethritis, prostatitis, and cystitis.

TABLE 14.3 Sources of Urinary Tract Infections

Structure	Source
Kidney	Incompetence of the uretervisical valve causes regurgitation of urine into the ureter
Bladder	Bacteria ascending from the urethra
Prostate	Ascending urethral flora
Urethra	Ascending bacteria

A structural abnormality, causing obstruction and slowing of urinary flow, results in urine stasis, which makes the kidneys more susceptible to bacterial infection and to abdominal discomfort. Other causes include the following:

Neurogenic bladder dysfunction.
Diagnostic testing.
Presence of foreign body, for example, indwelling catheter, stone.
Diseases of blood vessels, for example, diabetes mellitus, arteriosclerosis.
Lowered body resistance.

(See Table 14.3 for possible sources of urinary tract infections.)
Cystitis is an infection of the lower urinary tract involving the bladder, while *urethritis* is an infection of the urethra. Acute infections are usually caused by *Escherichia coli*. Cystitis is more common in women than in men, due to the length of the urethra and the anatomic proximity to the vagina and periurethral glands. Cystitis often occurs 36 to 72 hours after sexual intercourse.
Pyelonephritis is a bacterial infection associated with upper urinary tract infections. Pyelonephritis can be caused by the following:

Urinary obstruction.
Ureterovesical reflux.
Pregnancy.
Renal disease.
Trauma.
Metabolic disorders.

The infection usually begins in the lower urinary tract and progresses into the renal pelvis, tubules, and interstitial tissue of one or possibly both kidneys. A gram-negative enteric bacillus is usually responsible for the infection. An acute pyelonephritis is characterized by fever, chills, shaking, and pain in the costrovertebral region or flank. Chronic pyelonephritis has a typically insidious onset, caused by chronic renal insufficiency.

Clinical Manifestations
Symptoms of urinary tract infections may include the following:

SPECIFIC DISEASES CAUSING ABDOMINAL PAIN

Fatigue.
Headache.
Loss of appetite.
Weight loss.
Excessive thirst/polyuria.

Clinically, the patient will present with the following symptoms:

Dysuria.
Urgency.
Burning on urination.
Chills.
Fever.

Other presenting signs and symptoms may include the following:

Gastrointestinal disturbances.
Ileus.
Flank pain radiating to the groin.
Suprapubic pain.
Hematuria.

Diagnostic Studies
Diagnostic evaluation should include roentgenography, cystoscopy, and various laboratory studies. A flate plate and KUB (kidney, ureters, bladder) x-ray studies are made as a baseline and to visualize the size and shape of organ structures. Radiopaque urinary stones will be visible with these x-ray examinations. An intravenous infusion of a contrast material will produce opacification of the renal parenchyma and will completely fill the urinary tract. X-ray films are taken at several different intervals to study the filled and distended collective system.

A third diagnostic x-ray study used to evaluate the urinary tract system is the intravenous pyelogram (IVP). A radiopaque contrast media is introduced intravenously to visualize the kidneys, ureter, and bladder. The IVP is used to identify suspected urinary problems. The emergency department nurse should be careful not to overhydrate the patient, because dilution of contrast material can cause poor visualization.

In administering any invasive test, the emergency department nurse must check carefully to ensure that the patient is not allergic to the materials used during a diagnostic procedure. Emergency drugs should be available immediately to treat an anaphylactic reaction.

Another method used to evaluate urinary function is the retrograde pyelograph. An injection of opaque material is introduced through the ureteral catheter and passes up through the ureters into the renal pelvis. This test is used frequently in acute situations in which a nonfunctioning kidney is suspected.

Cystoscopy is the visualization of the urinary bladder with an instrument called a cystoscope. A cystoscopic examination is used to inspect the bladder for ulcer, tumors, or stones. This instrument can also be used to remove urinary stones from the urethra, bladder, and ureter. The emergency department nurse must force fluids to ensure a continuous flow of urine and to allow for the collection of a specimen during the procedure, if necessary.

Children are usually given general anesthesia for this procedure, since manipulation can be painful. A sedative, such as diazepam (Valium), and a narcotic, such as morphine sulfate or meperidine hydrochloride (Demerol), are usually administered one hour prior to examination.

Urine should be collected to identify the location and nature of the inflammatory process. A urinalysis and culture and sensitivity are performed to identify abnormalities and to establish a tentative diagnosis. The patient should be instructed to cleanse the meatus prior to collecting the urine in a clean container. The female patient is instructed to separate the labia and expose the urethral orifice. The area is then cleansed with an antiseptic solution. Urine is allowed to flow freely, and a midstream specimen is obtained in a clean container.

A multiple-glass test may be performed on the male patient. After the meatus is cleansed with an antiseptic solution, three specimens are collected. The first sample should contain any waste or sediment from the urethra and a sample of organisms that might be found. The second specimen is collected without stopping the stream and should contain organisms from the bladder and kidney. The patient will then stop voiding, and the prostate is massaged. The third specimen collected should contain secretions from the prostate. Each specimen should contain at least 100 ml of urine.

Nursing Care and Related Interventions
Nursing care should include identifying factors that contribute to the development of urinary tract infections. The patient should be made as comfortable as possible, and all procedures are explained prior to testing.

One medication prescribed for urinary tract infections, Pyridium, will turn the urine orange-red. The emergency department nurse should explain this occurrence to the patient to avoid alarming the person. Pyridium (phenazopyridine hydrochloride), excreted in the urine, exerts a topical analgesic effect on the mucosa of the urinary tract. This action helps to relieve pain, burning, urgency, and frequency. An antibiotic, such as Gantrisin, may also be perscribed, depending on the results of the urine culture. Normally 24 hours are required to obtain results from a urine culture. Sulfonamides are effective in the treatment of a urinary tract infection.

The patient should be encouraged by the emergency department nurse to increase his fluid intake to at least 2 to 3 l per day, unless contraindicated.

Discharge Planning
Patient education should include identifying precipitating factors, explaining drug therapy and the need for increased fluid intake, and follow-up instructions. The patient should return to the emergency department or contact his family physician, if symptoms are not relieved.

Personal hygiene should be reviewed to identify and correct inappropriate cleans-

SPECIFIC DISEASES CAUSING ABDOMINAL PAIN

ing habits, which may contribute to the development of a urinary tract infection. Sexual intercourse may have to be postponed during the infection.

Urinary Calculi

Pathophysiology
Urinary calculi, *urolithiasis*, refers to the presence of stones in the urinary system. This stone formation occurs in the presence of highly concentrated urine with the deposit of crystalline substances. Approximately 90 percent of the stones are calcium, 8 percent uric acid, and about 2 percent cystine.

Factors affecting urinary calculi formation include the following:

Obstruction.
Infection.
Dehydration.
Urine concentration.
Immobilization.

Immobilization causes the slowing of renal drainage and alters calcium metabolism.
Other factors contributing to urolithiasis include the following:

High concentration of blood calcium compounds.
Large amounts of calcium in the urine.
Excessive intake of vitamin D.
Alkalosis.
Uric acid.
Vitamin A deficiency.
Hyperparathyroidism.

Stone formation can be reduced by the following methods:

Filtered load.
Enhancing tubular reabsorption.
Diluting the concentration of urine.

Cystinuria is a disorder of the transport of amino acids. Cystine percipitates in acidic urine forming stones. Uric acid formation also occurs in acidic urine and may be the result of an anatomical defect. The etiology of calcium stone disease is unknown.

Clinical Manifestations
Pain and discomfort are experienced in the flank area, with sudden sharp pain radiating down the ureter. Severe pain (renal colic) is caused by obstruction or by the passing of a stone in the renal pelvis or in the ureter.

In men, pain is referred to the testicles, and in women, to the vulva. Pain may be experienced in the costrovertebral angle, resulting from distention of the kidney or hydronephrosis. Hydronephrosis results from an obstruction in the ureter, causing urine to fill the pelvis and calices of the kidney. The pain is excruciating as the stone moves along the ureter. Gastrointestinal symptoms may be experienced, such as nausea and vomiting.

Gross hematuria may be evident, if the stone has sharp edges. Symptoms of urinary tract infections may be present, including chills, fever, and dysuria.

Diagnostic Studies
An intravenous pyelogram (IVP) is performed to visualize the kidney, ureter, and bladder. The IVP may reveal dilation of a ureter above an obstruction or lodging of calculi. Several surgical procedures can be used to remove a stone, depending on its location.

Nursing Care and Related Interventions
About 85 to 90 percent of urinary calculi pass through the urinary system without assistance. All urine, therefore, should be strained to detect the passage of stones. Any stones found should be analyzed.

Urinary calculi are extremely painful. The emergency department nurse must take all necessary precautions to protect the patient during the intermittent, colicky pain. The episodic care of the patient suffering from urinary calculi should be aimed at relieving pain. Drugs such as morphine sulfate and meperidine hydrochloride (Demerol) are used for severe pain associated with movement of the stone. The average 70 kg adult may receive 2 to 3 mg IV and 7 mg IM of morphine sulfate. Fifty to 100 mg IM of Demerol may be ordered. An antiemetic may be given to control nausea and vomiting. The emergency department nurse should start an intravenous line for patients who experience nausea. Large amounts of fluid should be encouraged to dilute the concentrated urine and to assist in the passage of the stone through the urinary system.

Patients may be admitted to the hospital if they are febrile or dehydrated, or if the pain is severe and constant.

Discharge Planning
All patients being discharged from the emergency department should receive written instructions and follow-up care. The patient should be instructed to strain all of his urine, and any stones found should be returned to the hospital for analysis. Fluids up to 4 l a day should be encouraged. The patient should be instructed to return to the emergency department or to contact his family physician if he experiences the following symptoms:

Chills.
Fever.
Severe pain in the abdomen.
The inability to empty his bladder.
Blood in the urine.

SPECIFIC DISEASES CAUSING ABDOMINAL PAIN

Appendicitis

Pathophysiology
Appendicitis is an inflammation of the vermiform appendix, due to obstruction of its lumen. Appendicitis occurs more commonly among males between the ages of 10 to 20. The appendix may become edematous and/or necrotic, then rupture. Bacterial exudate is distributed throughout the abdominal area, causing irritation and pain. Pain is experienced in the epigastric region or in the periumbilical area. A pelvic examination should be done on all female patients to rule out inflammatory disease. Localization of pain indicates that abscess pockets have formed, usually in the right lower quadrant.

Clinical Manifestations
Appendicitis can be confused with other illnesses causing pain and tenderness of the abdomen, such as the following:

Cholecystitis.
Pancreatitis.
Ruptured follicular cyst.
Pelvic inflammatory disease.
Ruptured ectopic pregnancy.
Ulcerative colitis.

Pain may localize between the umbilicus and the right iliac crest, known as McBurney's point. The pain becomes constant, and the patient will lie extremely still and draw his legs up (fetal position) to relieve the tension on the abdominal muscles. Nausea, vomiting, fever, malaise, and anorexia are seen in children and adults due to the infectious process.

The onset of abdominal pain usually is gradual and lasts for 72 hours. Patients experiencing pain from retrocecal appendicitis will flex the right hip and knee in an effort to relax the right psoas muscle and relieve pain. Due to the infectious process, a mild leukocytosis, with a white blood cell count between 10,000 to 15,000, may be seen.

Diagnostic Studies
Diagnosis of appendicitis should be made based on clinical manifestations. If the patient is moving around well and does not appear to be in much discomfort, he probably does not have appendicitis. If, on the other hand, a history of epigastric pain, malaise, nausea, vomiting, and radiation of the pain into the right lower quadrant exists, the patient most probably has an acute inflammation of the abdomen.

Careful attention must be given to the initial abdominal examination and to all subsequent abdominal examinations. Localized right lower quadrant tenderness, together with peritoneal signs, probably indicate appendicitis.

Pain medication should never be given to a patient being evaluated for an acute abdomen, until a diagnosis has been made. Pain medication will mask all signs and symptoms and will interfere with treatment.

Nursing Care and Related Interventions

Patients suspected of having appendicitis are usually admitted to the hospital and placed on bedrest. Intravenous therapy is started, using Ringer's lactate to hydrate the patient. A nasogastric tube is passed and attached to low intermittent suction to empty the stomach. An ice bag to the abdomen may help to relieve some of the discomfort. Only after a diagnosis has been confirmed and the decision to operate is made may the patient be given an analgesic to relieve pain. The emergency department nurse should secure written signatures on all appropriate forms before an analgesic is given.

The patient will not be allowed to take anything by mouth, since this may cause nausea and increase peristalsis. Moreover, cathartics will also increase peristalsis and, therefore, should not be given. Vital signs, including temperature, should be taken for a baseline and as frequently as indicated to monitor the progression of the infection, at least every half-hour during the acute stage.

Perforation of the appendix will cause peritonitis and severe abdominal discomfort. Peritonitis is the inflammation of the peritoneal cavity caused by, in this case, exudate and pus from the infected appendix. After the appendix has perforated, abdominal pain becomes diffuse. The abdomen will be extremely tender with rigid muscles and pronounced rebound tenderness. The patient will be febrile, with an increased pulse rate and leukocyte count. Antibiotics should be started immediately.

In the adult, the body blocks the infection by forming adhesions, while the omentum helps to enclose the affected areas. In children, the omentum is not well developed, and peritonitis can spread quickly from a perforated appendix.

Discharge Planning

Patients being discharged from the emergency department should be instructed to return immediately if the following symptoms occur:

Pain becomes unbearable.

Pain is felt in the right lower quadrant.

Vomiting occurs.

Fainting occurs.

Temperature increases.

The patient should be instructed to take only clear liquids by mouth, rest, and not to take medication for pain, since it will mask symptoms. No laxatives or enemas are to be given, and the patient should take his temperature at least every two hours.

Pelvic Inflammatory Disease (PID)

Pathophysiology

Pelvic inflammatory disease is an infection that involves the cervix and endometrium, resulting in infection of the fallopian tubes and ovaries. Inflammation of the fallopian tubes is called salpingitis, and inflammation of the ovaries is called oophoritis. PID may be caused by staphylococcus, streptococcus, or venereal organisms.

The disease can be transmitted through the following ways:

Sexual intercourse.
Intrauterine devices.
Passed during childbirth.
Postabortive state.

PID can also be caused by tubercle bacillus, transmitted by the bloodstream from the pulmonary system. In most instances, the causative organism is introduced through the cervical canal into the uterus and then into the patient's pelvis via the fallopian tubes. After the pathogen lodges in the fallopian tube, purulent material collects, and strictures may occur.

Obstruction of the tubes may be partial or complete, causing infertility problems. A partial obstruction can predispose a woman to ectopic pregnancy. When adhesions are severe, a hysterectomy may be advised.

Clinical Manifestations
Symptoms are usually noticed during a menstrual cycle due to ovarian activity. Abdominal pain, pelvic pain, nausea, fever, and malaise are present. Leukocytosis and a vaginal discharge are also present. The patient will appear to have discomfort during ambulation causing a slow gait, sometimes called a shuffle, rather than walking.

Abdominal palpation elicits pain in the lower abdomen. On pelvic examination, pain and tenderness occurs with motion of the cervix. Tubo-ovarian abscesses may be felt in one or both lower quadrants. The vaginal discharge will be purulent and, depending on the causative agent, may be foul-smelling.

Chronic PID will present with a history of the following symptoms:

Chronic dull aching and discomfort in the lower abdomen.
Backache.
Low-grade fever.
Malaise.
Constipation.
Irregular menstrual cycles.

Occasionally an abscess forms in the cul-de-sac of Douglas.

Diagnostic Studies
A culture of the vaginal discharge should be taken, as well as cultures from the urethra, cervix, and anus on Thayer Martin media. A VDRL test should be done to identify the presence of any associated disease.

Nursing Care and Related Interventions

Treatment of PID may require hospitalization. Treatment includes controlling the infection and preventing it from spreading to others. Since PID is often caused by venereal disease, the emergency department nurse should be considerate of and supportive of the patient's emotional feelings regarding venereal disease.

A semi-Fowler's position is encouraged to promote dependent drainage and to decrease the possibility of an abscess forming high up in the abdomen. The causative agents can be identified from smears and cultures. Vital signs and physical, as well as mental, responses should be recorded by the emergency nurse.

Analgesics may be given for abdominal discomfort. Oral probenecid 1 g is given, followed in 30 minutes by procaine penicillin, 2.4 million units, IM in each buttock. Probenecid prolongs elevated blood levels of the penicillin. Patients allergic to penicillin receive spectinomycin 2 mg IM or tetracycline 500 mg orally every six hours for five days.

Discharge Planning

Discharge instructions should describe causes and preventative measures and the potential dangers PID poses to the reproductive organs. Heat to the abdomen may decrease pain. Douches should not be done, because they may spread the infection. A well-balanced diet should be maintained.

The control of infection should be emphasized and appropriate safeguards taken in handling contaminated articles. Instructions should also emphasize the need for continued evaluation by a physician, since PID can cause sterility, and to ensure that the patient does not have a resistant strain of gonorrhea. Sexual intercourse should be discouraged for at least two weeks.

If PID is caused by a venereal disease, the patient should be encouraged to report all contact individuals to the health department, because they may have been infected.

The patient should be instructed to return to the emergency department if the following symptoms occur:

Dizziness.
Chills.
Fever, higher than 101°F.
Increasing pain.
Persistent nausea.
Vomiting.

Bowel Obstruction

Pathophysiology

Major sites of bowel obstruction include the esophagus (hiatus hernia), duodenum, small bowel, and a hernia that has encarcerated. Bowel obstruction causes a catabolic state and a shifting of fluids and electrolytes to the intestinal lumen and peritoneal cavity. It also decreases the blood supply beyond the obstruction com-

SPECIFIC DISEASES CAUSING ABDOMINAL PAIN

pounding the problem. The most common cause of bowel obstruction is adhesions caused by previous surgery.

Hiatus hernia or esophageal hernia, which occurs usually in middle to later years, causes loss of function in the cardioesophageal sphincter and allows unneutralized gastric juices into the esophagus, producing inflammation and ulceration, leading to hemorrhage and fibrous tissue formation. Regurgitation can occur, causing pneumonitis.

Mechanical obstruction is often caused by hernia, adhesions, cancer, and intussusception or telescoping of a segment of the bowel within itself. Neurogenic obstruction interferes with peristalsis.

Intestinal obstruction in the newborn may result from a congenital defect or stenosis. Malrotation of the intestine is the most common cause of duodenal obstruction in children. Other anatomic abnormalities in the infant include the following:

Congenital hypertrophic pyloric stenosis.
Congenital duodenal obstruction.
Congenital annular pancreas.

Clinical Manifestations
Depending on the site of the obstruction, symptoms may vary from a feeling of heartburn due to hiatus hernia to abdominal distention, vomiting, diarrhea, and anorexia caused by lower bowel obstruction.

Small bowel obstruction will cause persistent vomiting that produces acute electrolyte imbalance and dehydration. The patient can become alkalotic due to the loss of hydrogen ions. Loss of water and sodium from the small bowel can cause severe dehydration and acidosis. Symptoms of small bowel obstruction include the following:

Colic cramps.
Some distention.
Vomiting.
Diffuse tenderness.
Increased bowel sounds.

Obstruction to the colon produces the following symptoms:

Cramps of the mid and lower abdomen.
Distention.
Vomiting/including fecal matter.
Fever.
Peritoneal irritation.

The white blood cell count increases, and the patient may show signs of toxicity with a rapid and weak pulse, decrease in blood pressure, and increase in temperature. A strangulated bowel will cause severe pain and localized tenderness.

Diagnostic Studies
The following tests should be done in the emergency department:

X-ray flat/upright of the abdomen.
Type/crossmatch.
Urinalysis.
Electrolyte profile.
Amylase.
Complete blood count.

X-ray studies may reveal fluid levels reflecting a mechanical obstruction or ileus. An upper gastrointestinal or barium meal and lower gastrointestinal or barium enema might be performed to visualize the gastrointestinal tract.

Nursing Care and Related Interventions
Since abdominal pain is similar for many disease entities, the emergency department nurse should assess the nature and location of the patient's pain accurately. Nursing care should be directed toward relieving discomfort and preventing complications. A nasogastric tube is passed to relieve distention. Ringer's lactate will correct interstitial fluid deficits, while dextrose and water will correct intracellular fluid deficits. Plasma substitutes, such as Na^+ and K^+, can be added if laboratory studies indicate their necessity.

Vital signs should be taken as often as indicated by the patient's condition, or at least every hour while the patient is in the emergency department. Accurate records should be maintained regarding intake and output. Stool should be examined for occult blood. Broad spectrum antibiotics may be given to fight infection.

The abdomen should be examined carefully to detect early signs of peritonitis. Bowel obstruction is corrected by surgical intervention. The patient should be prepared for a possible operation. Demerol and Phenergan may be given to relieve pain and to control postoperative nausea.

Aneurysm

Pathophysiology
An aneurysm is a localized enlargement or sac formed by the dilatation of the wall of an artery. Aneurysms occur more commonly in men over the age of 50, with a 30–50 percent mortality rate associated with the diagnosis. Aneurysms form when the wall of the vessel is weakened, causing a sac or pouch to develop. This area becomes weak, and it is extremely susceptible to rupture.

The most common site of an aneurysm is in the abdominal aorta, and atherosclerosis is the predominant cause. This condition is due to atrophy of the arterial tunica media, which is the middle layer of smooth muscle and elastic tissue. A dissecting aneurysm occurs when blood gains access to the media, causing the wall of the vessel to widen. Hemodynamic stress probably results in rupture. (The classification of aortic aneurysms is contained in Table 14.4.)

TABLE 14.4 Classification of Aortic Aneurysms

Type	Anatomical Placement
I	Extends from the ascending aorta to the arch and beyond
II	Involves the ascending arch only
III	Originates beyond the subclavian artery

Clinical Manifestations
The patient with an abdominal aneurysm frequently presents with the chief complaint of lower back pain. Aneurysm must be ruled out as a cause of back pain. Persistent or intermittent pain in the lower abdomen that radiates to the lower back may also indicate the presence of an aneurysm.

On inspection of the abdomen, a pulsating, expansile mass may be seen in the area of the umbilicus, primarily to the left of midline. Femoral pulses are usually present. Blood pressure may differ in each arm, and a murmur of aortic regurgitation may be present.

If the aneurysm is leaking, the patient may complain of dizziness, weakness, or syncope. If the aneurysm ruptures, it produces massive hemorrhage, and the patient will exhibit all the signs and symptoms of hypovolemic shock.

Diagnostic studies
Chest and abdominal x-ray studies may help in confirming the diagnosis of an aneurysm. Laboratory studies are extremely important and include type and crossmatch for at least six units of whole blood, a complete blood count, electrolyte values, glucose levels, blood urea nitrogen levels, and an urinalysis. An ECG is useful, particularly as a baseline before surgery.

Nursing Care and Related Interventions
If an aneurysm is suspected, the nurse must be ready to support the patient instantly in case of rupture. The patient's airway and circulatory status must be maintained at all costs. (Chapter 21 discusses in detail the care of the patient in hypovolemic shock.)

If rupture has not occurred, the patient will be stabilized in the emergency department prior to surgical intervention to prevent the possibility of rupture. At least two large-bore catheters (14 gauge) will be started with Ringer's lactate solution to support the circulatory system. A nasogastric tube will be placed to decompress the stomach. A Foley catheter is inserted to monitor closely the kidney function of the patient. Intake and output documentation is extremely important.

Nipride given via an infusion pump in a constant IV drip is the preferred drug to control hypertension associated with an aneurysm. Drug therapy is aimed at reducing the systolic blood pressure to 120 mm Hg.

The nurse must try to incorporate methods of stress reduction in the care of the patient. Stress plays a dominant role in increasing the chances of rupture. If the patient goes directly to surgery from the emergency department, the family must be allowed to see the patient before he leaves the emergency department. Both the family and the patient will require the emotional support of the emergency department staff. A chaplain or social worker also may help in this situation.

CONCLUSION

Patients present to the emergency department frequently with acute and chronic abdominal pain. An orderly assessment, a complete history, and appropriate diagnostic tests are necessary to determine the emergent nature of the situation.

Patients frequently are admitted to the hospital for further testing and/or surgery. Patients that are discharged from the emergency department must receive verbal and written instructions regarding their medication and follow-up care. The needs of both the patient and his family must be assessed and action planned to intervene for the benefit of the patient, as well as to provide quality patient care in every situation.

BIBLIOGRAPHY

Gonez, A., et al.: Acute appendicitis during pregnancy. *American Journal of Surgery* 137(2):180 (1979).

Hedberg, S.: Endoscopy in gastrointestinal bleeding: a systemic approach to diagnosis. *Surgical Clinicians of North America* 54:549 (1974).

Irving, G.: Pediatric Emergencies. In G. Schwaltz (ed.): *Principles and Practice in Emergency Medicine*. Philadelphia: Saunders, 1978.

Malasonos, L., et al.: Abdominal Assessment, *Health Assessment*. 2nd ed. St. Louis: 1981, pp. 348–375.

Nase, H.: The diagnosis of appendicitis. *American Journal of Surgery* 46:504 (1980).

Philbrich, T., et al.: Abdominal ultrasound in patients with acute right upper quadrant pain. *Gastrointestinal Radiology* 6(3):251 (1981).

Smith, G., et al.: Oral cholecystography in assessment of acute abdominal pain. *Archives of Surgery* 115:642 (1980).

Smith, L., and S. Thier: *Pathophysiology—The Biological Principles of Disease*. Philadelphia: Saunders, 1981, pp. 1612–1624.

Stamm, W., et al.: Causes of acute urethral syndrome in women. *New England Journal of Medicine* 303:409–415 (1980).

Stone, K., et al.: Ultrasound as the initial diagnostic study in patients with suspected gallstones. *American Journal of Surgery* 46:444 (1980).

Turck, M.: Urinary tract infection. *Hospital Practice* 15:49–58 (1980).

Washaw, A., et al.: Inhibition of serum and urine amylase activity in pancreatitis with hyperlipedemia. *Annals of Surgery* 182:72 (1975).

15
Epigastric Pain

Barbara Knezevich

After completing this chapter, the reader will be able to do the following:

1. Triage a patient experiencing epigastric pain.
2. List the common causes of epigastric pain.
3. Identify the clinical manifestations and diagnostic studies involved in caring for the patient with epigastric pain.
4. Discuss the nursing care of and related interventions for patients experiencing epigastric pain.
5. Discuss discharge planning, when appropriate, for the patient experiencing epigastric pain.

Epigastric pain is associated with many illnesses, and the epigastric area can be the site of major trauma and bleeding. This area involves the gallbladder, pancreas, and upper gastrointestinal system. Each organ or organ system manifests problems in somewhat different ways, even though the common presenting complaint is that of epigastric pain. The emergency department nurse must be aware of all the possible situations that must be handled to provide nursing care for the patient experiencing epigastric pain.

TRIAGE

Subjective Data

Collection of important data that begins with the first contact with the patient initiates the triage process. The patient's condition may be relayed to the emergency department nurse by a family member, friend, police, or ambulance personnel. Patients with epigastric pain, regardless of the cause, have similar complaints.

The nurse must collect, record, and analyze all information. Questions, such as the following, must be asked:

1. Where is the location of the pain?
2. Does the pain radiate?
3. How long does the pain last?
4. Is the pain relieved by food or antacids?
5. Is there a history of tension and anxiety?
6. Was there ingestion of an irritant or drugs?
7. Does the patient consume alcohol or smoke?
8. Are the symptoms more noticeable in the spring and fall?

Early in the examination the nurse establishes whether any vomiting or nausea exists, and whether the pain is related directly to the vomiting, as well as the color, frequency, and duration of the vomiting. A history of hurried and irregular eating habits is common.

Past medical history and knowledge of current health, allergies, and medications help the emergency department nurse to develop a plan of care.

Objective Data

Objective data is collected by inspection, auscultation, percussion, and palpation. These maneuvers are done on all patients who complain of epigastric pain. Inspection and palpation maneuvers are used to evaluate the history describing the nature of the pain, the site of the pain, nausea, vomiting, diarrhea, or constipation. The objective data collected is similar to the data collected for abdominal pain. (Chapter 14 contains further details on examining the abdomen and epigastric region.)

Assessment and Planning

After collecting and analyzing both the subjective and objective data, the nurse makes a diagnosis identifying all patient problems, then establishes and prioritizes a plan for care. Most patients with epigastric pain are triaged to the medical service and allowed to wait in the waiting room. Exceptions include patients with signs of shock or patients that are vomiting blood and exhibiting signs of unbearable pain. (Table 15.1 includes two examples of triage notes for patients experiencing epigastric pain.)

SPECIFIC CONDITIONS CAUSING EPIGASTRIC PAIN

Gastritis and Ulceration

Pathophysiology
Gastritis, an inflammation of the stomach, is associated with food poisoning; ingestion of corrosive material such as acid or alkali, alcohol; thermal or mechanical injuries; salicylates, and diseases that affect the gastric mucosal cells.

SPECIFIC CONDITIONS CAUSING EPIGASTRIC PAIN

TABLE 15.1 Examples of Triage Notes for Patients Experiencing Epigastric Pain

S: 52 yo BM with symptoms of "vomiting blood" for the past hour. Has epigastric pain, nonradiating, "gnawing in nature" over his left upper abdomen. "Vomited about two cups of bright red blood." PMH: ulcer disease, HTN, NKA, current meds Aldomet 250 mg q.d.

O: Weak, pale, skin moist and cool, P 100, thready, BP 100/72, vomited app. 150 ml bright red blood at triage desk.

A: Upper GI bleed, secondary to ulcer disease.

P: Medical evaluation, admit examination room immediately.

S: 40 yo WF with symptoms of right epigastric pain that goes through to the back for app. 2hrs, PTA. Pain increased "after I ate fried chicken for dinner." c/o nausea, no vomiting, no fever, anorexia, malaise. PMH: negative, NKA, no current meds.

O: Obese, fair-skinned, holding arm over upper abdomen. Grimace on face. T 99.6°F, BP normal, constantly fidgeting in chair.

A: Epigastric pain, R/O cholecystitis.

P: Medical evaluation, admit examination room ASAP.

During an acute stage of gastritis, inflammation is present due to polymorphonuclear cells, edema, and hemorrhage. Various pathologic changes can occur in the gastric mucosa. Gastric atrophy occurs when glandular cells are lost and then are replaced with a thin lining of cells that are histologically similar to the cells in the small intestine.

Pernicious anemia may result from the loss of gastric mucosa and diminished gastric secretions. Hypersecretion of gastric acid may be the cause of duodenal and gastric ulcers. An ulcer results from the sloughing of inflammatory necrotic tissue. A *peptic ulcer* (gastric ulcer) results from sloughing of the mucous membrane of the esophagus, stomach, or duodenum caused by the action of aciditic gastric secretions.

Duodenal ulcer is usually predisposed by emotional stress, poor eating habits, smoking, drinking alcohol or coffee, and takings drugs that are irritating to the mucous membrane lining. Duodenal ulcer usually is found between the ages of 25 to 40, and in men four times more frequently than in women.

Gastric ulcer occurs between the ages of 40 to 55, and in men two-and-one-half more times than in women. Approximately 15 percent of the population in the United States may have ulcers.

Gastric juice destroys and digests living tissue. Although the mechanism is not clear, in duodenal ulcers secretion of acid increases with a reduction in pancreatic and biliary bicarbonate concentrate. In gastric ulcers, however, a reduced amount of hydrochloric acid is secreted. Drugs such as salicylates, adrenal corticosteroids, indomethacin, Phenylbritazone, and reserpine seem to cause irritation of the mucosa.

Clinical Manifestations
Symptoms will depend on the nature of the gastritis and on whether it is acute or chronic. The acute patient presents with epigastric burning and pain due to transudation of plasma protein into the lumen of the stomach and ulceration of the mucosa. Other symptoms include nausea, vomiting, anorexia, or headache. Gastritis caused by alcoholism, aspirin, or food poisoning is usually short in duration.

Patients with chronic gastritis will have the following symptoms:

Loss of appetite.
Frequent belching.
Diffuse epigastric discomfort.
Nausea.
Vomiting.
A feeling of fullness.

Ulceration will result in the following:

Hemorrhage causing shock.
Perforation causing peritonitis.
Pyloric obstruction causing vomiting and alkalosis.

The patient presenting to the emergency department with hemorrhage resulting from an ulcer will exhibit signs and symptoms of shock. A patient with 20 to 25 percent blood loss will be thirsty and dizzy. The systolic blood pressure may be below 100 mm Hg. A patient with 40 to 45 percent blood loss will be diaphoretic and have cold extremities. The patient's blood pressure may drop to 70 mm Hg or below, and the pulse will be thready and rapid, probably 130 or higher.

Perforation of an ulcer can cause peritonitis (inflammation of the peritoneum). The patient will complain of severe upper abdominal pain. The abdomen will be extremely rigid and boardlike. The slightest palpation of the abdomen will cause severe discomfort. The patient also will have signs and symptoms of shock.

Pyloric obstruction may cause persistent vomiting resulting in the loss of acidic gastric juice, causing alkalosis.

Diagnostic Studies
Diagnosis is made by patient history, upper gastrointestinal (GI) series, gastric analysis, stool examination, and gastric biopsy. Questions asked by the triage nurse during assessment assist the emergency department nurse to formulate a nursing diagnosis. Blood should be drawn to include a complete blood count and electrolyte profile that will indicate any blood loss, infectious process, or electrolyte imbalances.

The upper GI series is a series of x-ray studies taken to visualize the upper gastrointestinal tract. This test usually requires the patient to fast and can be done on an outpatient basis.

The patient is required to ingest a contrast medium called barium, a tasteless insoluble powder. After barium is swallowed, fluoroscopy examination visualizes the esophagus, the stomach, and the small intestine. X-ray studies are made during the examination study for verification of possible abnormalities.

Gastric analysis can be achieved via the nasogastric tube. A nasogastric tube is inserted, and, the stomach contents evacuated for analysis. An increase in free hydrochloric acid suggests a duodenal ulcer. The absence of free hydrochloric acid may suggest gastric malignancy or pernicious anemia. Food particles with an increased amount of gastric secretions suggest pyloric obstruction.

Stool is examined for occult blood. Tarry black stool suggests upper GI bleeding, whereas bright red blood suggests lower GI bleeding. The emergency department nurse should remember that foods and medications affect the stool color. Barium, for example, will cause stool to turn milky white; beets will cause stool to turn red; and iron supplements cause dark tarry stools.

A gastroscopy is an examination used to visualize the esophageal and gastric mucosa. During the examination, the physician can obtain a tissue sample of an area that may appear diseased.

Any patient over the age of 40 should have an electrocardiogram done to establish the patient's cardiac status.

Nursing Care and Related Interventions

Nursing care is directed toward relieving the symptoms and preventing complications. Ulcers usually heal when the causative agent is removed. The emergency department nurse should discourage the use of alcohol, coffee, aspirin, steroids, and smoking, since they are factors causing the stimulation of gastric secretions.

Antacids may be given, since they work to reduce or to decrease discomfort by lowering the acidity of gastric secretions. Maalox and Mylanta are often chosen, since they are not easily absorbed from the stomach and, therefore, do not alter the pH of the blood. Antacids may be given every 30 to 60 minutes, depending on the patient's symptoms. Cimetidine (Tagamet) inhibits production of gastric acid and is frequently prescribed in the emergency department. Cimetidine can be given IV push, but IV piggyback is preferred, since rapid IV injection may cause cardiac dysrhythmias and hypotension. Cimetidine is not recommended for use in children under 16 years of age.

More aggressive measures will be indicated for the patient presenting to the emergency department with a bleeding ulcer. (The section on gastrointestinal bleeding contains more detailed information.)

Discharge Planning

The patient with gastritis should be instructed to take only ice chips until his vomiting has stopped. After the vomiting has ceased, the patient can begin to take clear liquids, such as tea, ginger ale, or broth. Solid foods can be added to the diet, when the patient begins to regain his appetite.

A regular exercise and rest program should be emphasized during discharge planning. Irritating drugs should be avoided. Smoking, alcohol, and highly seasoned foods should be discouraged.

The patient suffering from gastritis should be instructed to return to the emergency department if the following occur: vomiting does not stop after 48 hours; a fever of

TABLE 15.2 Bland Diet

Breakfast

Fruit	Grapefruit	½ medium
Cereal	Whole-grain	½ cup (cooked)
Egg	Soft-cooked egg	1
Bread	White toast	1 slice
Butter	Butter	1 tsp
Beverage	Coffee	1 cup
Half/half	Half/half	3 Tbs
Sugar	Sugar	1 Tbs

Lunch

Meat	Roast beef	2 oz
	Gravy	¼ cup
Potato	Mashed potato	½ cup
Vegetable	Buttered beets	½ cup
Salad	Sliced tomato	½ medium
Dessert	Vanilla ice cream	⅓ cup
Beverage	Milk	½ pint
Butter	Butter	1 tsp

Dinner

Meat	Cold sliced ham	2 oz
Potato	Baked buttered potato	1 medium
Vegetable	Buttered green beans	½ cup
Fruit	Sliced banana	1 medium
Half/half	Half/half	3 Tbs
Sugar	Sugar	½ Tbs
Beverage	Milk	½ pint
Bread	White bread	1 slice
Butter	Butter	1 tsp

100°F or more persists; blood, mucus or worms are found in the bowel movement; or, the epigastric pain becomes worse.

Patients being discharged from the emergency department with an ulcer may be instructed to stay in bed or rest at home, depending on the patient's condition. Prescribed medication should be explained to both the patient and appropriate family members. An ulcer diet should be provided in writing. (Table 15.2 contains an example of a bland diet that is appropriate for ulcer patients.)

The emergency nurse should emphasize the avoidance of anxiety-producing events and irregular eating and sleeping habits. The patient should be instructed to contact his family physician or to return to the emergency department, if his pain is not relieved by the prescribed treatment plan.

SPECIFIC CONDITIONS CAUSING EPIGASTRIC PAIN

TABLE 15.3 Sources of Gastrointestinal Hemorrhage

I. Upper Gastrointestinal Bleeding
A. *Inflammatory*
   Duodenal ulcer
   Gastritis
   Gastric ulcer
   Esophagitis
   Stress ulcer
   Pancreatitis
B. *Mechanical*
   Hiatus hernia
   Mallory-Weiss syndrome
   Hematobilia
C. *Vascular*
   Esophageal or gastric varices
   Aortointestinal fistula
   Hemangioma
   Osler-Weber-Rendu syndrome
   Mesenteric vascular occlusion
   Blue nevus bleb
D. *Neoplasma*
   Carcinoma
   Polyps-single, multiple, Peutz-Jeghers syndrome
   Leiomyoma
   Carcinoid
   Leukemia
   Sarcoma
II. Lower Gastrointestinal Bleeding
A. *Inflammatory*
   Ulcerative colitis
   Diverticulitis
	Enterocolitis, regional (Crohn's disease)
	   Enterocolitis, tuberculous
	   Enterocolitis, radiation
	   Enterocolitis, bacterial
	   Enterocolitis, toxic
	B. *Mechanical*
	   Diverticulosis
	C. *Neoplasms*
	   Carcinoma
	   Polyps-ademonatous and villous, familial polyposis, Peutz-Jeghers syndrome
	   Leiomyoma
	   Sarcoma
	   Lipoma
	   Metastatic (melanoma)
	D. *Anomalies*
	   Meckel's diverticulum
	E. *Vascular*
	   Hemorrhoids
	   Aortoduodenal fistula
	   Aortic aneurysm
	   Mesenteric thrombosis
	   Hereditary hemorrhagic telangiectasia
	   Blue nevus bleb
	F. *Systemic*
	   Blood dyscrasias
	   Collagen diseases
	   Uremia

SOURCE: Sleisinger and Fordtran, 1978, p. 227.

Gastrointestinal (GI) Bleeding

Pathophysiology

Gastrointestinal bleeding is a common medical emergency, causing physical weakness often not associated with pain. GI bleeding is not a disease entity, but rather the result of blood loss from the gastrointestinal tract. Many pathologic processes may cause a lesion that bleeds. (Table 15.3 contains a list of sources for GI bleeding.) The most common causes in adults are hemorrhoids, colonic diverticular disease, colon and rectal malignancies, and angiodysplastic lesions of the cecum.

In pediatric patients, bleeding may be caused by the following:

Varices.
Gastric or duodenal ulcers.
Ingestion of aspirin.
Alcohol.
Steroids.
Phenylbutaxone.
Reserpine.
Indomethacin.
Thrombocytopenia.
Hemophilia.
Disseminated intravascular coagulapathy.
Meckel's diverticulum.
Intussusception.

Clinical Manifestations
The patient may present to the emergency department with gross, bloody vomiting (hematemesis), indicating that the bleeding could be from the esophagus, stomach, or proximal duodenum. Melenemesis is blood that has been in the stomach and has come in contact with gastric acid. Melenemesis commonly is called "coffee grounds," because of its color and clumping. Melena or dark black, liquid stool is observed in patients bleeding from the proximal gastrointestinal tract. Hematochezia is bright red blood from the distal small bowel or from the colon or rectum.

Because of the acute loss of blood, the patient experiences a decrease in venous return and a decrease in stroke volume. The diastolic blood pressure will fall after the patient has acutely lost 20 to 25 percent of his intravascular volume. Coolness of the skin, diaphoresis, peripheral cyanosis, confusion, pallor, agitation, cardiac dysrhythmias, and oliguria may be observed. The chief complaint may be syncope and weakness.

Diagnostic Studies
Diagnosis involves using the following aids:

Gastroduodenal endoscopy.
Angiography.
Gastrointestinal barium studies.
Protoscopy.
Sigmoidoscopy.
Colonoscopy.
Laboratory studies.
X-ray studies.

SPECIFIC CONDITIONS CAUSING EPIGASTRIC PAIN

Upper GI bleeding can be evaluated with the fiberoptic gastroscope, while lower GI bleeding may be detected by barium studies, protoscopy, or sigmoidoscopy. Emergency endoscopy is a procedure used to visualize the esophageal and gastric mucosa. The procedure itself is not painful, but it may be frustrating, because the patient is unable to communicate during the procedure.

Laboratory studies may include a complete blood count, electrolyte profile, type and crossmatch, blood urea nitrogen levels, and clotting times. X-ray studies may include upright and flat plate of the abdomen, as well as a kidney, ureter, and bladder view.

Melena, stool stained with blood pigment, is normally associated with upper GI bleeding. During physical evaluation of the patient, care must be taken by the emergency department nurse to examine the patient for internal and external hemorrhoids. Bleeding internal hemorrhoids may be mistaken for upper GI bleeding.

Nursing Care and Related Interventions

Acute exsanguinating hemorrhage, evident in the patient with esophageal varies or duodenal ulcer, is an obvious emergency that requires an immediate plan of action. The airway must be evaluated, since vomited blood or food particles may obstruct the airway. Vital signs should be taken to establish a baseline and repeated every 15 minutes until stable.

Blood loss of 20 to 25 percent will require volume replacement. When a crystalloid solution is used for volume replacement, 3 ml of crystalloid solution is required to replace every milliliter of blood loss. Both peripheral and central intravenous lines should be started with large-bore needles. A central line will assist the emergency nurse to monitor volume replacement. When the patient history indicates liver disease, lactate should not be administered, since the patient will not be able to metabolize lactate. Lactic acidosis, therefore, may develop. Dextran interferes with cross-matching; therefore, blood should be drawn prior to the use of dextran.

An indwelling urinary catheter should be inserted to monitor actual urinary output. Urinary output will decrease in shock states, as the body attempts to conserve volume and increase blood pressure.

A nasogastric (NG) tube should be inserted to evacuate fluid and gas from the gastrointestinal tract. The emergency nurse may administer a continuous lavage through the NG tube with iced saline to stop the bleeding. Iced saline stimulates vasoconstriction. Vasopressors, such as vasopressin or levarterenol, can be instilled via the NG tube, causing local vasoconstriction. Emergency endoscopy may be performed to visualize the area of bleeding in the esophagus, stomach, and possibly the duodenum.

The patient experiencing gastrointestinal bleeding will become hypothermic. The emergency nurse, therefore, should make sure that the patient is kept warm with blankets.

During this stressful period, the patient will require psychological support from the emergency department staff. The emergency department nurse should attempt to decrease the amount of activity around the patient to provide a calm environment. An explanation of all procedures, medications, and treatments should help to relieve anxiety. The emergency nurse should display directness in all activity to ensure an environment of confidence.

Pancreatitis

Pathophysiology
Pancreatitis is an inflammation of the pancreatic gland. (The possible etiologies of pancreatitis are listed in Table 15.4.) One serious form of pancreatitis is hemorrhagic pancreatitis, which causes parenchymatous extravasation of lytic pancreatic enzymes. The release of these enzymes may lead to necrosis and possible infection.

Alcoholism and biliary tract disease have been associated with acute pancreatitis. Reye's syndrome, acute encephalopathy with fatty degeneration of the liver, occasionally is mistaken for pancreatitis in the pediatric patient. Pancreatitis may be confused with myocardial ischemia in the adult patient.

Clinical Manifestations
In pancreatitis, the patient experiences sudden, excruciating, epigastric pain in the back and chest. This pain is due to edema, extravasation of plasma and red cells, release of protein and lipids, and distention of the ductules. Back pain and flank pain may occur, because the enzymes released may stimulate the sensory nerves of the peritoneum and retroperitoneal space. Nausea, vomiting, jaundice, and abdominal distention are frequently observed.

Injury to the tissue and necrosis of the tissues establish an inflammatory reaction resulting in an increased body temperature. Cardiovascular symptoms may result from hypotension caused by exudation of plasma into the retroperitoneal space and accumulation of fluid in the intravascular and extravascular spaces, called "third space" fluid. (See Table 15.5 for a summary of pancreatic conditions with their signs and symptoms.)

Diagnostic Studies
Laboratory studies in patients with acute hemorrhagic pancreatitis may reveal glycosuria due to elevated beta cell destruction. Hyperglycemia is due to the increase in circulating levels of glucagon, the increased release of glucocorticoids, and the destruction of beta cells. Leukocytosis is observed due to the inflammatory activity. Normal serum amylase is 70 to 150 Somogyi units. With acute pancreatitis and increased cellular destruction, the serum amylase level can reach 600 to 800 Somogyi units in four to six hours. Serum calcium levels may decrease, while serum lipase levels will rise, along with serum amylase, but at a much slower rate.

Venous blood should be drawn to establish baseline values. Blood is drawn for a complete blood count, serum electrolyte profile, and levels of serum lipase, blood sugar, amylase, bilirubin, BUN, PT, and PTT. An electrocardiogram (ECG) should be done on all patients over 40 years of age, or on those patients with known cardiac disorders. A urinalysis is also obtained.

Nursing Care and Related Interventions
Relief of pain should be the primary objective in treating a patient who is suffering from acute pancreatitis. Merperidine hydrochloride (Demerol) is given by IM injection in doses of 50 to 100 mg in the adult patient. Opiates, such as morphine and codeine, are not given, because they may produce spasms of the biliary pancreatic ducts.

TABLE 15.4   Clinical Etiologies of Acute Pancreatitis

A. Most Common Associations
 1. Biliary disease (cholelithiasis)
 2. Alcoholism (?genetic factors)
 3. Traumatic-postoperative
 4. Duodenal ulceration
 5. Idiopathic

B. Infections
 1. Mumps
 2. Coxsackie viruses B2, B3, B5
 3. Hepatitis viruses
 4. *Salmonella typhi*
 5. Group A streptococci (scarlet fever)
 6. Staphylococci
 7. Enteroviruses: echovirus 6, 11, 22, 30
 8. Miliary tuberculosis, actinomycosis
 9. *Candida albicans*
 10. Role of *E. coli* in "biliary" group

C. Infestations
 1. Ascaris
 2. Hydatid cyst
 3. *Clonorchis sinensis*
 4. *Giardia lamblia*

D. Metabolic–Nutritional
 1. Hypercalcemia
    a. Hyperparathyroidism (especially perioperative)
    b. Multiple myeloma-lymphoma
    c. Bone metastases
    d. Hypervitaminosis D
    e. Tumor producing PTH-like hormones
 2. Hyperlipoproteinemias, Types 1, IV, V
 3. Hereditary
    a. ±leukopenia
    b. ±thrombocytopenia
    c. ±aminoaciduria
 4. Hemochromatosis-hemosiderosis
 5. Cystic fibrosis
 6. Kwashiorkor
 7. Pregnancy or oral contraceptives

TABLE 15.4 *(continued)*

    8. "Sprue"
    9. Postgastrectomy malnutrition
   10. Weber-Christian disease
   11. Obesity (hyperlipoproteinemia, diabetes)
   12. Whipple's disease
   13. Uremia
   14. Postrenal transplant (immunosuppression)
   15. Postextracorporeal circulation

E. Mechanical
    1. Pariampullary stone impaction
    2. Carcinoma of pancreas
    3. Metastatic carcinoma to pancreas
    4. Postsurgical (e.g., biliary, sphincterotomy)
    5. Periampullary diverticula
    6. Ascaris
    7. Pressure injuries (e.g., x-ray procedures)
    8. Afferent loop obstruction
    9. Superior mesenteric artery syndrome
   10. Crohn's disease, duodenal
   11. Congenital anomalies (e.g., annular pancreas)
   12. Polyposis, Peutz-Jeghers syndrome
   13. Dystonic sphincter, "papillitis"
   14. Postendoscopic pancreatography

F. Drugs
    1. Corticosteriods, ACTH
    2. Isoniazid
    3. Anticoagulants
    4. Diuretics, especially thiazides
    5. Thiouracil
    6. Oral contraceptives
    7. Furosemide
    8. Azathioprine
    9. Toxins
       a. Methanol
       b. Zinc
       c. Cobalt
       d. Saccharated iron oxide
       e. Mercuric chloride

TABLE 15.4 *(continued)*

G. Venom
   1. Scorpion, *T. trinitatis*

H. Vascular
   1. Myocardial infarction, atheromas
   2. Mesenteric infarction
   3. Collagen vascular disease
      a. Polyarteritis
      b. Disseminated lupus erythematosus
   4. Diabetic coma
   5. Eclampsia
   6. Electric shock

SOURCE: Sleisinger and Fordtran, 1978, p. 1418.

Pancreatic secretions should be decreased by giving nothing by mouth. Anticholinergic medications help to reduce pancreatic secretions by decreasing vagal activity.

An intravenous line of normal saline, with supplemental potassium, is started in the emergency department to correct electrolyte deficiencies. A nasogastric tube is passed to decompress the stomach and suction hydrochloric acid from the stomach.

The blood glucose level is tested and fractional urine specimens may be tested for sugar and acetone levels. Hyperglycemia is treated with small doses of a short-acting insulin.

Acute hemorrhagic pancreatitis is treated with whole blood and volume expanders. A central line should be started to monitor fluid replacement. A urinary catheter is inserted to determine output accurately. Any patient who is acutely ill with pancreatitis will be admitted for further observation and evaluation.

Discharge Planning

Patients with chronic pancreatitis and patients in stable condition may be discharged from the emergency department.

A bland, low-fat diet should be given to the patient. If the patient is aware of dietary restrictions, the emergency department nurse should try to determine why the patient has not followed the diet. Emphasis should be placed on avoiding rich foods that can stimulate pancreatic action. Substances to be avoided include the following:

Alcohol.
Coffee.
Spicy foods.
Heavy or large meals.

TABLE 15.5 A Summary of Pancreatic Conditions

Condition	Signs/Symptoms	Definition	Diagnostic Evaluation
Acute hemorrhagic pancreatitis	1. Abdominal distension 2. ↓ bowel sounds 3. May be jaundiced 4. Hypotension 5. Turner's sign 6. Cullen's sign 7. Excruciating epigastric pain 8. Nausea 9. Retching/vomiting	Parenchymatous extravasation of lytic pancreatic enzymes	1. Glycosuria 2. Hyperglycemia 3. Leukocytosis 4. ↑ serum amylase the first 24 hrs
Acute intestinal pancreatitis	1. Abdominal distention 2. Palpable firm mass under pancreas 3. Epigastric discomfort or pain 4. Fullness of the abdomen 5. Nausea 6. Vomiting 7. Jaundice	Related to acute alcoholism and infection	1. Leukocytosis 2. ↑ serum amylase 3. Glycosuria
Chronic pancreatitis	1. Abdominal distention 2. Jaundice 3. Recurrent epigastric pain 4. Nausea 5. Vomiting 6. Weight loss 7. Diarrhea	Chronic inflammation, pancreatic function associated with chronic cholecystitis	1. ↑ serum amylase 2. ↑ lipase 3. ↑ blood sugar 4. Foul-smelling stool

SPECIFIC CONDITIONS CAUSING EPIGASTRIC PAIN

Medication should be explained, including dosage and action of such drugs as oral hypoglycemics, antacids, anticholinergics, and analgesics. A crisis social worker from a community program on alcohol should interview the patient and family, if alcohol is a precipitating factor, and initiate a plan of rehabilitation.

The patient should be instructed to return to the emergency department, if the following events occur:

A significant increase in pain despite medication.

Significant development of new pain.

Evidence of blood in the stool or vomitus.

The patient should be encouraged to contact his family physician for further evaluation and treatment.

Cholecystitis

Pathophysiology

Cholecystitis is an inflammation of the gallbladder, usually associated with gallstones and with obstruction of the passage of bile. This disease is more rare in the pediatric than in the adult patient. Women acquire the disease more frequenty than men, in a ratio of about 3:1. It is more common in women in their 40's who are overweight.

Gallbladder disease can include three different types: cholecystitis (inflammation of the gallbladder); cholelithiasis (stones in the gallbladder); and, choledocholithiasis (stones in the common duct). The function of the gallbladder is to store bile, discharge stored bile into the duodenum during digestion, and stabilize bile pressure within the biliary system. When gallstones are forced into the biliary ducts, these functions are disrupted. Bacterial infection may reach the gallbladder via the bloodstream, lymph system, or the bile ducts.

Clinical Manifestations

Patients with acute cholecystitis will present with nausea, vomiting, and moderate to severe pain in the right upper quadrant. Their temperature, as well as their white blood cell (WBC) count, may be elevated. The patient may also experience an increased pulse rate and an increased respiratory rate.

Cholelithiasis, the lodging of stones or the passage of stones through the cystic or common duct, is usually associated with severe pain. The patient with cholelithiasis will have a history of the inability to tolerate fatty foods.

Presenting symptoms may include intermittent pain in the epigastrium or right upper quadrant that may be referred to the right shoulder. Nausea, with or without vomiting, may occur.

Signs may include fever and abdominal tenderness, with rigidity on palpation of the right upper quadrant and rebound tenderness. On percussion, tenderness may be elicited over the liver. The inability of the patient to take a deep breath, when deep palpation is done beneath the right costal arch below the hepatic margin, is known as Murphy's sign.

Diagnostic Studies

Cholecystography can be used to visualize the shape and position of the gallbladder. This test, however, is effective only if the liver cells are capable of excreting the radiopaque dye into the bile.

Ultrasonography also may be used in the emergency department. This test, which records the reflections of pulses of ultrasonic waves directed into the tissues of organs, makes visualization of the organs possible. Ultrasonography can detect calcifications in the abdomen, biliary stones, pancreatic pseudocysts, and pancreatic enlargement.

Leukocytosis is evident with disease of the biliary system due to the inflammatory response, as well as to an increased bilirubin in the plasma and urine. Conjugated bilirubin that acts directly with diazo-reagents increases in the presence of hepatocellular and obstructive biliary tract disease. Unconjugated bilirubin (requiring the addition of methyl alcohol) is eliminated with increased hemolysis of red blood cells.

No bilirubin is normally excreted in the urine. Urine with bilirubin is mahogany in color and has a yellow foam when shaken. Bilirubin levels greater than 0.4 mg/100 ml will be excreted in the urine and are indicative of obstructive biliary tract disease.

Blood may be drawn for a complete blood count, electrolyte profile, PT, PTT, and levels of glucose, creatinine, BUN, and serum glutamic pyruvic transaminase (SGPT). SGPT is found primarily in the liver. With necrosis of the liver cells, SGPT is released, and an elevated serum level will be found.

Nursing Care and Related Interventions

Most patients that present to the emergency department with an acute attack of cholecystitis are hospitalized for observation and treatment. Intervention can include medical or surgical procedures.

When medical intervention is employed, the emergency department nurse should try to relieve the patient's discomfort. The patient should be allowed to assume whatever position is the most comfortable for the person, without causing harm. An analgesic may be prescribed to relieve severe pain. Merperidine hydrochloride (Demerol) in doses of 50 to 100 mg IM is given. Phenobarbital, up to 100 mg IM, is given for sedation and to relax smooth muscles. A nasogastric tube is passed to decompress the stomach, relieve vomiting, and reduce gastric stimulation. Fluid and electrolyte balances are maintained by starting an intravenous solution of 1,000 ml normal saline in the adult, and 500 ml of 5 percent dextrose in normal saline in children. Intravenous antibiotics may be started in the emergency department. When acute symptoms persist for two to three days, surgical treatment is normally advised.

Discharge Planning

If the patient is being discharged from the emergency department, the nurse should review activities of daily living with the patient and family. Depending on the patient's condition and general health status, the patient may be instructed to rest at home for several days, before gradually increasing activity.

A written diet for fat control should be reviewed and included with any discharge material. A follow-up appointment should be made with the patient's physician or health care provider.

CONCLUSION

Epigastric pain is associated with many illnesses in both the adult and pediatric patient. The emergency department nurse must obtain complete data to help differentiate the causes of the epigastric pain. Appropriate nursing care includes making the patient as comfortable as possible while diagnostic studies are done to help pinpoint the cause(s). The nursing care must be continually evaluated to meet the changing needs of the patient, as new data are discovered. The total needs of the patient and his family must be assessed and action planned to intervene for the benefit of the patient, as well as to provide quality patient care in every situation.

BIBLIOGRAPHY

Burkhart, C.: Upper G.I. hemorrhage: The clinical picture. *American Journal of Nursing* 81:1817–1820 (1981).

Burnstein, A. V.: Peptic ulcer disease: Medical and surgical considerations. *Critical Care Quarterly* 5:1–7 (1982).

Danis, D. M.: Abdominal pain . . . Aftercare instructions. *Journal of Emergency Nursing* 8:200 (1982).

Getting aggressive with peptic ulcer. *Emergency Medicine* 13:88 (1981).

Kilarski, D. J.: Refocus on cimetidine: Prophylactic use in acute gastrointestinal hemorrhage and the stress ulcer. *Hospital Formulae* 15:453–455 (1980).

Lamphier, T., and R. A. Lamphier: Upper G.I. hemorrhage: Emergency evaluation and management. *American Journal of Nursing* 81:1814–1816 (1981).

McConnell, E.: Curtailing a life-threatening crisis: G.I. bleeding. *Nursing* 11:70–73 (1981).

Maltz, C.: A differential for diarrhea. *Emergency Medicine* 13:90–91 (1981).

Sleisenger, M. H., and J. S. Fordtran: *Gastrointestinal Disease: Pathophysiology, Diagnosis, Management.* Philadelphia: Saunders, 1978.

Slota, M.: Abdominal assessment. *Critical Care Nurse* 2:78–81 (1982).

Smith, L., and S. Their: *Pathophysiology: The Biological Principles of Disease.* Philadelphia: Saunders, 1981.

Wolf, S.: Gastrointestinal upset . . . nausea: what does it signal? *Consultant* 21:27–32 (1981).

16

Minor Wounds and Bites

Dorothy M. Kellmer

After completing this chapter, the reader will be able to do the following:

1. Identify the purposes of wound care.
2. Triage a patient experiencing minor wounds and bites.
3. Discuss the process of wound healing and recognize the implications for care and for health teaching.
4. Discuss the pathophysiology of the various types of injuries as a basis for determining appropriate nursing interventions.
5. Identify the appropriate nursing interventions for selected situations.
6. Describe approaches to discharge planning and follow-up care.

The management of minor wounds and bites includes enhancing healing, preventing infection, reducing scar formation, and assisting the patient in effectively managing major and minor life disruptions. Minor traumatic incidents generally rank low in treatment priority; however, the frequency of occurrence requires the emergency department nurse to understand clearly the mechanisms of injury, the underlying pathophysiological processes, the significant aspects of assessment, and the appropriate interventions, as well as the underlying theoretical rationale.

TRIAGE

Subjective Data

The initial assessment interview of the patient experiencing a minor wound or bite includes a description of the injury and the circumstances surrounding the incident, obtained from the patient, the family, or from other observers. Essential to data collection is a consideration of the etiology of the accident, the characteristics of the causative agent, and an estimation of the amount and direction of the injuring force. The amount of time elapsed since the injury occurred is noted, because healing begins almost immediately and treatment delays increase the potential for local and systemic complications. In addition, the amount, type, and quality of prehospital care provided to the victim is determined.

The nursing interview also solicits pertinent information regarding the age and the current health status of the patient. Disorders that significantly affect treatment and healing are diabetes, blood dyscrasias, bleeding disorders, and poor tissue perfusion. Hypovitaminosis should be identified, if possible, since Vitamin C deficiency, in particular, interferes with collagen formation resulting in nonhealing of wounds. Signs of Vitamin C deficiency include hemorrhages, loose teeth, and gingivitis. Severe obesity must be recognized as a form of malnutrition, since extremely overweight patients do not heal well. Drugs that patients are currently taking may be significant for wound treatment. Aspirin, the most frequently used over-the-counter medication, decreases platelet aggregation, thus prolonging bleeding time. A single dose (0.65 g) approximately doubles the amount of bleeding in normal persons for a period lasting from four to seven days. Determining whether cortisone or immunosuppressive drugs are used by the patient is also pertinent, since wound healing and tissue repair may be delayed.

Socioeconomic factors are assessed. The type of job the patient has may affect treatment. The dishwasher with a cut on his hand, for example, may be unable to return to work with a large dressing in place. The model with a facial cut may be more anxious than the elderly gentleman who is less concerned with his appearance. Furthermore, religious factors must be considered, if they affect treatment and care.

Additional aspects of the subjective assessment of the patient include obtaining a description of past related injuries, an allergy history, an evaluation of the patient's immunization status, and a description of any influencing psychological factors.

Objective Data

Objective assessment in the triaging of the patient with a minor wound or bite is also imperative. Noting the patient's general grooming, as well as observing the condition of the patient's hair and nails, may provide valuable indicators regarding the factors that contributed to the injury and the patient's potential for complying with treatment. Calluses, stains, scars, and needle marks must be noted. In addition to determining the circulatory and nutritional status, the triage nurse recognizes local and immune responses, including the body's normal inflammatory processes.

Inspection and palpation of the wound are included in the objective assessment. Color, temperature, and pain are noted, as well as location of the wound, underlying structures, thickness of the skin, and exposure of the body part. The presence of necrotic tissue and the extent of observable wound contamination may indicate the presence of bacteria in the wound. The effect of the injury on the function of the involved part is assessed, as well as blood vessel involvement, arterial and venous flow and lymphatic drainage. Reports of numbness are noted. A superficial pinprick in areas serving nerves located close to the injury site will reveal possible nerve damage.

PHYSIOLOGY OF WOUND HEALING

Associated injuries may affect the treatment and subsequent healing of the injury. Possible tendon injuries are determined by checking the adequacy of the flexion and extension of the part. Bone injury, indicated by pain, proximity to the wound, or restrictions of movement, is evaluated first by inspection, and then by light palpation of the area. Similarly, the possibility of a foreign body within the wound is considered and, if indicated, is evaluated further.

Objective assessment includes considering the size and stage of growth and development of the affected individual. Although a child's capacity for repair is greater than an adult's, children lack both the physiological and emotional reserves to handle traumatic situations. Infection prophylaxis must be handled quickly because children have a greater potential than adults for rapidly spreading infections and destruction of body tissues. Because children's emotional reactions vary at different ages, nursing explanations and interventions must be tailored to the child's specific developmental stage.

Assessment and Planning

Planning for care includes an assessment for associated injuries or complications. When the potential for infection is high, a culture of the wound drainage and antibiotic sensitivity determinations are indicated. Radiological studies are indicated for crush injuries and for wounds with possible bone involvement, as well as for determining the presence of selected foreign bodies.

The actual plan of care varies according to the patient and to the particular type of wound. General measures are surgical evaluation, application of a temporary dressing (a pressure dressing, if indicated), and the setting of care priorities. Wounds with arterial bleeding, as well as anaphylactic reactions from bites and stings, are emergent situations. Extremely contaminated wounds or injuries, such as wounds resulting from high-pressure paint guns, require immediate attention. Most other minor wounds and bites are classified as acute. (Table 16.1 contains two examples of triage notes for patients experiencing minor wounds or bites.)

PHYSIOLOGY OF WOUND HEALING

The skin, the largest organ of the body, is composed of three layers: the epidermis, the dermis, and the subcutaneous tissue. The epidermis plays a significant role in the healing process, because, in addition to the liver, it is one of the few types of tissue that can regenerate itself. An avascular cornified, cellular structure, the epidermis is stratified into layers or elements. The surface element is composed of dead keratinized cells, resulting from progressive maturation of deeper living cells. Below this layer is the stratum germinativum, where new epithelial cells are produced. Melanin, the substance that gives the cells color, is also produced at this level. A basement membrane separates the epidermis from the dermis.

Between the epidermis and the dermis is the junction, an area of irregular contour due to the downward extension of the skin appendages that consist of hair follicles, sweat glands, and the sebaceous glands. The bulk of the skin comprises the dermis—

TABLE 16.1 Examples of Triage Notes for Patients Experiencing Minor Wounds and Bites

S: 32 yo WF with c/o laceration to dorsum of right hand from glass while doing dishes approximately 20 min. PTA. PMH: HTN, NKA, tetanus toxoid app. 6 months ago.
O: 2 cm superficial lac., bleeding moderate, ROM nl, sensory nl.
A: Lac. of right hand.
P: Surgical evaluation, pressure dressing, waiting room.

S: 7 yo M with possible snake bite to lateral aspect of left ankle app. 45 min. PTA while playing on construction site. C/o pain in area, numbness and tingling of tongue and mouth extending to face and scalp. PMH: NKA, tetanus toxoid 2 years ago.
O: Two puncture wounds noted on lateral aspect of left ankle, mod. amount of local edema, alert and oriented, weak and diaphoretic, rapid shallow respirations, venous tourniquet in place on midcalf.
A: Snake bite of right ankle.
P: Surgical evaluation, elevation, admit exam room immediately.

a tough connective tissue that contains lymphatics and nerves and is highly vascular. Through storing fat, the subcutaneous layer regulates temperature.

The process of wound healing is essentially the same, despite the type of tissue involved or the particular form of injury. Research has demonstrated three general and overlapping stages of healing, characterized by differentiated cell activity within the wound. The three stages are inflammation, fibroplasia, and collagen maturation. The process of healing is a fascinating example of biological adaptation essential to survival and evolution of the individual. Consider, for example, the process of healing in an uncomplicated wound situation. After the initial injury to the skin, blood flows into the wound, fills the defect, and subsequently clots. Beneath this clot, a network of fibrinogen strands begins to form, tenuously uniting the wound edges. Fluid is gradually lost from the clot, while fibrin and the other proteins dry out. In about two hours, a hard scab forms that protects the wound from both further fluid loss and bacterial invasion. A pathway is also established for the fibroblasts that will soon arrive at the site. The inflammatory process then begins, as the wound becomes swollen and painful. At the same time, the dying and broken tissues produce substances that dilate the nearby uninjured blood vessels, causing them to leak serum protein containing albumin, globulin, and antibodies. This fluid normally is a sustaining environment for the white blood cells that will arrive later. If viruses exist within the wounds, however, they will be attacked by both the globulin and the antibodies. This inflammatory process results in local swelling, pain, redness, and sometimes generalized fever—all characteristics of the increased metabolism that facilitates the repair activity. White cell migration increases the swelling as these cells slip through the walls of the blood vessels and move into the area of the wound. Six hours after the injury, the white cells are beginning the work of disintegrating and removing the debris within the wound.

The first white blood cells to arrive at the scene are the neutrophils, characteristically simple and short-lived (a few days) cells, with two lines of defense. The first method of defense is phagocytosis in which bacteria are killed and ingested by the cells. As the cells degenerate and die, their outer membranes rupture and pour enzyme-containing granules into the wound, attacking the extracellular debris so that later it can be easily removed.

Twelve hours after the initial injury, the monocytes begin to arrive in the area of the wound through the bloodstream from the more distant bone marrow. These cells are macrophages, ingesting most of the remaining debris, then digesting the debris through continued production of enzymes and synthesis of protein. Monocytes survive longer than their predecessors, the neutrophils.

Twenty-four hours after the injury, sheets of epidermal cells migrate across the wound beneath the scab to reform the basement membrane so that the fibroblasts can begin reconstruction. This process continues until an unbroken layer is established. Meanwhile, the scab continues to dry and in a few days will slough off, leaving a new layer of epidermis.

On the inner side of the scab, the fibroblasts from the nearby connective tissue replicate and produce collagen and protein polysaccharides from which dermal scar tissue will be formed. The collagen gives the scar tensile strength. Fibroblast activity reaches its peak in about six days. In addition to collagen building, other damaged tissue, such as lymphatics, blood vessels, and supporting tissues, are replaced. Furthermore, during this period, capillaries, originating as budlike structures on the nearby blood vessels, grow into loops that move through the wound by cell division to form a vessel network. This network supplies large quantities of oxygen for cell protein synthesis. After healing is completed, many of these capillaries will regress. If the wound is disrupted, the new granulation tissue appears translucent, mucinous, grayish-red in color, and bleeds easily.

The collagen fibers within the wound regroup about two weeks after the trauma. These fibers, originally laid down in a random manner, now are separated and reorganized into thick bundles along stress lines. The amount of stress on the wound will determine the thickness of the scar; consequently, more scar tissue will form on an area of movement, such as on the leg or on the hand, than on a stationary area, such as on the chest. Heredity also affects this process, since increased amounts of scar tissue are frequently evident in individuals of Oriental, Mediterranean, or African descent.

Wound contraction continues throughout a period of weeks or even months. During this maturation phase of the healing process, wound and scar strength increases. This process, called remodeling, may continue for years, as collagen density increases, vascularity decreases, and the scar becomes pale. In addition, if the gap caused by the injury is not too wide to bridge, some nerve regeneration occurs.

A stimulus apparently present in each stage of the process of wound healing produces or triggers the next stage. If, for example, the inflammatory response is so inhibited that too few neutrophils appear, the fibroblasts will lag behind in releasing connective tissue proteins. An understanding by the emergency department nurse of this healing process is essential for the appropriate and effective management of patients with wounds and bites.

NURSING CARE AND RELATED INTERVENTIONS

Direct pressure applied over the wound will control the bleeding in the majority of the minor wounds seen in the emergency setting. Moreover, elevation of the body part, if possible, will also facilitate the control of bleeding. Ligation of major bleeding points is occasionally required. Masses of ligatures should be avoided, since a suture in a wound acts as a foreign body and may promote infection and delay healing.

Opinions differ regarding the importance of shaving the area around a wound. A basic rule is to remove as little hair as necessary. Direct application of a dry razor over a wound will facilitate removal of the short hairs that tend to remain on the edge of the cut. Eyebrows should never be shaved, since disruption of the hair follicles may occur and regrowth may be inhibited.

Wound Cleansing and Irrigation

Skin cleansing and wound irrigation are essential for preparing the wound for definitive treatment. Antiseptic soaps or skin preparations must be mild. Harsh germicides and solutions containing alcohol should be avoided because they tend to irritate and cause tissue damage. Colored antiseptics in particular should be avoided because they mask the color and condition of the tissues. Antiseptics should not be used within the wound itself because products that are capable of killing organisms also kill living tissue. Hydrogen peroxide should also be used cautiously because it tends to absorb the oxygen in the wound, is painful, destroys cells, and is not effective against anaerobes.

Mechanical irrigation is probably the most essential part of wound preparation. After thorough cleansing, the skin is flushed, then the wound itself is irrigated. A toomey or control syringe with an 18 gauge needle and normal saline or a prepared isotonic solution works well. A bottle of intravenous normal saline with attached tubing, a threeway stopcock, and a large syringe are extremely effective for prolonged irrigation. Except for superficial wounds, a bulb syringe does not provide sufficient force for adequate irrigation. Particles of foreign material caught in the wound may be removed with either a small brush or forceps and additional irrigation. Do not soak the wound because soaking does not accomplish the same objectives and tends to cause tissue maceration. An effective guide to wound irrigation is the Kirz rule: "Irrigate with 50 cc normal saline per inch of wound per hour of age of wound" (Lanros, 1983, p. 322).

Anesthesia Administration

Anesthesia for the wound area may be required prior to thorough cleansing and irrigation, if the patient is extremely uncomfortable. The most frequently used local anesthetics are lidocaine hydrochloride and procaine hydrochloride, administered in percentages of 0.5 percent to 2 percent. Lidocaine, however, has a wider diffusability and a lower sensitivity rate than procaine. Moreover, procaine is faster-acting, but its effects last for a shorter duration. Solutions containing epinephrine are useful in vascular areas due to the vasoconstrictive effect. The epinephrine prolongs the onset of the anesthetic response through delayed absorption, but the duration of the effect is extended. Local anesthetics containing epinephrine, however, are not used for wounds supplied by end arteries, such as the fingers, toes, ears, nose, or penis because local vascular spasm resulting in gangrene may occur. These anesthetics must be administered cautiously to the elderly, the hypertensive, persons with hyperthyroidism, and patients who are receiving antidepressant drugs because of epinephrine's effect on the blood pressure. Remember, too, that lidocaine for anesthesia is not interchangeable with lidocaine for cardiac use. Cardiac lidocaine does not contain a preservative and, therefore, deteriorates in an open bottle.

Injection of local anesthesia is performed with the use of a syringe and hypodermic needle, usually no larger than 25 gauge, preferably 27 gauge. The pain of injection is related to the amount and the speed (rate) of infiltration and to the size of the needle. Opinions vary regarding where to insert the needle in relation to the wound. Less pain is felt by the patient if the needle is inserted directly into the edges of the open wound. Contaminated material, however, may be forced into uninjured tissue, and the solution may also distort the tissues. Injecting through the skin next to the wound is another, well-recognized technique. Both techniques involve injecting the medication ahead of the needle and slowly moving forward into the anesthetized area. If withdrawing the needle to reenter the tissue at another site is necessary, the entry site should be in an area already anesthetized. The amount of anesthetic solution used for infiltration should be limited to approximately 20 cc in adults. Usually only 2-3 cc are needed. The maximum dose for children is 3 mg/kg. A common cause of inadequate anesthesia is insufficient waiting time after injection.

Side effects of local anesthetics include both central nervous system (CNS) stimulation and depression. Signs of CNS stimulation include shivering, tremors, and euphoria, while depression is manifested by convulsions, respiratory depression and arrest, vascular collapse, and cardiac arrest. Immediate treatment for side effects is the administration of high flows of oxygen, supportive measures, and intravenous diazepam (Valium) for convulsions.

Several alternatives are available for individuals who are allergic to the *caines*. Packing the affected area with ice for 10 to 15 minutes will provide short-term anesthesia. Diphenhydramine HCl (Benadryl) 50 mg diluted in 2-3 cc of sterile water or normal saline injected around the wound will also effectively reduce discomfort. Third, if the wound is extensive, narcotics and/or systemic anesthesia may be indicated.

Sedation as an adjunct to local anesthesia is an important consideration, particularly with young children. More frequent use of this combination, as well as the judicious application of restraints, would probably reduce the traumatic effects of the treatment experience. One sedation option is the use of pentobarbital 5 mg/kg. Another frequently used and available combination of drugs is the "lytic cocktail," which consists of Demerol 2 mg/kg, Phenergan 2 mg/kg, and Thorazine 2 mg/kg administered intramuscularly 45 to 60 minutes prior to the procedure. The total amount of these drugs in relation to body size should be evaluated carefully, with special consideration given to the obese child. The lytic cocktail is not appropriate for infants under one year of age because of the immaturity of the infant's liver, kidneys, and nervous system.

Topical anesthetic preparations are also used in the treatment of minor wounds. Available ointments are occasionally indicated, but they are not soluble in water. Jellies are used more frequently because they are water soluble, and they are useful prior to the cleansing of minor abrasions containing free-floating dirt. The duration of effectiveness of topical agents is about 20 minutes, and they can be reapplied if needed. They are also effective as preparation for local anesthetic injection, and they may be used exclusively during the repair of some minor lacerations.

Debridement and Wound Closure

Debridement, essential for effective wound management, involves careful removal of all foreign bodies and devitalized tissue with forceps, tissue scissors, and/or a small knife blade. Extreme care must be taken during the debridement process to avoid inadvertently removing viable tissue.

Three basic approaches are used for wound closure. Determine which approach to use by evaluating the entire situation. The first method is called closure by *primary intention*. The wound is initially closed at the first setting. Because minimal scarring and deformity result, this procedure is the preferred treatment method. The immediate application of a skin graft to an avulsive injury is a variation of closure by primary intention.

In closure by *secondary intention* no initial attempt is made to close the wound; instead, the wound is allowed to "granulate in"—in essence, the epithelial cells move from the periphery to cover the surface of the wound. Scar formation and scar contracture may occur, with possible deformity and/or function loss. This procedure is the preferred method, however, for infected or extremely contaminated wounds, or when a large amount of devitalized tissue exists.

The third approach is called *tertiary intention,* delayed closure, secondary closure, or third intention. Suturing is delayed for several days because of infection or extreme contamination. The wound is then carefully cleansed, irrigated and debrided, and subsequently closed. Scar formation with this approach is greater than with primary intention, but less than with secondary intention.

Application of Dressings, Bandages, and Splints

Eight basic purposes for the use of dressings on wounds include the following:

1. Protection of the wound from contamination.
2. Protection of the wound from trauma.
3. Compression of the wound to decrease dead space and promote drainage. Because drainage is promoted, the comfort of the patient will be increased by al-

leviating pressure from accumulated fluids on organs and tissues adjacent to the wound.
4. Maintenance of a dry wound site.
5. Immobilization and support of the wound site.
6. Debridement of necrotic tissue in infected and open wounds.
7. Provision of a vehicle for the application of medication to the wound.
8. Provision of important psychological benefits by concealing any disfigurement until the patient is ready to accept it.

Several approaches to wound dressing are currently being used, and the method chosen should be adapted to the particular situation. Dry dressings, used most frequently, involve a versatile three-layered approach. The initial layer, consisting of a porous, nonadhering material, placed directly over the wound, is designed to allow drainage to pass through it, so that the wound site, although moist, will not be wet, thus providing an appropriate environment for healing. Sterile absorbent materials, comprising the second layer, must be sufficiently thick to keep the area dry and, if indicated, to apply gentle pressure to reduce edema and provide control of bleeding. The depth and extent of this second layer will be determined by the size of the wound, the amount of drainage expected, and the desired amount of protection for the area. In addition, the dressing materials must conform to the body contours to avoid the formation of dead space or gaps. The final dressing layer, used for attachment purposes, consists of bandage material or tape or both and should conform to the body's contours to allow for mobility and flexibility. Care must be taken to avoid vascular compromise from constricting the body part during application, as well as to allow for possible swelling subsequent to treatment. Figure 16.1 illustrates the types of materials that may be used in a three-layered dressing.

Wet saline dressings are used primarily for open wounds and for debridement. Maximum debridement is obtained by applying the wet dressings to the affected area, allowing them to dry, and then removing them without remoistening. Patients and families can care for wet dressings easily at home with adequate instruction. Sterile

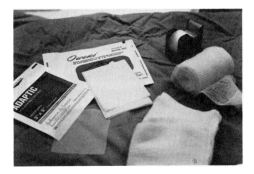

Figure 16.1 Types of materials that may be used in a three-layered dressing.

normal saline may be prepared at home by placing two teaspoons of table salt in one quart of water and boiling it for fifteen minutes.

A third method of wound care is the application of the semipermeable membrane. This dressing material was introduced in the United States after being developed in the United Kingdom. The actual dressing is an extremely elastic synthetic membrane that acts as a temporary second skin. Development of this synthetic membrane was based on evidence that moist, not dry environments, provide optimum conditions for rapid and effective healing. Research indicates that the rate of epithelialization can be almost doubled when the wound is covered with a membrane that is permeable to vapor and gases, but impermeable to liquids and bacteria. The membrane adheres to the dry, surrounding, undamaged skin, thus keeping the wound bathed in serous exudate that enhances healing, is removable without adherence, and minimizes scar formation. Immediate pain relief, ease of wound inspection, and increased patient mobility, including the freedom to bathe, are advantages to this approach. It is also used for some burn sites, decubitus ulcers, and for protecting donor sites of split thickness grafts.

Splints are occasionally used to treat minor wounds. Splints, generally applied to obtain partial immobilization of a part, may be constructed from a variety of materials.

DISCHARGE PLANNING

Discharge planning is an integral component of the treatment of patients with minor wounds and bites because most of these individuals are treated on an outpatient basis. Teaching begins with the arrival of the patient in the emergency care setting. For teaching effectiveness, the nurse must have an accurate theoretical knowledge base, an understanding of the teaching/learning process, and the ability to establish a relationship, as well as to communicate effectively, with the patient and/or the family. In addition, an assessment of the patient's and family's comprehension of the instructions, including their potential for compliance with treatment modalities, is crucial. Consideration must be given, however, to environmental and economic constraints in recommending particular medications and treatments.

Careful, thorough, specific written instructions are mandatory. The staff in many emergency settings have developed routine printed home-care sheets that provide specific essential information. This approach is particularly effective and efficient when additional space is provided for individual instructions. Figures 16.2 and 16.3 contain examples of discharge instruction forms used for routine problems.

Routine treatment measures for minor wounds and bites after discharge include elevation of the affected part, ice or heat, according to the particular problem and the amount of time elapsed since the injury, and Aspirin or Tylenol for discomfort. In addition, the patient and/or the family must be instructed to observe the wound site for signs of infection and other complications that would indicate the necessity to return to the emergency department for further treatment.

Arrangements must also be made or instructions given for follow-up care, either in a clinic or with a private physician, according to the policies of the particular health

WOUND / INCISION CARE INSTRUCTIONS

Your laceration ("cut") or incision has been treated by thorough cleansing, and sutures or a special tape have been applied to hold the skin edges together until healing has taken place.

The healing process usually takes a week to 10 days. During this time it is very important that you do all that you can to help the process and prevent infection.

Keep the wound dry and clean. If the present dressing becomes wet or dirty, you should:

a. Remove the old dressing carefully.
b. Wash your hands thoroughly.
c. Clean the wound with an applicator and hydrogen peroxide 3% or clean soapy water. An anti-bacterial soap is a good choice to use, such as *Dial*. Cover the wound with a new bandaid or gauze dressing.

If your wound is over 48 hours old and is not on a part of the body that will expose it to a great possibility of re-injury, you may leave the bandage off. However, if your work or play activities could cause reinjury or infection, keep a clean bandage over the wound.

Wounds on the face are usually not bandaged. An *antibiotic ointment* is generally recommended. This ointment is applied 3 to 4 times a day after the washing procedure has been done. These ointments can be purchased without a prescription. Examples are: Neosporin, Bacitracin, and Polymixin. Buy whichever is most economical.

SHOWERING OR BATHING:

Cover the dressing with a piece of plastic or saran wrap. Remove the plastic after your bath.

REMEMBER: Keep the wound clean and dry.

Infection can develop in a wound. Signs of infection are:

1. Redness or a red streak;
2. Excessive tenderness or pain;
3. Swelling;
4. Drainage or pus.

If you notice any of these signs, contact your physician or: _____

_____ , telephone # _____

RETURN APPOINTMENT

Please return to _____ Clinic on _____
                                                              DATE

at _____ AM ☐ Suture Removal;
       TIME   PM for: ☐ Dressing Change.

Figure 16.2 An example of a discharge instruction form for wound and incision care.

> Discharge Instructions
> Post-Animal Bites Instructions
>
> *General Measures:*
>
> Your animal bite has been treated by a physician. You may promote healing of the wound by following the instructions listed below:
>
> 1. *Cleanliness*—This is of primary importance; already there are germs or bacteria present in this wound introduced by the animal. Keeping this wound clean will help prevent the growth of this bacteria.
> 2. *Dry*—If you have stitches, keeping this wound dry is a must. Bacteria breeds in damp surroundings, so keep it dry.
> 3. *Dressings or Bandages*—If the doctor bandaged your wound, then leave it on for the prescribed length of time, unless it becomes wet or soiled. When it is time for the bandages to be removed, remember these tips:
>   a. If your bandage is stuck to the wound, use hydrogen peroxide to remove it. *Do not* tear the wound by pulling the bandage off.
>   b. *Always* dispose of your bandages in a small paper bag. Close the bag and then put it into the garbage.
>   *Signs of Infection*
>   a. *Redness/swelling*—Is there redness or swelling around the wound?
>   b. *Heat*—Is the area hot around the wound?
>   c. *Red streak*—Is there a red streak moving up the body from the wound?
>   d. *Pus/discharge*—Does the wound have pus or other discharges coming from it?
>   e. *Fever*—Are you running a fever?
>
> If the answer is *yes* to any of these questions, then your wound/bite is more than likely infected and you should return to the emergency department or to your private physician.
>
> *Reporting:*
>
> The local Public Health Department must be made aware of the animal that bit you. If the animal belongs to you, follow the directions of the Public Health Department in caring for this animal, If the animal belongs to someone else, make sure they are following the Public Health Department's instructions in caring for their animal. After all, animal bites can be fatal! It's your life you are dealing with. If you have questions regarding what procedures are correct in caring for an animal that has bitten you or someone in your family, call the Public Health Department at _____ or the twenty-four (24) hour number at the Dog Pound—

Figure 16.3 An example of a discharge instruction form for the care and reporting of animal bites.

NURSING CARE OF SPECIFIC INJURIES AND BITES

Lacerations

The laceration, probably the most common type of minor wound treated in emergency settings, is an open wound resulting from tearing or sharp cutting. The injury usually extends into the deep epithelial tissue, may involve underlying structures, and varies in depth and length. Nursing interventions include control of bleeding; careful assessment of the wound; appropriate shaving, cleansing, and irrigation; and, depending on institutional policies, administration of local anesthesia. Necrotic margins of the wound are then excised, edges approximated, and the wound closed with the use of either sutures or skin closure strips.

Suturing Considerations
Several considerations are essential before the nurse sutures a laceration, including an examination of the guidelines of the state nurse practice act, a determination of what is acceptable practice in the place of employment, and an assessment of the appropriateness of the repair of this particular wound to the nurse's skill level. The nurse generally should not repair a wound if any one of the following criteria exists (Lanros, 1983):

1. Presence of concomitant injuries requiring further evaluation.
2. Possible trauma to underlying structures.
3. Allergies to local anesthetics, epinephrine, antibiotics, and so forth.
4. Questionable tetanus immunization status, thus making the wound high risk.
5. Inability to adequately immobilize the patient or the wound.
6. Extent of required repair inappropriate to the skill of the nurse.
7. Face and neck wounds.
8. Wounds more than six to eight hours old.
9. Wounds with an extensive amount of crushed tissue.
10. Wounds that compromise circulation or affect sensory perception, motor function, or range of motion.

Types of Suture
The type of suture material used depends on the tissue being repaired and on individual choice. The area of the body requiring suturing and the amount of tension that will be placed on the wound edges are evaluated. Closure of a deep wound is done in layers to obliterate dead space and to prevent the collection of serum and blood that may act as a culture media and interfere with healing. Two general categories of suture material used for repairing minor wounds are absorbable and nonabsorbable sutures. Absorbable sutures, placed within the wound, reduce the tension on the skin

surface and decrease the problem of dead space. Some absorbable sutures currently available include plain gut, chromic, Vicryl, and Dexon. Nonabsorbable sutures for closure of the skin include silk, cotton, nylon, dacron, and steel.

While placing sutures in a wound area, the following principle should be considered: "The more tension on the wound, the closer the stitches should be to each other; the more tension on the wound edge, the closer the stitches should be to the wound edge" (Dushoff, 1973, p. 3). Skin edges must be slightly everted to ensure good healing and minimal scarring.

Suture Removal
The length of time sutures remain in place varies according to the body area, the circulation, and the degree of tension on the wound. (See Table 16.2 for the approximate number of days from placement to removal.) In preparing to remove sutures, always test the suture line to ensure that the wound will not separate. If any doubt exists regarding the adequacy of healing, apply skin closure strips between the sutures prior to removal of sutures. After removal, test and record range of motion and sensation of the affected area as a baseline for future evaluations.

Skin Closure Strips
Skin closure strips, used on superficial wounds, involve minimal tension. Advantages are that no anesthetic is required and the infection potential is less than with sutures, since no needle enters the tissues. Nevertheless, a greater potential exists for wound edge inversion, so wound edges must be joined carefully and smoothly. Disadvantages include a lack of strip adherence when wet and the potential for an allergic reaction to the adhesive.

Abrasions

An abrasion is a partial thickness denudation of a portion of the body's skin. Common and painful injuries, abrasions result from falls, scrapes, and, in particular, bicycle, minibike, and motorcycle accidents. The most important element in the management of these injuries is complete removal of dirt and debris. Particles that are allowed to remain embedded in the skin will cause permanent disfigurement,

TABLE 16.2 Approximate Number of Days From Suture Placement Until Removal

Body Part	Number of Days
Face	3–5 days
Scalp	6–8 days
Trunk	7–10 days
Extremity	7–10 days
Joint	12–16 days
Hands	7–10 days
Feet	7–10 days

similar to commercial tatoos. To prevent this problem, timing of treatment is essential. The pigmented material must be removed from an extremity within four to six hours; on the face, the increased vascularity in the skin allows about eight hours to effect removal.

Cleansing of the abraded areas must be done gently, without soap, but with a copious amount of normal saline. Local anesthesia in topical form or injectable solution may be required to minimize the discomfort. Scrubbing with a brush is frequently required; a sterile, hard, natural-bristle toothbrush works effectively. Forceps, a sterile needle, or a number 11 knife blade may also be used to lift out the tiny particles of asphalt or dirt.

To dress a facial abrasion, apply an antibiotic ointment and leave the area uncovered. Instruct the patient to wash the area four times a day and reapply the ointment. Healing generally occurs in two to three weeks. Direct sunlight should be avoided for six months, or the patient will risk developing pigmentary skin changes.

Avulsions

Loss of tissue that prevents approximation of wound edges characterizes avulsions and is commonly seen in fingertip and nose tip injuries. The problem requiring immediate attention is hemostasis. The area should be protected with sterile, saline-soaked gauze, and steady pressure applied. A small area of avulsion will usually heal by secondary intention, producing minimal scarring. Possible color differences in the affected tissue will fade in three to six months. Treatment of larger avulsed areas and of many digital avulsions often involves split thickness grafting, which may be performed in the emergency setting.

A large piece of avulsed tissue or an *amputated part* requires specific measures to prevent further damage and to preserve the tissue. At home or at the place of injury, the tissue should be rolled up so that the fat and the subcutaneous skin layer are inside and placed in a tight container to protect the part from drying in the air. Ice should be packed on the outside of the container if the travel time to the treatment facility is either prolonged or delayed. In the emergency setting, the tissue or part should be wrapped in gauze moistened with sterile normal saline, sealed in a plastic bag, and placed in a bath of ice saline or water. This procedure prevents the severed nerves, tendons, and vessels from becoming macerated so that they are more readily identifiable under the electron microscope. A part can be maintained in this fashion for six to ten hours. Surgical reattachment of the part may be attempted in the main operating area.

Contusions

Blunt trauma to superficial tissues, causing breakage of small blood vessels and extravasation of blood into the tissues, can produce contusions. General nursing measures involve local application of ice and elevation of the affected part. Three specific types of contusions include compartment syndrome, subungual hematomas, and wringer injuries.

Compartment syndrome is tissue compression within a fascial compartment due to increased content in the enclosed space, occurring most frequently in the area of the hand, the forearm, and the leg. Evaluation includes passive stretching of the involved segment to determine if pain can be elicited and palpation for local tenderness. In addition to the routine management of contusions, thorough instruction of the patient regarding the possibility of neurovascular changes is essential.

Subungual hematomas are injuries resulting from a blow to the fingernail or toenail. Blood collects beneath the nail causing increased pressure and throbbing pain. Treatment, which includes opening and draining the area, is done by using a small drill, a cautery set-up, or the tip of a heated paper clip briefly held against the nail to burn a hole through it. The patient should then soak the digit several times a day in warm water to promote drainage.

Wringer injuries, a combination of contusion and crush injuries, are caused by the drawing of a limb into the wringer of a washing machine or into an industrial machine and result in soft tissue and other structural damage. Deep burning of the skin may occur with severe contusions of the underlying musculature. In addition, extrication frequently involves the application of counter traction, leading to peripheral nerve damage. Less than five percent of these injuries result in bone fractures, but compartment syndrome may be a complication. Assessment of the injury includes the obtaining of data regarding the age, condition, and the type of wringer, the level to which the extremity entered, the duration of the exposure, and the measures used to extricate the part. Management consists of elevation, application of ice, x-ray studies to rule out bone injury, and continued observation for neurovascular damage.

Crush injuries of other types are caused when a heavy object falls on an extremity. Management generally involves procedures similar to those used for managing wringer injuries.

Puncture Wounds

Puncture wounds occur when the skin is pierced by a sharp or blunt object. Because these wounds bleed minimally, they tend to seal off, creating a high potential for infection. The characteristics of the injuring object, the length and/or depth of penetration, and the degree of contamination must be evaluated. Soaking, cleansing of the area, and observation for infection are usually adequate for wounds that are essentially clean. Contaminated puncture sites must be opened, debrided, irrigated, and packed. The use of local anesthesia should be limited because the additional fluid in the tissues causes engorgement, reduces blood supply, and may increase the infection risk. A rare complication of a puncture wound, if the instrument penetrates the deep fascia, is osteomylitis, a problem that may not be detected for several years. When fascial damage is suspected, however, exploration of the wound decreases the possibility that osteomylitis will develop.

Foreign Bodies

Foreign objects removed from various areas of the bodies of patients in the emergency department include wood and metal splinters, glass, clothing from gunshot wounds, rubber from tennis shoes, pins and needles, fishhooks, and other items. Radiologic examination is used for evaluating the foreign body and for determining its location and its accessibility. Wood splinters are not radio-opaque but, if paint is present on the wood, a shadow may form on the x-ray film. Steel particles, windshield glass, fish bones, and bony parts of fish fins will all appear on x-ray film; however, pieces of clothing usually do not appear.

A determination must be made regarding whether to remove the foreign body. Some wooden splinters, such as redwood, hemlock, and cedar, fulminate rapidly so they should be removed. Metal objects frequently become encrusted with scar tissue; thus, if the patient is experiencing no symptoms and removal is difficult, the object may be left in place. Needles are particularly difficult to find and may require removal under fluoroscopy. With any foreign body, the person must not move about after x-ray films are taken because the foreign body may change position within the tissues. Other precautions include the following:

Do not soak the part of the body containing a wooden splinter in water because the wood tends to absorb the liquid and disintegrate when removal is attempted.

Cutting a V-wedge in the fingernail will facilitate removal of a splinter that is beneath it. This procedure will also convert an anaerobic wound to an aerobic one, thus decreasing the danger of infection.

When the barb of a fishhook is deeply imbedded in the soft tissue of a digit, an incision can be made on the opposite side, and the tip forced through the tissue. The tip of the fishhook can then be cut off, and the shaft pulled out.

Missile Injuries

Superficial *stab wounds* are usually treated as lacerations or puncture wounds. Important initial assessment considerations include a verification of the type of instrument used (a knife, an ice pick, etc.), an estimate of the length of the instrument and the depth to which it was inserted, and a determination of the angle of entrance and direction of the force. A note of interest, with implications for evaluating the injury, is that men tend to stab in an underhand, upward direction, while women usually stab in an overhand, downward direction in an attack on another person.

Influential characteristics that are important in the assessment of *gunshot wounds* include missile ballistics: the movement of the bullet, tissue characteristics (because certain types of tissue are more resistant to injury), the type of weapon used, the distance of the victim from the weapon, and the characteristics of the bullet.

Three factors determine the extent of injury. The first factor relates to the actual laceration resulting from the penetration and direct cutting of the tissue. Handguns and rifles usually cause a small entrance hole and a large exit site. Shotgun injuries, particularly at close range, result in a large entrance hole with the lead shot lodging in the tissues.

The second factor that determines the degree and extent of injury is the cavity formation resulting from the energy shock waves. The severity of the wound relates to the amount of kinetic energy lost by the bullet to the tissue; thus, tissue located some distance away from the actual wound tract may also suffer severe damage.

Cavity formation and its effects are serious problems if the body was deeply penetrated by the missile.

Tissue and bone destruction by burning and expanding gases, the third factor, is a problem in close-range injuries. The combination of unburned and burning gunpowder causes a diffuse internal burn, particularly in shotgun injuries with large entrance sites. Close-range handgun wounds may also have gas trapped under the skin adjacent to the bullet entrance.

These three elements should be adequately evaluated in all gunshot injuries. Superficial wounds usually are treated as puncture wounds. The pellets or bullets may or may not be removed, depending on the location and on their accessibility. Removal of foreign bodies, such as bits of clothing and debris, must also be accomplished, and prophylaxis for infection considered.

Forensic considerations in the management of minor gunshot wounds are similar to those pertaining to major injuries. Appropriate reporting to law enforcement agencies, documentation of the condition of the patient, and the location of the bullet, as well as an accurate description of the entrance and exit sites, careful removal of clothing from around the wound, and appropriate handling and disposition of the bullet are all vitally important.

Other types of penetrating wounds reveal some of the same characteristics as missile injuries. A bolt from a high-powered machine or a rock thrown by a lawn mower may act as a bullet and lodge in the soft tissue. High-pressure injection wounds result when the nozzles of paint and grease guns blast their contents through the skin at a pressure of 600 to 7,000 lb/in.^{2}. The most common site of injury is the index finger of the nondominant hand. Serious problems result because the material, injected at the level of the fingers, spreads along the fascial planes, neurovascular bundles, and tendon sheaths, possibly reaching the wrist or elbow. Immediate treatment is required for this emergency. The tissue is usually opened, thoroughly debrided, and extensively irrigated. Nonetheless, amputation of the part may occasionally be required.

Bites

Human bites are potentially dangerous wounds with their seriousness being relative to the duration of time between the injury and the treatment. Types of human bites include self-inflicted injuries from nail biting, gum chewing, and epileptic seizures, accidental bites from poorly fitting dental prostheses, and person-to-person contacts during street fights, playground scuffles, and love-making. The most common site of injury is over the metacarpal phalangeal joint on the dorsum of the hand. This wound occurs when the fist hits the teeth of the opponent during an altercation so that the teeth tear the integumentary sheath, perforating the extensor tendon and exposing the joint capsule to bacteria.

Management of the human bite includes a culture of the wound, thorough cleansing, irrigation and debridement, and treatment with antibiotics. If sutures are required, they should be placed loosely. Frequently, delayed closure is the preferred treatment method. Individuals with wounds that are infected may require admission to the hospital and treatment with systemic antibiotics. Associated complications resulting from human bites include osteomylitis, abscess formation, pyarthrosis, and gangrene leading to subsequent amputation.

Ninety-five percent of the reported incidents of *animal bites* are caused by dogs. The victims are most frequently children or the animal's caretaker. The infection potential, except for the problem of rabies, is the same as that for human bites, but, fortunately, many of these injuries are superficial. Management is also the same as that used for human bites. In addition, rabies vaccine is administered if the index of suspicion is high. (See the section on rabies later in the chapter.)

The *gila monster* is a poisonous lizard found in Utah, Arizona, Nevada, New Mexico, and Gila river country. Coral and black in color, it is about 18 in. long. Venom glands located in the lower jaw supply ducts leading to about twenty grooved teeth. When the gila monster bites, it maintains a strong hold on its victim, and venom drools down the teeth. While forcibly jerking the animal's body to disengage the lizard from the victim, the lizard's teeth are often extracted.

The venom from a bite of a gila monster is essentially neurotoxic and anticoagulant. The wounds tend to bleed profusely with readily apparent edema and ecchymosis. If untreated, cardiac and respiratory failure may lead to death. Treatment is similar to that used for treating snake bites with an available antivenin (see the next section).

Snake Bites

Venomous snakes exist in all parts of the United States except in Hawaii, Alaska, and Maine. Several thousand snake bites occur each year, causing about 20 deaths. Ninety percent of the bites are on the extremities, and more than half occur in individuals under 20 years old, with 35 percent under 10 years old. The occurrence of a bite, however, does not always result in serious consequences because about 20 percent of the individuals bitten by snakes are not envenomated.

Snake venoms are complex mixtures composed primarily of proteins and enzymatic components. The enzymes were assumed to be the chief villains, and of course these elements do contribute to the problems that occur after a bite. The most serious effects, however, appear to result from certain peptide fractions affecting many of the body systems.

Pit vipers (family of Crotalidae) account for 60 percent of the snake bites in the United States and for nearly all of the deaths. This family of snakes is distinguished by the characteristic pit, a heat receptor organ that is a deep, easily recognized depression between the eye and the nostril. These snakes also have catlike elliptical pupils and triangular heads. They usually have two fangs (although more or fewer may be present); each fang is 0.5 to 2.5 cm long and functions on a swivel mechanism. The majority of pit viper bites are by rattlesnakes. Copperhead snakes account for most of the rest of the bites. Although copperhead snake bites result in gross edema, they are generally confined to the subcutaneous tissues and are not usually fatal unless a secondary infection results or the victim is a child. The cottonmouth water moccasin is also a pit viper, obtaining its name because it displays a white-walled oral cavity when threatened and has been mistaken for a ball of cotton. The bite of this snake is not particularly life-threatening, but may result in extensive swelling and ecchymosis.

Characteristic signs and symptoms of the bite of a rattlesnake are fang marks sometimes accompanied by a semicircle of teeth marks, instant burning pain, localized swelling (usually seen within five minutes with rapid progression), and numbness and tingling. Tingling is probably the most diagnostic sign and occurs in the tongue and mouth of a patient with a minor bite, extending to the face, scalp, fingers, and toes with increased severity of envenomation. Other signs include ecchymosis, vesiculation, thrombosis in the superficial vessels with sloughing and necrosis, diminished prothrombin activity, decreased serum fibrinogen levels, "burring" of the red blood cells, pulmonary edema, coma, convulsions, and respiratory paralysis.

Coral snakes (family of Elapidae) account for most of the rest of the venomous snake bites in the United States, with varieties being found in the south and west to Arizona and New Mexico. They are burrowing snakes that live in gardens and loose soil. Identifying characteristics include the presence of black, red, and yellow bands on the body with the black and yellow bands being wider than the red. The forepart of the heads of these snakes is black. They have slender bodies that are the same circumference as the head. Their length is usually under 50 cm, fangs are small and fixed, and eyes are round and black.

Characteristics of the bite of the coral snake are scratch marks or tiny puncture marks, with minimal to moderate edema, erythema, and pain. The victim may have paresthesia or may have no local reaction at all. Frequently, no symptoms appear for 12 hours after the bite, but when symptoms do occur, they progress rapidly and are usually paralytic. Although the venom of the coral snake is more toxic than venom from any other snake in the United States, a low incidence of death occurs because the snake has a small mouth, short fangs, and must chew to force the venom over the fangs and into the victim's flesh.

Variables to consider in assessing the severity of all snake bites include the size, sex, age, and health of the victim, the sensitivity of the victim to the venom, and the season of the year since snakes tend to be sluggish in the winter.

Prehospital care of the snakebite victim includes immediate immobilization of the individual followed by the application of a venous occlusive tourniquet about 2–4 in. proximal to the bite. The tourniquet should not be removed, but may be loosened slightly every 20 to 30 minutes and advanced as necessary to keep it above the swelling. If less than an hour has elapsed since the occurrence of the bite, a single linear cut through the skin should be made between the fang marks, and suction applied. No alcohol, stimulants, or depressants should be given to the victim because assessment then becomes difficult and these substances may interact with the toxins. If possible, a record should be maintained on the progress of signs and symptoms. Ice should not be applied to the site of the bite because unnecessary tissue destruction may result.

Immediate management of the snake bite victim in the emergency setting is basically supportive to deal with shock, fluid imbalances, and pain. No respiratory depressant drugs should be given. Baseline laboratory studies are conducted, including a type and crossmatch for possible blood transfusion. Antibiotics are usually administered. Surgical debridement of the wound may be indicated. Steroids, however, are contraindicated in the first six hours following the bite because they increase the possibility of gastrointestinal hemorrhage, enhance the action of the snake venom, and block the action of the antivenin.

The use of snake bite antivenin is somewhat controversial, and its use varies according to the physician's preference and the part of the country where the incident occurs. Some physicians feel that the antivenin should be reserved for life-threatening envenomations because of the risk of serious sensitivity reactions. If the drug is used, it should be given as soon as possible after the bite. Value appears to be minimal if the first dose is administered more than 12 hours after the bite. Intradermal skin or conjunctival testing must precede administration according to the manufacturer's directions. The dosage is calculated according to the severity of the reaction, rather than to the patient's weight, a particularly important factor in children, because the ratio between body size and the dose of snake venom is larger than in adults. Preparing for an anaphylactic reaction is recommended, even with a negative skin test. Antivenin is usually diluted in normal saline and administered piggyback to an intravenous infusion. It is given intramuscularly only if the intravenous route is not available. Antivenin should never be injected into the fingers or the toes, and direct infiltration into a snake bite wound appears to be ineffective.

Insect Stings and Bites

Insect stings become emergencies if a number of stings is incurred at one time or if the person stung develops an allergic response to the protein substance in the venom.

Types of stinging insects, classified into the *Hymenoptera group,* include bees, wasps, hornets, yellow jackets, and fire ants. Each species has its own distinct toxin, but similarities exist between the venoms. All Hymenoptera, except for the honey bee, have smooth stingers and can sting repeatedly. The honey bee has a stinger with barbs. The bee stings the victim, then the entire stinger apparatus is torn off as the bee flies away. The venom sac continues to contract, injecting serum, even though it has been separated from the bee. The stinger apparatus, therefore, must be removed as soon as possible. Squeezing the venom apparatus during removal will enhance the venom injection, thus, the best method is to scrape it away with a pocketknife or a fingernail.

The fire ant, native to South America, is now found in the southeastern United States. The sting of this insect produces a painful wound with a wheal in the center. The wheal expands into a large vesicle and progresses through the stages of purulence, reddening, scarring, and crusting, after reabsorption of the pustule.

The discomfort caused by the sting of a species of Hymenoptera may be relieved by the application of ice or by covering the affected area with a paste of Adolph's meat tenderizer, a commercial product that contains the proteolytic enzyme, papain. This enzyme, used for topical debridement, does not damage normal tissue. Continued management of stings of this type is mainly supportive and involves cleansing, application of an antiseptic, and rest and elevation of the limb. The use of antihistamines and steroids are effective for generalized reactions or for urticaria, but have minimal value for local responses.

About 25 percent of the world's population is hypersensitive to Hymenoptera venoms (Shires, 1979). A patient's and/or family's allergy history seems to be a predisposing factor. Reactions are more severe in individuals over the age of 30 and are rarely seen in children.

Anaphylactic Shock

Anaphylactic shock is the most serious complication of Hymenoptera stings. This systemic allergic response may also occur after the administration of various drugs, vaccines, or serums, if the patient has been previously sensitized either to these substances or to chemically related substances. Anaphylaxis results from the release of chemical mediators after antigen-antibody interactions, and its development depends on the presence of circulating, precipitating, gamma globulin antibodies.

The onset of anaphylaxis, an acute emergency, is usually immediate, although it may be delayed for 10 to 30 minutes. The clinical manifestations are similar to those occurring after an injection of histamine. Sudden anxiety, restlessness, and a feeling of doom are frequent, as well as spasms of smooth muscles, urticaria, profound respiratory distress, seizures, incontinence, and dramatic hypotension with circulatory collapse. Death may occur within 5 to 10 minutes.

Emergency management of the patient in anaphylactic shock includes the institution of basic life support measures. Intubation and positive pressure ventilation may be required, as well as the establishment of an intravenous line of dextrose 5 percent in water. Drug therapy includes aqueous epinephrine (1:1000) 1–2 cc intravenously to counteract the action of the histamine (aqueous epinephrine 1:1000 0.3 cc subcutaneously in less severe situations); antihistamines, usually diphenhydramine hydrochloride (Benadryl) 50–75 mg IV, to stop the action of the histamine as it affects the blood vessels and the bronchioles; and corticosteroids, hydrocortisone sodium succinate (Solu-Cortef) 100–200 mg or methylprednisolone sodium succinate (Solu-Medrol) 80 mg IV over one to two minutes for the anti-inflammatory action. Children's dosages of these drugs are aqueous epinephrine (1:1000) 0.01 cc/kg, diphenhydramine hydrochloride 1.25 mg/kg, and hydrocortisone 7 mg/kg. Metaraminol (Aramine) or levarterenol (Levophed) may also be indicated in a titrated drip if hypotension is extreme. Patients suffering anaphylactic reactions should always be hospitalized for at least 24 hours for adequate stabilization.

Discharge instructions regarding the prevention of future problems are essential. Precautionary measures to be observed by persons who are hypersensitive to bee or insect stings include avoiding the following:

1. Perfumes, sprays, and bright colors, because these attract insects.
2. Extensive skin exposure, especially around the neck.
3. Lying down or sitting in areas where there are many flowers, trees, and bushes.
4. Going barefoot.

Persons with known sensitivities should carry emergency insect bite kits when engaging in activities where the potential for bites or stings exists. It is also essential that both patient and family know how to use the equipment in the kit.

Arthropod Infestation and Bites

Infestation by *mites or chiggers,* sometimes called red bugs, is a fairly common problem resulting in localized skin irritation. These insects characteristically burrow into the skin, releasing a digestant that liquifies the epidermal cells and forms tubules. Macules with red centers appear on the skin surface and progress to vesicles. A medication used specifically for this irritating condition is gamma benzene hexachloride (Kwell). Additional treatment measures may also be required to relieve pruritus.

A *tick* is a species of arthropod that attaches itself to the host, secreting a cement-like material and burrowing into the skin to feed on blood. Because these insects are small and flat when not engorged with blood, the victim is frequently not aware of their presence.

A complication of the tick bite and subsequent attachment is tick paralysis, an acute flaccid condition that apparently results from the injection of a neurotoxin. The effects of the toxin start as a paresthesia and pain in the legs, followed by a symmetrically ascending paralysis. If untreated and the tick is not removed, the victim may die of respiratory failure. Upon removal of the tick, however, the condition clears spontaneously. An additional problem resulting from infestation is that some species of ticks carry the virus that causes Rocky Mountain Spotted Fever.

When removing the offending tick, care should be taken not to squeeze the tick because doing so can inject more toxin or virus into the victim. Various approaches are suggested for removal, including the application of a small amount of gasoline, ether, mineral oil, or touching the body of the tick with a hot (not burning) match. The tick will usually disengage itself within a few minutes of the applied treatment.

Approximately 30 species of *scorpions* are found in the United States. Although all are poisonous, the two species (Centruroides sculpturatus and Centruroides gertschi) that are considered deadly are found in Arizona and the other southwestern states. In Arizona, more deaths occur from scorpion envenomation than from rattlesnakes or from bites of other venomous animals. The scorpion does not actually bite, but stings by the flicking of its tail. The venom apparatus is at the end of the tail and consists of a pointed tip that is driven into the victim. The sting of the nonlethal species causes a sharp burning pain, with edema and discoloration. Anaphylaxis rarely occurs. The venom of the lethal species results in increased amounts of circulating catecholamines leading to myocardial damage and cardiac failure. No visible local effects of these stings exist, but immediate sharp pain and hyperesthesia are followed by hypoesthesia, numbness, and drowsiness. Itching of the nose, throat, and mouth, speech disturbances, jaw muscle spasm, nausea and vomiting, and convulsions may occur prior to death from the respiratory, circulatory, and cardiac failure.

Immediate application of a tourniquet, placed as near to the sting as possible, is done first, then ice is packed around the area well beyond the tourniquet. The tourniquet should be loosened in five minutes, but it may be reapplied. Continued care is supportive, including antivenin administration, if available.

Centipedes and millipedes cause discomfort and irritation. The centipede's bite is painful, with local swelling, redness, and occasional lymphangitis. Management involves the application of ice or a mild analgesic, wound cleansing, and the administration of antibiotics if indicated.

The millipede cannot bite, but, when handled, discharges a skin irritating toxin. Thorough washing of the affected area with soap and water and the application of a corticosteroid cream generally relieves the discomfort.

Spiders

Although most spiders are poisonous, only two species in the United States cause significant problems. These two species are the black widow and the brown recluse.

Black widow spiders (*Latrodextus mactans*) are found in all states, except Alaska. The female of the species is the offender and has a shiny black body with an hourglass or one or more triangles or irregular markings on the abdomen. It is about 15 mm by 10 mm in size. The poison is injected from venom glands through a pair of appendages near the mouth; the venom is histolytic and systemic and contains many protein fractions.

Patients frequently present for treatment with a vague history of a sharp pinprick, followed by a dull numbing pain. There may be slight swelling in the area and tiny fangmarks. If the bite is on a lower extremity, the individual will complain of localized pain, followed by pain and rigidity in the abdomen. An upper extremity bite results in pain and rigidity in the chest, the back, and the shoulders. This pain is fairly severe, beginning 15 to 60 minutes after the bite and increasing for 12 to 48 hours. Other clinical manifestations include dyspnea; nausea and vomiting; elevated temperature, blood pressure, and white blood cell count; hematuria; and paresthesias. Death occasionally occurs in the infant, the elderly person, or the patient with an allergic response from cardiac or respiratory failure.

Management of the patient following black widow spider envenomation involves application of ice to the area to slow absorption, treatment of the muscle spasms with muscle relaxants, such as Robaxin and intravenous 10 percent calcium gluconate, general supportive care recognizing that the venom is a respiratory depressant, and the administration of antivenin specifically for *Latrodextus mactans* bites. Symptoms usually subside within one to three hours after the administration of the antivenin. Without the use of antivenin, the symptoms, although severe, are usually self-limiting.

The *brown recluse spider* (*Loxosceles reclusus*) is found in Missouri, Tennessee, the midwestern and southwestern states, and also in the Pacific Northwest. This spider is smaller in size than the black widow and is brown or tan in color with a dark band on the dorsal cephalothorax, which is shaped like a violin, hence the common name *fiddler*. The initial bite of the brown recluse spider causes minimal pain, so frequently the diagnosis is only presumptive since the spider has not actually been seen. A local reaction begins in about two to eight hours, with pain in the area, and redness followed by blister formation and ischemia. Three or four days after the bite, the center becomes dark and firm. An ulcer forms in seven to fourteen days. Healing generally takes about three weeks, although grafting may be required for complete healing. Systemic responses include fever, chills, malaise, weakness, nausea, vomiting, joint pain and, on rare occasions, hemolytic anemia and thrombocytopenia.

Management of this bite is mainly supportive, although immediate excision of the wound area containing the toxins from the venom may enhance healing. Steroids, antibiotics, and antihistamines may be indicated. Antivenin is available in South America, but is not commercially purchasable in the United States.

Aquatic Organisms

Aquatic organisms do not usually prey on people, and injuries usually occur when the creature is disturbed. Antivenins for most aquatic bites and stings are available. Because the wounds frequently lead to secondary infections from the bacterial and viral pollution in fresh and salt water, antibiotics are usually administered after these injuries. Tetanus spores have not been found in water, but routine immunizations are given.

Marine creatures that bite include sharks, barracudas, moray eels, octopuses, sea snakes, sea lions, and killer whales. Sea snake and octopus venoms contain a neurotoxin, but lethal bites are rare. Management of these injuries is supportive with radiologic studies and surgical exploration and repair if the wound is deep or extensive.

Marine creatures that sting are coelenterates and include jelly fish, hydrozoans (Portugese man-of-war), anemones, and corals. Their stings occur by means of the firing of nematocysts that are capsules attached to the organism containing coiled, inverted, threadlike stingers. The stinging or firing of the nematocysts may occur immediately on contact with the skin or at a later time, set off by mechanical rubbing, exposure to fresh water, or a change in the pH. These capsules also break loose from the main body of the organism and may be found on beaches or in the water, still capable of firing. Clinical manifestations of these stings are burnlike welts, singularly and in clusters or in streaks. Initial pain is sudden and confusing, perhaps of such intensity as to cause shock and collapse and contribute to a number of drownings. The injected toxin may also be allergenic.

An acid wound is produced by this injury. Immediate treatment, at the scene if possible, is directed toward inactivation of the nematocysts by rinsing the affected area, first with sea water and then with a liquid such as alcohol, formalin, ammonia, or vinegar. Six to eight minutes after the application of the liquid, the area should be dusted with flour, baking powder, or sand to which the minute stinging cells can adhere and then be scrapped off with a knife and washed with salt water. The application of a corticosteroid analgesic balm will relieve the discomfort and irritation.

The stingray, the scorpion fish, the sea urchin, and the catfish are included in the group of *marine creatures with spines*. The spines produce a traumatic puncture wound, and the venom sacs from the spines release toxins that may produce cardiovascular, respiratory, or neurological complications.

The stingray is found along the U.S. coasts. When stepped on, this animal flips its tail into an arc, exposing a sharp spine. Immediate, intense pain occurs at the site of injury, in addition to bleeding, edema, and toxic responses due to the effects of the venom on the cardiovascular, respiratory, nervous, and urinary systems. Management involves immediate irrigation with cold salt water, removal of the parts of the integumentary sheath, and immersion of the affected part in hot water for one-half hour to neutralize the toxins. Antibiotics, antihistamines, and steroids may be indicated, in addition to thorough cleansing and possible surgical debridement. Severe toxic responses may require ventilatory support.

Scorpion fish include the California sculpin, the stone fish, and the lion fish. Each member of this species has venomous fin spines. Injury results in severe pain, edema, and possible acute toxic responses. Management is similar to that for treatment of injury by a stingray.

Another group of sea creatures in this category are the sea urchins. These animals have tiny fanglike organs along the spines called pedicellaries that break off on contact. The spine penetration of the skin causes pain, erythema, swelling, numbness, and paralysis leading to respiratory distress and death. The treatment again is similar to that for stingray injury. Soaking of the involved body part in vinegar may help to dissolve some of the spines. Radiological studies may be used to determine the location of the rest of the spines, but surgical removal is usually not attempted because granulomatous lesions often will eventually form around them.

The most prevalent poisonous fish in the United States is the catfish of which there are about 1,000 species. They are found commonly along the Gulf of Mexico. Fresh water catfish are found in the eastern rivers. Their sting results in an instant throbbing pain that usually subsides in a few hours. These wounds create an extremely high infection potential due to the life habits of the catfish. Management includes thorough cleansing, irrigation, debridement of deep wounds, and administration of antibiotics.

Wound Infections

Patients are seen frequently in the emergency department for the treatment of wound infections, either as the initial presenting problem or for follow-up care and continuing management of an injury. The cardinal signs of infection (pain, heat, redness, and swelling) are well known to all nurses.

Infections are usually easier to prevent than to treat. Several important principles apply to the care of all trauma patients in the prevention of infection. Rapid establishment of physiologic stability is the most vital. When the patient is in shock, the low cardiac output and the systemic hypoperfusion affects the bacterially contaminated wound. Rapidly restoring the peripheral, as well as the central, circulation is essential, therefore, to help prevent infection.

Further bacterial contamination of the wound must be avoided through the efficient use of dressings and sterile technique. Even if no time is available for definitive wound care, the simple covering of exposed wounds will reduce the incidence of continuing bacterial invasion.

The appropriate and timely use of antibiotics is the third principle. Antibiotic substances are most effective when they are present in the tissues prior to the arrival of the bacteria and become progressively less effective over the next few hours. Because, in most instances, administration of the medication prior to the injury is not feasible, the next best approach is to deliver the antibiotics to the tissues as soon as possible after injury. These drugs should be given with the initial fluid replacement at the same time that shock and acidosis are being reversed.

The final principle is the need for incision and drainage of localized wounds. This procedure is required, in addition to antibiotic therapy, because necrotic tissue and pus have no blood supply and also need an escape route.

Staphylococcus

Staphylococci are responsible for most of the human skin infections. The resulting abscesses usually are located in the superficial subcutaneous tissues and do not extend beyond the original site. If the body's defenses, however, are unable to control the bacteria, the infection may spread and become systemic. Whatever the location within the body, staphylococcal lesions necrose in varying degrees, tending to localize and to persist, despite antibiotic therapy, until the exudate is evacuated or can escape. Management involves incision and drainage of the wound, if indicated, and drug therapy. Penicillins and cephalosporins are among the most effective antistaphylococcal drugs available.

Pasteurella Multocida
Pasteurella multocida, caused by a species of small, gram-negative bacteria that is the normal inhabitant of the upper respiratory tract of mammals and birds, is a severe necrotizing infection associated with animal bites (particularly in cat and dog bites) and may follow cat scratches. The infection progresses rapidly leading to a cellulitis. Effective treatment in most instances is oral penicillin.

Clostridium Botulism (Wound botulism)
This rare wound infection is caused by the same anaerobic spore-bearing bacteria that results in food botulism and usually occurs with crush injuries or major trauma. The incubation period for wound botulism is 4 to 14 days. Symptoms, which are similar to those associated with botulism resulting from ingestion of contaminated food, include weakness, blurred vision, difficulty in speaking and swallowing, dry mucous membranes, dilated, fixed pupils, and progressive muscular paralysis as the cholinergic nerve fibers are affected. Ventilatory support may be indicated, in addition to other supportive measures.

Gas Gangrene
About 1,000 cases of gas gangrene caused by the anaerobic organism, *Clostridium perfringens,* occur each year in the United States. Occurrence has been noted after intestinal or gall bladder surgery, after certain hypodermic injections, especially subcutaneous epinephrine, and after minor trauma to an old scar containing clostridium spores. Symptoms begin one day to six weeks after the injury, with the rapid development of a woody-hard edema that interferes with the microcirculation and leads to hypoxia and the increased growth of anaerobic organisms. The result is thrombosis of the local vessels and the appearance of hydrogen sulfide and carbon dioxide in the tissues. Pain is severe and drainage consists of a thin watery brown or brown-gray liquid. Systemic symptoms include a low grade fever, increased pulse rate, anorexia, vomiting, diarrhea, coma, and death. Management involves general support, administration of penicillin or cephalosporins, excision of the affected tissue, hyperbaric oxygen, and the possible use of gas gangrene antitoxin.

Clostridium Tetanus
Tetanus is a disease of the neuromuscular system caused by exotoxins produced in an anaerobic environment by *Clostridium tetani,* a species of clostridium present in soil and in human and animal intestines. The organism also has been isolated in the air of operating rooms and in unsterile surgical supplies. Entry into the body is gained through a break in the skin, and the organism attaches itself to the cells of the central nervous system. The incubation period for tetanus is two days to several months, with an average of 6 to 14 days. Prodromal symptoms include restlessness, headache, and muscle spasms, with pain first being noted in the back, neck, or the face. Low back pain is commonly an early symptom. Progression of the disease is characterized

by extreme stiffness of the body, painful tonic spasms of the voluntary muscles, exaggeration of reflex activity, generalized convulsions, depression of the respiratory center in the medulla, and death.

Each year more than 100 cases of tetanus are seen in the United States, even with available effective immunization. At least half of these victims die. Wounds that are extremely contaminated or involve an anaerobic environment are tetanus prone. Prophylactic measures include the prompt, meticulous surgical care of all wounds, appropriate immunizations, and the use of antibiotics as ancillary measures because, even though these drugs have no effect on the tetanus spores, they will inhibit the co-infecting aerobic organisms, thus preventing anaerobic conditions. Obtaining an accurate immunization history is particularly important in the high-risk individual such as the addict, particularly the skin popper, young men and women whose immunity has waned, and older women who have never been immunized.

Immunity to tetanus, as well as to other diseases, occurs in one of two ways. The first is active immunity, whereby a vaccine containing a certain antigen is injected to stimulate the body to produce antibodies and to activate other cellular mechanisms. Passive immunity results from the administration of an agent containing antibodies produced in another host.

Toxoids are developed to provide active immunity and are prepared by chemical treatment of toxins that are secreted by bacteria. The manufacturing process destroys the pathogenic activity of the toxin, but the ability of the toxin to stimulate production of antibodies remains. The combination of diphtheria and tetanus toxoids (DT) is used routinely in most emergency departments throughout the country, according to the recommendations of the Immunization Practices Advisory Committee of the Center for Disease Control. (See Tables 16.3a, 16.3b, and 16.4.) When the initial immunization is administered in the department, follow-up instructions for the completion of the series of injections must be given. The avoidance of overimmunizing also is important because hypersensitivity reactions to tetanus toxoid are being in-

TABLE 16.3a Routine Diphtheria, Tetanus, and Pertussis Immunization Schedule Summary for Children Less Than 7 Years Old

Dose	Age/Interval	Product
Primary 1	6 wks or older	DPT 0.5 ml
Primary 2*	4–8 wks after 1st dose	DPT 0.5 ml
Primary 3*	4–8 wks after 2d dose	DPT 0.5 ml
Primary 4*	Approximately 1 yr after 3d dose	DPT 0.5 ml
Booster	4–6 years old, prior to entering kindergarten or elementary school	DPT 0.5 ml
Additional boosters	Every 10 yrs after last dose	DPT 0.5 ml

SOURCE: Recommendation of the Immunization Practices Advisory Committee, Center for Disease Control (MMWR, 1981, p. 395).

*Prolonging the interval does not require restarting series.

TABLE 16.3b Routine Diphtheria and Tetanus Immunization Schedule Summary for Persons 7 Years Old and Older

Dose	Age/Interval	Product
Primary 1	First visit	Td 0.5 ml
Primary 2*	4–8 wks after first dose	Td 0.5 ml
Primary 3*	6 months to 1 yr after second dose	Td 0.5 ml
Boosters	Every 10 yrs after last dose	Td 0.5 ml

SOURCE: Recommendation of the Immunization Practices Advisory Committee, Center for Disease Control (MMWR, 1981, p. 395).
*Prolonging the interval does not require restarting series.

creasingly recognized and seem to occur more frequently when the antibody titers are high. Signs of these reactions are rash, serum sickness, and anaphylaxis.

Immune serum globulins and antitoxins provide passive immunity. Human immune globulin is obtained from humans who are hyperimmune to the specific infection or disease. Human tetanus immune globulin (TIG) provides this passive immunity for individuals with tetanus prone wounds and gives immediate protection to persons never actively immunized. This agent has been shown to be quite safe, with few reported allergic reactions. No skin testing is required, and the product does not transmit serum hepatitis. Passive immunity is provided for one month with a dose of 250 units intramuscularly (500 units if the wound is extremely tetanus prone) in individuals over 10 years of age and 4 units/kg in children under 10 years (MMWR, 1981). The drug may be repeated at the end of the month if needed. The first dose of diphtheria and tetanus toxoid should be administered at the same time. Each drug must be injected into a different extremity, and TIG should not be given more than one hour before the toxoid, but either at the same time or one to two hours after to

TABLE 16.4 Tetanus Prophylaxis in Routine Wound Management

History of Tetanus Immunization (doses)	Clean, Minor Wounds Td	Clean, Minor Wounds TIG	All Other Wounds Td	All Other Wounds TIG
Uncertain	Yes	No	Yes	Yes
0–1	Yes	No	Yes	Yes
2	Yes	No	Yes	No*
3 or more	No†	No	No‡	No

SOURCE: Recommendation of the Immunization Practices Advisory Committee, Center for Disease Control (MMWR, 1981, p. 404).
*Yes, if wound is more than 24 hrs old.
†Yes, if more than 10 yrs since last dose.
‡Yes, if more than 5 yrs since last dose.

avoid competition or interaction. Patients who have disease processes that result in poor gamma globulin production should receive TIG even if they have been properly immunized. People requiring this protection include those with chronic lymphocytic leukemia, multiple myeloma, kidney transplants, or others who are receiving immunosuppressive drugs or corticosteroids.

Antitoxins contain antibodies from animals that have been immunized with the specific toxin. Skin testing is always recommended prior to administration due to the presence of foreign proteins that could result in allergic responses. Tetanus antitoxin (TAT) is rarely used today in the management of tetanus in the United States.

Treatment of the disease of tetanus includes respiratory support, muscle relaxants, and the administration of tetanus immune globulin in doses of 3,000–6,000 units. The drug is used primarily to neutralize circulating toxins because it is impossible to inactivate toxins that are already bound to nervous tissue.

Rabies

Rabies, also called *hydrophobia,* is an encephalitis due to a neurotoxic virus acquired from the saliva of a rabid animal. The incidence of rabies in humans has diminished significantly since the decline of the disease in domestic animals. Skunks in the midwest and California and raccoons in the southeast comprise the major reservoir of rabies virus. Nevertheless, rabid bats may be found in all areas of the country. The incubation period of rabies varies from ten days to several months. A history of a bite can usually be elicited from the patient. Information regarding the type of animal, the geographic area where the incident occurred, and whether the attack was provoked is essential to obtain. Clinical manifestations of the disease are general malaise, fever, headache, lymphadenitis, photophobia, muscle spasm, and coma. Children under the age of 12 seem to be more susceptible to rabies than are older children and adults. After the initial bite, routine, thorough wound care is implemented. Whether the wound should be sutured is subject to some controversy. Antibiotics are generally indicated.

Rabies prophylaxis is instituted if it appears that the animal causing the bite may have been rabid, and includes the quarantine or the pathological examination of the animal when possible. Several types of rabies vaccine are available for use. If antirabies treatment is indicated, both human rabies immune globulin (RIG) and human diploid cell rabies vaccine (HDCV) should be given as soon as possible (Eisenberg and Copass, 1982). The dose of RIG is 20 IU/kg, with approximately half of the vaccine injected directly into and around the wound, and the remainder given intramuscularly in the buttocks. If the human serum is unavailable, equine antirabies serum (ARS) in the recommended dose may be used. HDCV 1 cc intramuscularly is administered initially, and on days 3, 7, 14, and 28 following exposure. Serum is drawn to determine the antibody level two to three weeks after the last dose. If no antibody response occurs, an additional booster dose of the medication should be given. HDCV has proven to be highly immunogenic and to cause low reaction rates in recipients, and its use has replaced the previously used duck embryo vaccine (DEV) (MMWR, 1981).

Reporting of animal bites must be made to the appropriate local health authorities, either by the victim or by the care giver, depending on state and local policy.

CONCLUSION

This discussion of the management of the patient experiencing minor wounds and bites provides clear evidence that, although this type of problem is frequently treated in emergency departments, many factors require comprehensive, indepth assessment. Moreover, planning of nursing care and interventions involves individualization, according to the presenting situation, to enhance healing, prevent infection, reduce scarring, and offer assistance and support in a crisis situation.

BIBLIOGRAPHY

Budassi, S., and J. Barber: *Emergency Nursing: Principles and Practice*. St. Louis: Mosby, 1981.

Cain, H. D.: *Flint's Emergency Treatment and Management*. Philadelphia: Saunders, 1980.

Dushoff, I.: A stitch in time. *Emergency Medicine* 5(reprint), 1973.

Eisenberg, M., and M. Copass: *Emergency Medical Therapy*. 2nd ed. Philadelphia: Saunders, 1982.

Jaws that bite, things that sting. *Emergency Medicine* 10(7):24–59 (1978).

Howry, L., R. Bindler, and Y. Tso: *Pediatrics Medications*. Philadelphia: Lippincott, 1981.

Lanros, N.: *Assessment and Intervention in Emergency Nursing*. Bowie, MD: Brady, 1983.

Luckman, J., and K. Sorenson: *Medical Surgical Nursing: A Psychophysiological Approach*. 2nd ed. Philadelphia: Saunders, 1980.

Morbidity Mortality Weekly Report 30:392–396, 401–407 (1981).

Ross, R.: Wound healing. *Scientific American* 2–12 (1969).

Shires, G.: *Care of the Trauma Patient*. 2nd ed. New York: McGraw-Hill, 1979.

Turner, T.: Today's products and wound management. *Nursing Mirror* 149(25):i–xvi (1979).

Warner, C.: *Emergency Care: Assessment and Intervention*. 3rd ed. St. Louis: Mosby, 1983.

White, K: Evaluating the trauma of gunshot wounds. *American Journal of Nursing* 77:1589–1593 (1977).

Wolcott, M.: *Ambulatory Surgery and the Basics of Emergency Surgical Care*. Philadelphia Lippincott, 1981.

17
Orthopedic Trauma

Ann M. Van Hoff
Nancy L. Griffith

After completing this chapter, the reader will be able to do the following:

1. Triage a patient experiencing orthopedic trauma.
2. Understand the pathology of bone injury.
3. Correlate assessment data to help define patient problems.
4. Determine appropriate interventions.
5. Discuss the discharge planning appropriate for patients with orthopedic problems.

Orthopedic trauma can involve any of the 206 bones of the body, cartilage, ligaments, tendons, and muscle. In addition, trauma can occur to the neurovascular system. Approximately three-fourths of all orthopedic trauma involves the extremities, with fractures constituting the most common type. Although fractures may occur in anyone, regardless of age or sex, they tend to occur more frequently in the following groups: men, 20–40 years of age, are prone to fractures of the extremities; children frequently sustain fractures of the clavicle and supracondylar area of the humerus; middle-aged women commonly sustain fractures of the humerus and Colles' fractures of the wrist; and the aged have an increased incidence of compression fractures of the vertebrae and hip fractures (Gartland, 1979). These fractures usually occur due to activity level and to the physiological status of the body.

A thorough assessment and immediate, definitive treatment can facilitate the recovery process for the patient with orthopedic trauma.

TRIAGE

Subjective Data

Triage begins with an accurate history from the patient with suspected orthopedic trauma. Obtaining an accurate triage history involves determining the what, when, and how of the injury. Determining the time of injury assists in assessing the severity of the trauma and may affect the mode of treatment. Information obtained from the patient should include the location of the injury, precipitating event, factors that increase or decrease the severity of pain, and factors that relieve pain and concomitant symptoms (Emergency Department Nurses Association, 1980). Ascertaining the body posture at the moment of injury will assist in deducing the direction and degree of forces on the body and on the injured part. This assessment involves determining if there was direct or indirect force on the injured part associated with tensile, compression, or shearing motion. The family or emergency transport personnel should be questioned regarding the condition of the patient when found and treatment measures, if any, that were initiated.

The past medical history can reveal the immunization status, allergies, current medications, relevant medical illnesses, and the presence of recurring orthopedic injury. In the pediatric patient, the past medical history may reveal a chronic disease or unrelated illness of the recent past that may influence the mode of treatment.

Objective Data

The triage process continues with physical inspection. If extreme, life-threatening trauma does not exist, an initial skeletal survey is made. The skeletal survey will ascertain the extent of injury, provide a systematic pattern for assessment, and collect data that will assist in determining x-ray examinations required (Emergency Department Nurses Association, 1980). The survey, which moves from head to toe, uses inspection, palpation, and auscultation. The palpation process must be gentle to avoid causing further injury or pain. The survey involves the following steps:

1. Head
    a. Have patient open and close mouth.
    b. Palpate nose and cheek bones.
    c. Examine scalp.
2. Neck
    a. Note evidence of muscle spasm.
    b. Make sure cervical fracture has been ruled out.
    c. Palpate for bone point tenderness by moving spinous process (but do *not* move until cervical fracture is ruled out).
3. Chest
    a. Have patient deep breathe.
    b. Perform compression test for rib fracture. While supporting back, gently compress sternum (DeGowin and DeGowin, 1976). (Not used for pediatric patients; use careful palpation instead.)
4. Spine
    Carefully palpate spinous processes for point tenderness; (do not move the patient until all spinal fractures are ruled out; if movement is necessary, use the log roll technique).

5. Arms and hands
   a. Have patient move arms, hands, and fingers through range of motion.
   b. Palpate the fingers to check for phalangeal or metacarpal injury.
   c. Shake hands (elicits data on mobility, edema, skin temperature, and neurological functioning).
   d. Have patient turn arm when arm is straight and when it is partially flexed.
6. Legs and feet
   a. Have patient move each leg through range of motion.
   b. Have patient move toes and rotate feet outward against resistance.
7. Pelvis
   a. Gently compress iliac crests or symphysis pubis with patient supine (Gurd, 1981).
   b. Place clenched fist between knees and ask patient to squeeze knees together (Emergency Department Nurses Association, 1980).

The skeletal survey may identify abnormalities in other body systems.

Gentle firmness is required in handling the pediatric patient, who often hesitates to move voluntarily. Gathering objective data for a child with a suspected injury to the extremities involves looking for swelling and ecchymosis, gentle palpation of the extremity for point tenderness, and performing manual range of motion for the child (Emergency Department Nurses Association, 1980). The lability of a child in stressful situations requires vigilant observation to detect subtle signs of trauma. A child may react as strongly to being in a strange environment with unfamiliar people as to the injury itself.

The gathering of objective data continues with the assessment of the 5Ps (pain, pallor, pulses, paresthesia, and paralysis) of the injured extremity above and below the location of the injury. Assessment of circulation, sensory perception, and range of motion capabilities provides data necessary for determining the severity of the initial injury and the degree of continuing tissue compromise.

Assessment and Planning

The subjective and objective data enable the nurse to make a nursing diagnosis. In developing the plan of care, the nurse should consider the data collected and determine priority of care questions, which include the following:

1. What injuries endanger life and limb?
2. What injuries are particularly prone to produce shock?
3. What injuries have a poor prognosis when treatment is delayed?
4. What injuries are suitable for immediate immobilization or traction with definitive treatment implemented at a later time?
5. What injuries can be treated in a definitive manner without harm to a severely injured patient? (Kettelkamp, 1976)

TABLE 17.1 Examples of Triage Notes for Patients Experiencing Orthopedic Trauma

S: 40 yo M fell from ladder and cut right forearm 1 hr prior to admission. Wound wrapped with clean cloth. PMH: negative, no known allergies, last tetanus toxoid not known.

O: BP 140/90, P 78, ROM deferred. Able to move fingers and has sensation, prompt capillary refill, radial and brachial pulses WNL, facial grimacing present, jagged laceration 5 cm long and 1 cm deep with profuse bleeding, no obvious deformity.

A: Fractured ulna or radius with laceration.

P: Surgical evaluation with x-ray examination of Ⓡ forearm, splint with sling, sterile pressure dressing, admit to exam room as soon as possible.

S: 22 yo WM with "twisted left ankle" 2 hrs ago. Pain increasing. PMH: second injury to this ankle, first ankle sprain 2 months ago, NKA.

O: Unable to bear weight. Limited ROM. Swelling 3 inches above ankle on medial side, pedal pulses WNL bilaterally, ecchymosis over entire Ⓛ foot and ankle.

A: Injured Ⓛ ankle.

P: Surgical evaluation with x-ray examination, elevate, cold compresses, admit to exam room when possible.

S: 19 yo BF with c/o being involved in motor vehicle accident app. 3 hrs PTA. Passenger in front seat with seat belt, hit broadside on passenger side, thrown against center arm rest and dash. Transferred on back board. c/o extreme pain when moves hips, no other complaints. PMH: negative, NKA, tetanus toxoid 60 min PTA.

O: AAOx3, IV D$_5$RL infusing Ⓡ arm, Foley catheter in place with grossly bloody urine, ecchymosis around pelvic region. BP 132/68, P 82, femoral, popliteal, pedal pulses WNL bilaterally with Doppler.

A: Injured pelvis.

P: Surgical evaluation, admit to exam room now.

The plan of care will involve evaluation, immobilization, patient support, ice to the injury, elevation, ordering an appropriate x-ray examination, and referral to the surgical/orthopedic service.

Examples of triage notes related to orthopedic trauma are included in Table 17.1. A detailed discussion of nursing interventions for the patient with orthopedic injuries will assist the nurse in planning appropriate actions for the care of these patients.

ORTHOPEDIC INJURIES

The clinical manifestations of orthopedic trauma can involve structural, soft tissue, and neurovascular alterations. Assessment for the presence of these manifestations is essential for patients who have either known or suspected orthopedic trauma.

Neurovascular Alterations

Neurovascular trauma associated with orthopedic injury may involve circulation, motor function, and sensory perception. Initiated during triage, neurovascular assessment, using the 5Ps, should be an ongoing process.

Circulatory Status
Circulatory alterations include pallor, cyanosis, or pulselessness. Clinically, the normal body part is compared with the abnormal body part for paleness, mottled cyanosis, cool skin, and capillary filling time. Venous obstruction causes a bluish color to the skin, while decreased arterial supply causes pallor (Donahoo and Dimon, 1977). Arterial injury leads to cool skin, whereas venous injury can cause either warm or cool skin temperature (Sproul, 1983). Either sluggish capillary return or no return may indicate arterial insufficiency.

The rate and character of pulses distal to the injury are noted on a continuing basis. These pulses include the brachial, radial, and ulnar pulses of the upper extremity and the femoral, popliteal, posterior tibial, and dorsalis pedis pulses in the lower extremity.

Motor Function
Nerves may be bruised, lacerated, severed, torn, or stretched at the time of injury. In addition, ischemia and compression due to edema or hemorrhage for several hours after the injury can cause temporary loss of nerve function.

Assessing the motor component of nerve function necessitates considering the severity of the trauma. The movement required for assessment is minimal because excessive movement can be hazardous. The presence of paralysis in any of the muscle groups responsible for flexion, extension, abduction, adduction, or rotation must be determined. The functional evaluation of the major peripheral nerves is completed as follows (Conrad, 1979):

1. *Axillary*—abduction of the upper arm at the shoulder.
2. *Musculocutaneous*—flexion of the elbow.
3. *Radial*—dorsiflexion of the hand at the wrist.
4. *Median*—apposition of the thumb.
5. *Ulnar*—spreading and closing of the fingers.
6. *Femoral*—extension of the leg at the knee.
7. *Tibial*—plantar flexion of the foot.
8. *Peroneal*—dorsiflexion of the foot.

Sensory Perception
Assessing the sensory perception component of nerve function involves determining the nature of the pain experience and the presence of paresthesia. Assessment of sensory perception involves subjective and objective data.

Pain can be severe with orthopedic trauma due to disruption of the integrity of the periosteum and accompanying soft tissue injury. In addition, the degree of pain experienced by the patient is affected by the person's anxiety level. The actual nature of pain can be determined only through communication with the patient.

Sensory evaluation for paresthesia completes the assessment of nerve function. Patient impressions of sensory changes usually are reliable in evaluating nerve injury (Hoopes and Maxwell, 1979). Sensory evaluation includes the following major peripheral nerves (Donahoo, 1977; DeGowin and DeGowin, 1978):

1. *Radial*—Prick web between thumb and index finger.
2. *Ulnar*—Prick distal fat pad of little finger.
3. *Median*—Prick distal surface of index finger.
4. *Femoral*—Prick medial and anterior surface of thigh and knee.
5. *Peroneal*—Prick lateral surface of great toe and medial surface of second toe.
6. *Tibial*—Prick medial and lateral surfaces of the sole of the foot.

The assessment components for a child with orthopedic trauma are the same as those for an adult. Nevertheless, the responses of a child to trauma are different and must be considered during the evaluation of clinical manifestations. Communication with the child can be facilitated by talking slowly and in a low tone of voice, communicating at eye level with the child, and speaking truthfully in simple terms that the child can understand. Even if communication is established, the child may be unable to express his pain or to localize the area of pain. The child's inability to verbalize may be due to the child's age, language development, or confusion and anxiety related to the situation and/or environment.

Structural Alterations

Structural alterations refer to fractures in which the continuity of the bone is disturbed. Fractures may be either complete or incomplete. *Complete fractures* demonstrate discontinuity across the entire section of bone. *Incomplete fractures* involve discontinuity in only a portion of the bony structure.

Complete fractures are usually transverse, oblique, spiral, comminuted, multiple double–segmental, impacted, or pathological. *Transverse, oblique,* and *spiral* describe the direction of the line of fracture in relation to the long axis of the bone. Multiple, splintered fracture fragments constitute a *comminuted* fracture. A *multiple double–segmental* fracture involves two complete and separate breaks at different levels. A break in which one bone end is driven firmly into the other bone end is called an *impacted* fracture. A *pathological* fracture, which occurs in an area of abnormal bone, is caused by congenital, inflammatory, neoplastic, or metabolic conditions.

An incomplete fracture may be any one of the above types of fractures, except that it does not involve the entire cross-section of bone. The most common type of incomplete fracture is the *greenstick* fracture of the long bones in children. The trauma force bends the cortex on the compression side and breaks the bone on the distraction side (Brashear and Raney, 1978).

Bone Structure and Healing

Bone is living tissue that changes structurally in response to stress, as well as to vascular, endocrine, and nutritional influences. The primary functions of bone are to support the human body and to provide calcium. Bone also serves as a point of origin and insertion for muscles and as a protection for soft tissue structures. A fracture causes damage and death to the living cells of bone, as well as injury to the periosteum. Bleeding from damaged blood vessels causes a hematoma to form at the fracture site. As the phases of healing occur, a substance called *callus*—cartilage and new bone—is formed, which immobilizes the fracture fragments. The callus formation must be kept immobile by splinting and casting to enable mature bone to form. If the callus formation is not immobilized, it will remain fibrous and pliable. The last phase of the healing process is remodeling. Remodeling is the stage in which newly formed fiber bone is converted to lamellar bone. The process is primarily electrical (Heppenstall, 1980; Vaughn, 1981). This process, evolving for a period of months or even years, allows bone outside the stress lines to be removed and considerable deformity correction to occur. Fracture healing is unique because, when completed, it is almost impossible to distinguish healed bone from uninjured bone.

Unlike adults, children usually incur bone injuries that are relatively uncomplicated. The tough periosteum of children's bones often remains intact, which helps to prevent displacement. Special problems arise, however, in diagnosing and in treating *epiphyseal injuries*. The worst complication is growth disturbance. The two types of epiphyses are *pressure*—those at the end of long bones that contribute to longitudinal growth—and *traction* (apophyses) that are located at the origin or insertion of major muscles. Examples of apophyses are the greater and lesser trochanters of the femur. The problem is not the actual damage done to the epiphyseal plate, but whether the injury interferes with the blood supply. Although an accurate diagnosis depends on an x-ray examination, such an injury should be suspected when the child shows evidence of pain, swelling, tenderness, and spasm at a joint.

The best known description of epiphyseal injuries is the Salter classification (Salter and Harris, 1963). (See Fig. 17.1) In this classification, Type I is a simple separation of the epiphyseal plate with an excellent prognosis for complete recovery. Type II is a separation of the epiphysis with a fracture through the metaphysis, and it also has an excellent prognosis for complete recovery. In Type III, however, the plate itself slips, and a fracture through the epiphysis involves the articular surface. Open reduction is often required in this type of injury. Type IV is identified as an intra-articular fracture through the plate and the metaphysis, most commonly seen in the lateral condyle of the humerus. Type V in the Salter classification results from an impaction injury that crushes and destroys the epiphyseal plate. The prognosis is poor, and premature cessation of growth often occurs.

Osteoporosis is defined as a decrease in the total amount of bone mass to the point where fractures occur with apparently minor trauma. Approximately 70 percent of the patients with hip fractures are diagnosed as being osteoporotic (Larson and Gould, 1978). Generally associated with the aging process, osteoporosis reveals a decreased formation of protein matrix in which calcium is deposited. The condition has been considered to be a problem of calcium metabolism.

Clavicular Fractures

Pathophysiology
Clavicular fractures, the most common fractures of childhood, are often greenstick in nature and are usually caused by a fall on an outstretched hand. A less common

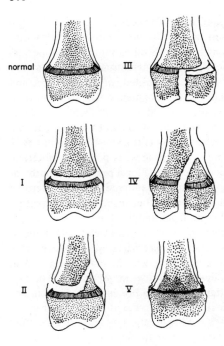

Figure 17.1 The Salter classification of epiphyseal injuries.

cause is a direct blow to the shoulder. About 80 percent of these fractures are of the middle third of the clavicle (Gurd, 1981).

Clinical Manifestations
The patient presents with tenderness and obvious deformity along the clavicular line with the arm often adducting and rotating forward and inward. There is point tenderness over the fracture site, in addition to swelling and crepitus. Because this position causes overriding of the bone fragments with subsequent pain, the patient usually supports the injured arm with the unaffected arm.

Vascular checks of the ulnar and radial pulses are imperative because of the location of the subclavian artery. Motor and sensory function of the affected arm also must be assessed because of the location of the brachial plexus. Symptoms of injury to this large, anatomically complex structure depend on location of the injury in the plexus; thus, a complete motor and sensory assessment is required.

Nursing Care and Related Interventions
Treatment includes reduction of the fracture and immobilization with the common figure-of-eight wrap. Immobilization should be for approximately two to three weeks in children, and five to six weeks in adults. Healing occurs in five to eight weeks.

Shoulder Injuries

The glenohumeral joint of the *shoulder* is a ball and socket joint consisting of the large humeral head and the glenoid capsule of the scapula. The joint, which is not mechanically stable, is supported by muscles, tendons, and ligaments.

Pathophysiology

About 90 percent of shoulder dislocations are anterior and usually occur in adults (Gurd, 1981). If an accompanying fracture exists, it is often located in the upper humerus. Fracture of the body of the scapula is rare. When it occurs, such a fracture usually results from the person falling on an outstretched hand in an attempt to brace a fall; or it results from a direct force to the posterior–lateral aspect, again usually from a fall.

Clinical Manifestations

The injured person presents with severe pain, with the arm rotated externally and abducted. The person usually refuses any attempts at movement and splints the injured shoulder with the other arm and hand. Neurovascular assessment of shoulder injuries is crucial.

Nursing Care and Related Interventions

Treatment is directed towards fast reduction and immobilization that prevents abduction and external rotation. Reduction is usually relatively easy to do, if accomplished before a reflex muscle spasm occurs. The majority of patients can be managed in the emergency department with intravenous use of analgesics and muscle relaxants. If reduction with simple sedation is not accomplished readily, a general anesthetic should be considered.

Four general methods are used to accomplish a closed reduction of the glenohumeral joint. In the oldest method, called the *Hippocratic* method, the patient is placed in a supine position at the edge of the table. Grasping the wrist and forearm, the physician places his or her foot in the axilla. Reduction is produced through gradual, gentle, longitudinal traction to the extremity and simultaneous countertraction with the foot. Extreme care must be used to avoid driving the heel of the foot into the axilla, which could cause neurovascular damage. With the *Kocher* method, traction in line with the humerus is applied to the elbow, which is flexed at a 90 degree angle. With the humerus in an adducted position to the thorax, slow, gradual, external rotation is applied until the extremity touches the examining table. Opponents to this method suggest that the leverage required to obtain reduction can result either in neurovascular damage or in associated fractures of the humeral shaft or the head. In a third method, called the *Stimson* method, the patient is placed in a prone position while the injured extremity hangs down. Skin traction weighing 10 to 15 pounds is applied and allowed to hang free. Reduction often is accomplished within 20 to 25 minutes. The fourth commonly used method is called *elevation*. With the patient placed in a supine position, the injured extremity is elevated gradually in forward flexion to a direct overhead position by applying gentle outward and upward traction at about 25 to 30 degrees of abduction. The operator's hand is placed under the patient's humeral head, gently lifting it into the glenoid fossa. The patient's cooperation obviously is required. If any paresthesia is experienced by the patient, the method should not be continued. A Velpeau or triangle sling is used for immobilization with tightening or reapplication every five or six days.

Humeral Fractures

The *humerus,* the most mobile long bone in the body, acts primarily as a lever. The subscapular artery anatomically branches off from the subclavian artery and wraps around the upper humerus, almost at the surgical neck. The brachial artery branches off the subclavian and enters the medial aspect of the shaft at the same level as the radial nerve. Because of this unique structure, interruption of arterial blood supply in humeral fractures commonly occurs. Consequently, humeral fractures are notorious for not healing.

Pathophysiology
Fractures of the proximal humerus involve either the anatomical neck (usually associated with a severe comminuted fracture of the area) or the surgical neck. They are commonly caused by a fall on the outstretched, pronated, upper extremity. This position can result in an impaction of the medial shaft into the central metaphyseal part of the humeral head. The most serious complication of an anatomical neck fracture is avascular necrosis, a common injury in the elderly woman who presents with swelling at the anterior aspect of the shoulder, severe pain, and inability to move the affected arm.

Clinical Manifestations
Patients may allow the injured arm to just hang because of motion pain, or they may attempt to provide splinting by supporting the injured arm with the unaffected limb. Ecchymosis may be evident on the axillary aspect of the arm and/or on the thoracic wall. In children these injuries are usually a Type II epiphyseal fracture.

A humeral shaft fracture may be caused either by the same mechanism of injury that caused a proximal fracture or by a direct blow from the side. The patient presents with pain and inability to move the arm. The deformity may be manifested by a bowing out of the upper arm and an overriding of bone fragments with subsequent tenderness and swelling.

Nursing Care and Related Interventions
The most important nursing actions are temporary immobilization of the arm to prevent further neurovascular damage and continuing neurovascular assessment. Immobilization is usually accomplished with a figure-of-eight wrap.

For any type of humeral fracture, the nurse evaluates the adjacent shoulder and elbow for injury, in addition to evaluating the distal neurovascular status of the affected extremity. Gurd (1981) states that five to ten percent of these patients have some degree of radial nerve damage. Severance of the radial nerve is evidenced by the immediate inability of the patient to raise the hand at the wrist. In addition to distal neurovascular assessment, interventions include cold packs and a sling to splint and support the injury.

Elbow Injuries

Pathophysiology
The *elbow*, a true hinge joint, is particularly susceptible to fractures and to dislocations in children and in young adults. Fractures of the elbow include fractures of the distal humerus and of the proximal radius and ulna (as, for example, in olecranon fractures) and are caused either by falls on the outstretched arm with the elbow

ORTHOPEDIC INJURIES

extended or by direct falls onto the elbow. Dislocations, which are most commonly posterior, result from the same types of forces that cause fractures.

Another common childhood injury is a pulled elbow, occasionally called a nursemaid's elbow. A sudden pull is exerted on the pronated forearm of the child when the elbow is in extension. In addition, the injury also can be caused by lifting the child when the arms of the child are extended, which can cause a temporary subluxation of the radial head.

Volkmann's contracture, the most devastating complication of elbow injuries, results from ischemia of the nerves and muscles. This injury can be caused by an artery being caught at the injury site. More commonly, however, the injury results because an artery was contused at the time of the injury with subsequent development of arterial spasms.

Clinical Manifestations
The patient with an elbow injury presents with severe pain, tenderness, rapid swelling that obliterates the normal triangular configuration, widening of the joint, a distorted, bulging appearance, and an inability to flex the arm. The patient usually supports the affected arm in a flexed position. The child with a pulled elbow refuses to move the arm and exhibits local tenderness over the radial head.

In a patient suffering from Volkmann's contracture, signs and symptoms that can occur shortly after the injury or within 48 hours include the following (Ross, 1979):

Constant burning pain in the forearm.

Swollen and cyanotic hand and fingers.

Radial pulse that is almost always absent.

Fingers and thumb that become numb if the condition is allowed to progress.

Pain in attempting to extend flexed fingers.

The resulting deformity is caused by tissue necrosis due to a deprivation of blood and oxygen to the muscle. The muscle is eventually replaced by fibrous tissue that contracts and shortens, causing the deformity.

Nursing Care and Related Interventions
In any elbow injury, immediate and continuous neurovascular assessment of the radial, median, and ulnar nerves, as well as the radial and ulnar arteries is necessary. The arm should be immobilized in the position presented and cold applications used to reduce edema.

Treatment of elbow fractures varies from open reduction with pinning to closed reduction and casting. A detailed discussion of the types of elbow fractures can be found in Heppenstall (1980). Dislocations are treated by reduction with full range of motion. The joint is usually immobilized for a week or two until the irritability has settled. For a pulled elbow, treatment is usually accomplished by immobilization with a sling for a few weeks to allow the ligament to heal.

Radius and Ulna Fractures

Pathophysiology
Fractures of the *radius and ulna,* which commonly occur in adults and in children, result either from a fall on an extended arm or possibly from a direct blow.

Clinical Manifestations
The patient presents with pain, point tenderness, and swelling. Obvious deformity usually exists with abnormal rotation and shortening of the arm. In children the midshaft fractures usually are greenstick in nature.

Nursing Care and Related Interventions
Immediate interventions should include a careful check of the distal neurovascular status because the deep branch of the radial nerve can be injured. Cold can be applied and a splint used to immobilize the reduced fracture.

Wrist Injuries

Pathophysiology
The *wrist,* the foundation of the hand, is the major shock absorber in falls on the outstretched hand. Fractures occur most frequently in the elderly, especially in women, while sprains and dislocations occur more frequently in the younger, more athletic person.

Force against the palm of the hand caused from a fall can result in the *Colles' fracture*—a fracture of the distal radius and ulna, creating the silver fork deformity (see Fig. 17.2). The wrist is angulated posteriorly, while finger movement is limited, and the fingers are flexed. In children, the fracture is usually of the distal radius with a Type II epiphyseal injury, and it is often associated with a greenstick fracture of the ulna.

Clinical Manifestations
Patients with wrist injuries present with pain, swelling, point tenderness, and deformity. Because of the minimal swelling associated with Colles' fracture, children are often seen two or three days after the injury. The persistent pain usually causes the child's parents to seek care.

Nursing Care and Related Interventions
The limb should be splinted in the presenting position and cold packs applied. Elevation will help relieve the pressure of the swelling. Although a neurovascular problem usually does not exist, the median nerve should be assessed for motor and sensory function and the radial pulse for circulation impairment. Reduction is usually accomplished by closed manipulation and the limb is most often placed in a short arm cast.

The key to assessment and planned interventions in *hand* injuries is knowledge of the functional anatomy of the hand. The initial assessment and history are important because the mechanism of the injury can indicate what structures might have been damaged. Moreover, preexisting deficits, as well as the patient's occupation and

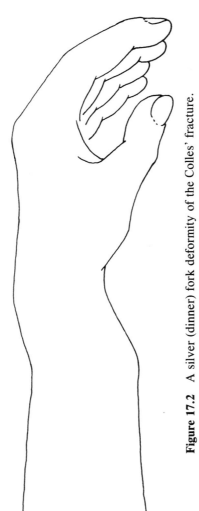

Figure 17.2 A silver (dinner) fork deformity of the Colles' fracture.

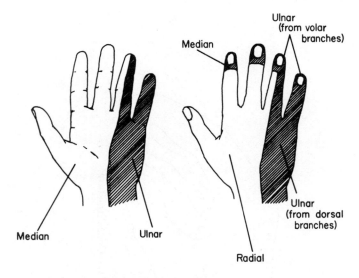

Figure 17.3 Sensory nerve patterns of the hands.

dominant hand, also should be identified (Adelman and Sarant, 1982). Assessment of motor and sensory functions are crucial in treating hand injuries (see Fig. 17.3).

Dressings and/or splints for hand injuries must provide proper positioning with subsequent support and stability. The proper anatomic (functional) position ultimately determines the outcome of emergency interventions (Adelman and Sarant, 1982).

Pelvic Injuries

Dissimilar to the shoulder girdle, the pelvic girdle is a relatively rigid structure that provides support and protection. The pelvic ring is formed by two innominate bones that posteriorly articulate with the sacrum and anteriorly with the symphysis pubis. The emergency nurse must be knowledgeable about the neurovascular supply to the lower extremities. The femoral nerve, arising from the lumbar plexus, enters the thigh anteriorly behind the inguinal ligament, while the sciatic nerve, which becomes the peroneal nerve, exits from the pelvis posteriorly through the greater sciatic notch. The obturator nerve, also arising from the lumbar plexus, exits from the pelvis posteriorly through the greater sciatic notch (see Fig. 17.4). The external iliac artery leaves the pelvis with the femoral nerve and becomes the femoral artery (see Fig. 17.5).

Pathophysiology
A *pelvic fracture* is most commonly seen in middle-aged and older adults. This injury is usually due to a car or motorcycle accident with a resulting crush injury or from direct trauma due to a fall. Any patient with a pelvic fracture should be assessed for other injuries because 65 percent are estimated to have associated injuries (Budassi and Barber, 1981).

ORTHOPEDIC INJURIES

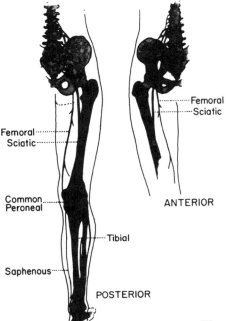

Figure 17.4 Nerves of the lower extremities.

Clinical Manifestations

The patient exhibits pain when a "springing action" is performed (exertion of downward pressure on the iliac crests or on the symphysis with the patient lying supine), muscle spasms, sacroiliac joint tenderness, perineal or scrotal hematomas, and even hematuria. Blood loss and shock can be severe, and an estimated 10 percent of patients with pelvic fractures eventually die.

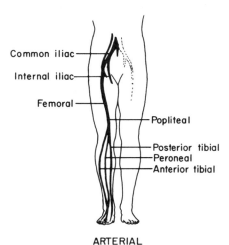

Figure 17.5 The arterial blood supply of the lower extremities.

Nursing Care and Related Interventions

Immediate treatment is directed toward physical stabilization, including immobilization of the spine and legs with flexed knees, which helps decrease pain. Oxygen administration, establishment of an intravenous line, and continual monitoring of vital signs are necessary. Distal neurovascular assessment must be continual. Hemorrhage is often extensive, with rarely less than 500 cc of blood loss. It is estimated that 60 percent of the deaths result from massive extraperitoneal bleeding (Heppenstall, 1980). Although not all pelvic fractures are this severe, the nurse must continually monitor the patient to detect signs of increasing severity.

Pelvic fractures are classified into four groups:

1. *Avulsion fractures* commonly occur at the anterior, superior iliac spine. Treatment is symptomatic with bedrest followed by return to full weight bearing as symptoms improve.
2. *Stable fractures* of the pelvic ring include fractures of the iliac wing, sacrum, coccyx, and the pubic rami. The treatment is bedrest for two to six weeks with a gradual return to weight bearing.
3. *Unstable fractures* include the "straddle fractures" in which the superior and inferior pubic rami are fractured bilaterally with severe pelvic disruption. Treatment involves skeletal traction with the patient placed in a pelvic sling. This position is maintained for six to eight weeks with nonweight-bearing for an additional six to eight weeks. Disruption of the symphysis pubis can be treated with a hip spica cast.
4. An *acetabular fracture* can involve either the rim or the central cup. This fracture frequently occurs when a pedestrian is struck along the trochanteric area by a bumper or fender of a car (Heppenstall, 1980). Dashboard injuries (a knee pushed against the dashboard) can cause a shattering injury of the acetabulum.

Hip Injuries

The *hip*, a ball and socket joint, is formed by the cup-shaped cavity of the acetabulum and the head of the femur creating an extremely stable joint. The femoral neck connects the head and body of the femur. Most of the blood supply to the femoral head lies close to the neck.

Pathophysiology

Dislocations of the hip frequently occur in car accidents in which the knee is jammed against the dashboard. They are usually posterior injuries. Fractures of the femur, commonly called hip fractures, are classified into four groups—head, neck, intertrochanteric, and subtrochanteric.

Fractures of the femoral head are common in people over sixty, especially in women who are frequently osteoporotic. The actual force involved in the injury is often slight, and, in most cases, the fracture occurs from a rotational movement. There are four types of femoral head fractures: impacted, stress, comminuted, and displaced. If no displacement exists, especially if the fracture is impacted, the history may be only a fall with groin pain. Often the person is able to stand up after the fall and to walk slowly. Impacted femoral head fractures are quite rare. *Stress fractures* most often occur in children and in athletic people. Femoral neck fractures do not commonly occur in children. When they do occur, caused by severe force, they constitute a major emergency.

Most *intertrochanteric* fractures result from a fall, and they occur more commonly in elderly women. *Subtrochanteric* fractures, the least common type of fracture, are caused by direct force. These fractures tend to occur in elderly patients with bone diseases, such as osteomalcia or Paget's disease. The fractures often produce considerable bleeding and are best repaired by open reduction and internal fixation.

Clinical Manifestations
The patient with a dislocated hip has severe pain upon active and passive movement, deformity due to the prominence of the greater trochanter, and a shortened leg. In most hip fractures, the patient presents with severe pain and an inability to bear weight on the injured leg. A noticeable deformity exists, as well as swelling in the immediate injury area and external angulation. Muscle spasm causes shortening of the limb, and the nurse may feel crepitus over the fracture site.

Nursing Care and Related Interventions
For a dislocated hip, the joint is reduced immediately with care taken to avoid either avascular necrosis of the femoral head or sciatic nerve damage. The possibility of avascular necrosis increases as the length of time increases between the time of the injury and the time of intervention.

Stress fractures are treated with nonweight-bearing and avoidance of strenuous limb exercises for six weeks with an additional six weeks of partial weight-bearing. In older people, internal fixation is preferable. *Comminuted neck fractures* in older people are treated with a prosthetic replacement. In younger people, open reduction with internal fixation is a common treatment. *Displaced fractures* are treated surgically by internal fixation.

Femur Fractures

Pathophysiology
The *femur,* the longest and strongest bone in the body, is the bone most subject to stress. A femoral shaft fracture occurs most often in a young adult who sustains a direct force either from an auto accident or from a traumatic fall.

Clinical Manifestations
Pain is often severe, with localized swelling and a shortened leg. The leg may be rotated or angulated.

Nursing Care and Related Interventions
The leg should be splinted in the position found. The patient must be observed for major blood loss. Because a femoral fracture can result in significant blood loss, the patient should have an intravenous line established. Continual monitoring of vital signs and extremity neurovascular status is also necessary.

Splinting should be done with an open splint, such as the Hare traction splint, instead of with the long leg air splint to enable the nurse to continue neurovascular assessment. Cold packs to the fracture site will help relieve pain and swelling. If Kirschner wires or Steinman pins are used for closed reductions and subsequent immobilization, they may be placed in position in the emergency department while using local anesthesia. Complete, balanced traction is usually not applied in the emergency department because of transportation difficulties.

Knee Injuries

The *knee,* not a pure hinge joint, depends almost entirely on its capsular and collateral ligaments for its posterior stability. The neurovascular structures lie close to the bone and are prone to injury. Injury to the popliteal artery endangers circulation to the distal leg. Data support the frequent occurrence of this injury because the amputation rate for the distal leg has not changed significantly during the past twenty years (Sternbach, 1979).

Pathophysiology
Knee injuries include fractures of the distal femur, fractures of the patella and proximal tibia, dislocations of the knee and patella, and soft tissue injuries to the extensor apparatus and the intra-articular structures of the knee.

Knee injuries usually result from a combination of indirect and direct forces that are often difficult to determine because the injury occurs so quickly. Severity ultimately relates to the damage in the popliteal space. Although the popliteal artery is bound down at either end of the space by membranous attachments, it also is strung like a bowstring making it quite susceptible to injury (Sternbach, 1979).

Clinical Manifestations
The patient with a knee injury presents with severe pain and a history of either a direct injury to the knee or a stumble, after which the knee collapses. Symptoms may include local point tenderness, inability to walk, swelling, hemarthrosis, and inability to straighten the leg.

Nursing Care and Related Interventions
According to Schneider (1980), the most critical factor in the assessment is determining whether the extensor mechanism is intact. Can the patient perform a straight leg raise against gravity while lying in a supine position? The optimal time to make an assessment is immediately after the injury before swelling and muscle spasms occur. Knee dislocations occur in all age groups, and the injury mechanism is severe trauma. The presenting symptoms are the same as those for a fracture. The joint should not be manipulated, but cold packs are applied to control swelling and pain, and the patient is cautioned to avoid any weight-bearing. The dislocation or fracture is reduced and splinted.

Tibia and Fibula Injuries

Pathophysiology

Tibia and *fibula* injuries are some of the most common orthopedic injuries. As the main weight-bearing bone of the lower extremities, the tibia is extremely vulnerable to fracture. It is also the most probable site for a compound fracture. The majority of fractures occur in the distal third of the bone where the shaft narrows and has less supporting strength. The head of the fibula articulates with the lateral portion of the tibia creating protection for the peroneal nerve. The abductor muscle group is located in the lateral compartment, which is the major everter of the foot. The posterior muscles are contained in two groups: the calf group and the deep flexor group located beneath the calf group. The posterior tibial artery and its peroneal artery branch also are contained in the lateral compartment. The extensor muscles, as well as the anterior tibial artery and the deep peroneal nerve, lie in the front of the leg in what is known as the *anterior compartment*. A specific syndrome, called *anterior tibial compartment syndrome,* develops when tissue pressure increases because of active bleeding and resulting muscle swelling, which produce ischemic changes in the musculature. The increased pressure results in a decrease in oxygen supply.

Tibial shaft fractures result from direct forces (such as gunshots or vehicular accidents) and indirect forces (either by a fall from a height in which the person lands on his feet, or by a rotational force trauma). If the tibial fracture is transverse, the fibula tends to fracture at the same level. Fibular fractures are produced by the same mechanisms that cause tibial shaft fractures. In some cases, only the fibula is fractured if there is direct trauma to the lateral side of the leg (Heppenstall, 1980; Gurd, 1981).

Clinical Manifestations

Symptoms of anterior tibial compartment syndrome include severe pain in the antero-lateral aspect of the lower leg, inability to dorsiflex the foot, pain on passive motion of toes, and diminished sensation across the dorsal first web space. Peripheral pulses do not provide an adequate assessment base because pedal pulses can be maintained by collateral flow. The best assessment clue is the capillary return to the toes.

The patient with a tibial fracture presents with pain that increases with movement and point tenderness. In fractures of the proximal tibia, there is immobility of the knee. These proximal fractures are not uncommon occurrences with knee fractures and/or with dislocations. The leg may vary in appearance from almost normal to severely angulated and swollen with limb shortening.

Nursing Care and Related Interventions

Nursing interventions for tibial and fibular fractures include immobilization of the injury. This type of fracture is suited for a pneumatic splint. The limb should be elevated, if possible, to promote venous drainage and to prevent swelling. Cold packs are applied, and neurovascular assessment is continuous. Casting is used for undisplaced fractures, while displaced fractures are usually managed by open reduction and casting. In children the treatment is directed toward obtaining correct length and alignment of the extremity. In anterior tibial compartment syndrome, fasciotomy is indicated to allow the muscle to expand with improved circulation (Sternbach, 1979; Heppenstall, 1980; Kuska, 1982).

Ankle Injuries

Pathophysiology
The *ankle,* a modified hinge joint with primary motions of flexion and extension, incurs fractures, fracture dislocations of the distal tibia, and injuries to its surrounding ligaments, as well as to the Achilles tendon. The ankle is particularly susceptible to injury because the foot is the only part of the body in contact with the ground when the person is standing and walking. The most frequent mechanism of injury is inversion of the foot and the leg with abduction or external rotation of the talus. A severe upward dislocation of the talus can cause a comminuted fracture of the distal tibia.

Ankle injuries commonly occur in all age groups. In adults, the injury can result in traumatic arthritis with severe motion disability. In children the epiphyseal growth plates of the tibia and fibula are open, which can result in premature closure followed by a varus or valgus ankle deformity (Schneider, 1980).

Clinical Manifestations
The patient presents with immediate pain and swelling, immobility, and inability to bear weight. A history of a "turned ankle" exists. The functional impairment increases as hemarthrosis and swelling increase. Point tenderness and obvious deformity exist. Patients presenting 24 to 48 hours after incurring a fracture will often have extreme edema with skin blebs and open blisters.

Nursing Care and Related Interventions
Immediate assessment of the neurovascular status and the condition of the skin overlying the bony prominences should be documented. The area should be immobilized, cold packed, and elevated. X-ray examination of the extremity may be used to determine the extent of the injury. A sprain, although never simple, can be managed with an ace bandage wrap and crutches. A more involved ligamentous injury may require a short, nonweight-bearing posterior splint and crutches. Undisplaced stable fractures heal with immobilization, accomplished with a short-leg weight-bearing cast. If the fracture cannot be reduced easily, skin necrosis can result due to displaced fragments beneath the skin (Schneider, 1980).

Foot Fractures

Pathophysiology
Fractures of the *foot* include those of the talar neck due to severe hyperextension of the foot that forces the talar neck against the distal tibia. These fractures frequently result from motorcycle accidents.

A calcaneus os fracture can be either minor or severely disabling. Frequently the result of a fall from a height in which the patient lands on his heels or from a sudden, forceful attempt to brake a car, this fracture often is associated with a compression fracture of the vertebral column.

The midfoot contains the navicular bone that can be dislocated. Comminuted fractures of the midfoot bones usually occur as the result of a twisting motion. The forefoot fractures of the metatarsals usually result from direct force or from repeated stress—for example, the "March fracture." Phalangeal fractures usually result from crushing forces or from direct trauma, such as stubbing the great toe.

Clinical Manifestations

Patients with a talar fracture present with severe pain and deformity. The distal neurovascular status must be assessed since avascular necrosis is not an uncommon occurrence.

With a calcaneus os fracture, point tenderness and some swelling will occur. The patient avoids weight bearing and tends to throw the foot outward. Injuries to the midfoot and forefoot exhibit similar symptoms.

Nursing Care and Related Interventions

Treatment for a talar fracture will vary depending on the classification of the fracture, particularly related to whether the fracture is displaced or stable. Immediate treatment of a calcaneus os fracture includes cold applications for the first 24 hours and elevation. A compression dressing or padded cast may be used. Intervention is often conservative in treating injuries to the midfoot and forefoot and includes cold packs, elevation, and support wraps. To reduce tarsal and metatarsal fractures, casting may be required. A fractured toe is usually splinted to the adjacent toe.

Soft Tissue Alterations

Soft tissue alterations may involve the skin, muscle, tendons, ligaments, and cartilage. Strains, sprains, dislocations, and fractures cause soft tissue trauma. *Strains* result from pulling trauma to the muscle, while *sprains* involve an incomplete tearing of the capsule and ligaments (Mock, 1979). *Dislocations* occur when forces producing the trauma separate the joint surfaces with resultant joint capsule and ligament injury (Budassi and Barber, 1981). An *open* fracture describes a break in which bone protrudes through the skin. A *closed* fracture does not penetrate the skin. Soft tissue trauma accompanies both open and closed fractures.

Clinically, soft tissue alteration is considered possible if swelling, ecchymosis, breaks in skin integrity, and changes in skin temperature exist. Swelling is due to hemorrhage, lymphatic drainage, and intracellular fluid escape that can increase rapidly during the first 12 hours after trauma. Initial swelling occurs due to lacerated vessels, while later swelling results from bone hemorrhage, and further swelling results from the accumulation of tissue fluid (Rodi, 1983). Soft tissue will lose elasticity and become indurated as the result of swelling. Massive swelling can create tissue and nerve ischemia by compression of vessels.

Assessment for skin integrity should ascertain whether the skin is intact with only swelling and ecchymosis, or whether the skin is lacerated with hemorrhage or oozing. When a wound is present, the inspection should include location, size, depth, condition of wound edges, and amount of bleeding.

Skin temperature above, below, and surrounding the trauma area provides information about vascular integrity. Temperature changes in the same extremity or differences between paired extremities can be detected within two or three degrees by the back of the hand (Sproul, 1983).

Sprains and Strains

Two of the most common injuries seen in the emergency department are sprains and strains of the ankle. Other areas commonly affected are the wrist and knee.

Pathophysiology
A sprain is defined as an incomplete tearing (in fact, a stretching) of the ligaments, capsule, and synovium of the affected joint. Degrees of sprains can vary from mild pain and swelling around a joint to a more serious disruption and loss of function of the joint.

A strain is trauma to a muscle or tendon due to excessive forced use or stretching. Strain injuries vary in intensity and exhibit clinical manifestations similar to those for a sprain.

Clinical Manifestations
Heppenstall (1980) classifies sprains into three degrees. A first degree sprain exhibits slight point tenderness, minimal hemorrhage, and swelling with little abnormal motion or disability. A sprain with greater loss of function (characterized by localized tenderness, additional joint reaction, some abnormal motion, and a partial tearing of the ligaments) is classified as a second degree sprain. The third degree sprain is more severe with significant abnormal motion and joint instability indicating a complete ligament tear. Some experts, in fact, identify a severe, third degree injury as a dislocation reserving the term sprain for an injury involving a stable joint (Schneider, 1980).

Symptoms of sprains and strains include localized swelling, tenderness, and pain. Muscle spasms result from tissue irritation and from the patient's *bracing* to help prevent pain and to effect some mobility. Depending on the degree of the injury, a tearing of the muscle fibers can occur with subsequent hemorrhage and a partial loss of function (Simon and Koenigsknecht, 1982). Prompt treatment is required to prevent severe hematoma formation and possible subsequent neurovascular damage.

Nursing Care and Related Interventions
Immediate nursing interventions include assessment of the neurovascular status of the area (especially distal to the injury), cold compresses, support, and/or elevation of the extremity to provide rest and to help reduce the swelling.

Ligament and Musculotendinous Injuries

Pathophysiology
Ligament and musculotendinous injuries occur in three major areas: the knee, the ankle, and the Achilles tendon. The damage, which is soft tissue in nature, occurs to the extensor apparatus of the Achilles and to the intra-articular structures of the knee and ankle (Gurd, 1981). Most of these injuries involve the ankle and knee. The possibility of an accompanying fracture, however, must also be considered. In similar incidents, the peroneal tendon can be dislocated by a twisting movement of the ankle.

A dislocation disrupts the joint. The two bones constituting the joint are completely separated, and their articular surfaces are no longer in contact. A subluxation is an incomplete separation of the joint in which the articular surfaces remain in partial apposition. A subluxation implies a stretching and loosening of the joint, but not necessarily a complete capsular rupture.

Clinical Manifestations
An Achilles tendon rupture may occur during aggressive physical activity, such as tennis. The person is aware of a snap and severe pain proximal to the ankle and in the calf. A flat-footed gait is exhibited, and the person is unable to walk on tip toe or to push off from a stance position. The patient presents with localized edema and ecchymosis over the posterior ankle. Symptoms are similar to those accompanying an ankle sprain.

With a peroneal tendon dislocation, symptoms also are similar to those for an ankle sprain. Symptomatology of a dislocated joint includes extreme deformity of the joint with almost complete joint immobility. The patient will not move the affected joint, nor will the patient allow anyone else to do so. Point tenderness exists around the disrupted joint, in addition to obvious swelling.

Nursing Care and Related Interventions
Treatment for an Achilles tendon rupture is often conservative with a short leg cast. Surgical repair is used in the younger, more athletic patient. Postoperative immobilization for three to six weeks in a long leg cast is a common procedure, followed by three weeks in a short leg cast.

For a peroneal tendon rupture, surgical repair is necessary due to the rupture of the tendon sheath located behind the fibula.

A dislocation usually constitutes a surgical emergency because the subsequent swelling and edema can cause soft tissue damage with changes in the involved joint preventing a facile reduction. After treatment, the joint is immobilized to permit reduction of swelling in the soft tissues. Immobilization is required for approximately three to six weeks.

Discharge Planning
Patients with joint and soft tissue injuries often are treated in the emergency department, then discharged. Discharge, therefore, necessitates appropriate planning and instruction for home care. Instructions should be in writing. Verifying that the patient or another responsible person understands the information is necessary.

Instructions should include necessary activity limitations, including the use of crutches if weight-bearing is ordered. (The fitting and use of crutches is discussed later in this chapter.)

Teach patients with sprains and strains how to use cold compresses and explain the need to replace cold compresses with warm compresses in 24 to 36 hours. Caution patients against using excessive heat, because the skin over the injured area is often less sensitive to heat than is skin over an uninjured site. The patient must realize that severe sprains and strains usually require four to six weeks to heal.

Caution patients against weight bearing. Moreover, for patients with Achilles tendon ruptures, no weight-bearing is allowed until after the cast is removed.

In addition to immobilization to treat dislocated joints, the patient should begin gentle range of motion exercises sometime after three weeks have elapsed. If the patient has been discharged, an appointment with a physical therapist should be made for initial teaching. Patients must continue to see the therapist on a regular schedule to ensure that the exercising is progressing. Daily, written schedules are useful for most patients. As soon as comfort allows, isometric exercises, with the joint sustained in the reduction position, can begin.

General Nursing Care Measures

Pain management in all orthopedic injuries should be individualized. To a large extent, the pain is caused by muscle spasm produced when the patient attempts to provide splinting. Swelling at the site of injury adds to the discomfort, and the nerve endings are further stimulated. The health care provider is often tempted to relieve the pain by immediately administering analgesics. A patient, however, who has experienced serious and sudden trauma is often in shock; thus, an intramuscular injection of analgesics has minimal value because of circulatory disturbance. In fact, repeated injections create a potential hazard after the shock condition is resolved and absorption of medication from the tissues improves. When sedation and/or analgesics are necessary for relieving severe pain, small amounts should be administered intravenously over an extended period of time. In closed reductions or dislocation manipulations, local anesthetics occasionally are used. In initial injuries, the application of ice or cold packs can reduce the swelling, and thus alleviate one cause of pain. Moreover, positioning the injured extremity at or above the level of the heart should also aid in reducing congestion and swelling. For any patient presenting with an open fracture or crushing tissue injury, the person's tetanus immunization status should be evaluated and appropriate action taken. Antibiotics also may be used.

Discharge Planning

Planning for discharge and teaching the patient and/or the family how to manage the injury at home begins when the patient is admitted to the emergency department. Instructions must be explained clearly, although caregivers realize that patients experiencing the stress of an injury often either do not hear or only hear selected parts of the conversation. Recall often relates to existing knowledge and previous experiences. Consequently, nurses should use written instructions that explicitly describe the patient's expected activities and what results are anticipated from these activities. The nurse must review the material with either the patient or with another responsible person. Explanations of why certain actions are necessary will help to emphasize the necessity for following the written instructions.

Furthermore, the home situation should be assessed. Who will assist the patient? Do any structural problems exist? Any patient dismissed directly from the emergency department probably won't have a serious disability. If the nurse perceives that a problem might arise, however, arrangements should be made for a home health or community health nurse to visit at least once to assess the situation in the patient's home territory. After the patient's home environment is assessed, alterations in the original discharge instructions might be required.

Patients are usually discharged with a mild analgesic and instructions to contact their physician if the pain is not controlled. Other mechanisms for controlling pain include ice or cold packs for 24 to 36 hours and elevation of the affected part. All patients are instructed in the signs and symptoms of circulatory interference with emphasis placed on reporting these symptoms to the attending physician.

Particular injuries will require specific instructions. Patients with fractures of the clavicle should be told that they may feel the bones move for a few days, but emphasize that this movement is not a cause for alarm. Finger exercises should be started as soon as comfort permits. Instructions should include seeing the physician to have the wrap adjusted at least five days after the injury.

Patients with shoulder dislocations and injuries of the proximal humerus require specific instructions in movement. Early shoulder motion is essential to prevent a "frozen shoulder," caused by scarring of the surrounding soft tissues and intraarticular adhesions. Neer (Gurd, 1981) recommends a rehabilitative process to include passive exercises for the first six weeks with emphasis placed on external rotation. Isometric exercises can be started three to four weeks after the injury, in addition to active exercises that emphasize external rotation and forward elevation. Wall-climbing exercises can help the patient with forward elevation. Furthermore, these patients are also instructed in neurovascular assessment, and they are told that they will probably have large areas of ecchymosis on the inner aspect of the upper arm and on the chest wall. In fractures of the humeral shaft, the patient should be instructed not to rest his arm on the elbow, to avoid excessive movement, and to try sleeping in a semi-Fowler's position. Emphasis is placed on frequent exercise of the wrist and fingers.

Active, gentle joint movement is encouraged to help prevent joint stiffness for patients with elbow injuries. To patients and/or to parents explain the symptoms of Volkmann's contracture and emphasize the need to report immediately such symptoms to the physician. For patients with injuries of the forearm and wrist, instructions should include finger exercises. Emphasize the importance of reporting pain and swelling, in addition to other circulatory interferences, such as tingling, numbness, and skin coolness. The angulation (residual deformity) of a wrist fracture should be discussed, including an explanation that the deformity will correct itself in three to four months through the process of remodeling.

Patients treated for fractures of the long bones of the lower leg and discharged must understand neurovascular assessment, as well as the incipient signs of compartment syndrome. They should be instructed to return the next day for professional neurovascular assessment. Moreover, instruction in exercises for the quadriceps is also provided. Patients with ankle fractures frequently are hospitalized. If patients with heel and foot fractures are discharged, they should be instructed on circulatory checks, the need to elevate, cold packs, and avoidance of weight-bearing. Explain and demonstrate support wraps, then schedule an appointment for the patient to return for rewrapping and/or adjustments.

Most patients with lower extremity injuries will require some type of assistive gait device. Emergency nurses should provide basic instructions in the use of these devices. If possible, the patient should return for additional assistance and reinforcement because too much information often is difficult for the patient to assimilate at once.

Crutch Walking
Axillary (wooden) crutches commonly are used for temporary assistance. To function adequately with crutches, the person must have normal upper extremity function (hand grasp, elbow extension), ability to extend the hip and knee normally, and adequate balance and coordination. Crutches must be fitted to each individual patient. Proper crutch fitting can be determined by having the patient stand erect. With the crutch tips placed 6 inches away from the lateral side of each foot, the crutch top should be two to three finger-breadths below the axilla. This placement will permit the proper angle of flexion—about 20 degrees. The patient must understand that his weight is sustained on the hands, *not* on the axillary region. Correct placement will help promote good balance and posture and will prevent radial nerve damage due to axillary pressure.

The most typical gait pattern is the three-point gait: in essence, three points are always on the floor, including both crutches and the uninvolved lower extremity. The injured extremity and both crutches are advanced; then, while the person bears his weight on both hands, the uninjured extremity is advanced beyond the crutches to maintain a tripod stance. This stance provides some stability for the patient. Three other methods of crutch use include the following: a four-point gait; a two-point gait; and, a swing-through gait. Walking with crutches is only the beginning. Patients must learn how to get in and out of chairs, move up and down stairs, and move through doorways. To move up stairs, a three-point gait is used by moving up with the uninvolved leg and following with the injured extremity. Moving downstairs is done with the same two basic steps. All of these activities require practice, and an actual demonstration might help the patient. Furthermore, initiate practice before the patient is discharged and request the patient to return on the following day for additional assistance. Walkers frequently are used instead of crutches for patients who lack strength, balance, and dexterity.

Cast Care
For patients dismissed with a cast, provide information about the care of the cast and explain possible circulatory interferences that might occur. Moreover, warn patients not to get the cast wet and to avoid damaging or destroying parts of it. Although the action of scratching beneath the cast may temporarily relieve itching, it can cause cuts and abrasions to the underlying skin that can be extremely difficult to heal. Placing foreign objects inside the cast, frequently done by children, can cause pressure areas, which can result in excoriation and ulceration of the skin. Joints above and below the cast must be exercised on a regular basis to prevent stiffness and to maintain muscle tone.

After patients have left the emergency department, they may want to resume their routine activity as quickly as possible. Explain to these patients that most casts, especially the larger leg casts, require 24 hours to dry. Care should be taken not to rest an extremity on the arms of chairs, table edges, and so forth. External dirt on a cast is not important, unless it is moist; however, some people may want to use stockinette to cover the dried cast to keep it clean. Using baking soda is one of the best ways to manage odors. Baking soda is sprinkled over the wet area and allowed to dry, then it is brushed away with a small brush such as a toothbrush. Powdered or spray deodorants are not particularly effective. Explain to the patient what signs and symptoms must be reported to the physician: for example, pain that is not relieved by the usual analgesics and other methods, swelling and discoloration of toes or fingers, pain with active or passive motion, and a burning or tingling sensation beneath the cast.

CONCLUSION

Emergency nursing care of the orthopedic patient requires assessment, not only of the bony injuries, but also of the neurovascular and soft tissue injuries. Appropriate treatment requires knowledge of regional anatomy, mechanisms of trauma, associated injuries, and the locally accepted emergency procedures. Ability to prioritize orthopedic injuries in the multiple-injured person is crucial. In the rush to treat severely injured patients, one might forget that the patients also have emotions and fears. The patients' concerns should be considered during any emergency treatment as well as in any instructions for home and follow-up care. The patients' anxiety level often will interfere with what they hear and remember. Moreover, the nurse should realize that patients require conditioning to accept the limitations placed on their usual activities and lifestyles. Understanding and support from the nurse will help make the patients' transition from the emergency department to an in-hospital service or to a home setting smoother and less traumatic. The entire recovery process will be facilitated.

BIBLIOGRAPHY

Adelman, R. and George Sarant: Hand Injuries. In Clark Chipman (ed.): *Emergency Department Orthopedics*. Rockville, Maryland: Aspen Systems Corporation, 1982, pp. 43–64.

Brashear, H. R., and R. B. Raney: *Shand's Handbook of Orthopedic Surgery*. 9th ed. St. Louis: Mosby, 1978.

Budassi, S. A., and J. M. Barber: *Emergency Nursing Principles and Practice*. St. Louis: Mosby, 1981.

Conrad, M. B.: Procedures on the Upper and Lower Extremities. In A. P. Klippel and C. V. Anderson (eds.): *Manual of Emergency and Orthopedic Techniques*. Boston: Little, Brown 1979, pp. 375–412.

DeGowin, E. L., and R. L. DeGowin: *Bedside Diagnostic Examination*. 3rd ed. New York: Macmillan, 1976.

Donahoo, C. A.: Orthopedic neurovascular chart. *The ONA Journal* 4:220–222 (1979).

———, and J. H. Dimon: *Orthopedic Nursing*. Boston: Little, Brown, 1977.

Emergency Department Nurses Association: *Core Curriculum.* Chicago: Emergency Department Nurses Association, 1980.

Friedenberg, Z. B.: Fractures of the Pelvis. In R. B. Heppenstall, (ed.): *Fracture Treatment and Healing.* Philadelphia: Saunders, 1980, pp. 611–629.

Gartland, J. J.: *Fundamentals of Orthopedics.* 3rd ed. Philadelphia: Saunders, 1979.

Gurd, A. R.: Injuries to the Bones and Joints of the Lower Limb. In Odling-Stone, W., and A. Crockard (eds.): *Trauma Care.* New York: Grune and Stratten, 1981, pp. 407–453.

———: Injuries to the Bones and Joints of the Upper Limb, In W. Odling-Stone and A. Crockard (eds.): *Trauma Care.* New York: Grune and Stratten, 1981, pp. 379–406.

———: Injuries to the Shoulder Girdle. In W. Odling-Stone and A. Crockard (eds.): *Trauma Care.* New York: Grune and Stratten, 1981, pp. 455–473.

Heppenstall, R. B.: Fractures and Dislocations of the Hip. In R. B. Heppenstall (ed.): *Fracture Treatment and Healing.* Philadelphia. Saunders, 1980, pp. 630–708.

———: Fractures of the Tibia and Fibula. In R. B. Heppenstall (ed.): *Fracture Treatment and Healing.* Philadelphia: Saunders, 1980, pp. 777–802.

———: Fracture Healing. In R. B. Heppenstall (ed.): *Fracture Treatment and Healing.* Philadelphia: Saunders, 1980, pp. 35–64.

———: Injuries of the Ankle. In R. B. Heppenstall (ed.): *Fracture Treatment and Healing.* Philadelphia: Saunders, 1980, pp. 803–838.

———: Injuries of the Elbow. In R. B. Heppenstall (ed.): *Fracture Treatment and Healing.* Philadelphia: Saunders Co., 1980, pp. 439–480.

Hoopes, J. E., and G. P. Maxwell: Soft Tissue Injuries of the Extremities. In G. D. Zuidema, R. B. Rutherford, and W. F. Ballinger (eds.): *The Management of Trauma.* 3rd ed. Philadelphia: Saunders, 1979, pp. 522–560.

Kettelkamp, D.: Orthopedic Emergencies, in C. Eckert (ed.): *Emergency Room Care.* 3rd ed. Boston: Little, Brown 1976, pp. 203–240.

Kuska, Barbara M.: Acute onset of compartment syndrome. *Journal of Emergency Nursing* 8:75–79 (Mar./Apr. 1982).

Larson, C. B., and M. Gould: *Orthopedic Nursing,* 9th ed. St. Louis: Mosby, 1978.

Mock, M.: Orthopedics in the emergency room: Sprains and strains. *The ONA Journal* 6:318–319 (1979).

Rodi, M. F.: Emergency Orthopedics. In C. G. Warner (ed.): *Emergency Care—Assessment and Intervention.* St. Louis: Mosby, 1983, pp. 361–374.

Ross, N.: Volkmann's ischaemic contracture: A complication following elbow injuries. *The ONA Journal* 6:211–215 (1979).

Salter, R. B.: Birth and Pediatric Fractures. In R. B. Heppenstall (ed.): *Fracture Treatment and Healing.* Philadelphia: Saunders Co., 1980, pp. 189–234.

———, and W. R. Harris: Injuries involving the epiphyseal plate. *Journal of Bone and Joint Surgery* 45-A:587–622 (1963).

Schneider, F. R.: *Orthopedics in Emergency Care.* St. Louis: Mosby, 1980.

Simon, R. R., and S. J. Koenigsknecht: *Orthopedics in Emergency Medicine the Extremities.* New York: Appleton-Century-Crofts, 1982.

Sproul, G.: Vascular Emergencies. In C. G. Warner (ed.): *Emergency Care—Assessment and Intervention.* St. Louis: Mosby, 1983, pp. 129–146.

Sternbach, G.: Fractures and dislocations. *Topics in Emergency Medicine* 1:119–132 (1979).

Vaughn, J.: *The Physiology of Bone.* 3rd ed. Oxford, England: Clarendon, 1981.

18

Facial Trauma

Judy Jo Wells-Mackie

After completing this chapter, the reader will be able to do the following:

1. Complete a triage history for the patient with facial trauma.
2. List initial priorities of assessment and care for a patient with facial trauma.
3. List special conditions of, as well as therapy for, facial wounds.
4. List conditions in which facial wounds are not sutured.
5. Describe cleaning and preparation of a facial wound.
6. List and describe the use of medications for anesthesia of facial wounds.
7. Describe the practice of applying dressings to facial and ear wounds.
8. List discharge instructions for a patient with facial wounds.
9. Describe the pathophysiology, clinical manifestations, nursing care and related interventions and discharge planning for the following: nasal fractures; mandibular fractures and temporal mandibular joint dislocations; zygomatic and orbital blow out fractures; maxillary fractures and dental trauma.
10. Describe injuries that may result from trauma to the eye, including the following: blunt trauma and sharp trauma; foreign bodies and burns.
11. List medications that may be used for examination or for management of ocular trauma.
12. Describe discharge planning for the patient with ocular trauma.

Facial trauma is a common problem resulting from automobile accidents, interpersonal altercations, child abuse or nonaccidental trauma (NAT), home accidents, athletic and work injuries, and animal and human bites. Fifty-four percent of the victims from motor vehicle accidents sustain significant facial trauma, usually from deceleration injuries (Schultz, 1977). Shatterproof glass and shoulder harnesses have decreased the incidence of facial trauma in automobile accidents (Cantrill, 1983). The incidence of facial trauma in motorcycle riders has increased because of their refusal to wear helmets.

Facial trauma is treated by physicians, including emergency physicians, plastic surgeons, oral surgeons, and ophthalmologists (Cantrill, 1983). The emergency nurse must initially triage, assess, and plan the care for all patients with facial trauma, including establishing priorities of care.

This chapter will discuss facial lacerations and soft tissue injury, facial fractures, dental trauma, and ocular trauma. This background of information will help the emergency nurse to care properly for patients with facial injuries.

TRIAGE

Subjective Data

A complete triage history of the patient with any facial trauma is important to help assess the severity of the injury, as well as to make a complete and accurate assessment. Patients with facial trauma, including children, often are able to tell the nurse the mechanism of injury. In addition, other important details that must be elicited from the patient, include the location of pain, the quality of pain, signs of any airway obstruction, when the trauma occurred, the speed in accidents, other descriptions of forces involved in the injury, the sensation of malocclusion of the teeth, sensation changes, partial or complete deafness or vision loss, tetanus status, a history of previous facial trauma, allergies, and any history of loss of consciousness.

Objective Data

Airway, breathing, and circulation must be checked initially in any trauma patient. After implementing initial intervention for these life-threatening conditions, the nurse begins a complete assessment of the extent of facial trauma.

Assess the patient in a semi-Fowler's position or in a sitting position if spinal injury is ruled out, and look for loose material and developing edema that may cause a potential airway problem. Displaced bone, cartilage, soft tissue, teeth, and blood clots commonly cause airway obstruction in facial trauma. Assess whether lacerations or edema might develop into life-threatening obstructions. (A more detailed explanation of airway assessment and management is included in Chapter 5.)

The patient with facial trauma appears acutely injured and is frightened because of hemorrhage secondary to the substantial vascularity of the face and scalp. Shock accompanying facial injuries alone is rare. If the patient's pulse or appearance indicates shock, less obvious trauma existing in the head, chest, or abdomen must be suspected as the primary cause (Cantrill, 1983). Bleeding from the face must be controlled with direct pressure. Always assume cervical spine trauma is present with facial trauma, and always protect the spine. (Techniques for protecting the spine while assuring an open airway are explained in detail in Chapter 5.)

Check for a closed head injury associated with facial trauma by evaluating the patient's level of consciousness. Evaluate the pupils for equality, reactivity, and a fluid line associated with a hyphema. Alcohol intoxication leading to an uncooperative patient and a nonaccurate history frequently is evident in the facial trauma patient. Document whether the patient responds readily and appropriately to verbal stimuli and whether the patient is alert and oriented to person, time, and place.

Analyze the forces involved in the injury and incorporate the history received into the assessment. Sharp trauma leads to lacerations, and blunt trauma leads to contusions and fractures (Cantrill, 1983). The apparent trauma should be consistent with the mechanism of injury.

Assessment and Planning

After the initial triage history, stabilization of life-threatening conditions, and general assessment of injury, the nurse develops a plan of care, including the treatment priority for the patient. Interventions, such as removing loose teeth that may cause airway obstruction, direct pressure on bleeding, positioning, oxygen administration, reassurance, and further assessment and cleansing of lacerations may be necessary.

Two examples of triage notes related to patients with facial trauma are included in Table 18.1. A detailed discussion of facial lacerations and soft tissue injury, facial fractures, dental trauma, and ocular trauma follows.

FACIAL LACERATIONS AND SOFT TISSUE INJURY

Pathophysiology

Facial lacerations and soft tissue injury frequently result from motor vehicle accidents and interpersonal altercations. In general, the face absorbs an impact if hit

TABLE 18.1 Examples of Triage Notes for Patients Experiencing Facial Trauma

S: 48 yo BM with c/o "I think I cut my cheek." Doesn't remember how or when he injured self. No pain or difficulty breathing, no loss of consciousness, unknown tetanus status, NKA. PMH: negative.

O: Walked in with ataxic gait and slurred speech, smell of alcohol on breath. 4 cm lac. over left cheek with no obvious recent bleeding, dried blood over entire face. Denies cervical spine pain with firm palpation, oriented to person and place, awakens easily but prefers to sleep when left sitting in chair.

A: 4 cm lac. of left cheek of questionable origin and duration, contaminated wound.

P: Surgical evaluation, initial cleansing of face and laceration, further assessment of depth and involvement of injury, investigation of alcohol problem with possible referral, to the waiting room.

S: 15 yo WM with c/o toothaches × 3 days PTA, no fever. "Unable to chew on the left side of my teeth." NKA, PMH: diabetic, 10 u reg. and 50 u NPH insulin q. a.m.

O: T 98.6°F, decayed first molar on bottom left, no signs of swelling or infection.

A: Toothache.

P: Surgical evaluation, to the waiting room.

directly instead of transferring the impact to the brain (Winspur, 1979). Serious facial injuries frequently occur without intracranial injuries; nonetheless, intracranial injuries must be suspected, until they are ruled out. Specialty physicians may be required to repair wounds that contain multiple layers or extensive debridement, nerve damage, and sensory, taste, hearing, or smell deficits (Budassi, 1981). Initially, however, the patient is triaged and assessed by emergency nurses and physicians.

Wounds are closed to prevent scarring and infection. An attempt to suture a laceration should be made in the first eight hours following infliction. If not sutured, the wound is prone to infection. In the presence of other life-threatening injuries, one may wait for a maximum of 24 hours to close a wound on the face, if it is properly cleansed, approximated, and dressed, and intravenous antibiotics are initiated (Cantrill, 1983; Constant, 1978).

Some wounds are never closed, including those that are more than 24 hours old, wounds with embedded foreign bodies, severely contaminated wounds (especially bites, unless they can be thoroughly cleansed and are less than six hours old), wounds overlying a fracture requiring treatment, and minor tongue and oral cavity lacerations. Many tongue and oral cavity lacerations are self-induced bites and are repaired only if deep. In some situations, it is preferable to cleanse and dress a facial wound and to wait for suturing if the patient is uncooperative due to alcohol intoxication (Cantrill, 1983).

The mechanism of injury may lead the nurse to suspect the possibility that a foreign body is embedded in a wound. Glass may be radio-opaque, while other foreign bodies may be palpated. Mouth burns are particularly prevalent in children who lick electrical outlets and chew electric cords. The nurse must be alert to the possibility of severe delayed bleeding of circumoral vessels with mouth burns (Cantrill, 1983). The high bacterial content in pores of the skin on the nose makes lacerations in this area more susceptible to infection. Ear trauma and soft tissue injury can cause a hematoma of the area below the perichondrium against the cartilage. If the hematoma is not incised and drained or aspirated, the cartilage may be reabsorbed and cause an ear deformity, sometimes called "cauliflower ear." A slapping injury or pressure changes to the ear may cause a rupture of the tympanic membrane.

Clinical Manifestations

A systematic assessment of any patient with facial injuries will enable a nurse to complete a thorough examination and to identify all injuries. First, inspect the face for asymmetry and obvious deformity, then gently palpate all areas to elicit point tenderness, bony defects, crepitus, and false motion. If the patient has sustained mouth trauma and complains of malocclusion of the teeth, grasp the maxilla between the thumb and index finger and gently test for anterior motion. Inspect the nasal septum and the tympanic membrane for intactness. Check nasal and ear drainage for the presence of cerebral spinal fluid. Check the mouth for excessive saliva from a possible laceration of the parotid gland or Stensen's duct. Note the presence of any lacerations and their length and depth. Note the presence of soft tissue injury, hematomas, and edema, and estimate the amount and size of area they cover.

If a wound is present from the tragus of the ear to the midcheek, suspect facial

FACIAL LACERATIONS AND SOFT TISSUE INJURY

nerve damage (cranial nerve VII) and carefully assess for motor function. Ask the patient to wrinkle his forehead, raise his eyebrows, smile, bare his teeth, and close his eyes tightly. In addition, prior to anesthesia for wound cleansing and suturing, test the trigeminal nerve (cranial nerve V) for face sensation and jaw movement.

Nursing Care and Related Interventions

Facial wounds are frequently dirty. Initial cleansing by copious irrigation with normal saline may help to preserve tissue viability. Replace tissue flaps in their proper position and put any avulsed parts, such as ears, nose, and teeth, in normal saline at room temperature. Effective wound cleansing prevents infection and tatooing (caused by dirt remaining under the skin).

After initial cleansing, examination, and anesthesia, scrub thoroughly for at least five minutes all abrasions and lacerations. Use a brush with iodine soap and water. Rinse the wound well after the scrubbing. Do not soak wounds unless they have existed for more than 12 hours. Do not use hydrogen peroxide to scrub a wound because it adversely affects tissue viability. Hydrogen peroxide may be used to remove dried blood from wound edges. To remove foreign bodies, loosen tissue, and irrigate any wound, especially puncture wounds, use either a velocity jet stream from a commercial appliance or a plastic intravenous catheter attached to a saline-filled syringe. Shave any area around a wound from one-half to 1 in. away from all edges so that the hair will not contaminate the wound during suturing. More shaving occasionally is necessary, but remember that hair grows back. Never shave eyebrows, however, because they may not grow back and accurate approximation is difficult without hair being present.

Some special considerations must be remembered for other facial wounds and facial trauma. The vermillion border of the lips must be marked before anesthetizing and prepping a laceration in that area because the anesthesia may cause blanching and edema. Exact approximation of the vermillion border can be done while suturing if a mark is made with a needle scratch, methylene blue, or a commercial marker.

Do not irrigate or instill drops in the ear unless the tympanic membrane is intact. If the patient complains of a foreign body in the ear, make sure that the tympanic membrane is intact. Instill mineral oil or isopropyl alcohol for insects. Irrigate cerumen gently with water jet stream, or instill liquid dioctyl sodium sulfosuccinate (Colace) to dissolve the cerumen. Never irrigate vegetable matter, such as beans or peas, that are commonly found in children's ears; because of their hydroscopic properties, the beans or peas will absorb the liquid and swell. Gentle suction or the use of forceps may be indicated for some foreign bodies. Use side rails if the patient is dizzy—a common occurrence with ear trauma. Tetanus immunization, as discussed in Chapter 16, must be considered because it is frequently a nursing responsibility.

Anesthesia for facial lacerations is usually accomplished by local infiltration using 1 percent lidocaine with 1:100,000 epinephrine. Epinephrine causes vasoconstriction that decreases bleeding and prolongs anesthesia. Never use epinephrine with ear or nose tip lacerations because excessive vasoconstriction in these areas can result in necrosis.

In using lidocaine, a maximum of 30 ml may be instilled safely in an adult without systemic effects. If more anesthesia is required, use 0.5 percent lidocaine. With extensive facial injury, a regional block, in addition to local infiltration, is used by injecting two ml of 1 percent lidocaine into the trigeminal nerve area. Two percent viscous lidocaine or 4 percent liquid pour lidocaine may be used topically for anesthesia prior to scrubbing (Cantrill, 1983).

A systemic anesthesia using a mixture of meperidine, promethazine, and chlorpromazine is especially recommended for children. Give 1 mg/kg body weight of meperidine up to a total of 50 mg and 0.5 mg/kg each of promethazine and chlorpromazine up to a total of 25 mg each. If this mixture is given, watch for respiratory depression. Naloxone (Narcan) intravenously can be administered to reverse the depression. Although it is used occasionally, diazepam (Valium) is a poor systemic anesthesia and is nonreversible.

Nitrous oxide used at a 50 percent rate of administration may be beneficial, especially in children with facial wounds (Cantrill, 1983). No major side effects result from the use of nitrous oxide. A patient who has received too much nitrous oxide will demonstrate the loss of lid reflex, relaxation with a loss of muscle tone, divergent eyes, and excitement or agitation. If these signs are evident, discontinue the nitrous oxide and administer oxygen at 2–3 liters per minute.

Properly positioning the patient with facial trauma is important to help obtain easy, close access for examination, prepping, and suturing. The nurse must also consider patient comfort and lighting when deciding about positioning. Many times children must be restrained on a papoose board. Another mechanism for restraint is the placement of adhesive tape on the forehead, being careful not to tape the hair, and soft gauze restraints, with a clove hitch on the hands so that circulation is not compromised. The nurse must remain with the restrained child in case of vomiting so that he can be released to prevent aspiration. Be alert to respiratory arrest in children from restraints that decrease chest expansion.

The nurse is responsible for preparing a patient for suturing and sometimes for suturing minor wounds. On the face, 4-0 or 5-0 absorbable (chromic) suture is used in deep layers, and 4-0 or 5-0 nonabsorbable synthetic (nylon) suture is used in the skin. Silk suture may promote scar formation (Cantrill, 1983). Dressings may or may not be used on facial lacerations depending on the practitioner's preference. The suture line must be kept soft with a topical antibiotic ointment. Never pack an ear or nose; simply cover it with a sterile dressing to absorb drainage. A significant ear injury must be splinted in anatomical position using fluffed gauze for support and wrapping the head. If a hematoma of the perichrondrium has been drained, apply a compression dressing to this area only.

Discharge Planning

Printed discharge sheets given to the patient should instruct the person to keep any facial wound clean, dry, and soft. The development of signs and symptoms of infection (redness, edema, tenderness, draining pus, tender lumps under the chin, chills, and fever) should alert the patient to call or return to the emergency department. Patients with mouth injuries should be instructed to rinse the oral cavity with one-half strength hydrogen peroxide and water at least three times a day. The patient should be instructed to have the sutures removed in four to six days and to elevate his head to promote drainage, decrease edema, and consequently decrease pain. Oral antibiotics and analgesics may or may not be ordered by the physician. Whatever the medications, the patient must understand their effect, route, dose, and potential side effects.

FACIAL FRACTURES

Facial fractures are classified by the impact required to cause the fracture. The frequency of occurrence of each fracture decreases as the force to create the fracture increases. Fractures that result from severe forces occur less frequently. Always consider nonaccidental trauma as a possible cause for fractures in children (Cantrill, 1983).

Nasal Fractures

Pathophysiology
The nose, with its central and protruding position, is the most frequently fractured appendage of the face but requires the least amount of force to fracture. A blunt blow to the face is the usual history causing a simple fracture if hit on one side or a comminuted fracture if hit with a frontal blow. A septal hematoma may result from a fracture. When the blood supply to the septum is decreased, necrosis, abscesses, and a permanent saddle nose deformity may result.

Clinical Manifestations
The diagnosis of nasal fracture is based on the patient's history and physical examination, not on x-ray studies. Nasal x-ray films are difficult to interpret. The patient presents with a decrease in the patency of the nasal airways, edema, and visual displacement of the nose. Epistaxis is common and usually stops on its own or after direct pressure is applied. Palpate the nose for false motion and crepitation and inspect it for a septal hematoma. Young children are susceptible to septal hematomas that present with a large purple swelling of the nose.

Nursing Care and Related Interventions
The nurse must ensure airway patency, consider and rule out cervical spine injury, and control hemorrhage with pressure. Continually watch for airway problems due to aspiration from epistaxis. If able, the patient should sit up and expectorate blood instead of swallowing it. Monitor the patient's pulse and blood pressure to detect hypotension from blood loss or epistaxis secondary to hypertension. If severe blood loss is evident, draw blood samples for a hematocrit, complete blood count, platelet count, and type and crossmatch.

Septal hematomas are incised and drained, then packed anteriorly, and the patient is given oral antibiotics. Anterior epistaxis is usually controlled with direct pressure for five minutes, and posterior epistaxis is controlled with posterior packs. Available equipment should include petroleum impregnated and antibiotic gauze packing, a good light source, nasal speculum, Frazier suction tip, and Bayonet forceps. Because the nasal packing procedure is uncomfortable for the patient, he will require reassurance. The packs are removed in 72 hours. If a nasal laceration is present with a fracture, the injury is treated as an open fracture, and antibiotics are prescribed.

In general, small fractures are monitored for complications, and large fractures are repaired when the edema subsides in approximately two to three weeks. Cold packs should be applied to all nasal fractures. Appropriate reassurance of the patient is an integral part of the role of the emergency department nurse because the patient will have temporary disfigurement.

A closed reduction of the nose may be performed in the emergency department for a patient with minimal nasal swelling. Ten minutes prior to the procedure a 5 percent cocaine solution is applied topically to the nasal mucosa as an anesthetic and manual pressure is applied. After relocation, the nose is packed with antibiotic gauze and dressed with an external protective splint.

Mandibular Fractures and Temporal Mandibular Joint Dislocations

Pathophysiology
Mandibular fractures, the second most common type of facial fracture, result from severe force applied to the jaw. Mandibular fractures frequently occur in sport injuries and temporal mandibular joint swelling and dislocation is frequently associated with the fracture. With temporal mandibular joint dislocation, the jaw is displaced forward and superiorly. Traumatic dislocation usually occurs secondary to opening the mouth too wide and from yawning. A spasm of the muscle prevents the jaw from returning to its normal position.

Clinical Manifestations
Even though fractures may occur in different areas of the mandible, assessment is the same. The patient will complain that pain exists in the mandibular area and that his teeth do not fit together properly. This misalignment of the cusps of the teeth is termed malocclusion. Until proven otherwise by x-ray examination, the patient with malocclusion of the teeth is considered to have a mandibular fracture (Cantrill, 1983). The nurse may be able to palpate the fracture upon examination; however, dental panoramic x-rays are diagnostic.

Nursing Care and Related Interventions
First ensure a patent airway for the patient with a mandibular fracture. Teeth that are out may be replaced in their sockets, if the patient is awake and alert. The patient is admitted for wiring and stabilization of his jaw in order to obtain occlusion. Intravenous antibiotics are usually ordered.

The patient with temporal mandibular joint dislocation will usually respond to manual relocation in the emergency department, and then the patient is discharged.

FACIAL FRACTURES

Zygomatic and Orbital Blow Out Fractures

Pathophysiology
Zygomatic fractures occur as isolated depressions of the zygomatic arch, depressions of the whole zygoma, and orbital rim or orbital floor fractures. The fracture may cause edema of the inferior rectus muscle of the eye leading to an abnormal consensual gaze. A fracture of the orbital floor, referred to as a blow-out fracture, is caused by pressure on the globe of the eye. The orbital contents may herniate into the maxillary sinus, and the inferior rectus muscle may become trapped, thus limiting upward eye movement. Entrapment of the optic nerve caused by this type of injury causes diplopia.

Clinical Manifestations
An examination of zygomatic fractures may reveal that asymmetry and a palpable deformity of the orbital rim exist before edema forms. Patients may have anesthesia of the infraorbital rim or persistent trismus, a chronic contraction of the chewing muscles. The patient with an orbital floor fracture will present with enopthalmos, periorbital edema, and/or hematoma, subconjunctival hemorrhage, an upward gaze, and a clouding of the maxillary sinus on x-ray examination.

Nursing Care and Related Interventions
Reduction of zygomatic fractures in the emergency department is rare and done only when infraorbital nerve problems are present. The patient is usually discharged following examination, with plans for hospitalization in approximately five days after injury for an open reduction.

Maxillary Fractures

Pathophysiology
Maxillary fractures are commonly caused either by automobile accidents or by blunt blows to the face. They are considered to be massive trauma. More force is required to create maxillary fractures than any other facial fractures (Cantrill, 1983). These fractures may occur in isolation, but check for other injuries, particularly cervical spine injuries, because of the forces involved. In addition, suspect massive soft tissue injury and edema. Maxillary fractures, classified according to increasing severity, are as follows: LeForte I, a fracture of the maxilla at the nasal fossa; LeForte II, a fracture of the maxilla, nasal bones, and medial orbits in a pyramid fashion; and LeForte III, a fracture of the maxilla, zygoma, nasal bones, and ethmoid creating a craniofacial dysjunction (Cantrill, 1983).

Clinical Manifestations
The patient with a maxillary fracture complains of severe pain and may present with objective findings of malocclusion of the teeth, epistaxis, cerebral spinal fluid rhinorrhea from a fracture of the cribiform plate, and midface mobility, evidenced by grasping the front teeth and moving them anteriorly. Diagnosis is based on anterior and lateral facial x-ray films.

Nursing Care and Related Interventions

The patient with maxillary fractures may require intubation or a cricothyroidotomy to ensure an adequate airway and to protect the person from aspirating blood from epistaxis. In all cases, the patient is admitted to the hospital for stabilization with open reduction and an external frame. After life-threatening injuries have been ruled out, the patient's head should be elevated and cold packs applied. Intravenous antibiotics are usually ordered. Because of the trauma involved, the patient must be continually observed for changes in his mental status and vital signs.

Discharge Planning for the Patient with Facial Fractures

The patient with any facial fracture who is discharged from the emergency department must be instructed to apply cold packs to his injury for at least 24 hours. If the patient understands that head elevation will decrease edema and decrease pain, the person may comply more readily with the instructions. The patient must be instructed to return to or to call the emergency department if any swelling or bleeding causes difficulty in breathing.

Warn the patient that significant flattening and disfigurement, permanent diplopia, and enopthalmos may develop without appropriate long-term repair. Be sure to inform the patient of follow-up appointments. If the patient has nasal packing, instruct the person when to return to have the packing removed. The patient must understand the dose, action, and side effects of any prescribed medications. Finally, instruct the patient about the hazards of visual impairment with diplopia while walking and driving.

DENTAL TRAUMA

Pathophysiology

Dental trauma is commonly associated with head, facial, and cervical spine injuries. In isolation, dental trauma occurs in sport injuries and in children who trip and fall on their faces. Because a chipped tooth may leave a nerve exposed, causing pain, it must be treated by a dentist as soon as possible. Blood supply to the tooth comes through the pulp. A completely avulsed tooth may be viable depending on whether the pulp is still patent.

Clinical Manifestations

The patient with a chipped or avulsed tooth will complain of pain or a missing tooth. Dental pain may also be produced by caries or abscesses. Dental caries cause sharp, shooting pain that persists for a short time. Irreversible abscesses produce more intense, persistent, throbbing pain (Ziter, 1975).

Nursing Care and Related Interventions

Thoroughly inspect the inside of the mouth for associated lacerations, additional pieces of the tooth, and bleeding from the gums.

Always rule out life-threatening injuries. Place an avulsed tooth in saline as soon as possible. If a missing tooth is not found, a chest x-ray is obligatory to rule out aspiration (Cantrill, 1983). If a tooth has been aspirated, it must be removed by bronchoscopy. An avulsed tooth out of the socket for longer than four to six hours may not survive. It should be replaced and wired in as soon as possible to increase the chances for success. Broad-spectrum antibiotics, for example, ampicillin, will be ordered to help prevent infection. If irreversible pulp damage from caries or abscesses is evident from examination, the tooth may be extracted in the emergency department. In many cases, analgesics are prescribed, and the patient is referred to a dentist.

Discharge Planning

A patient with dental trauma will require information regarding eating soft foods, as well as any pain medications he may be given. Follow-up appointments and a dental referral for increased pain must be provided for the patient. Emphasize that emergency care is rarely definitive; rather, it alleviates only immediate symptoms, and dental follow-up care is necessary. If the patient has had an extraction done in the emergency department, he should return to the emergency department if he experiences continued bleeding, difficulty in breathing, or unbearable pain.

OCULAR TRAUMA

Blindness is dreaded more than the loss of any other sense. Trauma is responsible for one-half of all cases of blindness in one eye (Anderson, 1983). Safety measures, such as safety glasses, have decreased the incidence of eye trauma. Trauma to the eye involving the eyelid is usually associated with a more serious injury.

Pathophysiology

Blunt trauma to the eye, usually from sport injuries (e.g., racquetball, handball, and tennis), causes considerable periorbital damage. The eye itself, however, is quite resistant. Blunt trauma will cause periorbital contusions, ecchymosis, edema, lacerations, and/or a fracture of the orbital rim or orbital floor. Hemorrhage into the anterior chamber of the eye, a hyphema, may also result from blunt trauma. A hyphema is serious and rebleeding leads to vision loss. Subconjunctival hemorrhages from ruptured capillaries in the conjunctiva occur commonly and appear worse than they are because of the contrast of red on white. Finally, blunt trauma that may rupture the globe of the eye is considered a severe injury (Anderson, 1983).

Foreign bodies in the eye and corneal abrasions from wearing contact lenses too long are common eye complaints in any emergency department. Unconscious patients with their contact lenses left in place may develop corneal abrasions leading to corneal ulcers, infection, and eventual vision loss. Superficial corneal abrasions heal without scarring. If a foreign body is metal and it is embedded, a rust ring may develop in a matter of hours that will have to be shelled out (Anderson, 1983).

Intraocular foreign bodies, usually embedded in the posterior chamber of the eye, may cause minimal pain and not reflect the seriousness of the injury. This condition, however, constitutes an emergency that necessitates surgical removal with the possibility of serious complications, such as infection, hemorrhage, and loss of vision (Budassi, 1981). Any injury to the lens of the eye may cause a catarac to develop later. Impaled objects lead to a loss of vitreous humor and other damage depending on their location.

Burns to the eye may be chemical, thermal, or radiant, and each must be handled as potential blinders. Because the cornea resists acid more than alkali, acid burns in the eye do not progress as rapidly and are usually more superficial than alkali burns. Alkali burns caused by lime, ammonia, lye, and mortar eat through the cornea and require emergency treatment. All burns may cause complications, such as adhesions, corneal ulcers, and eyelid damage.

Thermal burns are usually associated with facial and eyelid burns. Ultraviolet rays from welding, skiing, ice climbing, reading in the sun, and sunlamps cause radiant burns that may also be associated with facial and eyelid burns. Infrared burns from glass blowing and eclipse blindness are more severe than ultraviolet burns because of the damage to the lens of the eye (Budassi, 1981).

Clinical Manifestations

The patient's chief complaint usually points to ocular trauma because the patient understands the cause of his symptoms. Pain and decreased visual acuity cause the patient to seek help (Anderson, 1983). Information about ocular trauma that the nurse must obtain includes the following: what happened, names of the chemicals involved, type of foreign body, how it happened, where and when it happened, and the initial care received. Patients with foreign bodies, corneal abrasions, or burns will complain of the same subjective feeling of having something in their eye. Many times, anesthesia is required while examining the eye to decrease tearing, pain, and severe photophobia. Never use eye drops, however, before the ocular examination by the primary care provider.

Nursing Care and Related Interventions

In general, position the patient (flat or in semi-Fowler's position) and assure good lighting for examination, check for contact lenses, and ask about eye glasses. Perform a visual acuity examination, testing each eye separately. The best possible results are obtained by having the patient wear his contact lenses or glasses, if possible. As swelling increases, the ability to examine the eye properly decreases. Assess for the presence of photophobia, pupillary response, globe integrity, lacrimal duct integrity, tearing, and tetanus status. Irrigate eyelid injuries with normal saline.

If the lid margin is involved in the injury, intricate repair with careful approximation is necessary to restore function without tear problem complications.

Apply cold packs to the orbital rim, if traumatized. If a hyphema is present, the patient should be placed on a stretcher with side rails up in a semi-Fowler's position immediately. The patient will be admitted with bilateral eye patches and sedation for five days. Bilateral patching decreases movement, pain, and light. A hyphema that does not rebleed will probably clear spontaneously. A subconjunctival hemorrhage left untreated will resolve in two to four weeks. Be gentle and protect the eye with a metal shield for globe trauma. Do not give eye medications if there is any question about an open eye injury.

If the patient suspects a foreign body or thermal or radiation burn after the primary care provider examines the patient, instill anesthetic drops if ordered and test visual acuity. One-half percent tetracaine hydrochloride is a topical anesthetic that gives an initial sting when instilled but provides the best anesthesia. Proparacaine (Alcaine) is a rapid, short-acting anesthetic adequate for foreign body removal. Evert the patient's eyelid and irrigate the eye with a minimum of one liter of normal saline. Foreign bodies are usually easily removed with a cotton tipped applicator. If this technique is unsuccessful, a physician may use a sterile needle to remove the foreign body.

The same procedure for administering anesthesia is used for a suspected corneal abrasion without irrigation. For a suspected abrasion after the visual acuity test, the cornea is stained with individual-use sterile fluorescein dye strips, and a black light is used to visualize abrasions. The light delineates the dye that accumulates around the abrasion. After diagnosis, antibiotic drops are instilled and the eye is patched.

If an intraocular foreign body is suspected, the patient will require x-ray examination and must be prepared for emergency surgery. Intravenous antibiotics are usually ordered. Impaled objects are secured if possible with the patient's eyes bilaterally patched to decrease movement.

Chemical burns to the eye require immediate normal saline irrigation for 15 to 30 minutes. Check the ocular pH with nitrazine paper and continue irrigating until the pH is less than 8 (normal ocular pH is 7). A rarely needed antidote for acid burns is 2 percent sodium bicarbonate. Citric or boric acid is used as an alkaline burn antidote (Budassi, 1981). Topical antibiotic eye drops or ointment are instilled into the eye, which is then patched.

Ten percent sodium sulfacetamide (Sulf 10), sulfisoxazole diolamine (Gantrisin), bacitracin, polymixin, and neomycin (Neosporin) have a bacteriostatic effect against a wide range of gram-positive and gram-negative micro-organisms. They are used for patients with conjunctivitis, corneal ulcers, and superficial ocular infections. Steroid drops for the eye are rarely, if ever, used in the emergency department unless ordered by an ophthalmologist. If herpes is present in the eye, the steroids can cause a sudden proliferation.

Discharge Planning

Patients with eye trauma who are discharged from the emergency department require detailed instructions. If the patient has a unilateral eye patch, teach the person about the loss of depth perception. Caution the patient about his decreased visual fields and how this may affect his driving ability. Instruct the family and patient in the correct way to instill eye drops, apply ointment, and repatch the eye.

The patient must understand all side effects, route, and dose of any pain medication prescribed. Eye injuries can be painful, and the nurse must understand the need for adequate medication. Anesthetic eye drops are never dispensed to the patient to take home because continual anesthesia masks the course of pain in the eye that can indicate the development of complications.

The patient should keep from rubbing his eye and wear dark glasses to protect his eye from bright light or sunlight. The patient should call or return to the emergency department if pain increases, a fever over 39°C orally develops, or vision decompensates. Long-term maintenance should be coordinated with an ophthalmologist.

CONCLUSION

Facial trauma is common in emergency departments. The nurse must always perform careful triage to rule out life-threatening conditions associated with facial trauma and to examine the full extent of the injury. The nurse must understand and implement appropriate actions to provide quality care for the patient experiencing any type of facial trauma, including facial fractures, dental problems, and ocular trauma. Effective discharge planning will help the patient and family continue to provide quality care at home and to return for appropriate long-term care.

BIBLIOGRAPHY

Anderson, R.: Ocular Emergencies. In C. Warner (ed.): *Emergency Care: Assessment and Intervention*. St. Louis: Mosby, 1983, pp. 293–301.

Budassi, S., and J. Barber: *Emergency Nursing: Principles and Practice*. St. Louis: Mosby, 1981.

Cantrill, S.: Facial Trauma. In P. Rosen (ed.): *Textbook of Emergency Medicine*. St. Louis: Mosby, 1983.

Constant, E.: Trauma to the Face. In Schwartz (ed.): *Principles and Practice of Emergency Medicine*. Philadelphia: Saunders, 1978, pp. 627–646.

Ingram, N.: Trauma to the ear, nose, face and neck. *Journal of Emergency Nursing* 6:4 (1980).

Lanros, N.: *Assessment and Intervention in Emergency Nursing*. Bowie, MD: Brady, 1983.

Moore, L.: Emergency Management of Facial Injuries. In C. Warner (ed.): *Emergency Care: Assessment and Intervention*. St. Louis: Mosby, 1983, pp. 316–323.

Rea, R.: The Nursing Process in Eye Emergencies. In N. Holloway (ed.): *Emergency Department Nurses Association Core Curriculum*. Chicago: Emergency Department Nurses Association, 1980, pp. 101–111.

Schaefer, A.: Care of the Patient with Ocular Injuries. In J. Cosgriff and D. Anderson (eds.): *The Practice of Emergency Nursing*. Philadelphia: Lippincott, 1975, pp. 439–450.

Schultz, R., and R. Oldham: An overview of facial injuries. *Surgical Clinicians of North America* 57(5):987 (1977).

BIBLIOGRAPHY

Serio, J.: Emergencies Involving the Ear, Nose, and Throat. In J. Cosgriff and D. Anderson (eds.): *The Practice of Emergency Nursing*. Philadelphia: Lippincott, 1975, pp. 423–438.

Wells, J.: The Nursing Process in Ear, Nose, and Throat Emergencies. In N. Holloway (ed.): *Emergency Department Nurses Association Core Curriculum*. Chicago: Emergency Department Nurses Association, 1980, pp. 77–79.

Winspur, I.: Facial fractures and the emergency department physician. *Emergency Medical Service* (May–June, 1979).

Ziter, W.: Dental Emergencies. In J. Cosgriff and D. Anderson (eds.): *The Practice of Emergency Nursing*. Philadelphia: Lippincott, 1975, pp. 451–470.

19

A Burn Injury

Janet Gren Parker

After completing this chapter, the reader will be able to do the following:

1. Triage a patient experiencing a burn injury.
2. Discuss the pathophysiology of a burn injury, including local changes, cardiac changes, respiratory changes, and renal changes.
3. List the clinical manifestations of an inhalation injury.
4. Describe a method for estimating the extent of the burn injury according to body surface area and depth.
5. Discuss baseline diagnostic studies that are useful in the care of a burn patient.
6. Discuss the nursing care of a burn patient.
7. Explain the differences in care of a patient experiencing an electrical or chemical burn.
8. Discuss the discharge planning for a patient experiencing a burn injury.

Burn injuries are the third leading cause of accidental death in the United States. More than 2,233,000 burn injuries occur each year, with 10 percent of the injuries requiring admission into a hospital (Hummel, 1982). Approximately one-half of these injuries involve children, and 12,000 Americans die each year from a burn injury (Johnson et al. 1981). The actual burn itself is not the leading cause of death, but sepsis resulting from the burn injury is the main complication that leads to death. This chapter discusses in detail the care of a patient experiencing a burn injury in the emergency department.

TRIAGE

Triage is extremely important to help differentiate the seriousness of the burn injury and to establish priorities of care. Each emergency department must determine whether transfer to a burn facility is appropriate or whether the local hospital can handle the situation. Admission to a hospital is usually considered necessary when the burn encompasses 20 percent of the body surface area (BSA); it is a full-thickness burn; the age of the patient is either younger or older in nature; the burn involves the hands, feet, face, neck, or perineum; or previous chronic medical problems exist.

Subjective Data

The triage nurse must obtain as much history as possible relating to the nature of the injury. Where did it happen? How did it happen? When did it happen? Was the patient in an enclosed space or an open space? Did the house simply burn or was there also an explosion? What was the burning agent? Incidences of smoke inhalation have increased since the use of plastics and polyurethane foam in the manufacture of furniture and bedding. If a chemical was involved, the duration of contact, the amount of the chemical, and its concentration must be determined. Alkaline substances penetrate more deeply than acid substances and cause a more severe burn. If an electrical current was involved, what was the voltage of the current? Was it alternating or direct current?

The patient's past medical history is extremely important because chronic medical problems complicate the treatment of and survival rate for burn patients. Current medications and any known allergies must be documented as well as current tetanus immunization status.

Objective Data

The triage nurse begins a brief, immediate collection of objective data as soon as the patient arrives in the emergency department. Include in the initial assessment airway, breathing, and circulation status. If these are stable, do a more detailed examination. The depth of the burn as well as the amount of body surface involved must be documented. The "Rule of Nines" can be used to determine roughly the amount of surface area involved, but it is inaccurate for children under the age of 15. (This classification is discussed more thoroughly later in the chapter.)

The respiratory status of the patient is observed closely. Document any presence of soot on the tongue or mouth, singed facial or nasal hairs, and the quality and rate of the respirations. Is the patient using accessory muscles? Does the patient have a productive cough? If an extremity is burned, the peripheral pulses must be assessed, and capillary refill distal to the injury must also be documented. Describe the level of consciousness and check the pupils for equality and reactivity to light. The patient must be assessed for any associated injuries that may have occurred. Do not let the obvious injury of the burn detract from a more serious injury such as a tension pneumothorax. Document, too, any prehospital or pretransfer care the patient received, such as intravenous fluids (IV) or the use of sterile burn sheets.

Assessment and Planning

By analyzing the subjective and objective data collected, the triage nurse makes an assessment and develops an initial plan of care. This plan of care should include the

PATHOPHYSIOLOGY

TABLE 19.1 Examples of Triage Notes for Patients Experiencing Burns

S:	12 yo BM with c/o being involved in a house fire approximately 20 min PTA. Firemen found child in bedroom under bed with his clothes on fire. The entire house and contents were involved in the blaze. PMH: negative, NKA, no current medications, up-to-date on immunizations.
O:	Crying, PERL [pupils equal and react to light], 50% full and partial thickness skin burns over lower half of body from umbilicus downward. Face sooty with singed nasal hairs and soot on tongue. Quality of respirations normal, pedal pulses present in both feet.
A:	2° and 3° body burn with possible inhalation injury.
P:	Surgical evaluation, admit examination room immediately, protect airway, isolation techniques, social worker called to be with family.
S:	45 yo WM lab technician with c/o "spilled acid solution on my arm." App. 5 min PTA. c/o burning sensation to arm. PMH: negative, NKA, on PCN for ear infection, tetanus toxoid 3 yrs ago.
O:	Ⓡ forearm reddened with blister formation, burn circumferential in nature, radial and ulnar pulses strong and regular, cap. refill of fingers normal.
A:	Chemical burn, partial thickness to Ⓡ forearm.
P:	Surgical evaluation, admit to examination room immediately, water irrigation immediately, followed by cool compress dressing.

patient's priority of care and appropriate nursing actions, such as protection of the airway. The patient's family needs reassurance so that their anxiety will decrease to help them cope with the situation.

Table 19.1 contains two examples of triage notes for patients presenting to the emergency department with a burn injury. A thorough discussion of the pathophysiology of burn injuries, clinical manifestations, nursing care and related interventions, and discharge planning related to burn injuries follows. Knowledge of this material will aid the nurse in performing triage accurately and appropriately.

PATHOPHYSIOLOGY

The loss of skin due to injury creates many problems. Local changes that occur immediately include loss of the microbial barrier, loss of the fluid barrier, and loss of temperature control leading to hypothermia. In the emergency department, loss of the fluid barrier creates the most problems.

With the burning of capillaries in the skin, the permeability of the capillaries increases creating an isotonic fluid and plasma protein shift from the vasculature to the interstitial area. The increase in capillary permeability is related to the release of histamine throughout the body, not just at the site of the burn, which occurs primarily in the first 12 hours post burn, but can last for 18 to 36 hours post burn. It creates a decrease in the intravascular fluid volume which causes baroreceptors in the aorta, atria, carotid bodies and the kidneys to stimulate vasoconstriction. The autonomic nervous system stimulates the release of catecholamines, which increase the blood flow to vital organs and decrease it to peripheral tissues; this, in turn, leads to lactic acid buildup peripherally, which eventually creates a metabolic acidosis. Aldosterone is secreted from the adrenal cortex to conserve fluid via sodium reabsorption in the kidneys, which, in turn, creates a decreased urinary output with a decreased sodium concentration. This is called burn shock.

Cardiac output can decrease by 50 percent secondary to the hypovolemia from the fluid and plasma shift. DeSantis et al. (1981) have identified a myocardial depressant factor (MDF) that is present in patients with severe burns even after adequate fluid resuscitation. MDF is a cardiotoxic peptide produced by the ischemic pancreas in burn shock. MDF depresses the myocardial contractility, enhances splanchnic vasoconstriction, and exacerbates the impairment of phagocytosis by the reticuloendothelial system. It usually appears approximately four to five days after the burn injury (DeSantis et al., 1981). Because of MDF's effect on the cardiac output of patients, it has been postulated that MDF may contribute to the high mortality rate of burn patients.

The glomerular filtration rate is decreased due to hypovolemia and decreased plasma flow to the kidneys that can continue for 24 to 72 hours post burn. Acute renal failure (ARF) can develop secondary to tubular damage. Circulating red blood cells are destroyed from the burn injury itself, and the red blood cells that are not damaged decrease their life span by 50 percent. Consequently, free hemoglobin is released into the circulation that forms casts in the tubules of the kidneys causing ARF. Damage to muscle tissue releases myoglobin into the circulation, which also leads to tubular damage. Anemia may also develop due to the loss of red blood cells.

Carbon monoxide poisoning may be present because carbon monoxide has a greater affinity than oxygen does to hemoglobin. The epiglottis usually protects the lower airway from any actual burning. The superheated air inhaled usually results in burns to the pharynx and larynx with swelling that can produce an airway obstruction in four hours. The tracheobronchial mucosa is exposed to the toxic products of incomplete combustion (a chemical irritation) that can progress to pulmonary edema and eventually to a chemical pneumonitis. Pulmonary edema generally takes 36 to 48 hours to develop.

Infection develops as a complication because losing the microbial barrier of the skin allows bacteria from the surrounding air to invade the body. The burned, dead tissue provides an excellent medium for bacterial growth. The efficacy of systemic antibiotics is nil due to the poor circulation to peripheral sites where the bacteria flourish. A severe depression in the patient's entire immunologic system also occurs, including a decrease in the functioning of inflammatory cells, macrophages, and neutrophils.

CLINICAL MANIFESTATIONS

Most patients experiencing burn injuries arrive in the emergency department awake, alert, and oriented. If their level of consciousness is altered, it is probably due to an associated injury or to an inhalation injury. Always make sure the patient with a burn does not have associated injuries. The burn is such an obvious injury that other problems are frequently and easily overlooked. Suspect an inhalation injury if the

DIAGNOSTIC STUDIES

burn occurred in an enclosed space; there are burns around the mouth and face; singed facial hair, particularly hair of the nares; hoarseness; wheezing; carbonaceous-stained sputum; dyspnea; hemoptysis; and stridor or labored breathing.

Tobiasen et al. (1982) have developed an abbreviated burn severity index to help predict the prognosis of burn patients. This index is based on the variables of sex, age, presence or absence of inhalation injury, presence or absence of a full thickness burn, and the percentage of body surface area involved. Roi et al. (1981) have developed a nomograph for the computation of the mortality risk for a burned patient. The nomograph considers the patient's age, the size of the burn, and the presence or absence of a perineal burn. These tools are helpful in the triage of the burn patient, indicating which patients should be transferred to regional burn facilities. They can also be used in auditing the care of the burn patient in the emergency department.

Table 19.2 contains the classification of burn injuries according to the depth of the burn. Clinically, the burn is usually easily classified according to depth, except in cases of partial thickness superficial and partial thickness deep. It is difficult to determine clinically the degree to which the dermis is involved in the injury. In addition, the depth of the burn can increase over time due to the application of too much cold because cold can intensify the capillary damage and convert second degree burns to third degree. Development of infection can also convert the burn to a deeper depth classification.

It is extremely important to determine the amount of body surface area involved in the burn. The Rule of Nines can help in providing an initial, gross determination. The legs, the front of the trunk, and the back of the trunk each represent 18 percent body surface area (BSA). The arms and the head each represent 9 percent BSA, with the perineum representing 1 percent BSA. This classification is inaccurate in children due to their larger head size in proportion to the rest of their body. The Berkow burn chart (Christopher, 1980), shown in Figure 19.1, includes the proportional differentiation in its formula for estimating the body surface area involved in the burn.

The patient who is experiencing burn shock presents with tachycardia, a decreased blood pressure, decreased urinary output, poor peripheral circulation, metabolic acidosis, restlessness, and confusion. A paralytic ileus develops. Children, however, may become hypertensive after a severe burn (*Emergency Medicine,* 1980), a condition that may in turn cause seizure activity. Children are considered hypertensive if their diastolic pressure is above 90 mm Hg. A larger burned area means a greater incidence of hypertension. This drops off with a really severe burn injury due to hypovolemia. The cause of this phenomenon is unknown.

DIAGNOSTIC STUDIES

Diagnostic studies performed in the care of the burn patient in the emergency department are done to establish a data base used to determine the continual, ongoing care of the patient. Arterial blood gas values should be determined as well as an arterial carboxyhemoglobin level to help manage inhalation injuries. A carbon monoxide level as well as a cyanide level may also be helpful. The pH reading will help in the management of metabolic acidosis. A complete cell count, electrolyte values, glu-

TABLE 19.2 Classification of Burn Injuries According to Depth of Burn

Skin Layers Involved	Depth of Burn	Healing Time	Pain Perception	Skin Appearance	Healing Accomplished By
Epidermis	First degree: Superficial	3–5 days	Present, hypersensitive	Reddened, no blisters	Epithelialization
Epidermis and some dermis	Second degree: Partial thickness, superficial	10–14 days	Present, hypersensitive	Reddened with blister formation	Epithelialization
Epidermis and all dermis except basal layer (hair follicle still present)	Second degree, deep: Partial thickness, deep	30–60 days	Present, hyposensitive	Reddened with white center, blisters (hard to differentiate clinically from partial thickness, superficial)	Epithelialization from hair follicles that remain
Epidermis, all dermis, and some subcutaneous tissue	Third degree: Full thickness	Greater than 60 days	Absent	White, leathery, charred appearance, hard and dry with eschar	Grafts
Muscle and bone	Fourth degree	Never	Absent	Muscle and/or bone exposed	Excision of all dead structures; amputation

NURSING CARE AND RELATED INTERVENTIONS

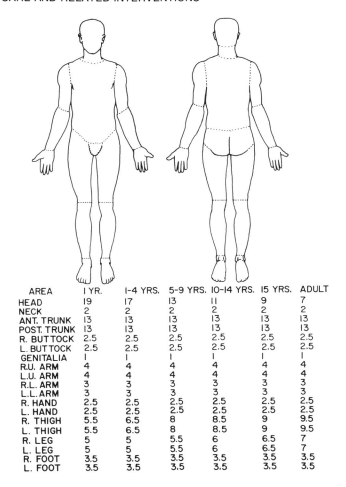

Figure 19.1 The Berkow burn chart.

cose levels, blood urea nitrogen levels, prothrombin time, creatinine levels, and blood cultures may be ordered. A urine sample should be obtained and sent for a complete urinalysis and myoglobin level. An electrocardiogram and chest x-ray film are also necessary for adequate baseline data. Other studies may be ordered if there are associated injuries.

NURSING CARE AND RELATED INTERVENTIONS

The first priority of care in the patient experiencing a burn is the maintenance of the patient's respiratory and circulatory systems. A patent upper and lower airway is essential with cardiopulmonary resuscitation instituted, if necessary. Humidified oxygen should be started immediately and delivered at 100 percent concentration if carbon monoxide poisoning is a possibility. Disrobe the patient entirely as soon as possible to stop any further burning. Place the patient on sterile burn sheets (such sheets are designed to absorb serous drainage without sticking to the actual wound). The health care providers should be gowned and gloved and the patient dealt with as aseptically as possible in the emergency department.

The second priority of care is the prevention of shock. Large-bore intravenous (IV) lines should be established, preferably in an unburned extremity or via a central line access. The catheter should be at least 16 gauge for an adult and an 18 gauge for a child. Several formulas have been developed to help guide the health care provider in fluid replacement. Table 19.3 contains the current formulas in use. The Parkland formula is the most popular because it is generally believed no colloid is necessary in

TABLE 19.3 Formulas for Fluid Replacement—First 24 Hours Post Burn

Parkland Formula (Also called Baxter or Ringer's Lactate)
Crystalloid: 4 ml Ringer's lactate/kg/% burn
Colloid: none
Water: none

One-half of total given in first 8 hrs post burn
One-quarter of total given in second 8 hrs post burn
One-quarter of total given in third 8 hrs post burn

Brooke Formula
Crystalloid: 1.5 ml Ringer's lactate/kg/% burn
Colloid: 0.5 ml/kg/% burn
Water: 2000 ml dextrose 5% in water

One-half of total given in first 8 hrs post burn
One-quarter of total given in second 8 hrs post burn
One-quarter of total given in third 8 hrs post burn

Evans Formula
Crystalloid: 1 ml Ringer's lactate/kg/% burn
Colloid: 1 ml/kg/% burn
Water: 2000 ml dextrose 5% in water

One-half of total given in first 8 hrs post burn
One-quarter of total given in second 8 hrs post burn
One-quarter of total given in third 8 hrs post burn

Hypertonic Resuscitation Formula
Hypertonic salt solution containing:
   300 mEq of sodium
   200 mEq of lactate
   100 mEq of chloride

Given at rate to maintain urinary outputs of 30–40 ml/hr

NURSING CARE AND RELATED INTERVENTIONS

the first 24 hours post burn until capillary permeability decreases. Remember that these formulas are only suggestions, and that altering fluid replacement may be required depending on the urinary output of the patient. The necessary urinary output is listed below.

Age	Output/Hour
Up to two months	5–20 cc (15 cc optimal)
Two months to one year	10–30 cc (20 cc optimal)
One year to five years	10–40 cc (25 cc optimal)
Five years to 15 years	30 cc
Fifteen years to adult	50–60 cc

The mental state in a child is extremely helpful in determining his hydration. A hypotonic solution (such as dextrose 5 percent in water) is contraindicated in children because it is likely to produce seizures as a result of hyponatremia. Ringer's lactate is used because it is a balanced sodium solution that most closely approximates the composition of extracellular fluid, has a pH of 7.4, and a sodium concentration of 130 mEq/l.

The Parkland formula is recommended for the first 24 hours post burn, with plasma being added in the second 24 hours at a rate of 0.3–0.5 ml/kg/percent burn and dextrose 5 percent in water replacing the evaporative free water loss to prevent hypernatremia. A Foley catheter must be inserted to monitor adequately the urinary output. If the urine contains myoglobin (appears red), be on guard for acute renal failure and make sure the patient maintains a urinary output of 75–100 cc/hour. A bolus of 25 g of mannitol may be ordered to help block tubular reabsorption. A maintenance dose of 12.5 g of mannitol added to every liter of fluid may be necessary to maintain urinary output.

The emergency department nurse must observe for signs of fluid overload, constantly monitoring the patient's respiratory status as well as the central venous pressure and the pulse and blood pressure readings. A record of the baseline weight of the patient, if at all possible, can help in long-term management. All rings and bracelets must be removed and distal circulation checked, sometimes with the aid of a Doppler to hear all the peripheral pulses.

A nasogastric tube should be inserted to help prevent gastric dilatation, abdominal distention, and nausea and vomiting. Later, in the course of therapy, it can be useful for tube feedings. The nutritional requirements of burn patients are dramatically increased in the days after a burn occurs. Total parenteral nutrition may be ordered, but it can create infection problems.

Wound Care

There is considerable discussion in the literature relating to wound care of the burn patient. Each burn care facility has its own beliefs and philosophies on treating burns. Two major areas of debate include sterile versus aseptic and open versus closed treatment.

TABLE 19.4 Topical Antibiotics in Burn Wound Management

Type	Advantages	Disadvantages
Silver sulfadiazine 1% (Silvadene)	Painless application Bacteriostatic Bacteriocidal No dressings needed No systemic complications	Slow penetration Resistant organism development May develop rash
Mafenide 10% (Sulfamyelon)	Bacteriostatic Fast penetration No dressings needed	Pain on application Metabolic acidosis Hyperventilation
Silver nitrate 0.5%	Effective against gram$^\ominus$ and gram$^\oplus$ bacteria No sensitivity reaction	Hyponatremia Hypocalcemia Hypokalemia Discolors everything it touches Very messy Must have dressing Pain on application
Silver nitrate chlorhexidine digluconate 0.2% (Cerium Nitrate)	Effective against gram$^\ominus$ bacteria Painless application No systemic effects	Only suppresses gram$^\oplus$ bacteria
Povidone iodine	Bacteriostatic Bacteriocidal	Elevates systemic iodine levels

In the emergency department it is difficult, if not impossible, to create a sterile environment for the patient. Health care providers should be as aseptic in their care as possible, wear gowns and gloves, and decrease the traffic into the patient care area as much as possible. Whether treatment is to be open or closed is determined by each burn unit according to the physicians' preference. The advantage of the closed method is that it prevents the exposure of the wound to microbes. Most burn care specialists believe, however, that contamination is unavoidable. The open method permits easier inspection of the burn; it is less expensive; and there are no dressings to inhibit joint mobility. (Table 19.4 contains the types of topical antibiotics available, with their advantages and disadvantages.)

The wound must be cleansed thoroughly with water and a mild soap in a warm room, preferably in some type of whirlpool tub. The warmth of the room is necessary to prevent hypothermia. Do not use hexachloraphene; its absorption may cause encephalopathy, especially in children. All dead tissue should be removed with forceps. This debridement includes removing blisters from around joint areas or from areas that would impede movement of the extremity to any extent.

An *escharotomy* is the incision of a full-thickness burn down to the subcutaneous fat layer. An escharotomy is performed in all circumferential burns to allow continued circulation distal to the burn. An escharotomy of the chest may be necessary to enable the lungs to expand when there has been a circumferential burn to the chest. No anesthesia is necessary because the skin is totally insensitive in a full-thickness burn. The hands, especially in children, are areas that may need escharotomies quickly to ensure adequate circulation to the fingers. An escharotomy has minimal risks and maximum benefits, so it should be done routinely whenever the development of circulatory compromise is considered a possibility.

Medications

Prophylactic antibiotics are not recommended for use in the care of the burn patient unless the health care provider suspects a streptococcal infection. If so, penicillin is the preferred drug. Antibiotics are used only when there is a positive culture result; otherwise the patient can develop organisms resistant to conventional antibiotic therapy. The blood vessels at the wound edge are occluded in deep partial or full-thickness burns, so systemic antibiotics have no effect on the localized bacterial colonization.

To relieve pain and anxiety in the burn patient, analgesics may be given. In fact, they should be given approximately 20 to 30 minutes prior to debridement if at all possible. The drugs of choice are morphine 2–4 mg every three to four hours in adults, 0.1–0.2 mg/kg every three to four hours in children, and Demerol 25–50 mg every three to four hours in adults, 1.0–1.5 mg/kg every three to four hours in children. These medications must be given intravenously, not intramuscularly, because the edema in the burned areas prevents the absorption of the medication. When the edema decreases, the sequestered medication may be absorbed all at once, causing a medication overdosage.

Sodium bicarbonate may be added to the IV fluids to correct the acid-base balance of the patient. Tetanus immunization must be ascertained. If needed, the tetanus injection is given intramuscularly.

Minor Burn Care

Partial-thickness burns of less than 15 percent BSA in adults and 10 percent BSA in children with less than 2 percent full-thickness burns are considered minor in nature. Electrical burns are excluded from this category as well as burns of the face, hands, feet, and perineum.

First aid treatment for the minor burn, as well as the major burn, involves cooling the burn and warming the patient. *Never apply ice* directly to a burn of any size because it can create further tissue damage and tissue death resulting in a frostbite injury to the skin. Covering the burn will decrease the pain involved because air currents of any kind seem to create pain in partial-thickness burns.

In the emergency department the minor burn is cleansed with soap and water, debrided as necessary, a topical antibiotic is applied (usually Silvadene), and the wound is dressed in a functional position. Tetanus immunization is documented.

ELECTRICAL BURNS

Burns caused by electrical currents present different challenges to the emergency department nurse. The damage actually visible is slight in comparison to the extent of internal involvement. One must assume that everything between the entrance and exit sites of the current is possibly damaged. High-voltage current burns create cardiac electrical problems often causing immediate death. Otherwise, injuries from high-voltage currents result in fourth degree burns involving blood vessels, nerves, and bones. Common household voltage (110–220 v) rarely causes death. The most common electrical burn in a child occurs in the mouth as a result of chewing an electrical cord at home.

In an electrical burn, the electrical energy is converted to thermal energy. This heat denatures the protein in tissue causing immediate cell death and occlusion of blood vessels, resulting in the death of tissue not directly exposed to the electrical current.

The cardiac status of the patient with an electrical burn should be monitored constantly. Even after normal sinus rhythm has been established, dysrhythmias frequently develop. Defibrillation may be needed repeatedly. Anyone with any cardiac dysrhythmias should be admitted for observation.

Fluid replacement is difficult to gauge in this type of patient. There is no formula for the computation because of the amount of unknown damage. The best gauge is the urinary output that should be maintained at 75–100 cc/hour for the adult. The release of myoglobin is prevalent in this type of patient. Mannitol is usually required to help prevent ARF, and sodium bicarbonate is used to combat metabolic acidosis.

Amputations, fasciotomies, and repeated surgery may be employed in the long-term management of the patient with an electrical burn. The extent of damage is impossible to estimate in the emergency department.

CHEMICAL BURNS

Chemical burns usually occur from surface contact with a chemical, but may also result from inhaling a chemical or ingesting a chemical. Injury in a chemical burn is usually not the result of heat but the result of a chemical reaction between the substance and the patient's skin.

Copious irrigation with large quantities of lukewarm water is the preferred method of immediate care. Antidotes are contraindicated in most cases because they, in turn, can burn the normal tissue surrounding the initial burn site. Lukewarm water is recommended, rather than cold water, to help prevent hypothermia. A shower, one large enough for a stretcher, is an ideal place to irrigate a patient's chemical burns for an extended period of time. Dry chemicals should be brushed from the skin surface before irrigation takes place in order to prevent the chemical and the water from producing a reaction that generates heat, thus creating further damage. Irrigation may continue for 15 minutes or for as long as several hours. A general guide to use is to stop the irrigation when the patient no longer feels any burning sensation. The resultant burn is treated similarly to a thermal burn injury.

Tar burns create special problems in emergency departments. Cold water applied to the tar (or ice) can harden the tar, and it can then be peeled off the skin. Be careful that hypothermia does not result from the continued exposure to the cold substances. But cold application does not always work. Another technique is to apply mineral oil to soften the tar so it can be peeled off. If all else fails, use ether to dissolve the tar. But be *careful*: Ether is an extremely volatile substance and must be used with utmost caution to prevent combustion and inhalation problems.

DISCHARGE PLANNING

Patients with minor burn injuries will be treated in the emergency department and discharged with follow-up care arrangements. These patients and their significant others must understand in detail how to care for the wound at home. The nurse can teach the patient while the wound is being cleansed and treated in the emergency department. Verbal feedback from the patient or family must illustrate their comprehension of the instructions.

Be sure to include the following steps in the instructions:

Assemble all the equipment necessary to change the dressing.

Wash hands in soap and water.

Take off the old bandage (soaking in warm water may help loosen it if it is stuck).

Wash the burn in soap (Dial or Ivory) and warm water.

Check the wound for infection (increased pain, red streaks going away from the burn, yellowish pus drainage, increased swelling, rash).

Reapply the antibiotic cream with a sterile tongue blade.

Rebandage the burn.

The patient should also understand that elevation of the affected part will help decrease pain and swelling. Range of motion exercises must be understood so that the patient does not immobilize the area, which could possibly create future positioning and mobility problems. A physical therapist could perhaps discuss appropriate exercises with the patient. The understanding of any prescribed medication should also be documented, including the understanding of side effects, route, times, dosage, and drug actions.

Follow-up care is particularly important for this type of patient. Return clinic appointments or doctor office visits should be understood, and appropriate transportation to the appointment ensured, before the patient is discharged from the emergency department. Prevention of similar accidents should also be discussed, emphasizing safety procedures in both work and home situations.

For the patient admitted to the hospital for further care, the psychosocial needs of the patient and significant others must be addressed in the emergency department before the patient is transferred. Social workers and chaplains, for example, can help the family and patient adapt appropriately and accept the implications of the injury. Because of the altered body image, everyone involved in the situation may need help coping with the sequence of events that has occurred in the emergency department and the ones that will continue in the hospital setting.

CONCLUSION

Care of the burn patient has improved dramatically during the last 20 years. The American Burn Association directs many of its activities toward prevention of burn injuries. The emergency department nurse must continue to provide excellent care and also become involved in public education efforts to help prevent the occurrence of burn injuries. Caring for the burn patient is an ongoing challenge for the entire health care team.

BIBLIOGRAPHY

Burns. *Emergency Medicine* 12:135–138 (Nov. 1980).

Burns and blood pressure. *Emergency Medicine* 12:99 (Sept. 1980).

Christopher, K. L.: The use of a model for hemodynamic balance to describe burn shock. *Nursing Clinics of North America* 15:617–627 (1980).

DeSantis, D., P. Phillips, M. A. Spath, and A. M. Lefer: Delayed appearance of a circulatory myocardial depressant factor in burn patients. *Annals of Emergency Medicine* 10:22–24 (1981).

Finlayson, L.: Emergent care of the burn patient. *Critical Care Update* 7:18–23 (1980).

Hummel, R. P.: *Clinical Burn Therapy—A Management and Preventive Guide.* MA: John Wright, PSG, 1982.

Johnson, C. L. E. J. O'Shaughnessy and G. Ostergren: *Burn Management.* New York: Raven, 1981.

Kenner, C., and S. Manning: Emergency care of the burn patient. *Critical Care Update* 7:24–33 (1980).

Kinzie, V., and C. Lau: What to do for the severely burned. *RN* 43:46–51 (April 1980).

Marvin, J. A., and L. E. Einfeldt: Infection control for the burn patient. *Nursing Clinics of North America* 15:833–842 (1980).

Rickham, P. P., W. Ch. Hecker, and J. Prevot: *Progress in Pediatric Surgery: The Management of the Burned Child.* Baltimore: Urban and Schwarzenberg, 1981.

Roi, L. D., J. L. Flora, T. M. Davis, R. G. Cornell, and I. Feller: A severity grading chart for the burned patient. *Annals of Emergency Medicine* 10:161–163 (1981).

Severely burned patients: anticipating their emotional needs—nursing grand rounds. *Nursing 80* 10:46–51 (Sept. 1980).

The systemic effects of a burn ointment: *Emergency Medicine* 12:159 (June 1980).

Tobiasen, J., J. M. Hiebert, and R. F. Edlich: The abbreviated burn severity index. *Annals of Emergency Medicine* 11:260–262 (1982).

Zuker, R. M.: The major and minor of burns. *Emergency Medicine* 12:93–98 (Oct. 1980).

20
Head and Spine Trauma

Judith "Ski" Lower

After completing this chapter, the reader will be able to do the following:

1. Triage a patient experiencing head and spine trauma.
2. Describe the significance of, and means for eliciting, data in establishing an immediate neurological baseline in an acutely ill patient: level of consciousness; pupillary, motor, and sensory responses; and vital signs.
3. State the pathophysiology of increased intracranial pressure and the resultant signs and symptoms.
4. Anticipate patients' needs based on knowledge of the pathophysiology of neurological insults commonly seen in the emergency department.
5. Determine priorities of care and provide appropriate emergency care for the patient with central nervous system trauma.
6. Describe the medical and nursing goals established in the management of patients with central nervous system trauma.
7. Describe the rationale for treatment of patients with central nervous system injury.
8. Describe and differentiate the specific types of traumatic insults to the central nervous system and the appropriate nursing interventions.
9. Develop discharge teaching plans for the patient with central nervous system trauma.

Trauma is the primary cause of death of people under the age of 40, and the number 4 killer in the nation. More than six million head injuries occur every year, of which one million are severe in nature. Mortality and morbidity remain high despite increased knowledge of pathophysiology, improved monitoring, and several new modes of therapy. The ultimate outcome depends on the initial evaluation and treatment.

Approximately 10,000 new spinal injuries occur each year. Vehicular accidents, falls, diving injuries, and other accidents account for most of these injuries. A spinal cord injury is one of the most devastating traumas and one of the most expensive in terms of long-term rehabilitation. More sophisticated methods of extrication and transportation from the scene of the injury, earlier recognition and management of complications, and better rehabilitation techniques and facilities have all contributed to a decrease in the overall mortality and morbidity. Unfortunately, little progress has been made in medicine's ability to alter the initial injury and the resultant loss of function.

TRIAGE

Subjective Data

The initial history, as well as the baseline physical assessment obtained from the ambulance personnel, the patient, or from family or friends accompanying the patient, begins the triage process. The patient's condition obviously dictates the amount of time required to obtain information. Check the patient's chief complaint and memory of events before and after the injury. Determine the mechanism of injury: motor vehicle accident, a fall, or personal violence. Determine the height of the fall, the position of the patient in the car, and the position in which the patient was initially found. Find out when the accident occurred, what time the first observer arrived, and when medical help was administered. Look at the impact, the speed of the vehicle, and whether forward motion was limited by a seat belt. If the patient is unconscious, determine the pattern and the length of coma. Question the patient's overall clinical course since the injury and any treatment received prior to arrival.

Review of past history should include known allergies, any contributing medical problems (diabetes, cerebrovascular or cardiovascular accident, dysrhythmias, chronic obstructive pulmonary disease (COPD), seizure activity, alcohol or drug usage, medications), any physical disabilities (hearing or vision), and handedness.

Objective Data

Assessment of the adequacy of the airway, of ventilation, and of circulation *always* takes priority. In addition, any patient with a significant head injury, with or without a decrease in the level of consciousness, or with a history suggestive of the potential, should be treated as a victim of spinal injury. Note the method and adequacy of stabilization used. A brief evaluation should be done of the following:

Level of consciousness—the ability to verbalize, to open the eyes, to be oriented, to remember, to pay attention, and to have insight.

Pupillary response—size, equality, reaction.

Motor response—ability to follow commands, to move purposefully, to have inappropriate posturing, the strength of the muscle groups and reflexes.

THE NEUROLOGICAL ASSESSMENT

Sensory response—ability to perceive pain, touch, pressure, and position sense.

Vital signs—blood pressure (hypo, hyper trends), pulse (rate, rhythm), and respiration (rate, pattern, effectiveness).

Palpate the head and feel for depressions or crepitus. Look for ecchymosis, lacerations, open wounds, or hematomas. If a spinal injury is suspected, check the ability to cough and clear secretions. Assess the peripheral pulses and skin temperature. Check for signs of concurrent injuries because spinal injured patients cannot perceive pain and will not express it. Palpate over the spinous process for deformities and tenderness. Look for swelling or ecchymosis.

Assessment and Planning

Note the potential for cardiac, respiratory, or neurological deterioration based on the data. Determine the priorities of care. Note any deviations and physical deficits. The neurological status of a patient cannot be evaluated until cardiovascular and respiratory status are restored. Resuscitation and stabilization of vital organs always take priority over specific treatment of head injuries or spinal injuries. If an altered level of consciousness is due to cardiac or respiratory compromise, the neurological status would be expected to improve. If it does not, the practitioner must be extremely astute in the subsequent neurological evaluation. If a spinal injury exists, specify the level of any sensory or motor deficit.

Plans should include the immediate resuscitation and stabilization of the patient, early recognition and surgical treatment of mass lesions, and aggressive intervention to prevent secondary injuries. Immobilization of the spine is of top priority in a spine injured patient. Crisis intervention for both the patient and the family remains an integral part of the overall plan and begins at the time of initial contact. (Table 20.1 contains two examples of triage notes pertaining to patients with head and spine trauma.)

THE NEUROLOGICAL ASSESSMENT

Always address the priorities first: adequate airway, ventilation, and circulation. The patient's neurological status is never valid until adequate ventilation and circulation have been restored.

The admission assessment of the neurologically injured patient is *the most* important evaluation. All further observations will be based on what was found initially and, as in any other system, change is the important factor. Therefore, it is critical to establish an accurate baseline assessment. The emergency department nurse is often the first person to see the patient. Frequently, it is that nurse's ability to observe, recognize, and interpret changes correctly that makes the difference between functional survival and a persistent vegetative state for the patient.

In establishing an accurate baseline assessment, remember that the examination is considered incomplete unless the examiner is assured that the *maximum* response

TABLE 20.1 Examples of Triage Notes for Patients with Head and Spine Trauma

S: 25 yo M brought in by police following an assault with a lead pipe ½ hr PTA. Questionable period of brief unconsciousness. PMH: negative, NKA.

O: BP 110/70, HR 120, RR 12. 7 cm laceration across right frontal area. Ecchymosis and edema across nasal area with drainage of clear fluid from right nostril. Drowsy but arousable with loud voice and shaking. Oriented × 3. No recall of fight. Pupils equal and react to light briskly, moderate size. Follows commands and moves all four extremities with equal strength. Alcohol on breath. Hematoma, occipital scalp.

A: Probable concussion, ETOH intoxication. Rule out skull fracture, rule out nasal fracture, rule out rhinorrhea.

P: Surgical evaluation, admit exam room now.

S: 17 yo M brought in by paramedics after diving into a shallow lake. Removed immediately from the water by friends. No loss of consciousness. Spine immobilized at the scene, IV started, O_2 6 liters by mask. Patient c/o neck pain and loss of movement. PMH: negative, NKA.

O: BP 90/60, HR 56, RR 12 abdominal and shallow. No motor movement except upper extremity flexion. Awake, oriented. Pupils 6 mm, equal, react briskly. Skin warm and dry.

A: Probable midcervical spine injury, potential for respiratory compromise, probable spinal shock, R/O other injuries.

P: Trauma room for immediate evaluation/resuscitation.

---

the patient is capable of achieving has been elicited. If the baseline assessment does not reflect the patient's maximum capabilities, all further assessments will be based on false or inaccurate information. The consequences of inaccurate assessment are costly. Many of the clues given early in a compensated deteriorating state will be missed, and early treatment may be delayed.

Use the least amount of stimulation required to elicit an appropriate response always proceeding from lesser to greater stimulus. A good rule of thumb is to begin with the spoken voice, then proceed to shouting, shaking, and painful stimulation as needed. There are several acceptable ways to stimulate a patient, all of which result in sufficient pain to arouse the patient without causing unnecessary trauma. These methods include supraorbital pressure (pressure applied over the supraorbital notch by the examiner's thumb), trapezius squeeze (pinching 1 to 2 inches of the muscle just above the clavicle close to the neck), sternal rub (a grinding of the knuckles into the patient's sternum), and any other centrally induced pain.

The neurological examination in the emergency department should be detailed enough to cover the essentials, yet quick and concise enough to allow for rapid determination of the status of predictive areas. The essential components of the examination are the level of consciousness, pupillary and motor responses, cranial nerve check, and vital sign evaluation.

The Glasgow Coma Scale is an excellent predictor of outcome, but it is not intended to replace the minute-by-minute neurological evaluation. Other parameters should not be neglected because the coma scale is in use (Bruce, 1978).

Level of Consciousness

The level of consciousness is the most important indicator of the patient's brain function and the earliest and most sensitive indicator for detecting increased intracranial pressure. *Consciousness* is defined by Plum and Posner (1980) as an awareness of self and environment. Consciousness consists of two components: arousal and awareness. Clinical indication of arousal is simple awakefulness, a function of the reticular activating system in the brainstem, and is demonstrated by eye opening. Clinical indication of awareness involves many cortical functions, such as orientation, memory, intelligence, language, and goal-oriented behavior, and is a function of the cerebral hemispheres.

Unfortunately, there is no general agreement on which terms to use in describing levels of consciousness, nor is there universal interpretation of the terms already in use. There is full agreement, however, on what constitutes an awake, alert, and oriented patient versus a comatose patient, but in between these conditions there is a large gray area that is open to a variety of terminology (lethargic, drowsy, somnolent, stuporous, semiconscious, obtunded). It is therefore more important to describe what is seen and to paint a picture with words rather than merely labelling a behavior. A clear, concise description of what the patient does in response to the examiner leaves no room for doubt.

Orientation

To ascertain orientation, *specific* questions must be asked. Orientation has three spheres: person, place, and time. Patients lose orientation in a characteristic way, first to time, then to place, and last to people. For the patient to respond to a simple, "What year is it?" is sufficient. To ask, "Are you in a hospital?" allows a choice of "yes" or "no" and a 50–50 chance of answering correctly, whether he really knows the answer. Patients who are intubated or unable to verbalize an answer may be given a series of multiple choice questions to answer: "Are you at home, at a friend's house, in a motel, in a hospital?" The purpose is to ascertain the patient's ability to integrate the question and answer with an appropriate response. It is not a test of the ability to say "yes" or "no." Make the patient think. Children may be asked the same questions, although their answers will depend on their age. Time questions should focus on the seasons, holidays, or schooltime.

Memory

Memory is assessed in both recent and remote spheres. Recent memory is ascertained by asking the patient what happened to him, what events have occurred in the past four to six hours, or about events that may be easily validated, such as the latest national news event or the name of the president. The patient's ability to recall new information should also be tested; to do this, ask the patient to learn and retain your name, for example, or a series of three items (e.g., cat, dog, apple). Test his ability to repeat any of that information correctly after three to five minutes.

Remote memory is a function of the temporal lobe and is assessed by such questions as, "Where were you born?, In what year?, or What are the names of your children?" Children, depending on age, may be asked about family members, pets, or playmates.

Loss of memory for the period immediately after recovery of consciousness is termed *posttraumatic amnesia*. Pretraumatic or retrograde amnesia is loss of memory for the period immediately preceding the injury.

Language

Dysphasia, or *aphasia*, is the acquired deficit in any one of the areas of listening, speaking, reading, or writing. Aphasia represents damage to the cortical speech centers and is seen in an expressive, receptive, or mixed form. Language is not tested in the child under age two.

Expressive aphasia is also called *motor aphasia* or *Broca's aphasia*. It involves the inability to produce meaningful words. Patients frequently know what they want to say, and have the muscle power and nervous innervation to produce speech, but cannot say whole words. The speech is nonfluent.

Receptive aphasia, also called *sensory* or *Wernicke's aphasia*, is characterized by the inability to comprehend the written or spoken word. Frequently, these patients will exhibit fluent spontaneous speech but with impaired comprehension. They also lack insight into their problem and are prone to anger.

Aphasia should be differentiated from dysarthria, or the inability to manipulate speech musculature with precision, which results in the inability to articulate. It is the result of paralysis, paresis, or incoordination of the articulatory musculature (facial), the resonatory muscles (palatopharyngeal), and the phonatory muscles (laryngeal). Dysarthria is characterized by slurring of words and unclear or unintelligible speech. The muscles involved may be tested by asking the patient to say "me me me" (lips), "la la la" (tongue), and "ga ga ga" (soft palate). The pathology of dysarthria derives from interruption of the cranial nerve innervation producing a motor deficit involving the lips, tongue, and palate.

Clues to Altered Condition

The real challenge is keying into the subtle changes that occur *before* the patient's condition becomes obvious or advanced. Most of the clues are subtle, but if a picture has truly been painted with words in describing the patient these clues should easily be identified. Look for the patient who reveals the following symptoms:

Was oriented and now cannot identify what year it is.

Had been able to recall and now asks repetitive questions.

Had clear verbal responses that are now less clear and slightly delayed.

Loses insight.

Is now showing less interest in his environment.

Has an attention span that is more difficult to capture and maintain.

Does not think as quickly as before.

Had coherent speech that is now less distinct.

Three critical clues are the following:

1. The awake, quiet patient who suddenly becomes restless. Restlessness is always a strong danger clue and usually means hypoxia. In the absence of hypoxia and in the presence of a head injury, restlessness may mean a deterioration in consciousness.

2. The restless patient who suddenly becomes quiet. It could be that he is tired, but it could also be that his level of consciousness has slipped. Go back and thoroughly repeat the assessment to be sure, using maximum stimulation if necessary.
3. The patient who requires more and more stimulation of increased intensity and duration to elicit the same response.

Pupillary Response

The pupils are examined for size, equality, and reaction and provide a valuable guide to the location of brainstem disease causing coma. The pupils are relatively resistant to metabolic insult, unlike the level of consciousness, so the presence or absence of pupillary response is the most important *physical* sign distinguishing structural coma from metabolic coma.

Size and Equality
Note any deviation in size or shape of pupils. Ascertain if the patient is, or has been, on any medications that may affect pupillary size. Remember that pupillary size varies with the amount of surrounding light. Overhead, direct light makes it difficult to visualize pupils in people with brown eyes. It is helpful to use only the overbed light or indirect lighting. In assessing equality, a slight difference, less than 1 mm, exists normally in about 20 percent of the population. Gross inequality is called *anisocoria*.

Reaction
Reaction is best tested by asking the patient, if he is able, to focus on an object in the distance. The room does not need to be darkened unless the pupils are very small. Darkening the room will cause a natural pupillary dilatation, allowing the examiner to observe any constriction in response to light. Pupils are tested for both the direct response to light (or constriction in the same eye) and consensual response (constriction in the opposite eye). Direct response is tested by opening only the eye of the pupil to be tested to avoid confusion with accommodation, the normal constriction and adduction of the eyes when changing the visual focus from a distant to a near object. Normally, the pupil constricts and remains constricted as long as the light source remains. One might also observe a sluggish response or no response (a fixed pupil). The test is then repeated in the other eye.

Potential Pitfalls

1. The blind eye, if not checked for consensual response, may be falsely recorded as unresponsive due to an intracranial event, rather than due to the inability to see the light stimulus.
2. Local eye trauma may negate the pupillary response.
3. Glass eyes, far more common than many people realize and difficult to detect, will be fixed to light response.
4. Drugs and emotions may influence pupillary response.

Clues/Critical Assessment Factors
Be alert for a unilateral, dilating, sluggish or fixed pupillary response presenting as a change from the baseline or for unequal pupils, especially accompanied by changes in the level of consciousness and motor responses. Both are potential emergency situations and require immediate attention and intervention.

Motor Response

Determine whether the patient moves spontaneously or requires stimulation to move. Patients move spontaneously in obvious or subtle ways. If the patient is able to shift his weight to move off a needle cap left under him, he is capable of feeling a stimulus, integrating that feeling, and directing his body to move away from it. If the patient has not been observed to move spontaneously, ask him to move. Some patients do not move because they are afraid or they think they are not supposed to move.

Appropriate or Inappropriate Response
When the patient does move, is the movement normal (appropriate) or abnormal (inappropriate)? The highest level of motor achievement is the ability to follow commands. An objective command is better to use to help prevent a possible subjective misinterpretation of the patient's ability. The evaluation of the response to the classic command of "squeeze my hand" is extremely subjective. It is often so weak that one cannot tell if a response has occurred, or it is so firm that the examiner's hand must be pried from the patient's grasp. Besides the subjectivity, another pitfall is the grasp reflex. This reflex, present in infants, is inhibited in the adult by higher centers in the frontal lobe. If there is an injury in that area, the inhibition of that reflex is no longer active, and the reflex returns in response to objects placed in the hand. To validate following commands rather than a grasp reflex response, ask the patient to "let go now." This may be used for both adults and children. If the patient lets go, he is following commands. A more objective command is to ask the patient to "hold up two fingers." Try both sides if one side does not respond.

The next highest level of response is localizing pain or purposeful movement. Localizing is often difficult to differentiate from decortication because both involve a flexion response. It is helpful to apply the painful stimulus *above* the nipple line (use the trapezius squeeze or supraorbital pressure; do *not* pinch the nipple) to prevent confusion. The patient should attempt to find or localize the stimulus and remove it. In localization, the arms will move *above* the nipple line, whereas in decortication, they will remain at or below the nipple line.

All of the following responses are considered abnormal.

GEGENHALTEN
One of the earliest hemispheric signs of motor dysfunction that precedes changes in muscle tone and paralysis in expanding mass lesions in the anterior motor cortex is *gegenhalten,* or paratonia. The word *gegenhalten* means "go and stop." The condition is characterized by an increase in muscle tone detected on passive movement of the extremity, regardless of its starting position. To the examiner, it feels as if the

THE NEUROLOGICAL ASSESSMENT

patient is opposing the effort to move him. Paratonia is thus a hint of motor regression.

RIGID FLEXION/DECORTICATION
Rigid flexion/decortication is characterized by flexion of the arms with the upper arms held tightly against the side, flexion of the wrists and fingers, and extension of the legs with internal rotation. The feet are plantar flexed. The intensity varies from a fine tremor to intense stiffness. The term decortication means "without cortex" and implies moderate to severe injury above the brainstem.

RIGID EXTENSION/DECEREBRATION
Decerebration is seen in brainstem injuries and implies a more severe neurological condition than decortication because the person is functioning without a cerebrum. It may be seen as spontaneous, intermittent, or in response to a stimulus. Fully developed decerebration is characterized by arms fully extended, teeth clenched, and opisthotonous. This condition usually indicates a poor prognosis. In acute lesions, decerebration is often accompanied by waves of shivering and hyperpnea.

NO MOVEMENT/FLACCID
Lack of any response to central pain implies severe central nervous system damage and is associated with a poor prognosis.

All responses should be assessed for symmetry. Abnormalities are described as an incomplete paralysis or weakness (paresis) or a complete paralysis (plegia).

Potential Pitfalls
Any one of the following may alter the patient's ability to carry out normal motor function:

A fractured extremity.

Nerve damage (brachial plexus).

Deafness (inability to hear commands).

Communication barrier (does not speak English).

Coma.

Reflexes

Babinski's Reflex
Babinski's reflex is tested by applying a firm, but not painful, stimulus to the lateral aspect of the sole of the foot. The stimulus is then run in a stroking movement from the heel to the toes, moving across the ball of the foot to the great toe. A normal response is plantar flexion. An abnormal response is a dorsiflexion of the great toe with a fanning of the remaining toes. Babinski's reflex is normal in children under the age of two, but in adults it represents a lesion of the upper motor neurons.

Clonus

If the patient has hyperreflexia, test for clonus. Clonus is the rhythmic series of contractions that occur in response to maintained tension in a muscle. Briskly dorsiflex the patient's foot, sustain the pressure, and observe any repetitive contraction of the muscle. The foot will look as if it is flapping. A few beats of repetitive contractions may be normal in a patient with brisk reflexes. Sustained clonus indicates an upper motor neuron lesion. In the unconscious patient, unilateral hyperreflexia with pathological reflexes indicates hemiparesis.

Oculocephalic Reflex—Doll's Eyes

Normally, this reflex is present to allow the person to fix the vision voluntarily on a point while the body is moving. This reflex is not present in an awake or conscious patient, and it appears involuntarily when there is damage to the higher brain centers. This reflex is *never* tested until cervical x-ray examination has ruled out any spinal injury. To test for this reflex, the examiner holds the eyelids open and turns the patient's head rapidly to one side. If the brainstem is intact, the eyes will move in the direction opposite to the direction in which the head is turned; the movement is followed by a slow return of the eyes to midposition. This reflex is absent in deep coma and severe brainstem injury.

Oculovestibular Reflex—Cold Calories

This test covers the same basic anatomical pathways as does the previous one, but it is more sensitive and is safer to perform on a patient with the potential for a spinal injury without bony evidence on x-ray film. After ensuring an intact tympanic membrane by otoscopic examination, the patient's head is elevated to 30 degrees and 50 cc of iced water is introduced into the auditory canal by a soft catheter. With an intact brainstem, the eyes move together toward the irrigated ear. Dysconjugate eye movement or no movement is abnormal.

These last two tests are done on comatose patients to test the integrity of the brainstem and are frequently used as one component of the brain death evaluation.

Vital Signs

Vital sign changes associated with increased intracranial pressure usually develop after an alteration in the level of consciousness and represent a compensatory response to perfuse and preserve the brain.

Blood pressure is taken in the same arm to provide consistency. *Closed*-head-injured patients do not present in a hypotensive state as a result of the head injury except as a terminal event. With the exception of infants, hypotensive head-injured patients have a blood volume loss from an injury to some other system. Infants whose fontanels have not yet closed can lose a large amount of circulating blood volume from a closed head injury, enough to cause a decreased blood pressure.

The *pulse* may present in a variety of ways. Tachycardia accompanies pain, anxiety, fear, anger, or hypoxia. A critical finding is a full bounding bradycardia that often appears before any blood pressure change. Sinus dysrhythmias commonly occur.

Respiratory assessment is extremely important, because it not only helps in identifying the patient's respiratory capabilities, but it is also useful as a diagnostic tool. *Respirations* should be observed for a full minute to allow identification of the various patterns. The rate, the rhythm (describe the pattern if it cannot be named), the depth, and the muscles used should be noted. The nurse must be aware of several respiratory patterns including the following:

Cheyne Stokes.
Kussmaul.
Central neurogenic hyperventilation.
Apneustic.
Cluster.
Ataxic.

Do not be fooled by normal respirations occurring between any of these patterns, assuming that the intracranial pressure has been relieved, because this is part of the pattern as the pathology progresses down the brainstem.

The *temperature* usually falls immediately after an injury and then rises. The route—oral, rectal, or axillary—is determined by the patient's level of consciousness and any accompanying injuries. Note a spike or a gradual trend upward. Be aware of any environmental factors that contribute to the patient's temperature.

Vital signs should be checked a minimum of every 15 minutes and preferably more frequently if other injuries exist or if the patient's condition is changing. Cushing's triad (increased systolic pressure, decreased pulse, and abnormal respirations) is a *late* sign and occurs as an emergency means of perfusing the brain.

Cranial Nerves

The 12 cranial nerves are picture windows of the brain because each nerve follows a specific pathway and may be an important localizer for intracranial lesions. A few minutes should be taken to assess superficially the cranial nerves. Any gross deviations found dictate a more thorough evaluation.

Cranial Nerve I—Olfactory
This sensory nerve is responsible for the sense of smell. The most common causes for inability to smell (anosmia) are rhinitis, sinusitis, or the common cold. The evaluation of this nerve may be deleted on the initial superficial examination.

Cranial Nerves II, III, IV, and VI: Optic, Oculomotor, Trochlear, and Abducens
These four nerves are considered to be the "eye signs" and collectively are responsible for vision, extraocular movements (EOMs), pupillary constriction (direct and consensual), accommodation, and elevation of the upper lid. The six fields of vision are tested. Any unusual eye movements or failure of the eyes to move together in any of the six fields should be communicated to the physician.

Cranial Nerves V and VII—Trigeminal and Facial
These mixed motor and sensory nerves are broadly tested by ascertaining the ability of the patient to perceive the sensation of light touch and/or pain over the face and the person's ability to use the facial muscles symmetrically to smile, frown, wrinkle the brow, show the teeth, or raise the eyebrows. The corneal reflex is a function of these nerves and is tested by lightly touching the cornea with a wisp of cotton, then watching for a bilateral blink response. The patient's inability to protect his cornea must be identified early to allow institution of measures to prevent corneal abrasions.

Cranial Nerve VIII—Acoustic
This nerve is responsible for hearing and for vestibular functions of balance, orientation in space, and body position.

Cranial Nerves IX and X—Glossopharyngeal and Vagus
These mixed motor and sensory nerves are responsible for the gag reflex and the ability to swallow. Patients who are able to cooperate should be asked to swallow. If the patient is unable to swallow, the gag reflex must be assessed to determine the ability to protect the airway. Inability to protect the airway requires protective intervention. These nerves also innervate the carotid sinus, which is responsible for reflex control of blood pressure, pulse, and respiration.

Cranial Nerves XI and XII—Spinal Accessory and Hypoglossal
If the patient's level of consciousness allows this assessment, ask the patient to stick out his tongue while observing for any deviation, to elevate his shoulders against resistance, and to move his head against resistance. Note any asymmetry.

Cerebrospinal Leaks

Cerebrospinal fluid (CSF) leaks happen when a fracture occurs causing a tearing of the dura and arachnoid layers of the meninges allowing CSF to leak from the subarachnoid space.

Rhinorrhea is CSF discharged from the nose and is characterized by a thin, clear, watery discharge that usually ceases spontaneously in 48 hours. To differentiate between mucus discharge and rhinorrhea, if there is no blood present, Tes-Tape is used to test for sugar. Rhinorrhea contains glucose; mucus does not. The reliability of this test is not 100 percent because the patient with heroin withdrawal or one with a recent cold may have a positive Tes-Tape result with mucus alone.

Otorrhea is CSF from the ear and is almost always found in combination with a bloody discharge. The drainage is suspiciously thin, may be profuse, and is usually self-limiting. To differentiate between a purely bloody discharge and bloody otorrhea, allow some of the drainage to fall on a gauze pad. Blood will produce a single bloody ring, whereas bloody otorrhea will produce a bloody drop surrounded by a pinkish CSF ring, sometimes called a halo. The CSF halo test is also appropriate for bloody rhinorrhea evaluation. Recall that only 150 cc of CSF circulate in the system at any one time, so a large volume of "otorrhea" may indicate a bleed as well.

SPECIFIC NEUROLOGICAL INJURIES

Neurological trauma is divided into parenchymal injuries (injuries to the brain tissue itself); hemorrhages (involving the potential spaces of the brain); and injuries to the bone, or fractures. They can vary from mild, such as a concussion or linear skull fracture without complication, to severe, such as a brainstem contusion.

Parenchymal Injuries

Concussion
PATHOPHYSIOLOGY

A *concussion* is an immediate and transient loss of neurological function due to a mechanical force from which there is usually rapid (within 12–24 hours) and complete recovery without neurological residual. The brain does not demonstrate any damage; however, the electrical activity of the reticular activating system is disturbed resulting in loss of consciousness.

CLINICAL MANIFESTATIONS

Clinically, the patient may present with a history of short-term loss of consciousness, vomiting, or amnesia. Even without a history of loss of consciousness, loss of memory is sufficient criteria to diagnose a concussion. The duration of the loss, rather than the severity, determines the prognosis. Headache, dizziness, or nausea may be present. It is not an uncommon occurrence for some patients to present initially with a superficial picture of hypovolemic shock: elevated pulse; shallow respiratory rate; unresponsiveness; cool, pale skin; and dilated pupils. The blood pressure is usually normal. In addition, children may appear fine initially, only to become lethargic and somnolent in a few hours and then fully recover.

DIAGNOSTIC STUDIES

Diagnosis of concussion is strictly by clinical evaluation and repeated observations. There are no x-ray, laboratory, or pathological findings to validate a concussion.

NURSING CARE AND RELATED INTERVENTIONS

Continued evaluation and reassurance of the patient and family are essential. It is frightening for patients to be unable to recall what happened to them. The almost continuous, repetitive questioning by the nurse should never be treated as a game, no matter how humorous it may seem. Repeated reinforcement of reality, with reassurance, is appropriate.

DISCHARGE PLANNING

Disposition of patients with concussions is an eternal source of question and doubt. Most patients with minor loss of consciousness who present with a normal neurological examination in the emergency department will be discharged within several hours. Those patients who are normal except for a loss of memory may be discharged if retrieval of recent memory is intact. Home discharge should be to the care of a responsible adult, one who will stay with the patient, who understands the discharge instructions and has access to transportation should a return visit be necessary. The suggested list of which patients should be admitted for observation is varied indeed and, unfortunately, sometimes depends on bed availability. Preschool age children whose neurological course is often atypical should be admitted, as well as any symptomatic patient.

Discharge planning must include teaching the patient and family assessment parameters, frequency of examination, and critical findings that would necessitate a return to the hospital. Those findings include a change in the level of consciousness, unequal pupils, weakness on one side, projectile vomiting, and seizures. The phone number of the emergency department is a reassuring aid to provide in case of questions. Patients and families should be told of the potential for postconcussion syndrome that may include headache, dizziness, irritability, fatigue, inability to concentrate, and memory impairment. Duration of this syndrome may be several days to several months.

Contusions
PATHOPHYSIOLOGY

Contusions, which are structural alterations of the brain characterized by small hemorrhages and edema, are more severe and recovery is not guaranteed. Causes include contre-coup injuries, high-velocity blows or missiles, and/or acceleration-deceleration injuries.

CLINICAL MANIFESTATIONS

Clinical manifestations vary with the area affected and severity of the injury. Patients with frontal lobe contusions often present with restlessness and combative, bizarre, or irrational behavior. Cursing is a common occurrence, as are challenging statements made to caregivers. Amnesia and disorientation usually accompany temporal lobe contusions in the awake patient. Brainstem contusions are quite severe clinically with profound coma, devastating neurological deficits, and decorticate or decerebrate posturing.

DIAGNOSTIC STUDIES

Diagnosis is usually made by computerized axial tomography (CAT scan), which is able to demonstrate size, position, and content of the ventricles, the density of the brain, and the presence of bleeding.

NURSING CARE AND RELATED INTERVENTIONS

Once the diagnosis is made, it implies potential neurological consequences of edema and/or mass lesion. These patients are hospitalized. They need support, reassurance, and a sense of security given by unhurried, soft-spoken, gentle caregivers who can ignore their behavior and concentrate on their needs. Nursing care is aimed at observation for, and the prevention of, cerebral edema and a mass lesion.

Hemorrhages

Subdural Hematoma
PATHOPHYSIOLOGY

The accumulation of blood between the dura and the arachnoid layers of the meninges is a *subdural hematoma*. The bleed is usually venous in origin and may be

SPECIFIC NEUROLOGICAL INJURIES

bilateral or unilateral. Subdurals may occur after relatively mild trauma in which acceleration-deceleration movement causes the brain to glide within the skull. The bridging veins beneath the cortical surfaces and the dural sinuses tear, allowing blood to flow freely and quickly into the subdural space.

Subdural hematomas are classified into three groups based on the delay of onset of symptoms after the initial injury. Acute subdurals occur within 48 hours of injury, subacute subdurals occur from within 48 hours to two weeks posttrauma, and chronic subdurals present anytime after two weeks posttrauma. In addition to classification, subdural hematomas are now also divided into two types: simple and complicated. The simple subdural is defined as blood in the subdural space with no underlying injury to the brain. Some of these patients never lose consciousness. They remain lucid the entire time. The complicated subdural involves a contused or lacerated brain beneath the bleed. The mortality for the simple subdural is approximately 25 percent, for the complicated subdural it is approximately 60–80 percent.

CLINICAL MANIFESTATIONS
Clinical manifestations are due to the mass effect of the expanding bleed and to the accompanying cerebral damage. If the level of consciousness is altered, it remains so; there is no secondary lucid period. The level of consciousness at the time of surgery correlates well with outcome. Diagnosis is made by CAT scan or arteriogram.

NURSING CARE AND RELATED INTERVENTIONS
Treatment varies and is currently a source of controversy. Surgical removal, if the hematoma is large enough or if a significant shift is seen on diagnostic testing, is one possibility. The treatment may also be medical, allowing the hematoma to gradually reabsorb and treating only the cerebral edema. The problem arises with the complicated subdural hematoma. Some practitioners believe the bleed is the priority and will surgically remove it. Others believe the edema from the contusion is the priority and should be medically treated, since surgery will only exacerbate the brain swelling and lead to increased intracranial pressure.

Epidural Hematoma
PATHOPHYSIOLOGY
An *epidural hematoma* is the accumulation of blood between the skull and the dura. This condition represents a true surgical emergency because arterial bleeds, unlike venous bleeds, do not tamponade. The most common cause of an epidural hematoma is a fracture that crosses one of the branches of the middle meningeal artery located in the temporal area. In children, the middle meningeal artery is not incorporated into the bone as it is in adults, so children can have epidural hematomas without fractures. Venous bleeds are rarer and come from a tearing of the transverse sinus in the posterior fossa. Although accounting for less than 5 percent of all head injuries, epidural hematomas carry a 25–50 percent mortality rate.

CLINICAL MANIFESTATIONS
Clinically, the course of the hematoma is usually short, less than 12 hours. Despite its billing as "classic," only 30 percent of patients with epidural hematomas present with a classic history: a brief loss of consciousness (a concussion), followed by a

lucid interval that may last five minutes to five hours (a recovery from the concussion), and then the onset of a severe headache and a rapid loss of consciousness. Once the headache and loss of consciousness become obvious, a secondary rise in intracranial pressure has already occurred, and a significant mass effect is present. This condition indicates that the compensatory capabilities of the brain have been exhausted and a rapid deterioration usually follows. In children, bradycardia and early papilledema may be the only warning.

NURSING CARE AND RELATED INTERVENTIONS
Diagnosis is made by CAT scan and the bleed is surgically removed.

Fractures

Attention has traditionally been placed on fractures that cross the major vascular channels of the skull, particularly the temporal area, the sagittal and transverse sinuses of the vertex, and the occipital areas. The findings of such a fracture should alert caregivers to the increased potential for subsequent intracranial hemorrhage and the need for careful observation of the patient.

The most common of all skull fractures, especially in children is the *linear* skull fracture, which is a break in the continuity of the cranial vault. These fractures are readily diagnosed by x-ray examination and usually require no treatment.

Depressed skull fractures are breaks in the continuity of the bone with part of the bone depressed below the outer layer. The parietal and frontal bones are most commonly affected. They may be complicated by edema, venous congestion, or bleeding. Diagnosis is suggested by physical examination and confirmed by x-ray study. Frequently, the examiner may mistake a marked contusion of the scalp or a subgaleal hematoma, with its soft distendible feel on palpation, for a depressed skull fracture. If the scalp overlying the fracture is intact, the surgical elevation of the bone may be done electively. Children frequently have this type of fracture. If the scalp is lacerated, the debridement of the wound and surgical repair is done as an emergency procedure to repair the dural laceration, control bleeding, and/or to remove loose bone fragments or necrotic brain.

Fractures occurring at the base of the skull, or *basilar skull fractures,* occur most frequently in the anterior or middle fossa and are more frequently diagnosed by clinical signs and symptoms than by x-ray examination. CSF leaks occur in approximately 5–10 percent of the patients.

Fractures occurring in the *anterior fossa* frequently present with conjunctival hemorrhage, CSF rhinorrhea, and periorbital ecchymosis or "raccoon's eyes." *Middle fossa* fractures present with bleeding from the ear and/or CSF otorrhea. The CSF may go into the eustachian tube and be swallowed if the tympanic membrane is intact and will not be visible without an otoscopic examination. Occasionally, a hearing loss with associated vestibular dysfunction may accompany a petrous bone fracture. This loss is usually correctable if treated early, which suggests that all awake patients with this diagnosis be tested. Battle's sign, or mastoid process ecchymosis caused by the petrous fracture, will not be present until at least 24 hours after the injury. Ecchymosis at the base of the neck and behind the mastoid along with blood in the pharynx suggests a *posterior fossa* basilar skull fracture.

Basilar skull fractures are not repaired surgically but are treated symptomatically. CSF leaks usually heal spontaneously. Antibiotics may or may not be given prophylactically to prevent infection. These patients should be watched for signs and symptoms of infection and cranial nerve palsies.

The two major consequences of cerebral injury are cerebral edema or mass lesion, both of which may lead to increased intracranial pressure. The assessment is designed to help find early clues of increasing pressure so that therapy can be started as soon as possible.

INCREASED INTRACRANIAL PRESSURE

The Box Theory

The brain is surrounded by a nondistendible bone called the *skull*. The brain is "boxed in"; hence, the name *Box theory*. There is very little room for expansion of any of the intracranial contents. Within the cranial confines, there are three fluid compartments that allow for some give: the cerebrospinal fluid, the cerebral blood volume, and the water in the brain tissue. The CSF accounts for approximately 10 percent, the blood volume for 2–11 percent, and the brain tissue for the other 80 percent. Any increase in one of these volumes will be compensated for by a decrease in one or both of the remaining volumes. The purpose of this compensatory ability is to maintain the normal pressure within the cranium by balancing these three fluids. A more formal way of describing this is the Monro Kellie doctrine:

$$V_{ICV} = V_{CSF} + V_{CBV} + V_{BRAIN}.$$

Intracranial volume = volume CSF + blood volume + brain volume.

Nothing can take up space in the cranium without subtracting volume from one or both of the other fluids.

One would assume that as the total intracranial volume increased, the intracranial pressure would rise in a parallel fashion, but this is not always the case. The brain, through its ability to compensate via the three fluids, will show little change in the intracranial pressure over a range of volume increase, because as long as these fluids can be displaced the intracranial pressure remains within normal limits. Initially, compensation is achieved by increasing the absorption of CSF. When this buffer is exhausted, cerebral blood volume is decreased by compression of the low-pressure venous system. This compliance, or the ability to "give" to increases in pressure, is limited and represents the ability of the intracranial contents to tolerate further increases in intracranial volume. The compliance becomes less and less as the brain becomes tighter. When the compensatory mechanisms are fully used, only a small increase in volume is required to increase intracranial pressure quickly.

The pathophysiology of increased intracranial pressure and the resultant clinical manifestations will be discussed in terms of anatomical disruptions. (See Fig. 20.1 for anatomical reference.)

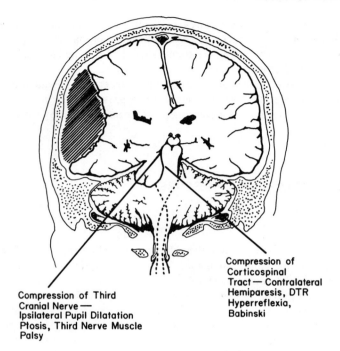

Figure 20.1 Uncal herniation.

Alterations in the Level of Consciousness

Full consciousness requires continuous and effective interaction between relatively intact cerebral hemispheres and the reticular activating system (the arousal center found in the brain stem). Impulses to and from these areas may be decreased or abolished by increased intracranial pressure through direct compression that disrupts the system, its blood supply, or associated pathways.

The reason cited for the early alteration in levels of consciousness (Jimm, 1974) is that the most highly specialized cortical cells of the body are the most sensitive to the lack of oxygen, which occurs with increased intracranial pressure. The cortical cells are supplied by terminal arteries rather than by large vessels, which supply the brainstem.

Alterations in the Motor Response

The motor strip is located in the frontal lobe. Impulses travel from the motor cortex through a tentorial opening where they cross over to the opposite side in the medulla before traveling down to the spinal cord. As a result, abnormalities of weakness or paralysis will be demonstrated on the side opposite to the lesion's site. Initially, intracranial pressure increases will cause increased tone or *gegenhalten*. As pressure increases to involve more of the brainstem, the response will change to decortication, then to decerebration as it travels to the midbrain. Thereafter, the patient lacks the ability to make any response.

Alterations in Pupillary Response

Parasympathetic fibers, which originate in the midbrain, travel up through the tentorial opening on their way to the pupillary constrictor muscles. In increased intracranial pressure, the oculomotor nerve is compressed and the ability of the pupil on that same side to constrict to light and hold it is affected. Initially, the pressure may cause irritation that may lead to constriction or to *hippus* (an initial constriction of the pupil followed by a dilatation). Hippus, although seen normally in some persons, may also be a clue to early parasympathetic irritation. Later, the pupil will dilate as the sympathetic fibers go unopposed by the parasympathetic fibers that are rendered inactive by the pressure. Sympathetic fibers do not pass through the tentorial opening but, rather, follow a different route to the eye.

Alterations in Vital Signs

As the pressure builds, it begins to choke off the blood supply to the brain tissue. The central nervous system, in response, alerts the body to pump the blood under more pressure so it can reach the ischemic areas. The arterial, or systolic pressure, will increase until blood flow is restored. As a result, one may observe a steady upward trend of the systolic pressure as the body fights to overcome the pressure within the brain to open up its vessels and perfuse the brain.

In a compensatory move, the body will also increase its stroke volume, the amount of blood that leaves the heart with each beat, by dropping its heart rate. This is thought to be due to pressure on the nerve centers in the medulla supplying the inhibitory fibers to the vagus nerve.

Pressure on the diencephalon and midbrain creates pressure on the medulla and lower pons, which control respiration. Depending on the area of pressure, characteristic respiratory patterns will emerge.

Other Alterations

Vomiting is due to compression of the emetic center in the medulla. It is usually spontaneous, projectile, and not associated with or preceded by nausea. Headache is caused by traction and distortion of the pain-sensitive structures (the dura and blood vessels) and the stretching and kinking of the larger arteries. With increased intracranial pressure, the pressure of the CSF in the subarachnoid space around the optic nerve gives rise to edema. This condition leads to decreased venous return, congestion, and distortion of the vein and altered vision. Clinically, this is known as papilledema. The threshold for seizures is usually lowered in increased intracranial pressure, making the patient more prone to seizure activity.

HERNIATION

The ultimate disastrous event of increased intracranial pressure, which carries a high mortality and morbidity, is *herniation,* or a protrusion of a part of an organ through structures that normally contain it. There are several types of herniation, with those occurring across the tentorium being seen most commonly in trauma.

The tentorium is an extention of the dura, the tough outer layer of meninges known as the "tough mother," which surrounds the brain and spinal cord. The tentorium separates the cerebral hemispheres from the brainstem and cerebellum by forming a tough membranous shelf between them. There is an opening, the tentorial opening, through which pass the blood vessels, nerves, and brainstem.

When the uncal portion of the temporal lobe is forced through the tentorial opening by a bleed or mass lesion in the outer middle fossa, *uncal herniation* has occurred. It is characteristically seen with a decreased level of consciousness, contralateral hemiparesis, and an ipsilateral fixed and dilated pupil.

Central herniation occurs when the hemispheres are displaced downward, usually due to a lesion in the frontal, parietal, or occipital lobes. It is frequently seen with massive cerebral edema. Characteristically, diencephalon dysfunction is seen—for example, decreased level of consciousness, constricted but reactive pupils (initially), positive Babinski's reflex, *gegenhalten* or decorticate posturing, and Cheyne-Stokes respirations.

NURSING CARE OF THE NEUROLOGICALLY INJURED PATIENT

Care of the neurologically injured patient is aimed at the prevention of secondary insults because after the initial injury has occurred any one of a series of events may follow that further compromises the patient in terms of increased mortality and morbidity. These events must be approached from a preventative aspect because their role in further cerebral compromise is well established. The secondary events are hypoxia, hypercarbia, hypotension, hypertension, and hyperthermia. Intervention is also aimed at the medical or surgical decompression of the brain.

Prevention of Hypoxia

There is increasing evidence that the final common denominator in irreversible brain damage and death in the head-injured patient is hypoxia from respiratory insufficiency and ischemia.

Establishing and maintaining an adequate airway is *the most* important aspect in the care of head-injured patients. Cerebral oxygenation problems can be minimized by providing adequate oxygen carrying capacity and adequate oxygen delivery to the brain as determined by arterial blood gas studies and cardiovascular parameters. A Pa_{O_2} higher than 70 mm Hg and preferably greater than 100 mm Hg, if no preexisting disease or coexisting injury prevents it, should be the goal. Adequacy of ventilation must constantly be assessed by the nurse. Suctioning, although known to increase intracranial pressure, must be done when indicated. Suctioning should be preceded by hyperoxygenation with 100 percent oxygen and the event itself limited to less than 15 seconds. Pulmonary edema, which may be of neurogenic origin, is a potential complication. Any neurological deterioration should prompt arterial blood gas determinations to rule out hypoxia and/or hypercarbia as the cause.

Prevention of Hypercarbia

Two common causes of hypercarbia are a partially obstructed airway and hypoventilation. Proper positioning of the patient with frequent assessment of the airway is a necessity. The arterial carbon dioxide level is the most accurate predictor of the adequacy of alveolar ventilation and should be monitored carefully.

Maintenance of Normotension

In everyday functioning, the brain has the ability to alter the size of its blood vessels to maintain normal cerebral blood flow despite changes in intracranial pressure and/or in the systemic arterial pressure. This ability is called *cerebral autoregulation*. Cerebral autoregulation has an upper limit for vasoconstriction and a lower limit for dilatation believed to occur at mean readings of 160 mm Hg and 45 mm Hg, respectively. Above or below these ranges, blood flow to the brain is passively dependent on the blood pressure and the intracranial pressure. As a result, cerebral blood flow will rise or fall with changes in the blood pressure; therefore, it is imperative to control blood pressure in a normotensive range.

Hypotension in the head-injured patient must be rapidly treated to prevent further compromise of the brain. Remembering the limits of cerebral autoregulation, it is important to note that a patient with normal intracranial pressure, but in a severe hypotensive state, can have inadequate cerebral perfusion that will lead to ischemia and only exacerbate the injury with edema.

The treatment for hypotension is determined by the cause and may take any one of the following forms:

1. *Fluid resuscitation*. Fluids may be crystalloids (only isotonic to prevent cerebral edema) or colloids depending on the degree of hypovolemia and blood loss. If hypotension is due to hemorrhage, vasoconstriction from the sympathetic response will shunt blood to the brain. But in severe cases, unless blood is used as a resuscitative fluid, hemodilution will occur, which decreases osmotic pressure and favors the development of cerebral edema.
2. *Pharmacological support*. Dopamine, titrated as needed, is the drug usually used.
3. *MAST Trousers* (Military Antishock Trousers). The use of MAST trousers is suggested for patients with a systolic pressure of less than 80 mm Hg. In the past, there was concern that use of the MAST trousers, by virtue of their autotransfusion effect to the chest and head, might increase intracranial pressure. It is now known that patients with intravascular volume deficits requiring MAST trousers

support *need* this autotransfusion to assist with adequate perfusion to the brain. The trousers prevent cerebral ischemia and thus cerebral edema that may lead to increased intracranial pressure.

The main danger with sudden spontaneous *hypertensive* states in the head-injured patient is an increased cerebral flow and volume that can be ill tolerated by a "tight" brain. It is important to differentiate the hypertension of a Cushing's response from the hypertension of an intensive systemic vasoconstriction. The former should not be treated with antihypertensives, whereas the latter should. Cushing's shows an elevation only in the systolic pressure with a low diastolic and a widening pulse pressure accompanied by a bradycardia. Systemic hypertension is usually accompanied by a normal pulse and a high diastolic as well as systolic pressure.

Treatment of hypertension is directed toward control of the cause, if known, or is controlled by the use of antihypertensive agents. Shivering, central hyperthermia, hyperkinesis, spontaneous inappropriate motor responses, and suctioning may all precipitate a hypertensive event. Morphine sulfate, chlorpromazine, or Pavulon, titrated to the individual patient, are all effective. Morphine and chlorpromazine are both vasodilators and can precipitate a hypotensive event in the patient who is not adequately volume resuscitated. Intravenous Arfonad or hydralazine may be used to control the hypertension.

Maintenance of Normothermia

Temperature should be kept within normal limits so that nutrition available to the brain will not be used at a rate faster than it can be supplied. The use of hypothermia to decrease cerebral oxygen demand is infrequent at present except in conjunction with barbiturate therapy in children. On the opposite end, hyperthermia is an event that should not be taken lightly and should not be underestimated. For every degree above normal that the body temperature rises, the oxygen requirements of the brain increase by 6 percent on the Farenheit scale and 13 percent on the Celsius scale. In the patient whose oxygenation is borderline and in whom cerebral injury is severe, hyperthermia can be critical and must be treated aggressively.

Shivering, which often accompanies efforts to drop a patient's temperature or which may occur in conjunction with spontaneous decerebration, significantly increases metabolic demands of the brain and must be treated. Chlorpromazine, with dose adjustments based on the individual and the severity, is the preferred drug.

The nurse's role in the control of temperature consists of frequent temperature checks—at least every one-half to one hour—with *early* initiation of antipyretic measures when the temperature shows an upward trend and/or acutely spikes to higher than 101°F. Sponge baths, a hypothermia blanket, or Tylenol may be used.

Medical Decompression of the Brain

The patient arriving in the emergency department in a severe state of injury as demonstrated by decerebrate posturing or signs of herniation or visible deterioration is usually treated with the triad of hyperventilation, steroids, and osmotic diuretic therapy. Each hospital has its own protocols and methods of treatment that have been found successful. There is no one "right way." Each patient situation must be evaluated individually.

Hyperventilation

The first method of producing medical decompression of increased intracranial pressure is by producing a hypocarbic situation. Manipulation of carbon dioxide levels is accomplished through hyperventilation. The Pa_{CO_2} is an important determinant of cerebral blood flow. As the Pa_{CO_2} rises, cerebral blood vessels dilate in response causing an increase in cerebral blood flow and volume and an increase in intracranial pressure. When the Pa_{CO_2} is decreased to 25–30 mm Hg, cerebral vasoconstriction occurs, decreasing cerebral blood flow. An increase in cerebral blood volume is one of the major causes of increased intracranial pressure in the early phases of acute head injury. The absence of responsiveness to changes in Pa_{CO_2} is invariably associated with an unsatisfactory patient outcome of either death or a persistent vegetative state (Marshall, 1980). A secondary benefit of hyperventilation is the respiratory alkalosis produced, which may be useful in combating brain tissue acidosis. Hyperventilation also decreases end capillary pressure and may allow a decrease in edema formation and increased fluid removal from brain tissue itself (Bruce et al., 1977). Hyperventilation may be done manually by bag mask or mechanically by ventilator.

Nursing responsibilities include monitoring arterial blood gas results to ensure maintenance of therapeutic levels and frequent reassessment of respiratory rate and depth of the spontaneously ventilating patient. Care should be taken not to allow the Pa_{CO_2} to fall too low, for it may cause not only too severe a vasoconstriction, but also an increase in pH beyond 7.50 that will shift the oxyhemoglobin curve to the left and decrease the amount of oxygen released to the tissues.

Patients who cannot be adequately ventilated or hyperventilated because of restlessness or decerebrate posturing may be sedated if *absolutely* necessary. Pavulon and morphine are the two drugs used most frequently.

Steroids

The role of steroids in the treatment of head injuries remains controversial. Despite the fact that steroids have been used to treat increased intracranial pressure and cerebral edema for years, their effect on cerebral perfusion pressure and their mechanisms of action are as yet undetermined. It has been suggested that steroids stabilize cellular and intracellular membranes and help to control cerebral edema. Dexamethasone is also known to decrease CSF production.

Some questions are now being raised about which dosage offers the best results. Recently, the use of high dose, or megadose, steroids in the first 24 hours has shown some promise in decreasing mortality and improving the quality of survival, although these reports are, at present, still conflicting. Megadoses are defined as 1.5 mg/kg of dexamethasone in both adults and children. Megadoses of methylprednisolone are 2 g in the adult, 1 g in the child ages 5–15 and 0.5 g in the child under five years of age (Bruce et al., 1977; Tyson et al., 1979). Conventional therapy calls for a loading dose of 12–15 mg of dexamethasone IV or 125 mg of methylprednisolone IV in the emergency department.

Osmotic Diuretics

The effectiveness of osmotic diuretics lies in their heavy concentration of particles in contrast to the intracellular contents. An osmotic pressure gradient is created. Striving for equilibrium, water moves from normal cerebral cells to the intravascular system effectively reducing intracranial volume. The increased intravascular volume is then diuresed out through the kidneys. This therapy is most useful when the increased pressure is due to cerebral edema.

Caution is now being urged in the use of mannitol, an osmotic diuretic, in the emergency department without knowledge of the *cause* of the patient's deterioration. The reason for this caution is that if the cause is a bleed, normal tissue is allowed to "shrink," potentially allowing for expansion of the intracranial bleed. Clearly, in a rapidly deteriorating patient, all rules are flexible and the patient should be treated with all therapy available to decompress the brain medically until surgery can be done.

In addition to questioning the blind use of mannitol, the dosage is also being reviewed by some practitioners. Studies have shown that smaller doses of 0.25–0.5 g/kg, rather than the standard 1 to 2 g/kg are as effective in decreasing intracranial pressure without the extreme fluid and electrolyte imbalances of the higher doses. Mannitol may be given by a 20 percent IV drip or by a 25 percent IV bolus and is usually given over a ten-minute period. This dosage helps to ensure that a rapid increase in systolic pressure does not occur with the additional added volume resulting in loss of autoregulation and a resultant increase in cerebral blood volume. A response is seen within ten minutes of infusion, with a peak response in about 20 minutes. In stressful situations, there is sometimes a tendency to give more mannitol if no response is noted. This is a dangerous practice, for the body will soon be placed in a hyperosmolar state that further compromises the cerebral state. The serum osmolarity should not exceed 330 mosm/l. Keep in mind that alcohol, as well as hyperglycemic or hypernatremic states, will contribute to a hyperosmotic state.

Caution is also being discussed in the use of mannitol in pediatric patients. Bruce (1978) found that 50 percent of head-injured children have diffuse brain swelling due to *hyperemia,* not cerebral edema, and recommends caution with the use of mannitol during the first 24 hours after injury. Injudicious use of mannitol in children whose deterioration is due to hyperemia and cerebral vascular congestion could lead to disastrous increases in intracranial pressure.

Mannitol is contraindicated in patients with accompanying hypovolemia, shock, congestive heart failure, dehydration or neurogenic pulmonary edema.

The nurse must carefully monitor the blood pressure, urinary output via Foley catheter, and central venous pressure of the patient, along with obtaining baseline serum osmolarity levels and monitoring serum electrolyte balances. The use of an IV filter with mannitol to catch unseen, undissolved crystals is indicated. Never use solutions with crystals. The solution may be heated until the crystals dissolve and then administered.

Mannitol, with its resultant diuresis, can decrease the total circulation volume, which is *not* the goal in the management of increased intracranial pressure. Excessive shrinkage of the patient's blood volume causes an increased aldosterone production with a secondary hypernatremia. Maintenance intravenous (IV) fluids should be isotonic crystalloids in sufficient volume to restore adequate circulating blood volume without raising the central venous pressure. Serum sodium should be kept between 140–150 mEq/l and the serum osmolarity, without mannitol, between 290–300 mosm/l.

Recently, attention has been given to some of the tubal diuretics, specifically furosemide and ethacrynic acid, as possible adjuncts to osmotic diuretic therapy. Studies have shown that these diuretics, when administered just before mannitol infusion, potentiate both the rate and duration of intracranial pressure reduction. The profound fluid and electrolyte imbalances produced by mannitol do not occur with the simultaneous use of these diuretics. Both furosemide and ethacrynic acid reduce CSF production and may or may not decrease intracranial pressure. There is a suggestion that both of these drugs have ototoxic and nephrotic side effects and should therefore be administered at a rate of no more than 10 mg/minute. Onset of action is between 20 and 60 minutes.

Surgical Decompression of the Brain

Burr holes may be done on a rapidly deteriorating patient as an emergency means of surgically decompressing a tight brain. Ideally, the procedure is done in the operating room, but may be done in the emergency department if the patient's condition warrants immediate action.

Bleeds or surgical mass lesions are removed in the operating room. Rarely is the removal of brain tissue to allow for expansion of a swollen brain justified.

Other Interventions

Control of Seizures

Carol et al. (1979) suggest that acute anticonvulsant therapy is indicated in the following circumstances:

Penetrating head injuries, with or without seizures.
A single posttraumatic seizure but with no postictal signs of neurological recovery.
A seizure concomitant with neurological deterioration.
Depressed skull fractures near the motor cortex.
Multiple seizures.
Glasgow Coma Scale of less than 8.

Acute seizures after head injuries are treated with the intravenous administration of diazepam (Valium). Adult dosage is 5–10 mg IV, which may be repeated two or three times at ten-minute intervals. Pediatric doses are given slowly in a dosage not to exceed 0.25 mg/kg IV, with the initial dose repeated after 15–30 minutes. Diazepam should be administered no faster than 5 mg/minute to avoid hypotension and respiratory depression. Large veins should be used whenever possible.

After the seizure is controlled, the patient will usually be given a loading dose of phenytoin (Dilantin) of 10 mg/kg IV in adults. Phenytoin must be administered only in normal saline solution or in an IV line flushed well with normal saline solution before and after the drug administration, or else the drug will precipitate and clog the line. The rate of infusion should not exceed 50 mg/minute. The patient's electrocardiogram should be monitored continuously during the infusion. Hypotension and bradycardia with prolonged QRS or PR intervals dictate discontinuance of the infusion. The administration may be restarted once the vital signs have returned to their preadministration state. Phenytoin is contraindicated in patients with sinus bradycardia, sino-atrial blocks, or Adams-Stokes syndrome.

The incidence of posttraumatic epilepsy in closed head injuries is approximately 5 percent and increases to 50 percent in open head injuries.

Cerebrospinal Leaks
The drainage of any CSF should not be impeded in any way, either by plugs or dressings. For rhinorrhea, elevation of the head of the bed, if not contraindicated, will facilitate drainage. The nasal route should not be used for passage of airway adjuncts, nasogastric tubes, or suction catheters. Coughing, sneezing, and nose blowing is to be avoided. A folded gauze pad may be fitted over the upper lip (moustache area) to catch any drainage that may be upsetting to the patient.

The patient with otorrhea should be turned on the same side as the otorrhea, if not contraindicated. The outer ear should be kept clean and any clots that may impede flow should be removed. A *loose* gauze pad dressing may be placed over the outer ear to catch any drainage.

SPINAL CORD INJURIES

Spinal cord injuries overwhelm the majority of health care professionals. The goal in the initial management of spinal injured patients is to preserve the remaining neural function and to prevent further damage to allow for maximum rehabilitation potential. Injuries may be mild or severe and involve bony anatomy, muscles and tendons, and the spinal cord and/or nerve roots. Deficits may or may not be present. Severe or potentially severe injuries will be discussed and limited to cervical and high thoracic injuries.

From an *anatomical* perspective, injuries may be limited to the vertebrae only, to the spinal cord, or to a combination of the two. *Functionally,* injuries are classified as complete or incomplete. Complete injuries present with an absence of voluntary muscle activity and the absence of sensation below the level of injury. A severed or transsected spinal cord is an example of a complete injury that is *not* reversible. The validity of the presence or absence of reflex activity in diagnosing a complete lesion remains controversial. Incomplete lesions show a sparing of *any* motor or sensory ability. This implies partial cord sparing and the potential for some degree of recovery.

Types of Injuries

Spinal Cord Contusion/Concussion
Spinal cord contusion/concussion involves a jarring of the spinal cord with a temporary alteration of spinal cord function. Recovery usually begins within eight hours

SPINAL CORD INJURIES

with total return of function within 24–48 hours after injury. Diagnosis is strictly clinical and is made retrospectively once the patient recovers. All patients, therefore, should be treated as if they had a complete lesion—with maximum aggressive therapy—because practitioners are unable to distinguish between the two initially.

A Central Cord Injury

A *central cord injury* most frequently occurs as the result of severe hyperextension injuries. It is not a surgical lesion because it represents injury to the spinal cord alone. The injury is characterized by disproportionately more motor impairment in the upper than in the lower extremities and in the distal more than in the proximal muscles. Bladder dysfunction with urinary retention and varying degrees of sensory loss below the level of the lesion also occur. The degree of recovery varies and is significantly influenced by the amount of accompanying edema. When recovery does occur, lower extremity function returns first, then bladder, and finally upper extremity function.

Anterior Cord Syndrome

Anterior cord syndrome is the result of a flexion injury that may result in a herniated disc. Pathophysiology is of a dual nature: the impingement of the cord by bony fragments or herniated disc and the vascular insufficiency produced by occlusion of the anterior spinal artery, which deprives the anterior two-thirds of the cord of its blood supply. As a result, the patient presents with complete paralysis below the level of the lesion, along with loss of pain and temperature. Touch, pressure, and vibration are spared because the posterior third of the spinal cord housing the posterior column functions is not supplied by the anterior spinal artery.

Brown-Sequard Syndrome

Penetrating injuries are the cause of *Brown-Sequard syndrome*. As the name implies, one-half of the spinal cord is rendered nonfunctional, which results in loss of motor function and sensations of position, movement, vibration, touch, and pressure on the same side of the lesion. The opposite side shows loss of pain and temperature perception. Few lesions are truly hemisections, but rather present as a partial Brown-Sequard syndrome.

Root Syndromes

Presentation of *root syndromes* depends on the area supplied by the root. Paresthesia, paralysis, and radicular pain are all common occurrences.

Assessment

Respiratory and Circulatory Evaluation

The initial assessment must center on the patient's respiratory and cardiovascular status. The adequacy of ventilation cannot be overemphasized. Spine-injured patients should be *expected* to deteriorate in respiratory function dictating frequent assessment to allow for early interventions. Injuries above the level of C_6 will result in partial or complete inability to breath due to loss of the phrenic nerve. Low cervical or high thoracic injuries, due to loss of intercostal muscles, result in the inability to take a deep breath or to cough effectively. The latter group of patients are breathing entirely with their diaphragm with some help from the accessory muscles. Mid and lower thoracic spinal injuries usually do not result in respiratory failure, but may be accompanied by pulmonary or chest wall injury, which can interfere with the adequacy of ventilation.

Patients presenting in a state of shock may do so as a result of hemorrhagic shock from accompanying injury or from spinal shock due to loss of sympathetic tone. Careful monitoring of blood pressure trends and pulse is critical. The two types of shock can be differentiated on the basis of the pulse. Tachycardia accompanies the hypotension in hemorrhagic shock, while bradycardia and hypotension are the hallmarks of spinal shock. The skin is warm and dry in spinal shock and cool and clammy in hemorrhagic shock.

Assessment of the Neck
Look for physical signs of trauma, such as edema, ecchymosis, and lacerations. Palpate over the spinous processes for separation or deformity. Subjectively, the patient may complain of pain, neck stiffness, muscle spasms, or guarding. Any of these symptoms should alert the nurse to a possibility of spinal injury until it is ruled out by further evaluation.

Motor Ability
The presence or absence of voluntary motor activity must be ascertained. Just asking the patient to move might allow some subtle weakness to go undetected. Each major muscle group in the upper and lower extremities should be tested individually for voluntary motor movement, reflexes, and for strength. Strength is graded as follows:

> 0 None
> 1 Trace
> 2 Movement with gravity removed
> 3 Movement against gravity
> 4 Movement against resistance
> 5 Normal

Sensory Evaluation
The sensory examination gives added information regarding the level of the lesion and will also help to localize a thoracic lesion that could be missed on motor examination (Carol et al., 1979). Always begin in the area of deficit and proceed upward. The sensory examination of the upper extremities will give information about roots C_5 to T_1, whose dermatones are not present on the trunk. (Refer to Figure 20.2.)

A clean safety pin is used to gently prick, not puncture or scratch, the skin to ascertain the patient's ability to perceive pain. Note any lack of symmetry and record the anatomical area of deficit (e.g., 2 in. above the umbilicus).

Touch is difficult to assess because of the subjectivity of the response and the patient's anxiety. Using a wisp of cotton, test grossly at first using large skin areas. Keep the testing area wide enough to allow the patient to discriminate. Then use the pin to test specific areas of deficit identified.

SPINAL CORD INJURIES

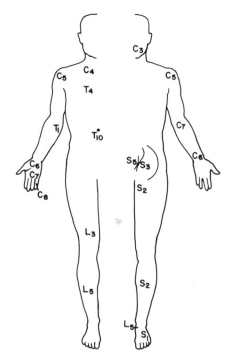

Figure 20.2 The location of dermatones for the sensory evaluation of the patient with an injured spine.

Proprioception is the knowledge or awareness of posture, movement, and changes in equilibrium. Testing is carried out by asking the patient to identify if the part being tested (finger, toe, wrist, or ankle) is moved up or down.

Any progression of a deficit in either motor or sensory ability should be brought to the attention of the physician at once, especially if it represents a significant change from the patient's condition immediately after injury.

The rectal examination offers the key to complete or incomplete lesions. The preservation of sensation in the buttocks, perineum, and genitalia or the presence of some anal sphincter tone is often the only sign of an incomplete lesion.

Observe for signs of autonomic dysfunction, such as a lack of sweating, vasomotor instability, loss of bladder and rectal control, and priaprism in the male.

Listen for bowel sounds, the absence of which may indicate an ileus commonly seen in the spine-injured patient. Resultant gastric distention may lead to vomiting with aspiration or impairment of respiratory effort.

Diagnostic Studies

Even if the patient arrives without a neurological deficit, significant instability of the spine may be present that, if stressed, could produce a cord lesion. Therefore, all patients with a decreased level of consciousness, head injury, or the potential for a spinal injury based on the history *must* have a cross-table lateral cervical x-ray film *before* they are moved in any way. Means of stabilization are not removed until the film is judged to be normal and all seven vertebrae are visualized. If those conditions are not met, stabilization methods remain until more definitive diagnostic tests can be carried out. Twenty percent of patients suffering trauma have more than one spinal injury, so it is wise to obtain a complete spinal x-ray series. Baseline electrolyte levels, arterial blood gas (ABG) studies, coagulation studies, and blood alcohol levels should be obtained. Blood is ordered for type and crossmatching and used as needed.

Nursing Care and Related Interventions

Damage to the spinal cord results from two pathophysiological factors—intrinsic and extrinsic. Intrinsic factors include hemorrhage, edema, ischemia, and hypoxia that are dealt with by oxygenation, steroids, and occasionally osmotic dehydration. Extrinsic factors include bony or soft tissue injury that disrupts the cord or spinal canal lesions. Surgical alignment or surgical correction must be done immediately to reverse or limit the resultant intrinsic pathological process.

Similar to treating head injuries, the ABCs—adequate airway, breathing, and circulation—are always the first priority. Adequate oxygenation and blood flow to the injured cord should be immediately addressed. Ventilatory decline should be anticipated and preparations made to handle the decline. Shock must be anticipated and handled appropriately.

Spinal Shock

Spinal shock is the result of the loss of sympathetic control. The sympathetic system, or the fight or flight response, comes off of the thoracic and lumbar cord at the level of T_1 to L_3. In stress, this system's major functions are that of vasoconstriction to maintain adequate blood pressure and tachycardia to increase cardiac output and oxygen delivery. In high thoracic cord injuries, as well as in cervical injuries, this sympathetic response is interrupted or cut off. As a result, vasoconstriction is lost and massive vasodilation occurs below the level of the injury. Blood pools in the abdomen and lower extremities, venous return to the heart is decreased, cardiac output drops, and a shock picture emerges. Because the sympathetic system is disrupted, the parasympathetic system goes unopposed. Bradycardia, often severe, hypotension, warm dry limbs, atonic bladder, and areflexia comprise the clinical picture.

Treatment modalities should be selected on the basis of the presence or absence of clinical compromise and not merely on the blood pressure or the pulse rate. Fluid resuscitation to increase circulating blood volume must be done with caution to prevent fluid overload. The resultant potential for pulmonary edema with increased mortality and morbidity is high. Hemodynamic monitoring may be necessary to monitor the fluid status adequately. Pharmacological support with alpha adrenergic drugs (Neo-Synephrine, Levophed or alpha-range dopamine) may be needed. Milder cases may be helped by supporting venous return with elevation of the lower extremities or with ace wraps. The bradycardia is treated with atropine sulfate 0.5 mg IV initially for up to 2.0 mg total in adults. Some practitioners prefer to await nodal or ventricular escape rhythms before administering atropine. Pediatric doses are as follows: 17–24 lb = 0.15 mg, 24–40 lb = 0.2 mg, 40–60 lb = 0.3 mg, and 65–90 lb = 0.4 mg.

A Foley catheter is inserted to prevent distention that may alter muscle tone in the bladder and affect future rehabilitation potential. Patients in spinal shock do not have the ability to regulate their temperature through sweating or vasoconstriction to the skin (both sympathetic responses) and need to have their environment made conducive to normothermia.

Other Interventions

Immobilization of the spine should have been carried out at the scene of the accident. If not, do it *immediately* upon arrival.

Additional interventions are primarily supportive and preventative with the main goal being to optimize conditions for spinal cord recovery. The main thrust of support is respiratory and cardiovascular stabilization. In addition, steroids are used by most practitioners, although their value is still being debated. Steroids do decrease the amount of damage done in incomplete lesions. The use of drugs to dehydrate the tissues is debatable and generally not recommended for use in the emergency department.

ALIGNMENT: NONSURGICAL AND SURGICAL

The purposes of alignment are to decompress the spinal cord, to relieve pain, to prevent further damage to the neural tissues, and to relieve nerve root compression. Realignment does not result in a reversal of the damages already done. Nonsurgical alignment is tried first and consists of the application of skeletal tongs and traction. Gardner-Wells or Crutchfield tongs are used most frequently. The initial weights applied are calculated at 2–3 lb per vertebrae (e.g., a C_4 fracture would take 8–12 lb of weight initially). Weights are readjusted once alignment has been verified by x-ray examination. Most physicians recommend that all patients with injuries between C_1 and T_1 be in traction before they leave the emergency department. If adequate realignment cannot be achieved by traction or with the addition of muscle relaxants (diazepam) and countertraction, surgical reduction is necessary. Surgical decompression may be done after a myelogram to remove herniated discs, bone fragments, or foreign materials that may be impinging on the cord.

Muscle spasms accompanying most cervical spine injuries are intense and combine with the discomfort of the tongs. While caution must be exercised to prevent respiratory compromise, pain relief must be adequately addressed.

PSYCHOLOGICAL SUPPORT

Initially, the patient will be in some degree of shock and will probably not comprehend what has happened or the magnitude of it. Denial is a common and necessary response for one whose entire life, in a matter of seconds, has been totally altered—physically, emotionally, socially, sexually, and vocationally. It is not necessary to reinforce the denial, nor is it appropriate to snatch away all hope. An honest answer of "We don't know at this moment what you will be capable of doing, but there is a strong possibility you won't walk again," is fine. Reality is presented, hope is maintained, and, most important, lies are not initiated. This is important, for as Pepper (1977) states, the needs of the spinal injured patient with quadriplegia can be compared with Erickson's eight stages of life. The quadriplegic will regress back to stage one, that of infancy, with the developmental task being that of learning to trust or mistrust. The patient, like the infant, is totally dependent on caregivers and must have his needs met consistently in order to learn to trust and begin anew. The goal is to provide dependability and consistency in his care and his environment, along with an attitude that will allow trust to develop.

A patient's family usually is told the suspected outcome, even if the patient is not. Remember that they too will regress, experience denial, and vent anger. Anger may be displaced onto the medical profession for their inability to "do something." Keep this in perspective, recognize the source, and do not respond with personal anger. This is a difficult time for both patient and family. Chaplains and social workers trained in crisis intervention and family counseling are excellent resources.

THE PATIENT WITH ACUTE BACK PAIN

Frequently seen in the emergency department is the patient suffering from an acute attack of back pain. Although a seemingly minor injury, this type of pain can be extremely difficult to cope with and its treatment regime almost encourages noncompliance because patients want an "active" cure, not rest and heat.

In planning discharge instructions, a few minutes taken to elicit *how* the patient spends a typical 24 hours will allow the instructions to take on some specific meaning rather than just giving general hints. Having one attack of acute back pain due to trauma or "overdoing it" does not mean the patient will be saddled with back pain forever. But, if he has mistreated his back or if he is out of condition and this has been a warning from his body, the likelihood is high that it will become a recurrent problem. The nurse's role is not only to impart discharge instructions, but also to impart *preventative* education. Consider several of the following aspects as the specific plan is being developed:

1. The foundation of back pain treatment is rest.
    a. Is the purpose understood?
    b. Given the home and job situation, is rest realistic for this patient?
    c. Is outside intervention necessary?
    d. Is family education required to encourage compliance?
    e. What is the sleep pattern (position, number of pillows used, and type of mattress)?
    f. How much sitting, standing, driving, walking, and lifting is done by the patient in a typical day at home and at work?
    g. Are modifications in home and work environment necessary?
2. Moist heat is the second mainstay of treatment.
    a. Is the principle understood?
    b. Is moist heat available?
    c. Are precautions and safety understood?
3. The avoidance of further strain is the last major component of discharge instruction.
    a. Is posture correct?
    b. Does the patient's height encourage improper sitting?
    c. Is there an awareness of how to provide relief if standing for any length of time cannot be avoided?

d. Can a redemonstration (verbal is sufficient) of proper lifting, sitting, or standing be given?
   e. Is overweight contributing to the problem?
   f. Are shoes flat, or with medium or spiked heels?
   g. Is the role of heels understood? Is there a willingness to modify foot wear temporarily?
   h. Have sexual activities and positions of comfort during the acute attack of pain been discussed?
   i. Are exercises a part of the patient's daily routine?
   j. Is there a willingness to accept an exercise regime to strengthen back muscles once the pain subsides?
   k. Are the *consequences* of noncompliance *fully* understood?

There are more than 80 million sufferers of acute back pain with some 10 million being acutely treated for *chronic* low back pain. This number is increasing every year. There is no magic cure for most low back pain; it requires an *active* effort on the patient's part to keep his back healthy. It is the nurse's job to teach him how.

CONCLUSION

The emergency department nurse must be capable of caring efficiently and effectively for a patient experiencing head and spinal trauma. The emergency department nurse must demonstrate a thorough understanding of all types of head and spine problems to ensure adequate patient care beginning with triage, progressing to stabilization of the patient with appropriate nursing care, and ending with adequate discharge teaching or patient and family support to help provide the highest level of care possible.

BIBLIOGRAPHY

Bordeauz, M.: The intensive care unit and observations of the acutely ill with neurological disease. *Heart and Lung* 2(6):884–888 (Nov./Dec. 1973).

Bruce, D.: Resuscitation from coma due to head injuries. *Critical Care Medicine* 6(4):254–270 (July/Aug. 1978).

———., et al.: CSF pressure monitoring in children: Physiology, pathology, and clinical usefulness. In L. Barnes (ed.): *Advances in Pediatrics*. Chicago: Yearbook Medical Publishers, 1977, pp. 233–290.

Carol, M., et al.: Acute care of spinal cord injury. *Critical Care Quarterly* 2(1):7–21 (June 1979).

Dagrosa, T: Brainstem damage associated with cerebral injury. *Journal of Emergency Nursing* 2:9–14 (Sept./Oct. 1976).

Erickson, R: Cranial check: A basic neurological assessment. *Nursing 74* 4:67–72 (Aug. 1974).

Jimm, L.: Nursing assessment of patients for increased intracranial pressure. *Journal of Neurosurgical Nursing* 6(1) (July 1974).

Lipe, H: Positioning the patient with intracranial hypertension: How turning the head rotation affects the internal jugular vein. *Heart and Lung* 9(6):1031–1037 (Nov./Dec. 1980).

Marshall, L.: Lecture notes prepared for the Conference of Intensive Care for Neurological Trauma and Diseases—A new decade. Miami, FL, January 1980.

Mastrian, K.: Of course you can manage head trauma patients. *RN* 44:45–51 (Aug. 1981).

Mitchell, P.: Intracranial hypertension: Implications of research for nursing care. *Journal of Neurosurgical Nursing* 12:145–154 (Sept. 1980).

Pepper, G.: The person with a spinal cord injury: Psychological care. *American Journal of Nursing* 77:1330–1335 (Aug. 1977).

Plum, F., and J. B. Posner: *The Diagnosis of Stupor and Coma*. 2nd ed. Philadelphia: Davis, 1980.

Rameriz, B: When you're faced with a neuro patient. *RN* 42:67–76 (Jan. 1979).

Shapiro, H: Intracranial hypertension. *Anesthesiology* 43(4)(Oct. 1975).

Simmons, S: Evaluating hidden intracranial bleeds. *Journal of Emergency Nursing* 4:9–17 (Sept./Oct. 1978).

Snyder, J., and D. Power: Care of the neurologically impaired patient. *Heart and Lung* 8(6)(Dec. 1979).

Tyson, G., et al.: Acute care of the head injured patient. *Critical Care Quarterly* 2(1):23–44 (June 1979).

21

Hypovolemic Shock, Septic Shock, or Disseminated Intravascular Coagulopathy

Cathy Bremer

After completing this chapter, the reader will be able to do the following:

1. Triage a patient experiencing hypovolemic shock, septic shock, or disseminated intravascular coagulopathy (DIC).
2. Identify the etiologies and/or predisposing factors associated with hypovolemic shock, septic shock, and DIC.
3. Describe the clinical manifestations of hypovolemic shock, septic shock, and DIC.
4. Relate pathophysiologic processes of hypovolemic shock, septic shock, and DIC to the clinical manifestations of each.
5. Describe and interpret diagnostic studies indicated in these disorders.
6. Identify appropriate nursing interventions in the emergency management of the patient with hypovolemic shock, septic shock, and DIC.

Hypovolemic shock, septic shock, and disseminated intravascular coagulopathy (DIC) are clinical entities that result from a number of underlying pathologic conditions. The clinical manifestations of these entities result in hemodynamic and hematologic abnormalities that are potentially life-threatening. This chapter will discuss the pathophysiology, clinical manifestations, and emergency nursing interventions of each of these conditions.

TRIAGE

Recognizing these life-threatening conditions in the emergency department is often the nurses' responsibility because they usually see the patient first. An organized and efficient approach to assessment, therefore, is necessary. Data collected during the assessment provide the framework for the planning and delivery of nursing care.

Subjective Data

The collection of subjective data usually begins with the presenting complaint. In other words, ask, Why did the patient come to the emergency department? or What is the history of the present illness? The patient with hypovolemic shock, septic shock, or DIC may relate a typical history of injury and blood loss, infection and fever, or severe bruising. On the other hand, the patient may describe vague signs and symptoms requiring the nurse to exercise well-honed interviewing skills. The nurse should be alert to the possibility of hypovolemic shock if the patient complains of weakness, fatigue, dizziness, syncope, thirst, and anxiety.

Septic shock should be suspected in the patient on immunosuppressive agents or on prolonged antibiotic therapy or with a history of an indwelling urinary or intravenous catheter who complains of fever, chills, or feeling hot and flushed. The quadriplegic patient with a tracheostomy or decubitus ulcers and patients on home hyperalimentation are also at risk.

DIC should be considered in the diagnosis of a patient with a history of a recent obstetrical or surgical procedure, massive blood transfusions, or malignancy.

Information should be obtained concerning past medical history, current medications, and allergies.

Objective Data

Objective data is obtained during the physical examination through observation, percussion, palpation, and auscultation. Using these skills, the nurse may observe a pale, dyspneic, anxious patient with bleeding from a chest wound. The nurse may palpate a weak, thready pulse and auscultate a decreased blood pressure. Percussion might reveal an area of dullness over a lung field.

Objective data also include baseline vital signs, inspection of skin and mucous membranes, and notation of any treatment the patient received prior to arrival in the emergency department. The nurse is able to integrate this information with the subjective data to formulate a nursing diagnosis and plan of care for this patient.

A rapid head-to-toe assessment should be done on all patients and must include level of consciousness, pupillary responses, skin color and temperature, limb mobility and sensation, and peripheral pulses.

Assessment and Planning

Using the foregoing example, the nursing diagnosis would be hypovolemic shock due to hemothorax. The plan of care would include such measures as initiation of intravenous fluid therapy, supplemental oxygen, position with legs elevated, sterile nonocclusive dressing to wound, and assembling equipment for chest tube insertion. (Table 21.1 contains triage notes for patients experiencing hypovolemic shock, septic shock, and DIC.)

HYPOVOLEMIC SHOCK

Simply defined, *shock* is a state of inadequate tissue perfusion. The three interrelated hemodynamic components of tissue perfusion are blood volume, vascular tone, and cardiac function. A condition affecting any one of these components can cause inadequate tissue perfusion—that is, shock. The adjective that precedes the word *shock* usually indicates which component has failed. Thus, *hypovolemic* shock refers to inadequate tissue perfusion due to the loss of circulating blood volume.

Circulating blood volume may become inadequate because of the loss of either whole blood, plasma, or extracellular fluid. Acute loss of whole blood is commonly called *hemorrhage,* and the bleeding can be external or internal. Traumatic injury is one of the most common causes of external bleeding. Hematemesis, epistaxis, and vaginal bleeding are also major sources of external blood loss.

Occult or internal whole blood loss can result from bleeding into any one of the body's contained cavities or spaces. Many of these cavities are large enough to accommodate a quantity of blood sufficient to cause hypovolemic shock. Bleeding into the peritoneal cavity can occur after intra-abdominal injury, aortic aneurysm rupture, or ectopic pregnancy rupture. The pleural space can accommodate more than one liter of blood. The gastrointestinal tract, both lower and upper, is often the site of occult bleeding. Retroperitoneal bleeding occurs quite commonly in the presence of a fractured pelvis because of the vascularity of the involved area. Large amounts of blood can also accumulate in the tissue planes of the thigh after fracture of the femur.

Loss of extracellular fluid is most often seen as simple dehydration, which can result from inadequate intake or excessive output. Vomiting, diarrhea, diaphoresis, diuresis, and fistula drainage are causes of excessive output and, if untreated, can progress to hypovolemic shock.

Sources of plasma loss are sometimes grouped together and collectively called *third space loss.* Third space loss is actually a shifting of fluid from the circulating volume to areas where it is unavailable to the effective circulation, thus creating the potential for hypovolemic shock. The sites of fluid accumulation or *sequestering* depend on the cause, but the most common locations are the peritoneal cavity, intestinal lumen, pleural space, and interstitial space. The causes include peritonitis, ascites, pancreatitis, intestinal obstruction, pleural effusion, burns, and traumatic injury (Johansen, 1980).

Pathophysiology

In hypovolemic shock, every system of the body is affected. The clinical manifestations of shock are reflections of the initial and progressive responses of these systems to decreased tissue perfusion.

TABLE 21.1 Examples of Triage Notes for Patients Experiencing Hypovolemic Shock, Septic Shock, or DIC

S: 18 yo WM in motor vehicle accident 1 hr prior to admission. Complaining of abdominal pain, weakness, and thirst. PMH: neg., no current meds.
O: P 120, BP 90/80, RR 28. Pale, anxious, diffuse abdominal tenderness, LUQ ecchymosis.
A: Possible intra-abdominal hemorrhage due to blunt abdominal trauma.
P: Surgical evaluation, admit trauma room immediately.

S: 76 yo BM transferred from nursing home with history of fever and hypotension. Past history of recurrent urinary tract infections. Digoxin 0.25 mg qd. PMH: CVA 2 yrs PTA.
O: T 103°F rectal, P 116, BP 80/60. Skin flushed and warm to touch. Anxious and confused. Indwelling Foley catheter draining small amounts of cloudy urine.
A: Septic shock, infection originating in urinary tract.
P: Medical evaluation, admit examination room immediately.

S: 24 yo Spanish woman 2 weeks postpartum, complains of heavy vaginal bleeding, generalized bruising, digital pain. PMH: neg., no meds.
O: P 100, BP 110/80, RR 24. Active vaginal bleeding, ecchymotic areas on limbs, fingertips cyanotic, oriented × 3.
A: Possible DIC.
P: Medical evaluation, admit examination room immediately.

Cellular anoxia is the common denominator of all shock states. At the *cellular level,* pathophysiologic responses begin with decreased oxygen delivery and the conversion from aerobic to anaerobic metabolism.

Normally, under aerobic conditions, glucose is metabolized to pyruvate and then enters the Krebs cycle with carbon dioxide and water as the end products. For each mole of glucose metabolized, 38 moles of adenosine triphosphate (ATP) are liberated. When oxygen does not reach the cells, they must undergo anaerobic glycolysis. In this situation, glucose is converted to pyruvate with only 2 moles of ATP formed per mole of glucose. Pyruvate cannot enter the Krebs cycle in the absence of oxygen and is converted to lactate and 2 more moles of ATP are liberated, for a net gain of only 4 moles of ATP per mole of glucose (Guyton, 1981). Continued lactate formation will eventually result in a metabolic acidosis (Rothstein, 1979).

The combination of acidosis, hypoperfusion, and hypoxia results in significant dysfunction of the intracellular structures. The most important of these structures are the mitochondria and lysosomes. Because intracellular respiration and energy production are the function of the mitochondria, the ultimate consequence of depressed mitochondrial activity is reduction of tissue levels of ATP.

Lysosomes function as the digestive system of the cell and, similar to other cellular structures, are fueled by adenosine triphosphate. When the level of ATP generated is insufficient, lysosomal membrane disruption occurs, and powerful enzymes are released into the cell. The end result is cellular autolysis and eventual release of these enzymes into the circulation where they can have detrimental effects on other structures (Shatney, 1981).

Sodium pump dysfunction also occurs as a result of insufficient ATP production. As the sodium pump fails, intracellular water and sodium increase, and intracellular potassium decreases.

In early hypovolemic shock, the response of the *respiratory system* is tachypnea. While the respiratory rate (RR) is increased, tidal volume (TV) is decreased, thus increasing the work of ventilation. The patient will nevertheless have an increased minute volume ($RR \times TV = MV$) that will be reflected in the arterial blood gas analysis as respiratory alkalosis.

As shock continues, hypoxia and decreased tidal volume combine to produce decreased surfactant production and increased atelectasis. The net result is a progressive intrapulmonary arteriovenous shunting that, in late shock, is reflected in the arterial blood gases as a respiratory acidosis (Rothstein, 1979).

The responses of the *endocrine and renal systems* to hypovolemic shock are compensatory in nature. One of the earliest events after a loss of circulating volume is the release of catecholamines—epinephrine and norepinephrine—from the adrenal medulla and the sympathetic nerve endings.

Norepinephrine has a predominantly alpha effect that results in excitation of smooth muscle, specifically vascular smooth muscle. The resultant vasoconstriction is most pronounced in the skin, skeletal muscle, mesenteric vasculature, and kidneys. Blood flow is diverted from these less essential organs to the heart, brain, and lungs.

Epinephrine, a beta stimulator, produces a chronotropic and inotropic effect on the heart, thereby increasing heart rate, stroke volume, and cardiac output. Epinephrine is also responsible for the release of adrenocorticotropic hormone (ACTH).

As a result of hypoperfusion of the pancreas and catecholamine effects, insulin secretion is decreased in shock (Shatney, 1981).

Decreased renal blood flow from hypovolemia causes an increase in the secretion of renin. This increase in turn causes the conversion of angiotension I into angiotension II, which causes vasoconstriction. These substances also promote secretion of aldosterone, a potent mineralocorticoid, which enhances sodium and water reabsorption. Water reabsorption is further enhanced by the secretion of antidiuretic hormone (ADH) from the posterior pituitary in response to hypovolemia (Guyton, 1981).

The initial response of the kidneys is to concentrate urine and to decrease water excretion. If hypovolemia and the concomitant decreased renal blood flow persist, renal ischemia can lead to tubular necrosis and oliguric renal failure.

The earliest responses of the *cardiovascular system* to hypovolemia are compensatory in nature and mediated through the sympathetic nervous system. When more than 10–15 percent of the circulating volume is lost, norepinephrine is released. The release causes vascular smooth muscle contraction, which results in an increase in peripheral vascular resistance. In general, this increase is sufficient to restore adequate tissue perfusion if the fluid loss is arrested (Porth, 1981).

As fluid continues to be lost, pressure decreases, and the baroreceptors of the aortic arch and carotid bodies are stimulated, resulting in an increased release of catecholamines. Increased amounts of norepinephrine cause marked vasoconstriction of the skin, skeletal muscle, kidney, and splanchnic bed. The blood from these organs is shunted to the heart, lungs, and brain. Epinephrine acts directly on the heart muscle, increasing both the rate and strength of contraction. This in turn increases cardiac output and arterial pressure (Guyton, 1981).

When fluid loss exceeds 30 percent of the circulating volume, the compensatory responses of the cardiovascular system are no longer adequate. Vasoconstriction and increased cardiac output can no longer maintain an adequate arterial pressure to perfuse the organs that had earlier been spared. Specifically, myocardial perfusion decreases, and cardiac function begins to deteriorate. The contractile ability of the heart decreases as a result of profound ischemia. Contractility is further depressed by the presence of myocardial depressant factor (MDF) in the circulation. MDF is thought to be released from the ischemic pancreas in late shock. In the microcirculation, a stagnant hypoxia occurs in prolonged shock because of arteriolar dilation in the presence of continued venule constriction (Guyton, 1981).

In early shock, there is a rather rapid movement of extracellular fluid from the interstitial to the intravascular space. This *fluid shift* occurs because of reduced hydrostatic pressure in the capillaries. Hydrostatic pressure is reduced not only as a result of volume loss, but also as a result of arteriolar constriction in the precapillary area. In prolonged shock, these losses from the interstitial space must also be replaced. This initial fluid shift is self-limiting as the interstitial fluid becomes depleted. Intravascular colloid oncotic pressure is reduced due to the dilutional effects of the fluid shift (Zamora, 1979).

As shock continues, cellular damage resulting from anoxia contributes to the movement of fluid out of the intravascular space. The dysfunction of the sodium pump in the cell membrane allows sodium to move into the cell. Water passively follows the sodium, causing swelling of the cell and reduction of extracellular volume.

Altered capillary membrane permeability contributes most significantly to the reversed fluid shifts in late shock. As the permeability increases, protein molecules can move through the membranes. This movement further decreases colloid oncotic pressure intravascularly and increases it in the interstitial fluid, thereby drawing fluid out of the vascular compartment (McSwain, 1981).

Late shock is sometimes called the stage of *decompensation*. During this stage, many of the pathophysiologic responses are actually detrimental to the body and are considered preterminal events.

Clinical Manifestations

When the loss of circulating volume does not exceed 15 percent in a normal individual, clinical manifestations will be absent (Rothstein, 1979). Compensating mechanisms are capable of maintaining a normal blood pressure at this point.

If the losses are between 15 and 20 percent, the patient will exhibit the signs of early hypovolemic shock. Skin will be pale, cool to the touch, and it may be slightly diaphoretic. Anxiety and nervousness are the typical behavioral manifestations at this stage. The child may exhibit irritability. The patient's vital signs will reveal a mild tachycardia, a decreased or "narrowed" pulse pressure, a decreased central venous pressure (CVP), and an increased respiratory rate. Orthostatic vital signs will be present. Urinary output will be decreased.

As loss approximates 30 percent, the patient begins to manifest more pronounced symptoms of shock. In addition to pale and cool skin, the patient will have poor capillary refill. Behaviorally, he may be restless and confused or even combative. Typically, the patient will complain of extreme thirst. The tachycardia will be more severe and the pulse will feel thready. The pulse pressure will be even narrower with both systolic and diastolic blood pressure beginning to fall. Central venous pressure will be further decreased. Urine volume will be scant and extremely concentrated.

As volume loss approaches 50 percent, the patient will be in a severe, and possibly irreversible, state of hypovolemic shock (Guyton, 1981). The patient's skin will be quite pale, or it may even have a mottled appearance and it will feel cold to the touch. If the mucous membranes are inspected, they will be cyanotic. Behaviorally, the patient will be weak, obtunded, or moribund. Hemodynamically, the patient may be either extremely tachycardic or he may be bradycardic if myocardial contractility is depressed. Severe hypotension will be present and cuff blood pressure may be unobtainable. The respiratory pattern will be shallow or agonal. There will be no urinary output (McSwain, 1981).

Diagnostic Studies

Shortly after admission, and at appropriate intervals thereafter, blood samples should be drawn to determine the hematocrit (Hct), hemoglobin (Hg), and the arterial blood gases (ABGs). The initial results will serve as a baseline against which subsequent results can be compared.

In early shock, if blood loss is acute, there is no change in either the Hct or Hg because the ratio of cellular components to plasma remains the same. If the blood loss has been chronic, Hct and Hg are decreased because compensatory mechanisms have shifted extracellular fluid into the intravascular compartment diluting the cellular components of the blood. Arterial blood gas studies at this point reflect a respiratory alkalosis resulting from the increased respiratory rate of early shock (Porth, 1981).

In moderate shock, the Hct and Hg are usually decreased, reflecting compensatory fluid shifts. However, if the blood loss has been extremely rapid, these values may still be normal. Arterial blood gas studies will show a mixed respiratory alkalosis and mild to moderate metabolic acidosis.

In severe or prolonged shock, the Hct and Hg will be decreased. Because of severe ischemia, arterial blood gas studies will reflect both a respiratory and a metabolic acidosis.

In addition to these tests, blood samples should be sent for complete blood count, platelet count, type and crossmatch, electrolyte values, glucose level, coagulation profile, and levels of creatinine and blood urea nitrogen (BUN). Additional blood tests may be indicated depending on the patient's condition. A urinalysis should be obtained, preferably prior to the insertion of a Foley catheter to avoid misdiagnosing the source of any red blood cells in the urine. If indicated, or if the patient has any doubts, a pregnancy test should be done.

For the patient in hypovolemic shock certain x-ray films may be required as part of the initial assessment and stabilization. Most often these x-ray studies include cervical spine, skull, and chest films. Further radiographic evaluation can usually be delayed until the patient is stable.

A 12-lead electrocardiogram (ECG) should be done as soon as the patient's condition permits. During hemorrhage, it may show nonspecific ST segments or T wave changes due to reduction of coronary blood flow (Zamora, 1979).

Nursing Care and Related Interventions

Similar to treatment of any seriously ill or injured patient, ensuring a patent *airway* with adequate ventilation is the top priority. If the patient is ventilating adequately, medium- to high-flow supplemental oxygen may be all that is required. Most patients can tolerate nasal prongs better than a mask. Nevertheless, a mask adequate in size to cover the nose and mouth should be used in children. Nasal cannulas may be used in neonates. In the patient who is apneic, in ventilatory failure ($Pa_{CO_2} > 50$ Torr or $Pa_{O_2} < 50$ Torr), or has an injury affecting the respiratory system, intubation and mechanical ventilation are indicated.

Restoring *circulation and perfusion* are the main goals in the treatment of hypovolemic shock. External bleeding should be controlled with the application of pressure over the site. Tourniquets are usually contraindicated, except perhaps for patients with complete amputation injuries with massive bleeding.

Pneumatic or *military antishock trousers* (MAST) can be applied to both adults and children to translocate blood from the lower extremities to the central circulation. In adults and children more than six years old, criterion for use is a systolic blood pressure below 80 mm Hg. In children under six years old, the criterion is a systolic blood pressure below 60 mm Hg (Walkerle, 1980). The garment (see Fig. 21.1) consists of three radiolucent compartments, one abdominal and two legs, which inflate separately. Once the garment is properly applied, inflation is begun in the leg compartments and proceeds to the abdominal compartment. Inflation is adjusted according to the patient's clinical problem and hemodynamic response. Deflation begins with the abdominal compartment and proceeds to the legs while the blood pressure is constantly monitored. If the blood pressure drops 5 mm Hg, deflation should be stopped while intravenous fluid administration is increased. If uncontrolled internal hemorrhage is suspected, deflation should not be attempted until the patient is in the operating room (Walkerle, 1980). The use of pneumatic trousers is contraindicated in patients with congestive heart failure and pulmonary edema. Controversy exists concerning their use in patients with chest injuries (Hoffman, 1980). In the pregnant patient, only the leg compartments are inflated. If pneumatic trousers are unavailable, the patient's lower extremities can be elevated to augment circulatory restoration.

Access to the circulatory system is established with the insertion of at least two large-bore intravenous (IV) catheters. This activity should be occurring simultaneously with the other life-saving measures. Types and location of any injuries

HYPOVOLEMIC SHOCK

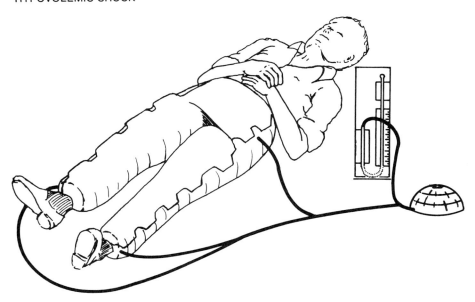

Figure 21.1 Pneumatic or military antishock trousers.

should be taken into consideration when IV sites are chosen. In small children and infants, a saphenous vein cutdown provides a fast and easy route for administering large volumes of fluid (Crone, 1980). A central venous line should be inserted if possible, but not at the expense of delaying treatment. In the adult and in older children, insertion sites are subclavian, basilic, and internal and external jugular veins. In infants and small children, the femoral vein is cannulated (Rucker, 1981).

Because of their immediate availability, crystalloid solutions are the fluids initially used for volume replacement. Ringer's lactate, a balanced electrolyte solution, is the preferred crystalloid solution used for treating hypovolemic shock. In the adult, infusion should be as rapid as necessary to maintain adequate hemodynamic parameters. In the child, an initial bolus of 20 ml/kg is given. If there is no response, this bolus should be repeated (McSwain, 1981).

Colloids are almost always used as an adjunct to fluid therapy in hypovolemic shock. Colloid solutions include volume expanders, whole blood, and blood components. The use of synthetic blood is being initiated in some centers.

Volume expanders are solutions that, because of their oncotic properties, draw fluid from the interstitial to the intravascular space. Those solutions used most frequently are serum albumin, plasma protein fraction, and dextran. Serum albumin, although quite expensive, is considered the safest (Shoemaker, 1981). Numerous side effects have been associated with dextran including allergic reactions, coagulopathies, and altered blood study results. Fresh or whole blood is the ideal replacement fluid when blood loss has been rapid and severe because all components are being lost at the same rate. Stored blood is less than ideal because platelets and many of the clotting factors are inactivated during storage.

Blood component therapy is fast replacing the use of whole blood for several reasons. The most compelling reason is that component therapy can be deficit-specific, which eliminates the risks to the patient from those components of whole blood the person may not need. In addition, component therapy helps to conserve blood because several patients may benefit from one unit of whole blood. Those components most commonly used are packed red blood cells (see Table 21.2), plasma components (Table 21.3), and plasma derivatives (Table 21.4).

Synthetic blood is experimentally available in three forms at the present time. Stroma-free hemoglobin is human hemoglobin that has been stripped of elements that clog capillaries. It functions at low oxygen levels and exerts colloid pressure, but it can cause iron toxicity and hypervolemia in certain patients. Oxygen-binding chelate, another blood substitute, is an iron-based material that binds oxygen similar to the way hemoglobin does. The major disadvantage is iron toxicity. The final product, a perfluorochemical, is the only one available for use at this time. Advantages include a tremendous oxygen-carrying capacity and low cost, and certain brands retain osmotic pressure as well. Disadvantages are the necessity for high oxygen concentrations and thrombus formation because of altered platelet membranes (Leser, 1982).

In certain patients, autotransfusion can be used to supplement volume replacement. In the emergency department, autotransfusion is indicated for the patient with a massive hemothorax or for the patient with massive bleeding from an uncontaminated source in the chest cavity. Autotransfusion can be a readily available source of fresh, compatible blood. Benefits should outweigh risks, but autotransfusion has been associated with microthrombi, coagulopathies, and sepsis (Thurer, 1982).

Restoration of circulating volume alone will not be effective treatment unless the adequacy of perfusion is assessed. Since cardiac function is a determinant of perfusion, the patient should be attached to continuous cardiac monitoring.

Urinary output is an excellent indicator of perfusion and should be monitored carefully. An indwelling urinary catheter should be inserted for this purpose. In the adult patient, 30–50 cc of urine output per hour is considered adequate. A minimum urine output of 0.5–1.0 cc/kg/hour for children is considered acceptable (Lyon, 1981).

Maintenance of hemodynamic stability of the patient in hypovolemic shock depends on continuous monitoring. Careful *monitoring* of hemodynamic and other critical parameters allows for evaluation of medical and nursing interventions as well as the early detection of a change in the patient's condition.

The physical examination of the patient should be repeated at appropriate intervals as part of the monitoring process. Noninvasive monitoring should include measurements of blood pressure, pulse rate and quality, respiratory rate and pattern, cardiac monitoring, level of consciousness, and skin color and temperature. The frequency of these measurements is determined by the patient's condition.

In the more critically ill patient, invasive monitoring is frequently necessary. Central venous pressure reflects circulatory adequacy and right heart function. It is especially accurate in children and adults with healthy cardiorespiratory systems. Arterial blood pressure can be directly monitored by insertion of an arterial catheter connected to monitoring equipment. This method has the advantage of continuous monitoring and provides access to arterial blood samples.

A balloon-tipped pulmonary artery catheter can provide considerable information

TABLE 21.2 Red Blood Cells

Preparation				
Fresh	*Stored*	*Washed*		*Frozen*

Characteristics

270–300 cc/unit, Hct: 60–85%, 1 unit raises Hct 3% →→ Refrigerated up to 21 days after processing →→ Washed with saline to remove leukocytes →→ Treated with glycerol and frozen, washed with saline × 3 during thaw, most leukocytes and plasma proteins removed, use within 24° of thawing

Indications

Decreased Hct or Hg, anemia or chronic blood loss, acute blood loss if used with other volume expanders →→→→→→ Allergic individuals, potential organ transplant recipients →→ Individuals with rare types, autotransfusion

Benefits

Less fluid overload, decreased risk of reaction to plasma antigen, more viable RBCs →→→→→→ Decreased leukocyte reaction, decreased rejection risk →→ 2–3 yr storage, stockpile blood, almost hepatitis-free, decreased plasma citrate

Risks

Incompatibility, infection, contamination →→→→→→→→→→

TABLE 21.3 Plasma Components

Preparation	Fresh	Stored	Fresh Frozen	Cryoprecipitate	Platelets
Characteristics	Processed and administered within 4 hr. of collection, platelet-rich, contains plasma proteins	Separated but not frozen until after 6 hours, no platelets, contains factors VII, IX, X	Frozen within 4 hr. of collection, no platelets, contains factors V, VIII, IX, X, XI	Precipitates out of FFP during thawing, rich in factor VIII	Separated from plasma by centrification. Single donor: 1 unit; concentrate: 4–10 units. Stored at room temp. up to 72° with agitation, retains hemostatic effectiveness 24–72 hrs. posttransfusion
Indications Volume expansion, thrombocytopenia	→	Treatment of bleeding from vitamin K deficiency	Correct coag. deficiencies from liver disease, hemophilia, defibrination, fibrinolysis	Hemophilia A, prior to surgery with potential for massive blood loss	Thrombocytopenia, aplastic anemia, bone marrow depression
Benefits	Clotting factors present, platelets present, cross-matching unnecessary	Some clotting factors	All clotting factors, stores for 1 yr	Treats specific deficiency, less fluid overload	Less fluid overload
Risks Hepatitis			→	Give group specific for large amounts →	Can't use microfilters

406

TABLE 21.4 Plasma Derivatives

Preparation	Albumin	Plasma Protein Fraction	Gamma & Immune Globulin	Factor VIII Concentrate	Factor IX Concentrate
Characteristics	Pasteurized, 5–25% solution, no clotting factors	⟶	Prepared from pooled plasma, nonspecific or specific antibodies from human blood	Lyophilised, factor VIII concentration 100 × that of plasma, made from pooled plasma	Lyophilised, made from pooled plasma
Indications	Volume expansion, severe protein loss, hypoalbuminemia	⟶	Hypogamma-globulinemia, prophylaxis for infection, hepatitis, rubiola, mumps, pertussis, rabies, tetanus	Hemophilia A	Hemophilia B
Benefits	No hepatitis risk, store at room temp. 1 yr, refrigerated 3 yrs	⟶		Store up to 1 yr	⟶
Risks	Infuse undiluted 25% slowly	⟶		Hepatitis	⟶

about the patient's cardiovascular status. Pulmonary artery and pulmonary capillary wedge pressures are reliable measurements of left heart function. In addition, cardiac output can be measured and mixed venous blood samples drawn. This sophisticated type of hemodynamic monitoring, however, is usually not initiated until the patient is admitted to an intensive care unit.

Serial hematocrits and serial ABG determinations are essential for the hypovolemic patient. Urinary output and urine specific gravity should be measured hourly. Nasogastric aspirant and all other drainage (chest tubes, wounds, fistulas) should be documented frequently.

Medications

The primary treatment of hypovolemic shock is restoration of circulating volume. Therefore, pharmacologic intervention should not be instituted until the patient is normovolemic. If the normovolemic patient remains hypotensive, the etiology of the problem may be cardiogenic and a *vasodilative, inotropic agent* may be given to aid in tissue perfusion. Table 21.5 contains the vasoactive drugs used in the treatment of late hypovolemic shock. Vasoactive agents should be administered via an infusion pump while the patient's arterial pressure is being directly monitored.

The use of pharmacologic doses of *corticosteroids* has been, and continues to remain, controversial. Nonetheless, their use is relatively commonplace and advocated because of their positive cardiac inotropic effect, peripheral vasodilatory effect, and lysosomal membrane stabilization properties (Zamora, 1979).

Sodium bicarbonate should be given in appropriate amounts if the patient's ABG studies reveal acidosis.

The patient will either go to surgery or be admitted to an intensive care unit (ICU). Both the patient and the patient's family will need reassurance and an explanation of what has happened and what will happen in the future. The nurse in the emergency department must accurately and objectively communicate all information concerning the patient to whomever will be assuming responsibility for the person's care when he leaves the emergency department.

SEPTIC SHOCK

As its name implies, the underlying cause of *septic shock* is an infective process. The causative organisms, sources of contamination, and predisposing factors of septic shock are contained in Table 21.6.

Historically, the etiology of septic shock has shifted from gram-positive to gram-negative organisms due to the development of antibiotics specific against common gram-positive bacteria. When septic shock does result from gram-positive septicemia, it usually originates as pneumonia in very young and very old people.

Pathophysiology

At one time it was believed that the physiologic response to septic shock differed in gram-negative and gram-positive sepsis. Recent investigations, however, have

SEPTIC SHOCK

TABLE 21.5 Vasoactive Agents in the Treatment of Late Hypovolemic Shock

Drug	Dose (Adult and Children)	Effect
Dobutamine	2–10 µg/kg/min	↓ systemic vascular resistance, ↑ cardiac output
Dopamine	2–5 µg/kg/min	↑ renal and splanchnic blood flow, ↑ cardiac output
Isuprel	5–10 µg/kg/min 0.05–0.5 µg/kg/min	↓ systemic vascular resistance, ↑ cardiac output
Nitroprusside	3 µg/kg/min	↓ peripheral resistance

shown that the responses are essentially the same and that the differences reflect the stage of shock (early or late) and underlying etiology rather than the organism (Wiles, 1980).

The hypoperfusion of septic shock is a result of a defect in the vascular component of the cardiovascular system. The basic problem is a diffuse peripheral vasodilation that creates a *relative hypovolemia*.

A lipopolysaccharide complex, known as *endotoxin*, is responsible for initiating the process that results in the decreased peripheral resistance. Endotoxins are found in the outer layers of the bacterial cell wall and are released into the circulation during lysis of gram-negative organisms. When the endotoxins interact with infected tissue, blood vessels, and white blood cells, vasoactive substances are released. One of these substances, kallikrein, when released from leukocytes, causes the produc-

TABLE 21.6 Septic Shock

Causative Organisms	Sources of Contamination	Predisposing Factors

Gram-negative
  E. coli
  Klebsiella
  Enterobacter
  Serratia
  Pseudomonas
	Exogenous
	  Foreign body
	  Clothing
	  Environmental elements
	  Ingestion
		Immunosuppression
		Chronic illness
		Malnourishment
		Age

Gram-positive
  Staphylococcus
  Streptococcus
  Pneumococcus
  Clostridium
	Endogenous
	  Perforated GI viscous
	  Perforated GU viscous
	  Respiratory tract	

Fungi
  Candida
	Nosocomial
	  Indwelling tubes & catheters
	  Invasive testing or monitoring	

tion of kinins, alters the action of epinephrine and norepinephrine on blood vessels, and causes release of histamine from mast cells (Eskridge, 1980). Histamine causes vasodilation and decreased peripheral resistance, which, in turn, decreases arterial blood pressure. Similar to reactions in hypovolemic shock, the baroreceptors are stimulated and cause the release of catecholamines. The cardiac response is the same—increased heart rate and cardiac output. However, the presence of the endotoxin causes venules and arterioles to be unresponsive to the vasoconstrictor effects of catecholamines. This pnenomenon is referred to as *hyperdynamic shock.*

If the diffuse vasodilation and relative hypovolemia are not corrected, or if underlying cardiac disease exists, the patient will progress to a hypodynamic state that physiologically resembles hypovolemic shock. Coagulopathies and metabolic disturbances are also associated with septic shock (Sugarman, 1981).

Clinical Manifestations

The clinical manifestations of septic shock in the early and late stages may differ significantly. In early septic shock, chills and fever are present with mild hypotension and slight tachycardia. Unlike hypovolemic shock, the skin is dry, warm, and flushed. Other early manifestations include oliguria, glycosuria, tachypnea, and high cardiac output. A change of sensorium may be one of the earliest signs of septic shock.

As septic shock progresses to the point where decompensation occurs, the clinical manifestations resemble those of hypovolemic shock. Hypotension, tachycardia, and tachypnea become more pronounced. The patient is usually hypothermic with cool, moist skin. Central venous pressure is decreased and the patient may be anuric (Shatney, 1981).

Diagnostic Studies

Diagnostic studies in septic shock are aimed at identifying the foci of infection and the responsible organism as well as assessing hemodynamic stability and oxygenation.

Specimens for culture and sensitivity should be obtained. These specimens should include blood, urine, sputum, stool, fluid from wounds, and spinal fluid, when appropriate. A complete blood count, blood and urine glucose, electrolytes, BUN, urinalysis, coagulation profile, and platelet count should be done. Thrombocytopenia is a frequent finding in septic shock and may, in fact, be the most valuable indicator of sepsis in the infant (Sugarman, 1981). When indicated, lumbar puncture, abdominal paracentesis, and culdocentesis may provide diagnostic information if pus is aspirated. An electrocardiogram should be done and x-ray examinations taken as indicated. ABG studies should be completed as well.

Nursing Care and Related Interventions

Nursing care of the patient with septic shock begins, of course, by ensuring a patent airway and adequate ventilation. Management guidelines are the same as those outlined earlier. While patients in septic shock may be normovolemic, they are "relatively hypovolemic" and must be given intravenous fluids to restore perfusion. Large-bore intravenous catheters should be inserted and an infusion of Ringer's lactate or normal saline initiated. Colloids are usually unnecessary unless an underlying condition dictates their use (Sugarman, 1981). Response of the arterial blood pressure, central venous pressure, and pulmonary artery and capillary wedge pressure (when possible) should be the determinants in selecting the amount and rate of infusion.

Further treatment includes the removal of all catheters and tubes that the patient arrived with because they may be the foci of infection. The tips of these may be sent for culture and sensitivity. All wounds should be cleansed and debrided. A rectal temperature should be taken, and a Foley catheter and nasogastric tube inserted.

Monitoring of the patient with septic shock follows the same guidelines described for hypovolemic shock.

Medications

Sodium bicarbonate is given to correct acidemia as indicated by the patient's ABG studies.

Vasoactive drugs are usually not used unless the patient has deteriorated to the hypodynamic state despite fluid resuscitation. When this occurs, dopamine is the preferred drug, given at doses between 2 to 5 μg/kg/minute.

Rapid digitalization may be beneficial to the patient whose septic shock is complicated by heart failure. The dose is 0.75 to 1.5 mg of digoxin IV for the adult patient. For the child between 2 and 10 years of age, the dose is 0.03–0.044 mg/kg IV. The dose for the child more than 10 years old is 0.3–0.6 mg IV (Hazinski, 1981).

Antibiotics should be started immediately in the patient with septic shock. Table 21.7 provides guidelines for their administration.

Corticosteroids in pharmacologic doses are advocated in the treatment of septic shock. The recommended dose of methylprednisolone is 30 mg/kg given intravenously during a 10 minute period. This treatment may be repeated every four hours (Sugarman, 1981).

After the patient is stable and the diagnosis has been made, the nurse must remember to protect both personnel and other patients from unnecessary exposure to infection. The appropriate infection control procedure should be instituted as soon as the patient's condition permits.

The patient in septic shock will be admitted to a hospital bed. Documentation should be complete, and the appropriate information should be communicated to those assuming the care of the patient.

DIC (DISSEMINATED INTRAVASCULAR COAGULOPATHY)

Disseminated intravascular coagulopathy (DIC), also known as *consumptive coagulopathy* or *defibrination syndrome,* is a condition in which excessive coagulation and ultimately inadequate hemostasis occur.

DIC is almost never seen as a separate entity, but usually occurs as a complication

TABLE 21.7 Antibiotic Therapy in Septic Shock

Suspected Organism	Antibiotic	Dose (IV)
E. coli	Amikacin (Amikar)	7.5 mg/kg q12h (adult & children)
Pseudomonas Klebsiella	Gentamicin (Garamycin)	1–1.5 mg/kg q8h (adult) 2–2.5 mg/kg q8h (children)
Serratia Proteus	Nebcin (Tobramycin)	1–1.5 mg/kg q8h (adult & children)
Bacteroides Staphylococcus	Clindamycin (Cleocin)	400–600 mg q8h (adult) 8–12 mg/kg q8h (children)
Klebsiella	Cephalothin (Keflin)	1–2 g q4h (adult) 20–30 mg/kg (children)
Pseudomonas Staphylococcus Streptococcus Clostridium	Ticarcillin (Ticar)	200–300 mg/kg q4–6h (adult & children)

SOURCE: *PDR*, 1981.

of or in association with other conditions. It may occur in conjunction with multiple organ failure including the following: hypovolemic and septic shock, abruptio placenta, neoplastic growths, massive blood transfusions, trauma, snake bite, prolonged extracorporeal circulation, malaria, and hepatic diseases (Jennings, 1979; Mant, 1979).

Pathophysiology

Although the exact mechanism is not known, several events can trigger the process of excessive intravascular coagulation. As illustrated in Figure 21.2, activation of the coagulation mechanism through the intrinsic or extrinsic pathway leads to the formation of fibrin. Fibrin then combines with the formed elements of the blood to produce a clot. In DIC, this process occurs rapidly and excessively. These clots, or fibrin thrombi, are deposited in the microvasculature of various organs producing tissue ischemia. At the same time, circulating clotting factors are being depleted. The formation of these clots activates the fibrinolytic system, again in excess. This activation results in the presence of large amounts of fibrin degradation products (FDPs) in the circulating blood. FDPs act as anticoagulants, and this, combined with fibrinogen depletion, accounts for the excessive bleeding seen in DIC (Steedman 1981; Guyton, 1981).

In addition to tissue ischemia and hemorrhage, DIC results in a microangiopathic anemia due to red cell fragmentation by fibrin strands in the peripheral vasculature.

DIC (DISSEMINATED INTRAVASCULAR COAGULOPATHY)

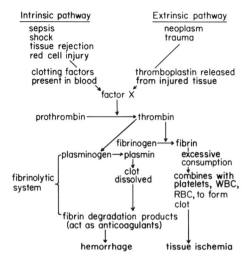

Figure 21.2 The clotting mechanism in disseminated intravascular coagulopathy (DIC).

Clinical Manifestations

The clinical manifestations of DIC reflect both hemorrhagic and thrombotic effects of the condition. Occasionally, the patient simply presents with purpura, petechiae, or ecchymosis; but, more often, the bleeding is more significant. The gastrointestinal and genitourinary tracts are common sites of massive bleeding. Surgical wounds and internal sources are other sites. The patient can rapidly progress to hypovolemic shock when hemorrhage is severe.

Thrombotic manifestations reflect the organs that are affected. When the skin is affected, the patient will exhibit acrocyanosis and thrombotic lesions. Hematuria and renal shutdown may occur in the affected kidney. Gastrointestinal manifestations include distention, ileus, vomiting, and diarrhea. Central nervous system manifestations may range from an altered sensorium to coma and convulsions (Birch, 1978).

Diagnostic Studies

Diagnostic studies in DIC are those that provide information concerning the blood's clotting ability and oxygen-carrying capacity.

The platelet count and fibrinogen level will be decreased because of the consumption of these during clotting. Prothrombin time and partial thromboplastin time will be prolonged reflecting the inactivation of certain clotting factors by the FDPs. FDPs, as expected, would be increased because of the rapid fibrinolysis that occurs in DIC. A lowered hematocrit and hemoglobin are the result of both the bleeding and hemolytic anemia that occur in DIC. The urinalysis will reveal concentrated urine with either gross or microscopic hematuria (Jennings, 1979).

While blood is being drawn for diagnostic studies, the patient's blood should be typed and crossmatched, since whole blood or some blood component is usually needed.

Nursing Care and Related Interventions

Airway and circulatory management follow the guidelines previously discussed. The special consideration in circulatory management is to avoid unnecessary needle punctures. The practitioner with the most expertise should perform a single venipuncture for both fluid therapy and blood sampling. A Foley catheter and a nasogastric tube should be inserted, ideally with minimal trauma to surrounding tissues. The patient should be placed on continuous cardiac monitoring. Hypovolemic shock should be corrected as outlined previously, and therapy should be initiated to correct the underlying disease and eliminate the triggering event (Birch, 1978).

Heparin, though controversial, is the drug most frequently used in the treatment of DIC. Heparin is given in an attempt to stop microthrombosis. Its major action is to prevent thrombin formation that decreases fibrin and FDP formation. To be most effective, it should be given early in the disease. If given late, it can contribute to severe hemorrhage (Mant, 1979). The usual dose is 100 units/kg (50 units/kg in children) every two to four hours intravenously (Hazinski, 1981).

Heparin treatment is monitored by measuring clotting time (Birch, 1978). Its effect can be neutralized by giving 0.75 to 1.0 mg of protamine sulfate for each 100 units of heparin estimated to be in the circulation.

Replacement of consumed clotting factors and platelets is often necessary in severe DIC associated with bleeding. Those components richest in clotting factors are fresh and fresh frozen plasma and cryoprecipitate. In children, hemostatic levels of clotting factors can be achieved with 10 ml/kg of plasma. Platelets may also have to be replaced and generally hemostatic levels are reached with 1 unit/6–8 kg of body weight.

Whole blood, packed red blood cells, or cryoprecipitate may also be indicated. (See Table 21.2 and Table 21.3.) In neonates and small children, exchange transfusion may be the most efficient therapy. The patient with DIC will always be admitted to the hospital. People involved in transporting the patient should be advised of the need for gentle handling, and pertinent information should be communicated to those assuming the patient's care.

CONCLUSION

Not only are hypovolemic shock, septic shock, and DIC sometimes related by their etiologies, but they share many of the same pathophysiologic defects. Consequently, nursing interventions interrelate and overlap.

This chapter prepares the nurse to recognize the emergent nature of these conditions and to make appropriate interventions. An understanding of the content will be reflected in the quality of nursing care rendered.

BIBLIOGRAPHY

Birch, C.: Disseminated intravascular coagulation. *Nursing Times* 74:15-6 (1978).
Buickus, B.: Administering blood components. *American Journal of Nursing* 79:937-941 (1979).
Campbell, C.: *Nursing Diagnosis and Intervention in Nursing Practice*. New York: Wiley, 1978.
Cohen, S.: Nursing care of patients in shock, Part I: pharmacotherapy. *American Journal of Nursing* 82:943-964 (1982).
Crone, R.: Acute circulatory failure in children. *Pediatric Clinics of North America* 27:525-38 (1980).
Eagle, M.: Septicemia proceeding to disseminated intravascular coagulation. *Nursing Times* 74:17-21 (1978).
Eskridge, R.: Septic shock. *Critical Care Quarterly* 2:55-60 (1980).
Estrada, E.: Triage systems. *Nursing Clinics of North America* 16:13-24 (1981).
Franco, R.: Acute DIC. *Critical Care Update* 8:17-20 (1981).
Greene, G.: Management of the child with fever and infection. *Topics in Emergency Medicine* 3:19-42 (1981).
Guyton, A.: *Textbook of Medical Physiology*. Philadelphia: Saunders (1981).
Hardaway, R.: Expansion of the intravascular space in severe shock. *American Journal of Surgery* 142:258-261 (1981).
Hazinski, M.: Critical care of the pediatric cardiovascular patient. *Nursing Clinics of North America* 16:671-97 (1981).
Hoffman, J.: External counterpressure & the MAST suit: Current & future roles. *Annals of Emergency Medicine* 8:419-21 (1980).
Jennings, B.: Improving your management of DIC. *Nursing 79* 9:60-7 (1979).
Johansen, B. L.: Third space loss. *Focus AACN* 7:34-36 (1980).
Leser, D.: Synthetic blood; a future alternative. *American Journal of Nursing* 82:452-6 (1982).
Lyon, S.: Critical care of the child with multi-trauma. *Nursing Clinics of North America* 16:657-70 (1981).
Mant, M.: Severe acute DIC: A reappraisal of its pathophysiology, clinical significance, and therapy based on 42 patients. *American Journal of Medicine* 67:557-63 (1979).
McSwain, N.: Objective approach to the management of shock. *Comprehensive Therapy* 7:7-13 (1981).
Miller, H.: Therapy for septic shock. *Comprehensive Therapy* 5:26-32 (1979).
Physicians' Desk Reference. 35th ed. Medical Economics, 1981.
Porth, C.: *Pathophysiology: Concepts of Altered Health States*. Philadelphia: Lippincott, 1981.
Robinson, W.: Fluid therapy in hemorrhagic shock. *Critical Care Quarterly* 2:1-13 (1980).
Rothstein, R.: Hemorrhagic shock in multiple trauma. *Topics in Emergency Medicine* 1:29-40 (1979).
Rucker, R.: Monitoring critically ill children. *Topics in Emergency Medicine* 3:1-6 (1981).
Shatney, C.: Pathophysiology and treatment of circulatory shock. In D. Zschoche (ed.): *Comprehensive Review of Critical Care*. St. Louis: Mosby, 1981, pp. 713-53.
Shoemaker, W. C.: Fluid therapy in emergency resuscitation: Clinical evaluation of colloid and crystalloid regimes. *Critical Care Medicine* 5:367-72 (1981).
Sugarman, H.: Gram negative sepsis. *Current Problems in Surgery* 18:(1981).

Steedman, R.: Postoperative complications in the adult cardiac surgical patient. In D. Zschoche (ed.): *Comprehensive Review of Critical Care*. St. Louis: Mosby, 1981, pp. 379–99.

Thurer, R.: Autotransfusion and blood conservation. *Current Problems in Surgery* 3:100–56 (1982).

Walkerle, J.: Antishock garments. *Critical Care Quarterly* 2:15–25 (1980).

Wiles, J.: The systemic response: Does the organism matter? *Critical Care Medicine* 8:55–61 (1980).

Zamora, R.: Management of hemorrhagic shock. *Hospital Medicine* 15:7–29 (1979).

22

Chest Trauma

Judy Jo Wells-Mackie

After completing this chapter, the reader will be able to do the following:

1. Triage a patient experiencing chest trauma.
2. Give discharge instructions for the patient with rib injuries.
3. List the usual cause of sternal fractures and two commonly associated injuries.
4. Describe the pathophysiology of a pneumothorax and how that injury can progress to a tension pneumothorax.
5. Describe how a nurse assists with chest tube insertion.
6. List the nurse's responsibilities in monitoring a patient with a chest tube.
7. Define *flail chest* and describe the breathing pattern of a patient who has this injury.
8. Describe the major injury associated with a flail chest and the clinical manifestations of this injury.
9. Describe the clinical manifestations that lead to the diagnosis of tracheobronchial and esophageal injuries.
10. Describe the injury and clinical manifestations of a patient with a myocardial contusion.
11. Describe how a pericardial tamponade interferes with the pumping action of the heart and the signs and symptoms that result.
12. List the nurse's responsibilities in performing a pericardiocentesis.
13. Describe the usual presentation of a patient subsequently found to have major tears or holes in the myocardium or great vessels.

Chest trauma is one of the most urgent problems dealt with by the emergency department nurse. All patients with chest trauma must be considered critically ill until proven otherwise. Structures in the thoracic cavity that may be traumatized include the heart, lungs, airway, great vessels, sternum, and ribs. Gunshot wounds, stabbings, and injuries from high-speed motor vehicle accidents are common causes of chest trauma. Chest trauma is the major cause of death in 25 percent of all trauma cases and a factor contributing to death in 25–50 percent of accidents (Dougall, 1977).

Chest injuries that are life-threatening and considered emergent include sucking chest wounds, pneumothorax, tension pneumothorax, hemothorax, flail chest, pericardial tamponade, penetrating heart wounds, and great vessel rupture or tears. Chest injuries that are life-threatening, but may not present with immediate problems with airway, breathing, or circulation, include tracheobronchial tree rupture, esophageal rupture, diaphragmatic rupture, pulmonary contusion, and myocardial contusion (Kohn, 1979).

TRIAGE

Subjective Data

The patient with major chest trauma is often unconscious or unable to relate information about his injury. If the patient cannot answer questions, the nurse should obtain history about the injury and the patient from the patient's relatives, paramedics, or the police. Information about the incident, the vehicle, the instrument used, or anything contributing to the trauma is pertinent.

If the patient is awake, listen to the person's own account of the incident to obtain detailed information about the mechanism of trauma and the forces involved. Ask the patient about breathing difficulty and pain on inspiration or expiration, and note the presence or absence of coughing, choking, hematemesis, hoarseness, and dysphagia.

Objective Data

The patient with immediate life-threatening chest trauma is identified by major alterations in the basic vital signs of respirations, pulse, or blood pressure. Life-threatening chest injuries and the underlying physiological causes of those injuries are not always immediately obvious. A patient with potentially life-threatening chest injuries may not initially have major alterations in vital signs. As the injury develops and pathophysiological changes occur, however, major alterations in basic vital signs appear. Examples of these injuries are a gunshot wound in which the bullet is lodged near a major vessel, a developing pericardial tamponade, or a myocardial contusion.

To ensure that the patient has an adequate airway, assess chest movement, including rate, rhythm, depth, and symmetry of respirations. Check the carotid or femoral pulse for rate and quality, and assess the skin for cyanosis or diaphoresis, which signals respiratory or cardiovascular compromise.

After ensuring stabilization of the airway, breathing, and circulation, the nurse makes an additional, detailed assessment to assess the structures injured that will require treatment. Wound size, location, associated ecchymosis, abrasions, and lacerations suggest the possibility of internal injuries. Inspect the chest and neck, looking for distended neck veins, tracheal deviation, substernal and intercostal retractions, and accessory muscle breathing. Respiratory sounds should be auscultated and documented, but they may be deceptive in chest trauma. Decreased sounds, for

TRIAGE

example, may indicate a pneumothorax or hemothorax or merely the patient splinting from pain. Listen in particular for stridor, sucking, and the presence or absence of bilateral and equal breath sounds. Heart sounds are also auscultated for extreme abnormalities and to obtain a baseline for future assessment.

The chest is palpated for the presence of subcutaneous emphysema, which indicates an air leak from the pulmonary tree or esophagus. Gently palpate to elicit any point tenderness and stress the rib cage manually with firm pressure laterally and anteriorly-posteriorly to elicit instability and pain.

Assessment and Planning

The ABCs—airway, breathing, and circulation—are the immediate priorities. Each injury has some influence on the heart's ability to pump blood or the lungs' ability to exchange air or oxygenate blood (Kohn, 1979). Conditions that do not permit normal cardiac or pulmonary functions must be corrected immediately. Secure the airway (for more detail, see Chapter 5). In chest trauma, never hesitate to administer oxygen, especially for the combative patient who may be hypoxic.

Patients with chest injuries are given highest priority, including arrangements for immediate care. Immediate interventions such as covering open chest wounds, splinting a flail chest, or stabilizing any penetrating object must be instituted. (Table 22.1 contains two examples of triage notes for patients with chest trauma.)

TABLE 22.1 Examples of Triage Notes for Patients Experiencing Chest Trauma

S: 30 yo WM states, "A car hit me on my arm and chest" app. 20 min PTA, c/o pain in Ⓛ chest area with movement, breathing, and coughing. States he coughed up pink sputum, denies loss of consciousness. NKA, PMH: smokes two packs a day × 10 yrs. History by paramedics of a small car falling from 2 ft height onto chest and Ⓡ arm, removed after 5 min.

O: Arrives by ambulance, awake, alert, oriented × 3, pale, diaphoretic, RR 36 shallow. Able to move Ⓡ arm but splinting because of pain, no paradoxical chest movement, bilateral breath sounds with wheezing, monitor en route = NSR. P 110 regular, BP 96/60.

A: Blunt chest trauma, R/O myocardial and pulmonary contusion, rib fractures, pneumothorax.

P: Surgical evaluation, O₂ 6 l/min nasal prong, cardiac monitor. Admit exam room now.

S: Paramedics relate history of app. 36 yo WM with gunshot wound to chest app. 6 min before their arrival on scene. PMH: unknown, allergics unknown.

O: GSW Ⓛ chest third intercostal space, RR 6 shallow, carotid pulse weak, 180, BP unobtainable. Unconscious, diaphoretic, pale and cool to touch.

A: GSW Ⓛ chest.

P: Surgical evaluation, immediate resuscitation.

FRACTURED RIBS

Pathophysiology

Normal ventilation depends on an intact chest wall. Minor chest trauma can lead to fractured ribs; however, trauma that fractures more than three ribs is considered significant (Vukich and Markovchick, 1983). Most commonly, the fourth through ninth ribs are fractured; if simple fractures, they heal spontaneously in three to six weeks. In the elderly, the lower ribs are frequently fractured in a fall because of inelasticity of the bones. If the first or second ribs are fractured, suspect injuries of adjacent structures. Severe forces are necessary to fracture the first and second ribs because they are protected by the clavicle and scapula. Any fractured rib is a clue to search for signs of associated injuries, such as a subclavian artery laceration, hemothorax, pneumothorax, lung contusion, or myocardial contusion.

Clinical Manifestations

The diagnosis of rib fracture is made by patient history and physical findings that include point tenderness, ecchymosis, crepitus, muscle spasm over the injured area, pain at the fracture site from anterior-posterior stress pressure, and increased pain with deep inspiration. Many single-rib fractures are not noticeable on x-ray films; therefore, if done, x-ray examinations are used to rule out complications, such as pulmonary contusions, pneumothorax, or hemothorax. Patients with rib fractures can maintain adequate oxygenation by using their respiratory reserve, unless other pulmonary injuries exist. If the patient's history mentions a preexisting pulmonary disease such as emphysema, respiratory reserve may not be sufficiently able to compensate. The patient with a costochondral separation presents as though he had a rib fracture; however, his pain will persist for weeks longer because of poor vascularity and the extended healing time of cartilage. The differential diagnosis between a rib fracture and costochondral separation is rarely made. Because the patient with a costochondral separation will not exhibit evidence of injury on a chest x-ray film, the diagnosis is made by findings on physical examination and the absence of a rib fracture on the chest x-ray film.

Nursing Care and Related Interventions

Completely undress the patient, observe the person's respiratory effort, and count the person's respirations. The patient with a rib fracture is usually most comfortable in a Fowler's position. Palpate and inspect the chest wall and apply manual anterior-posterior and lateral pressure to elicit pain. If the patient has a history of pulmonary disease, supplemental oxygen may be ordered. A chest x-ray film is usually obtained.

Patients with simple, nondisplaced fractures are usually discharged from the emergency department with analgesics. If a jagged or misplaced fracture is palpated or if the patient has a history of pulmonary disease, the person may require temporary hospitalization for observation of possible complications and for pulmonary therapy. Chest binders or tape dressings may decrease pain, but they are rarely applied because they promote hypoventilation by restriction of chest wall movement. This restriction leads to atelectasis and pneumonia.

Discharge Planning

Upon discharge, the patient with a rib fracture must be instructed about the use of analgesics prescribed. When used properly, analgesics should minimize pain, promote rest, and permit normal breathing. The need for adequate pulmonary function and instructions to cough and deep breathe while splinting the chest must be stressed. The patient should be told to return to the emergency department if pain either increases or is unrelieved by the analgesics prescribed; if the person is coughing up blood or thick yellow-green sputum; if the person is short of breath or unable to catch his breath; or if the person has chills and fever.

STERNAL FRACTURES

Pathophysiology

Sternal fractures rarely occur because of the tremendous force required to create them. The usual history is of a patient who hits his chest directly on a steering wheel in a high-speed deceleration accident. Sternal fractures rarely occur alone without an associated injury. Mortality results from the associated injuries, such as myocardial contusion, pulmonary contusion, cardiac rupture, or cardiac tamponade.

Clinical Manifestations

The patient who presents in the emergency department with a probable history for a sternal fracture will have point tenderness, extreme pain with inspiration and expiration, and possibly sternal ecchymosis. Additional signs and symptoms will be consistent with the associated injuries (see the following sections for more detailed information). The diagnosis of sternal fracture is confirmed with chest x-ray examination.

Nursing Care and Related Interventions

After initial resuscitation and stabilization, nursing care consists of careful monitoring of vital signs and cardiac rate and rhythm. Fowler's position will ensure the most comfort and maximum respiratory excursion. The patient will be admitted for observation of associated injuries, such as myocardial contusion, which may produce cardiac dysrhythmias.

PNEUMOTHORAX AND TENSION PNEUMOTHORAX

Pathophysiology

A *pneumothorax* is defined as air in the pleural space of the lung causing a loss of the normal state of negative pressure. When the pressures inside and outside the pleural space are equal, the lung is unable to expand normally, so that it partially or totally collapses. A pneumothorax may develop spontaneously or because of trauma to the lung, tracheobronchial tree, or esophagus.

A pneumothorax that progresses by continually allowing air to enter the pleural space on inspiration, but not allowing that air to escape on expiration, is a *tension pneumothorax*. Flap-type injuries often allow air to flow in only one direction. As the tension progresses, intrathoracic pressure increases, the lung collapses, and the heart vessels and trachea are compressed to the unaffected side of the chest creating a mediastinal shift. With this shift of the heart, great vessels, esophagus, trachea, and lungs, venous return to the right atrium and ventricle decreases, and blood is not adequately circulated. The patient experiences hemodynamic and respiratory compromise.

Clinical Manifestations

The patient with a pneumothorax will complain of dyspnea, pain, and the inability to catch his breath. Upon examination, the patient will have unequal or decreased breath sounds on auscultation, hyperresonance on percussion, and decreased fremitus on palpation. The patient may be cyanotic depending on the percentage of collapsed lung, the person's ability to compensate, and associated injuries. The chest x-ray film shows a collapsed lung.

In addition to these classic signs and symptoms of a pneumothorax, the patient with a tension pneumothorax will demonstrate hemodynamic and respiratory compromise manifested by distended neck veins, shock, and extreme shortness of breath. The patient may also exhibit extreme dyspnea, possible paradoxical chest movement, tracheal deviation to the unaffected side, and cyanosis. A chest x-ray film reveals a mediastinal shift.

Nursing Care and Related Interventions

Place the patient with a pneumothorax in a semi-Fowler's position. Administer approximately 5 l of oxygen via nasal cannula or mask. If the patient is stable after assessing the amount of respiratory distress demonstrated by his vital signs, the diagnosis is confirmed by chest x-ray examination. A small pneumothorax is best seen on an end expiration x-ray film. If the patient is unstable, decompensating, and a pneumothorax is suspected from physical examination before x-ray examination, a chest tube is inserted by a physician in the affected pleural space and is attached to a water seal chest drainage device, which recreates the intrathoracic negative pressure and allows the lung to reexpand.

Explain the procedure of chest tube insertion to the patient and provide emotional support. If sufficient time exists and the patient's condition is stable, written consent must be obtained. The skin is prepped with iodine soap, and a local anesthesia is infiltrated. A size 24 French-scale chest tube is used for most adults with a pneumothorax and smaller sizes for children. Silk suture, petroleum-impregnated gauze, adhesive tape, and an instrument tray for a closed thoracotomy are also required. The nurse is responsible for setting up a chest tube drainage system to underwater seal with 15–20 cm of water suction. A follow-up chest x-ray film is always obtained immediately after placement of the chest tube.

If a patient complains of shortness of breath after the lung is reexpanded, an arterial blood gas reading may be obtained. This test will determine whether the shortness of breath is the result of a low partial pressure of oxygen caused by the pneumothorax. If a patient has an altered level of consciousness or is unconscious in combination with a pneumothorax, an arterial blood gas (ABG) study should be obtained. This procedure is necessary because in the unconscious patient mentation cannot be assessed to judge adequate oxygenation.

If the patient presents with tension in the thoracic cavity causing hemodynamic and respiratory compromise and near cardiorespiratory arrest is observed, the tension must be relieved immediately or the patient will indeed suffer arrest. The tension is relieved by inserting a 16-gauge or larger gauge needle over the top of the fifth rib at the anterior axillary line or over the top of the third rib at the midclavicular line on the affected side. With relief of the tension, air will rush out, and the patient's condition, as evidenced by vital signs, should immediately improve. If the patient's condition does not improve, repeat the procedure on the other side. After relief of the tension, a chest tube is inserted to reexpand the lung and to prevent reformation of the tension pneumothorax. Oxygen is administered, and the patient is prepared for admission.

HEMOTHORAX

Pathophysiology

A hemothorax is the collection of blood in the pleural space of the chest cavity usually in combination with air, a hemopneumothorax. The amount of blood may vary from 50 cc to a near exsanguinating hemorrhage of 1,000–2,000 cc, depending on the type of injury. A hemothorax is a common cause of hypovolemic shock in chest trauma, and it also creates many other problems because of the pressure placed on the lung.

Clinical Manifestations

The patient with a hemothorax presents with the same symptoms as though he had a pneumothorax and, if extreme, a tension pneumothorax. In addition, the patient may show signs of shock from hypovolemia. On percussion, dullness is elicited because of the presence of blood. The chest x-ray film shows a fluid line if the patient is upright when it is taken.

Nursing Care and Related Interventions

Initial resuscitation includes oxygen administration, fluid replacement through establishment of several intravenous life lines, reexpansion of the lung through chest tube placement, and drainage of the blood. A size 36 to size 40 French-scale chest tube for an adult or smaller size appropriate for a child is inserted in the fifth or sixth intercostal space on the midaxillary line to drain blood.

If the injury causing the hemothorax is potentially life-threatening or vital signs indicate deterioration, maintain two intravenous lines in the upper extremities with at least size 16 gauge or larger angiocaths. (Cardiac dysrhythmias are managed as described in the chapter on medical cardiac illnesses.) Consider the possible development of acidosis with shock and administer sodium bicarbonate if needed.

In addition, most important is the serial documentation of vital signs, which may include central venous pressure monitoring. Obtain an immediate baseline hematocrit, then monitor cardiac rate and rhythm and urine output. Consider hypothermia with massive fluid resuscitation; obtain a rectal temperature; use warm blankets, warm crystalloids, and warm blood.

Chest tube placement may be the only treatment required to decrease active bleeding because of the pressure on the pleural surfaces (Kohn, 1979). In addition to assisting with insertion of the chest tube, it is the nurse's responsibility to measure and record the amount and character of chest drainage. If there is an initial 1,000 cc of blood in the chest (Kohn, 1979) or 200 cc of blood drainage per hour for 24 hours (Budassi, 1981), a thoracotomy is required to stop the bleeding. If, after insertion of the chest tube, the bleeding is severe and the patient continues in shock despite crystalloid and colloid fluid resuscitation, an open thoracotomy may be performed in the emergency department by qualified physicians to identify and stop the source of bleeding (Kohn, 1979). Autotransfusion is used, for example, to treat the patient exsanguinating from a hemothorax. The blood is collected in a sterile fashion from the chest, treated to prevent coagulation, and retransfused into the patient. The patient is then prepared for the operating room for a thoracotomy to be performed so that the bleeding source may be identified and the bleeding stopped.

FLAIL CHEST

Pathophysiology

A *flail chest* is defined as having two or more ribs fractured in two or more places. This multiple fracture results in a free-moving or floating segment of the rib with subsequent paradoxical movement of the chest wall during respiration. The flail segment responds to intrathoracic forces created during respiration and does not aid in respiration. On inhalation, the intrathoracic negative pressure or vacuum increases, drawing the flail segment inward. On exhalation, the intrathoracic positive pressure pushes the flail segment outward. This movement, called *paradoxical,* increases the work of breathing. Ventilation and subsequent oxygenation of blood are significantly hampered. Tremendous forces are required to create a flail chest, and an associated pulmonary contusion is almost always present. Some researchers claim that the respiratory compromise with a flail chest is from the underlying pulmonary contusion, not from the paradoxical movement. Trinkle (1975), for example, supports this conclusion with his studies on dogs, where flail chests were surgically created without the underlying lung trauma that failed to cause severe respiratory disturbance. This phenomenon is also shown postsurgically in a patient with a pectus excavatum repair in which a flail segment is created with little or no resulting pulmonary compromise (Vukich and Markovchick, 1983).

In addition to the pulmonary contusion associated with the flail chest injury, the patient experiences pain with breathing. Consequently, the patient hypoventilates leading to hypoxemia from decreased tidal volume and atelectasis.

Clinical Manifestations

A muscle spasm over the flail segment may initially splint the paradoxical movement, and many flail chest injuries are missed in the emergency department. In addition, a flail chest injury may also be missed when practitioners focus on other aspects of the resuscitation, or if the patient is not completely undressed and insufficient time is taken to observe respirations and the classic paradoxical movement. The patient with a flail chest will have symptoms of hypoxia, which include a rapid shallow respiratory rate, pallor, cyanosis, diaphoresis, and confusion. Subcutaneous emphysema may be present around the fracture sites.

Nursing Care and Related Interventions

After maintenance of the airway, breathing, and circulation, the patient with a flail chest should be placed on high-flow oxygen and a large-bore intravenous line should be established with Ringer's lactate (RL) or normal saline (NS). The initial treatment for a flail chest is to stabilize the chest wall by placing the patient on his injured side in a semi-Fowler's position, or by applying manual pressure, or by securing sandbags to the flail segment to reduce the paradoxical movement. The patient should be constantly monitored for the possible development of a pulmonary contusion or pneumothorax.

Internal stabilization of the flail segment may be done by intubation and mechanical ventilation. Some controversy exists about the appropriate time to intubate the patient with a flail chest. In general, the patient is intubated if there is extensive chest wall damage in which eight or more ribs are fractured, a poor respiratory effort, associated hypovolemic shock, previous pulmonary disease, or the patient is older than 65. The patient is not intubated if arterial blood gas studies show that the patient's Pa_{O_2} remains above 60 mm Hg on 100 percent oxygen (at sea level) and blood pressure and pulse are stable (Vukich and Markovchick, 1983; Wilson, 1977).

External stabilization, frequently used in the past, is rarely used now. External stabilization is done by fixation of the flail segment with towel clamps and weights. The patient with a flail chest is admitted and monitored closely for complications and decompensation.

TRACHEOBRONCHIAL INJURIES

Pathophysiology

Tracheobronchial injuries, most commonly involving the mainstem bronchus, are caused by blunt trauma, or by a penetrating gunshot wound, or by a stab wound. Because these injuries are uncommon, to be found they must be suspected. If a tension pneumothorax does not respond to chest tube insertion, a tracheobronchial tear is likely. This injury can also occur with the fracture of one of the first three ribs (Kohn, 1979; Wilson, 1977).

Clinical Manifestations

The patient with a tracheobronchial injury will exhibit any combination of the following signs and symptoms in association with chest trauma: partial airway obstruction, atelectasis, hemoptysis, progressive subcutaneous emphysema, or a tension pneumothorax.

Nursing Care and Related Interventions

Oxygen is administered, an intravenous line of RL is established, and the patient is placed in a semi-Fowler's position. Diagnosis of the injury is done most effectively with a bronchoscopy, which may be done either in the operating room or in the emergency department, and the nurse must reassure the patient and assist with this procedure. After a diagnosis is made, surgical repair is completed as soon as possible. The patient and significant others must be reassured and the patient prepared for surgery.

ESOPHAGEAL INJURIES

Pathophysiology

The esophagus is protected by its position deep in the mediastinum and by surrounding structures. It may be ruptured with blunt chest trauma, or perforated from gunshot wounds or, less commonly, from stab wounds. Esophageal rupture is rarely an isolated injury and, therefore, is frequently overlooked. Perforation of the esophagus is rapidly fatal because of infection of the mediastinum leading to shock and respiratory failure.

Clinical Manifestations

Because the injury rarely occurs in isolation, the symptoms of esophageal rupture are frequently masked by other chest trauma. The patient will complain of pain along the course of the esophagus, coughing and choking, hematemesis, hoarseness, dysphagia, and dyspnea. During examination, subcutaneous emphysema may be found. The patient develops a mediastinitis and eventually sepsis with cardiovascular collapse (Hurst, 1983). On chest x-ray examination, the signs of esophageal rupture are mediastinal widening, pneumomediastinum, pulmonary contusions, and subcutaneous emphysema.

Nursing Care and Related Interventions

Suspecting an esophageal rupture, performing an examination, and completing studies, such as laboratory analysis of pleural fluid, chest x-ray examination, esophagram, and endoscopy to rule out a rupture, are the main activities of emergency care. Performing careful nasogastric suction to minimize additional trauma to the esophagus, establishing an intravenous lifeline, monitoring vital signs, administering antibiotics, and preparing the patient for surgery are the functions of the emergency department nurse in the care of the patient with an esophageal rupture.

PULMONARY CONTUSIONS

Pathophysiology

When the lung is traumatized, extravasation of blood into the lung parenchyma causes anoxia and increased tissue permeability. This damage occurs within minutes of the injury and is localized to a lobe or segment of the lung. Frequently the result of deceleration motor vehicle accidents, pulmonary contusions are usually associated with rib or sternal fractures or a flail chest. The hypoxia and CO_2 retention cause the patient with a pulmonary contusion to be symptomatic (Vukich and Markovchick, 1983). Intravenous overhydration in resuscitation can increase the size of the contusion.

Clinical Manifestations

Because the onset of symptoms from a pulmonary contusion is insidious, the nurse must constantly monitor the patient for any developing signs or symptoms. The patient may have dyspnea, tachycardia, tachypnea, cyanosis, hypotension, chest contusions, hemoptysis, rales, and a cough. The diagnosis is made on the basis of suspicion. The chest x-ray film ultimately shows an infiltrate.

Nursing Care and Related Interventions

If a pulmonary contusion is suspected, intravenous fluid volume should be limited to 1,000 cc maximum during resuscitation (Budassi, 1978). The need for volume replacement supersedes, of course, this limitation. After resuscitation, a maximum of

50 cc per hour of intravenous fluid should be administered. The patient should be placed on high-flow oxygen on arrival, and arterial blood gases checked. If the Pa_{O_2} is not greater than 80 mm Hg (sea level) when oxygen is administered, the patient should be intubated and ventilated with positive pressure (Vukich and Markovchick, 1983; Trinkle, 1975). Diuretics such as furosemide and, less commonly, steroids, such as methylprednisolone sodium succinate, may be ordered. Analgesics, such as morphine sulfate, are important; however, the dosage must be titrated to avoid respiratory depression. Monitor the respiratory rate and effort so that analgesia will improve respirations, not depress them.

CARDIAC CONTUSIONS

Pathophysiology

Similar to many other chest injuries, a cardiac contusion must first be suspected to be discovered. Consider the possibility of cardiac contusion in blunt trauma directly to the sternum from steering wheel injuries in motor vehicle accidents, sternal and first rib fractures, and external cardiac compressions in cardiopulmonary resuscitation. Actual pathophysiological changes in a myocardial contusion range from hemorrhage into the heart muscle leading to myocardial cell necrosis and capillary damage, to coronary artery thrombosis and pericardial effusion. Diagnosis of myocardial contusion is made on the basis of the electrocardiogram and on the basis of serum glutamic-oxaloacetic transaminase (SGOT), serum glutamic-pyruvic transaminase (SGPT), and lactate dehydrogenase (LDH) levels. The changes, however, may not be present for 12 to 24 hours post injury. This injury leaves the patient subject to dysrhythmias and to the risk of cardiogenic shock, as though he had suffered an acute myocardial infarction (Budassi, 1978).

Clinical Manifestations

Suspect myocardial contusion in any patient with blunt chest trauma. The condition is often missed because of low suspicion, the presence of other life-threatening injuries, and delay in the onset of symptoms. The patient may have an imprint of the steering wheel and ecchymosis on his chest and sinus tachycardia without hypovolemia or hypoxia (Kohn, 1979).

Electrocardiogram (ECG) changes are the same as those seen in myocardial ischemia, including ST-T wave changes, conduction abnormalities, and dysrhythmias. The most common dysrhythmias are premature ventricular contractions (PVCs), atrial fibrillation, or atrial flutter (Tucker and Markovchick, 1983). The location of the chest injury as it relates to the position of the heart in the thorax determines the type of dysrhythmia. The anterior surface of the right atrium and right ventricle are close to the sternum along with the sinoatrial (SA) node, atrioventricular (AV) junction, bundle of His, and left and right bundle branches. If the right chest is injured, atrial dysrhythmias, SA block, and high-degree AV block result. If the left chest is injured,

PVCs and left- and right-bundle branch blocks can result (Tucker and Markovchick, 1983).

Nursing Care and Related Interventions

Treatment of a patient with a myocardial contusion is the same as treatment of a patient with an acute myocardial infarction. Oxygen should be administered, an intravenous lifeline established, the patient placed in a semi-Fowler's position, the patient's cardiac rate and rhythm monitored, and drug therapy instituted, including supportive drugs and analgesics. A baseline 12-lead electrocardiogram and cardiac enzyme levels are extremely important because these studies will be done serially while the patient is being treated in the intensive care unit.

PERICARDIAL TAMPONADE

Pathophysiology

The mechanism of injury causing a pericardial tamponade is usually penetrating trauma. Any chest injury may result in a pericardial tamponade, which may not manifest itself for a week or more after the injury. A relatively minor wound of the heart may bleed into the pericardial space. The blood either cannot escape or cannot escape as fast as the bleeding occurs, interfering with the pumping action of the heart and with ventricular and atrial filling during diastole (Budassi, 1978). The resultant decreased stroke volume decreases cardiac output and arterial blood pressure. To compensate, the heart rate and vasomotor tone increase, resulting in respective increases in cardiac output and central venous pressure. Finally, compensatory mechanisms fail, causing decreased arterial blood pressure and central venous pressure, which leads to imminent cardiac arrest (Markovchick, 1977).

Clinical Manifestations

The signs and symptoms of pericardial tamponade are similar to those of a tension pneumothorax and may be difficult to recognize in a major resuscitation. The patient will be cyanotic and dyspneic, and a chest x-ray film will show a widened mediastinum. A paradoxical pulse and a drop in the systolic blood pressure greater than 10 mm Hg during normal inspiration will be auscultated. Classically, the patient with a pericardial tamponade has three symptoms, together called *Beck's triad:* (1) elevated central venous pressure greater than 15 cm of water with distended neck veins; (2) hypotension; and (3) tachycardia not due to hypovolemia with muffled heart sounds. Suspect a pericardial tamponade in any patient with a high central venous pressure, hypotension, and trauma to the chest. The patient with these symptoms can deteriorate within minutes.

Nursing Care and Related Interventions

After initial stabilization of airway, breathing, and circulation, a pericardial tamponade should be highly suspected, depending on the location of the penetrating wound or a poor response to vigorous volume resuscitation. Oxygen, a high Fowler's position, and pericardiocentesis are the life-saving treatments.

To buy some time before performing a pericardiocentesis, the adult patient may respond to a 200–300 cc crystalloid fluid challenge or to the application and inflation of pneumatic trousers, which increase venous filling and cardiac output (Kohn, 1979). Increasing cardiac preload can increase cardiac output only to a certain point; after that point, increasing preload will significantly decrease cardiac output.

To assist with the pericardiocentesis, the anterior chest and abdomen must be prepped with an iodine solution. Equipment to assemble includes a 3-inch, 18-gauge spinal needle with a metal hub, a 50 cc syringe and a 12-lead electrocardiogram machine with the four extremity leads attached to the patient and the chest lead attached to the needle hub with an alligator clip. For children, the size of equipment must be adapted to the size of the child.

When the procedure is performed, the spinal needle is inserted toward the apex of the heart. The removal of 10–20 cc of fluid or blood will cause a rapid improvement in the patient's condition as evidenced by an elevation in blood pressure. In performing the procedure, if the electrocardiogram shows ST elevation or PVCs, more than likely the myocardium has been entered. Watch for signs and symptoms, such as dyspnea, chest pain, and cardiac dysrhythmias, indicating complications from the pericardiocentesis. Complications include a laceration of a coronary artery or the lung. Eventually the patient will require an operation for definitive treatment via thoracotomy, and the pericardiocentesis may have to be repeated prior to the operation. Performing a thoracotomy in the emergency department is indicated for the chest injured patient with no vital signs and electromechanical dissociation on the cardiac monitor upon arrival.

MYOCARDIAL OR MAJOR VESSEL RUPTURE

Pathophysiology

Myocardial rupture refers to rupture of the atria or ventricles, pericardium, intraventricular or intra-atrial septum, chordae, papillary muscles, or the valves with the ventricles being the most commonly ruptured (Tucker and Markovchick, 1983). Rupture is caused by blunt trauma and compression of a blood-filled chamber (end of diastole or early systole) and may be delayed after cardiac contusion necrosis or an infarcted area forms. Usually a rupture is immediately fatal, although some patients may make it to the operating room for repair, especially with atrial rupture. In fact, myocardial rupture is the lesion most commonly found at autopsy after fatalities due to nonpenetrating chest trauma (Liedtke, 1973).

Deceleration motor vehicle injuries can cause a rupture or tear of the aorta that most commonly occurs distal to the subclavian artery from shearing forces.

Clinical Manifestations

Depending on the extent of the injury, the patient with a myocardial or great vessel rupture may present in full cardiac arrest with hypovolemia and a hemothorax or with symptoms of a pericardial tamponade. The sternum will be contused and pulmonary edema may be evident. A chest x-ray film will show a widened mediastinum.

Nursing Care and Related Interventions

As initial interventions for airway, breathing, and circulation are carried out, keep in mind the possibility of the diagnosis of myocardial or great vessel rupture. Monitor the central venous pressure. If the patient is near cardiac arrest or has arrested, an emergency thoracotomy may be done to control hemorrhage with digital pressure, until the patient is taken to the operating room for repair. The size and location of the wound determines the prognosis. Even under ideal therapeutic conditions, most cases are fatal. Some physicians believe that a pericardiocentesis before surgery may help to control hemorrhage in myocardial rupture, while others claim it has no value (Tucker and Markovchick, 1983).

PENETRATING CARDIAC OR GREAT VESSEL TRAUMA

Pathophysiology

Stab wounds most often penetrate the myocardium or great vessels; however, the incidence is increasing with gunshot wounds (Kohn, 1979). Many of these patients do not live long enough to make it to the hospital alive because of hemorrhage or ventricular dysrhythmias.

Clinical Manifestations

The patient with a penetrating wound of the myocardium or great vessels will present in impending or frank shock with evidence of a stab or gunshot wound on the anterior or posterior thorax.

Nursing Care and Related Interventions

Aggressive fluid therapy replacement must be started to treat the patient's shock. The airway and breathing, of course, are always checked and supported initially. If signs of a pericardial tamponade are present, a pericardiocentesis should be performed. If fluids do not support the patient in terms of producing a palpable carotid pulse, an emergency thoracotomy is performed. This procedure is necessary to attempt to cross-clamp the aorta or to repair temporarily a major injury to the heart or great vessels. Chances of survival without a thoracotomy are virtually zero. A major thoracotomy tray with the necessary supplies, kept in the emergency department, must always be ready for use.

After a quick prep of the anterior chest with an iodine solution, an incision is made on the side of the injury in the anterior lateral fifth intercostal space, and the ribs are held open with sterile rib spreaders. The descending thoracic aorta is cross-clamped in all thoracic-abdominal injuries associated with massive blood loss. A hole in the heart is blocked with a gloved sterile finger until it can be temporarily sutured with 2-0 silk and a long, thin cardiovascular needle. Bleeding from a pulmonary artery or vein can often be controlled by clamping across the entire hilum (Baker, 1980; Lim, 1981; Moore, 1979).

CONCLUSION

The urgent nature of chest injuries is evident due to the number of life-threatening injuries and organ damage that may occur. When the patient presents in the emergency department, the nurse knows only the potential injuries possible, as assessment and initial treatment to establish the airway, breathing, and circulation are performed. After the patient is stabilized, assessment and treatment of more obscure or delayed onset chest injuries that may also be life-threatening are initiated. It is through suspicion, discernment, obtaining a complete history, and performing a complete physical assessment that many chest injuries are discovered and treated to promote comprehensive emergency care.

BIBLIOGRAPHY

Baker, C.; A. Thomas; and D. Trunkey: The role of the emergency room thoracotomy in trauma. *The Journal of Trauma* 10:848–855 (1980).

Bayer, M., and D. Burdick: Diagnosis of myocardial contusion in blunt chest trauma. *JACEP* 6:238–242 (1977).

Budassi, S.: Chest trauma. *Nursing Clinics of North America* 13:533–541 (1978).

———, and J. Barber: *Emergency Nursing Principles and Practice*. St. Louis: Mosby, 1981, pp. 349–364.

Dougall, A.: Chest trauma-current morbidity and mortality. *Journal of Trauma* 17:547–558 (1977).

Hurst, J.: Esophageal perforation. In P. Rosen (ed.): *Textbook of Emergency Medicine*. St. Louis: Mosby, 1983.

Kohn, M.: Management of chest injuries. *Topics in Emergency Medicine* 1:79–94 (1979).

Liedtke, A., and W. DeMuth: Nonpenetrating cardiac injuries. A collective review. *Heart Journal* 86:687–697 (1973).

Lim, R., and C. Baker: Assuming responsibility for emergency thoracotomy. *The Practical Journal for Primary Care Physicians* 6:23–26 (1981).

Markovchick, V.: Traumatic acute pericardial tamponade. *JACEP* 6:562–567 (1977).

BIBLIOGRAPHY

Moore, E.; J. Moore; A. Galloway; and B. Eiseman: Postinjury thoracotomy in the emergency department: A critical evaluation. *Surgery* 4:590–598 (1979).

Moore, J.: Traumatic asphyxia. *Chest* 62:634–636 (1972).

Patrick, V.: The patient with cardiovascular trauma. *Emergency Nursing* (Update Series) 1:5 (1979).

Simoneau, J., and D. Wolf: Nursing process in cardiac trauma emergencies. In N. Holloway (ed.): *Emergency Department Nurses Association Core Curriculum,* Chicago: EDNA, 1980, pp. 43–54.

Symbas, P.: Chest and heart injuries. In G. Schwartz (ed.): *Principles and Practice of Emergency Medicine.* Philadelphia: Saunders, 1978, pp. 653–673.

Trinkle, J.: Management of flail chest without mechanical ventilation. *Annals of Thoracic Surgery* 19:355–363 (1975).

Tucker, J., and V. Markovchick: Myocardial contusion, myocardial rupture, aortic rupture. In P. Rosen (ed.): *Textbook of Emergency Medicine.* St. Louis: Mosby, 1983.

Vukich, D., and V. Markovchick: Chest wall injuries, pneumothorax, pulmonary contusion. In P. Rosen (ed.): *Textbook of Emergency Medicine.* St. Louis: Mosby, 1983.

Wilson, R.: Nonpenetrating thoracic injuries. *Surgical Clinics of North America* 57:17–35 (1977).

23
Abdominal Trauma

P. Howard Cummings
Sally Pahnke Cummings

After completing this chapter, the reader will be able to do the following:

1. Triage a patient experiencing abdominal trauma.
2. List examples of two basic categories of abdominal trauma.
3. Identify types of blunt and penetrating abdominal trauma, describe their pathophysiology and signs and symptoms, set priorities for triage, and name the initial life-saving interventions.
4. Delineate specific complications resulting from abdominal trauma.
5. List diagnostic studies used for patients experiencing intra-abdominal trauma.
6. Discuss nursing interventions for managing patients who are experiencing abdominal trauma.
7. List routine medications used in the treatment of patients experiencing abdominal trauma.
8. Incorporate teaching in discharge planning for patients who experienced abdominal trauma.
9. List diagnostic studies used for patients experiencing specific types of abdominal trauma.
10. Determine priorities of care for patients experiencing specific types of abdominal trauma.

In the United States, trauma is still the number one cause of death for people under the age of 40. Although the 55 miles per hour speed limit established in 1972 has reduced the total number of injuries, automobile accidents still remain one of the major causes of abdominal trauma (Bouterie, 1981). In fact, the decrease in the speed limit may have contributed to an increased incidence of abdominal trauma, since more victims of accidents prior to the decrease in the speed limit were killed because of high speed during impact.

Abdominal trauma is usually categorized into one of two types of injuries: penetrating or blunt. Penetrating injuries caused by stab wounds or low-velocity missiles create little tissue damage, whereas shotgun and high-velocity missiles cause extensive tissue destruction. Blunt injuries, caused by crushing or shearing forces, usually involve extensive tissue damage (Frey, 1976). Since the major threat to life in abdominal injuries is hemorrhage, prehospital personnel should complete an immediate, brief evaluation of the patient's injuries in relation to the circumstances of the event because these victims are often semiconscious or unconscious when they present to the emergency department. Trained prehospital personnel should also anticipate the need for application of military antishock trousers (MAST) and the administration of intravenous fluids, as well as continuous monitoring of the patient's status enroute to the hospital. The mechanism of injury, surrounding clues concerning other possible injuries, continued patient assessment, and efficient prehospital intervention for immediate life-threatening emergencies are imperative to ensure proper assessment, treatment, and survival of the victim in the emergency department.

TRIAGE

Patients who present to the emergency department with multiple trauma that might involve abdominal organs or with either blunt or penetrating abdominal trauma of any type require a rapid initial assessment. The first priority in any triage assessment is ensuring that interventions for life-threatening emergencies are initiated immediately. All patients who present to the triage area must be rapidly assessed for adequate airway and respiratory and cardiac status. They should also be assessed for external signs and symptoms of internal hemorrhage. In addition, patients eliciting signs and symptoms of shock should be triaged as emergent, and interventions to correct the life-threatening conditions should be initiated immediately.

Subjective Data

An accurate history relating to the patient's injury is vital in assessing whether important complications might develop. If the patient is alert and conscious, the triage nurse identifies as much specific information as possible relating to the circumstances of the injury. Victims of multiple trauma, automobile accidents, fights, explosions, and falls should automatically be suspect for blunt abdominal trauma, even if there are no external signs of injury.

When *automobile accidents* are the cause of injury, the triage nurse attempts to determine whether the victim was driving the car, whether seat belts were worn, whether the victim was thrown from the car, and any history of previous injuries or illnesses involving the abdomen. Victims of *gunshot wounds* are questioned concerning the type of gun and bullet used, their distance from the gun, the bullet direction, and protective clothing worn by the victims. Victims of *stab wounds* are questioned concerning the type of object used, their distance from the assailant, the length of the weapon, and the stabbing direction. Victims of *falls* or *jumps from high places* are questioned concerning the distance they fell, how they landed and on what surface, whether anything was hit while falling, and why the fall occurred (e.g., the victim passed out, was pushed, etc.) (Luckmann and Sorensen, 1980). If the patient cannot give the nurse these details, attempts should be made to acquire the information from a family member, a rescue squad member, a highway patrol person, or anyone else who may know the specific details.

If the patient is conscious and alert, identify precisely how, where, and why the person is seeking assistance in the emergency department. If the patient is disoriented or confused, attempt to identify from a family member why the patient has sought care in the emergency department. This information is often useful in identifying what the patient's priorities are in relation to his injuries and his expectations of the priority of care and treatment implemented by the emergency department nurse.

The triage nurse attempts to assess the patient's current pain status by identifying the location, onset, duration, description, and radiation of the patient's pain. The patient is also assessed for nausea and vomiting. If vomiting has occurred, the number of times, amount, duration, and contents (bile, blood, feces, digested or undigested food) are noted. Identifying the last time and amount the patient ate is also important to know in case surgery is necessary.

Objective Data

The triage nurse should perform a rapid, but adequate, patient assessment that will ensure proper identification of abdominal injuries. *Vital sign measurements* identify the patient's blood pressure, pulse, respiration, and temperature. The patient is *inspected* for signs and symptoms of ascites, distention, Turner's sign (purplish discoloration on the loin), Cullen's sign (purplish discoloration around the umbilicus), old scars, external hernias, visible or pulsating masses, hematomas, abdominal discoloration, ecchymosis, contusions, anal bleeding, abrasions, and entrance and exit wounds. The position currently being assumed by the patient should also be noted. The patient's abdomen is *auscultated* for normal, hypoactive, hyperactive, high-pitched or absent bowel sounds, bruits, and friction rubs over the liver. *Palpation* of the abdomen is completed by performing light, then deep palpation in all four quadrants. The triage nurse identifies the point of most pain, rebound tenderness, direct tenderness, referred pain, guarding, palpable masses, subcutaneous emphysema, organ enlargement, and aortic pulses or masses. The abdomen is *percussed* for liver size and span, abdominal distention, shifting dullness, fixed dullness, bladder size and fullness, and evidence of kidney flank pain.

Assessment and Planning

From the information obtained, the triage nurse should be able to identify any abnormal findings that might indicate intra-abdominal injury. Specific organ injuries might continue to be difficult to determine, but a triage decision or strong suspicion of intra-abdominal trauma of any type requires that the patient be triaged as emergent for further assessment and treatment. (Table 23.1 contains two examples of triage notes for patients experiencing abdominal trauma.)

TABLE 23.1 Examples of Triage Notes for Patients Experiencing Abdominal Trauma

S: 26 yo WM with c/o motor vehicle accident app. 1 hr PTA. Driver of car, wearing lap-type seat belt. Hit head on windshield. "Stomach hurting alot," no LOC, holding abdominal area with hands, and c/o "severe, sharp" RUQ [right upper quadrant] pain radiating to right shoulder, no N/V. PMH: none, NKA, no current meds.

O: Awake, alert, oriented × 3, PERRLA, spontaneous movement all extremities. Abdomen slightly distended with ecchymosis and abrasions across lower abdomen. Bowel sounds hypoactive, no bruits or friction rubs over liver. Intense pain with light palpation of RUQ, no pulses or masses identified. BP 96/60, P 120, RR 24 regular, T 98.2°F oral.

A: Blunt abdominal trauma.

P: Surgical evaluation, admit examination room immediately.

S: 19 yo BF with c/o "Boy friend hit me in my stomach" app. 3 hrs PTA. c/o N/V and pain in LLQ [left lower quadrant], nonradiating and "crampy" in nature, without hematemesis, states she is 4 months pregnant, with vaginal bleeding. PMH: G_1 P_0 AB_0, NKA, vitamins.

O: Awake, alert, oriented × 3, no observable signs of injury upon exam. BP 120/80, P 92, RR 16 regular, T 98.6°F oral. Bowel sounds normal. FHR 180.

A: Blunt abdominal trauma.

P: Surgical/OB evaluation, admit examination room as soon as possible, social worker referral.

PENETRATING ABDOMINAL TRAUMA

Pathophysiology

Penetrating injuries commonly result from stabbing (ice pick, knife), impalement, gunshot (handgun), flying missiles (wires, stones), and shotgun (rifle). Penetrating abdominal injuries are not normally associated with multiple system injuries, but should be evaluated according to the mechanism of injury and the delineation of multisystem involvement. The location of the wound and the angle and relative speed of trajectory provide valuable clues about the amount of intra-abdominal injury. Stab injuries, for example, enter the peritoneum in about two-thirds of the victims, but inflict visceral damage in less than one-third. In contrast, gunshot wounds penetrate the peritoneal cavity more than 80 percent of the time and produce injury to abdominal organs in more than 95 percent of these cases (Moore, 1981). The pattern of injury in relation to the type of weapon causing the abdominal penetration is important to consider, therefore, when evaluating the extent of injury. Examining the victim thoroughly for entrance and exit points is also important when the penetrating missile enters the abdomen at high velocity. High-velocity missile penetration to any part of the trunk or proximal extremities may also ricochet off bones and cause possible intra-abdominal penetration and injury. Suspect ricochet especially if there is no exit wound or if the exit wound is in a precarious location that is not relatively parallel to the entrance wound.

Clinical Manifestations

Emergency department personnel must perform a detailed physical examination while recognizing the possible existence of penetrating abdominal trauma in all trauma patients. Obvious trauma, such as deformed limbs, bleeding, lacerations, burns, abrasions, and altered sensorium, often result in faster interventions from emergency department personnel because they are the most obvious injuries. It is imperative that the "not-so-obviously," masked, or subtle clues in the patient's signs and symptoms not be overlooked. A stone or wire penetrating the abdomen during an automobile accident, for example, is very likely, but also difficult to detect, especially in an unconscious or semiconscious patient; yet this type of injury could easily lead to serious complications for the patient, depending on the amount and type of intra-abdominal injury suffered from the penetration. Obscure injuries within the abdominal cavity may cause a variety of physiologic derangements without producing overt clinical symptomatology.

It is difficult to discuss specific signs and symptoms expected in a victim with a penetrating abdominal injury. Signs and symptoms depend entirely on the type of injury, the involved intra-abdominal organs, other related injuries, and the patient's age and state of health at the time of the injury. The emergency department nurse must observe the patient continuously and closely for any obscure or progressively visible clinical manifestations that may indicate worsening of the person's condition. Meanwhile, appropriate diagnostic studies can be performed to rule out or confirm specific organ injury.

BLUNT ABDOMINAL TRAUMA

Pathophysiology

Blunt abdominal trauma, which usually occurs from a crushing or shearing force, is often associated with extensive tissue damage. The most common cause of blunt abdominal trauma is the automobile collision. Other causes may include blows to the abdomen, falls, or being struck by large-diameter objects. DiVicenti, et al. (1971) concluded that automobile accidents and pedestrian accidents combined accounted for 74 percent of blunt abdominal trauma, blows to the abdomen 14 percent, falls 9 percent, and miscellaneous causes the remaining 3 percent. The study also concluded that the most common type of injury associated with blunt abdominal trauma was a splenic rupture, while a ruptured hollow viscus (most frequently the small bowel) was the second most common type of injury, a ruptured urinary bladder third, kidney lacerations fourth, ruptured diaphragms fifth, and pancreatic injury the least identified type of injury in patients experiencing blunt abdominal trauma.

Another common cause of blunt abdominal trauma is the improper use of lap seat belts. Properly worn, such belts rest low over the anterior iliac spines and should not result in intra-abdominal trauma (Sube et al., 1967). Patients receive trauma from lap seat belts when they are suddenly decelerated in an automobile accident. The force of deceleration causes the body to flex suddenly from the waist, compressing the abdominal contents. The injury occurs either by direct compression between the seat belt and posterior abdominal wall or by entrapment of a short segment of intestine by the seat belt, creating an acute, closed-loop obstruction with resultant circumferential bowel transection or perforation (Williams and Kirkpatrick, 1971).

Clinical Manifestations

Blunt abdominal injuries, which are often insidious, are present in many asymptomatic patients. These injuries, frequently associated with injuries to other organ systems, may obscure the diagnosis and complicate the treatment and physical findings that are often not noticeable until long after the injury has been sustained (Wilkins, 1978). Since the majority of blunt abdominal trauma is also associated with other injuries, the emergency department nurse must always be aware of the likelihood of an insidious or asymptomatic abdominal injury. When external bruises, lacerations, lower rib fractures, or contusions are present, they frequently correlate with internal organ involvement (Perdue, 1981). Automobile accident victims wearing a lap seat belt often present classic signs of abdominal trauma that may signal intestinal or mesentery injuries. These signs include a transverse band of contusion, abrasion, or ecchymosis across the lower abdomen (Perdue, 1981). Other significant signs and symptoms include diminished or absent bowel sounds, pain, hematuria, tenderness, or rebound tenderness, muscular rigidity, and hypovolemic hypotension. The emergency department nurse should suspect major injury even if the patient exhibits few symptoms or signs. When blunt abdominal trauma is suspected, the patient must be carefully observed at frequent intervals, even though the person's condition may appear stable.

DIAGNOSTIC STUDIES

Patients who present to the emergency department with obvious signs and symptoms of shock that are unexplained by other injuries, an enlarged abdomen, or other objective signs of intra-abdominal injuries are often candidates for surgical intervention. Patients with marginal signs and symptoms of intra-abdominal injury, however, require additional diagnostic studies to confirm the presence or absence of injury. Of all the available diagnostic procedures for attempting to identify intra-abdominal trauma, a detailed physical examination repeated at frequent intervals remains the most important step in making an accurate assessment of intra-abdominal injury. The patient who is conscious will be able to relate subtle changes that will indicate a need for further observation and assessment prior to admission or discharge. If the patient is not able to describe his pains, pressures, and feelings to the emergency department nurse, however, other diagnostic adjuncts may be required.

Peritoneal Lavage

Peritoneal lavage is probably the simplest, safest, and most useful diagnostic procedure in both adults and children to help identify the presence or absence of blood in the peritoneal cavity. This procedure has essentially replaced the four quadrant tap because it is considered to be both more accurate and less dangerous for the patient. In addition, this procedure should be used cautiously for all pregnant women, and it is contraindicated if pregnancy has progressed for longer than three months. If abdominal hemorrhage is strongly suspected in a woman who is more than three months pregnant, exploratory surgery is usually indicated.

Precautions must be taken to ensure that the urinary bladder is empty prior to initiating the peritoneal lavage. Thus, a urethral catheter is inserted into the patient prior to beginning the procedure. A nasogastric tube must also be inserted to decompress the stomach and to prevent the possibility of penetration.

Peritoneal lavage is performed by introducing a peritoneal dialysis catheter through a midline intraumbilical incision. After the peritoneal catheter has reached the base of the abdomen (where dependent drainage will collect), it is aspirated. If the return is bloody, the test is positive for intraperitoneal bleeding. If the return is negative, 1,000 ml of Ringer's lactate (RL) solution or normal saline (NS) is instilled into the abdomen of an adult through the catheter. In children, 10 ml/kg body weight of the same fluid is instilled into the abdomen. The patient is then turned from side-to-side, if his other injuries allow. The fluid, which drains from the peritoneal cavity via gravity, is placed into a clear container for visual observation. Traces of blood will often be identified in the returned peritoneal fluid due to the likelihood of invasive trauma during the procedure, but it is considered positive only if newsprint placed behind the clear container *cannot* be read through the fluid (see Fig. 23.1). Flint (1978) reported that diagnosis of significant intraperitoneal injury was confirmed by positive peritoneal lavage in 97 percent of patients harboring such injuries, but he identified only a five percent complication rate, with an acceptably low incidence of false positive and false negative examinations.

Peritoneal lavage fluid may also be examined microscopically to determine whether it is positive or negative for intra-abdominal injury. Lavage fluid that contains more than 100,000 red blood cells/mm^3; and/or contains more than 500 white blood cells/mm^3; and/or contains any bile, intestinal contents, or bacteria; and/or contains amylase in the lavage fluid more than 1.5 times the patient's serum amylase is considered to be positive (Flint, 1978). Most authorities agree that peritoneal lavage will probably *not* detect injuries to the genitourinary system, colon, or extraperitoneal portions of the duodenum and pancreas (Moore, 1981).

Radiography

Radiography of the abdomen has limited use in diagnosing intra-abdominal injuries. It is useful in identifying the presence of free air in the peritoneum or under the diaphragm and is usually completed as a baseline study in case of a ruptured viscus. Radiography of penetrating abdominal trauma is important in attempting to ascertain the direction, depth, location, and possible organ injury resulting from a penetrating

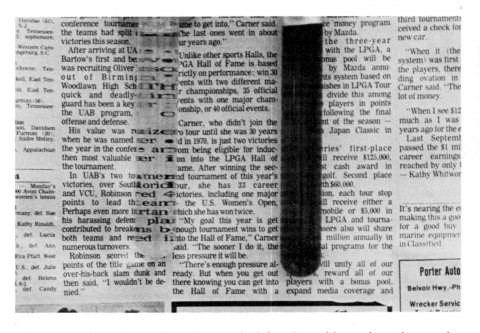

Figure 23.1 A negative peritoneal tap on the left and a positive peritoneal tap on the right.

object, especially if the object is still in place during x-ray examination. X-ray exposure of pregnant patients should be as limited as possible, with the uterus being shielded when x-ray films are required.

Laboratory Studies

Laboratory studies obtained immediately upon the patient's arrival at the emergency department usually are useful only for establishing a baseline. Even with intra-abdominal bleeding, changes in the patient's hematocrit (Hct) and white blood count (WBC) usually occur several hours after the trauma. An initially low Hct, in the absence of chronic anemia, means severe hemorrhage. A normal Hct, however, should not be considered definitive because prior to equilibration the blood remaining in the vascular space may have the same Hct as that leaving it (Moore, 1981). In addition, a high WBC in the range of 20,000–30,000 mm^3 occurs frequently in the multiple-injured patient, so white counts of this magnitude may have little significance (Moore, 1981). A blood sample should also be typed and crossmatched for possible transfusion in case surgery or blood replacement is required. An elevated amylase normally indicates injury to either the pancreas or duodenum, but this elevation takes one to two days to occur and may not be conclusive for or against an intra-abdominal injury. Baseline amylase values will be useful for recognizing a subsequent rise that would be positive for pancreoduodenal injury.

Other Studies

Celiac angiography is useful for diagnosing major liver injuries, but it may not detect some of the peripheral bleeding. When angiography is implemented, it is a specific procedure and has a low incidence of false results (Flint, 1978).

Radionuclide scanning may also be used to diagnose intra-abdominal trauma. This procedure has the advantage of being noninvasive, but it is also time consuming. Large defects of the kidney, liver, and spleen are normally assessed with this procedure.

Blunt trauma to the back and flanks can cause severe retroperitoneal bleeding. Sequential hematocrit determinations and *intravenous and/or retrograde pyelograms* are frequently used in assessing injury to the kidneys, ureters, and urinary bladder. *Cystourethrograms* are also frequently used to aid in diagnosing injury to the urinary bladder, urethra, and ureters.

A *culdocentesis* may be indicated for female patients for the purpose of detecting free intra-abdominal blood that gravitates to the cul-de-sac, the most dependent portion of the peritoneal cavity (Barber and Budassi, 1979). Aspirated fluid is evaluated in the same manner and for the same tests as peritoneal lavage fluid aspirant.

Local Wound Exploration

Local wound exploration is a fairly common procedure in small penetrating abdominal stab wounds. This procedure can easily be performed in the emergency department under local anesthesia. It was widely taught that a penetrating wound to the abdomen required abdominal exploration, regardless of its type. This philosophy is not shared by all. When other diagnostic studies are negative for intra-abdominal trauma, local exploration of the wound may be performed to identify the depth and the possibility of peritonitis or bleeding. If the wound penetrates deeper than the posterior rectus fascia or the internal oblique muscle, peritoneal penetration is presumed and intra-abdominal injury highly suspected (Flint, 1978). If no objective findings of intra-abdominal injury are present, the patient should be admitted for observation for 12 to 24 hours after injury. Any findings of positive intra-abdominal injury or bleeding require exploratory surgery for final diagnosis and treatment.

Most patients who present with gunshot wounds, as well as patients with stab wounds of the back and flanks, frequently require exploratory laparotomy for assessment and treatment. Local wound exploration of these penetrating injuries rarely proves practical because of the increased likelihood of organ damage from extensive missile tracts and deflection of bullets and the close proximity of the liver, spleen, and kidneys to the back and flank. (Fig. 23.2 and Fig. 23.3 present guidelines developed to help the nurse care for a patient with penetrating or blunt abdominal trauma.)

NURSING CARE AND RELATED INTERVENTIONS

Emergency department nurses play a vital role in the initial care and treatment of the patient experiencing abdominal trauma. The nurse must first ensure that life-support

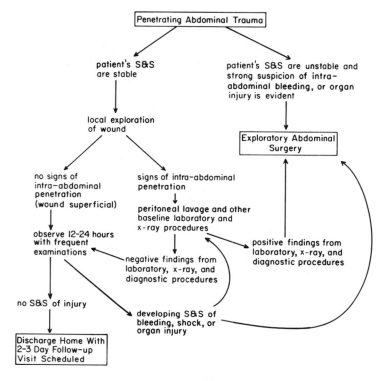

Figure 23.2 An algorithm for penetrating abdominal trauma.

measures initiated in the prehospital setting are continued or immediately implemented when the patient arrives at the emergency department. An immediate and rapid evaluation of the patient's physical condition is vital for determining appropriate life-saving measures to initiate, what physicians to alert, and the urgency of the patient's condition. After the emergency department nurse has ensured the maintenance of or assessed the adequacy of a patient's airway, proper circulation, and adequate oxygenation, additional plans should include an assessment of the patient's trauma in relation to the possibility of internal hemorrhage. Intra-abdominal hemorrhage often accompanies blunt abdominal trauma, especially if the liver or spleen has been traumatized. Take care with multiple trauma patients to avoid excessive movement until a detailed assessment has been performed.

Control of external hemorrhage from wounds is most important. If a patient is experiencing hypovolemic shock, do not allow his blood volume to be depleted from external wounds. Blood volume must be increased with rapid infusion of a Ringer's lactate (RL) solution or albumin until the patient's blood can be typed and cross-matched. It is imperative that two or more intravenous lines using large-bore needles (14 gauge or 16 gauge) be inserted to ensure the rapid infusion of fluid and blood. At this point, whole blood and/or packed cells are administered to replace the estimated amount of blood loss. Hypotension from moderate hemorrhage (500 ml in adults and

NURSING CARE AND RELATED INTERVENTIONS

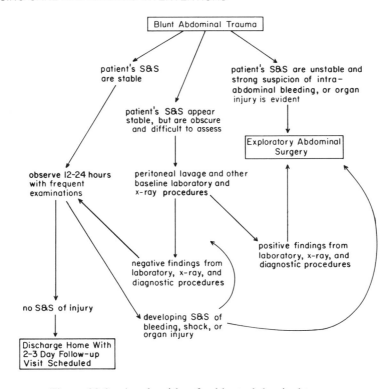

Figure 23.3 An algorithm for blunt abdominal trauma.

250 ml in children) can usually be corrected with the rapid administration of a balanced salt solution during the course of 15 minutes. Blood loss exceeding 500 ml in adults and 250 ml in children requires infusion of whole blood to correct the hemorrhagic hypotension. Antishock (MAST) trousers may also be required to help control intra-abdominal hemorrhage by autotransfusion until fluid deficits can be replaced. Autotransfusion occurs with the application of antishock trousers by shifting the patient's blood to vital organs during the shock phase.

Protruding abdominal viscera are covered with sterile saline dressings to prevent their drying. Never manipulate protruding viscera or make any attempt to replace them in the abdomen; handling the viscera enhances the danger to the patient of infection (peritonitis) and the danger of additional trauma and shock.

An indwelling urethral catheter should be inserted as soon as possible. This procedure allows the nurse to identify and to examine the urine for the presence or absence of blood, which would indicate an intra-abdominal injury to the urethra, bladder, ureters, or kidneys. If an injury to the urethra or bladder is suspected, the physician may consider performing a cystourethrogram prior to inserting an indwelling urethral catheter. It can be performed quite rapidly and may prevent further trauma to an already injured urethra or bladder. The insertion of an indwelling urethral catheter also allows the nurse to monitor the patient's urinary output frequently. The procedure also drains the bladder of fluid, preventing possible penetration of the bladder during peritoneal lavage.

A continuous record of the patient's treatments, fluid therapy, medications, vital signs, assessments, and changes in condition must be kept by the emergency department nurse. Many patients experiencing abdominal trauma do not initially present overt signs and symptoms of intra-abdominal injury. In order to monitor any changes, it is imperative that baseline data be collected when the patient arrives at the emergency department. Data usually include a detailed and repeated physical examination, abdominal and chest x-ray films, complete blood count, urinalysis, serum amylase, type and crossmatch, arterial blood gas and electrolyte studies, serum glutamic-oxaloacetic transaminase (SGOT), total bilirubin, coagulation studies, blood urea nitrogen (BUN), and serum creatinine.

A nasogastric tube is inserted through the patient's esophagus and into the stomach to allow for gastric decompression via suctioning. This procedure helps alleviate the chances of the patient aspirating vomitus in case the person becomes unconscious, or if surgery is necessary.

Continual observation of the patient by the emergency department nurse is mandatory to identify any changes in the patient's condition. A continuous, systematic assessment will allow the nurse to remain alert to changes in the patient's condition that may require quick, decisive, immediate intervention (Perdue, 1981).

For patients experiencing any open wounds from trauma, tetanus prophylaxis must not be overlooked. If wounds are especially dirty, or if the abdomen is contaminated by fecal material from hollow organ rupture, the patient must not only be administered tetanus toxoid but should also receive an injection of tetanus immune globulin—human serum.

Broad spectrum antibiotics (e.g., penicillins, aminoglycosides, and cephalosporins) are frequently ordered to help prevent infection (Cummings, 1983) because bacterial contamination is a common occurrence in patients experiencing abdominal trauma. Complications from infections are significantly decreased if antibiotic therapy is initiated as soon as possible after intra-abdominal injury is suspected.

DISCHARGE PLANNING

One vital aspect of emergency department nursing is patient/family teaching. Patients and families who are informed about the progress and continuance of care in the emergency department consistently demonstrate more patience, understanding, and trust, as well as less apprehension concerning the care and treatment instituted by the emergency department nurse. The nurse must not only be aware of the patient's apprehension and anxiety concerning the necessary procedures, machines, and treatments, but must also consider the apprehension and worry being experienced by the patient's relatives and significant others in the waiting area. Angry and hostile feelings expressed by patients and families toward the care and treatment received in the emergency department often result from their lack of knowledge and information. Reassurance, information, explanation, and instruction are considered constant and vital aspects of the emergency department nurse's role.

Patients who are *admitted for surgery* must be aware of the circumstances surrounding the necessity of the procedure. Patients and/or families must also be in-

DISCHARGE PLANNING

formed of the procedure and possible complications of the surgery prior to their granting signed permission. The emergency department nurse should be assured that the patient or family member signing the operative permit thoroughly and fully understands the reasons for and consequences of the surgery previously explained by the physician. This procedure is especially important for people who speak little English and for people of limited education.

Patients *admitted to the hospital for observation* after penetrating or blunt abdominal trauma must be informed of the reasons for their admission. They should be made aware of the hospital routines, including visiting hours, visitor ages, and the number of visitors allowed in hospital rooms at one time, and they should be provided with directions their visitors will need to locate the hospital. Patients should be told to expect frequent visits by nurses and physicians for repeated physical examinations during the observational period, as well as informing them of other routine procedures that normally occur on the hospital unit to which the patient is being admitted.

Patients who will be *discharged from the emergency department* after abdominal trauma must be taught various signs and symptoms to watch for once they are home. The nurse must be reassured that someone will be staying with the patient for at least 24 to 48 hours after the person's discharge from the emergency department. The patient, as well as the person staying with the patient, must be informed of all possible complications, progressive signs and symptoms of injury, and what to do if the patient's condition begins to worsen. These signs and symptoms include the following:

Significant increases in pain in the abdomen, chest, shoulders, or back.

Persistent abdominal cramping, swelling, rigidity, or tenderness.

Unusual epigastric or back pain.

Difficulty in breathing.

Persistent nausea or vomiting.

Vomiting that contains blood, bile, feces, or undigested food.

Blood in the urine or feces.

Unusual pain when attempting to urinate or to defecate.

Inability to empty bowel or bladder.

Temperature higher than 102°F.

Unusual dizziness or fainting when sitting up or standing up.

Increasing disorientation.

Decreased level of consciousness.

The nurse must make sure that the patient is scheduled for a follow-up visit in two to three days. The patient and family must have arrangements made for transportation for the follow-up visit or for any other emergencies that might arise after the patient has been discharged.

Any prescriptions or medications given to patients should be reviewed with them prior to their discharge. Patients should be encouraged to fill their prescriptions and to take all of their prescribed medications even if their symptoms subside. The use of pain medication should be explained to prevent either underuse or overuse.

Finally, the emergency department nurse should make certain that all discharge instructions are understood, that any questions from the patient and the family have been answered, and that they have a mechanism for seeking more information prior to their leaving the emergency department facility. Only when this planning and teaching is used by the emergency department nurse can it be assured that the role of patient advocate has been met and that the possibility of complications occurring after penetrating or blunt abdominal trauma are detected early enough for the patient to seek further care and intervention.

SPECIFIC ORGAN INJURIES

Liver and Spleen

Pathophysiology
Two of the most common intra-abdominal injuries are those to the spleen and liver. Causes include motor vehicle accidents, blunt trauma, and penetrating trauma. Mortality for spleen and liver injuries ranges from 10 to 20 percent (Dickerman and Dunn, 1981). Mortality is usually caused by exsanguination. Mortality rates are on the decline because of aggressive prehospital care, treatment of shock, advances in postoperative nutrition, and hemodynamic support (Dickerman and Dunn, 1981).

Clinical Manifestations
During assessment, *hepatic injury* is characterized by hypotension, signs of peritoneal irritation, including right shoulder pain and right upper quadrant tenderness, spasm, and guarding. Liver injury should be suspected if these signs and symptoms occur and if lower right rib fractures are present.

Splenic injury should be suspected if left side rib fractures are evident or if a left pneumothorax is present. Symptomatology includes severe upper left quadrant pain, rapidly developing hypovolemic shock, referral of pain to the left shoulder (Kehr's sign), and neck pain related to irritation of the phrenic nerve (Saegesser's sign) (Dickerman and Dunn, 1981). Physical assessment reveals areas of ecchymosis in the upper left quadrant, tenderness and a mass in the splenic region, and percussion dullness that changes with the patient's position (Ballance's sign). Laboratory data reveal a decreased hematocrit (Hct) and an increased white blood cell (WBC) count (Barber and Budassi, 1979).

Diagnostic Studies
Diagnosis of hepatic injury is made based on signs and symptoms as well as on peritoneal lavage that is positive for blood. Peritoneal lavage should be considered along with plain abdominal x-ray films, especially if the patient has multiple injuries and a decreased level of consciousness (Dickerman and Dunn, 1981). Other types of useful diagnostic studies include nuclear scanning, ultrasonography, and angiography.

Diagnostic studies for splenic injury include abdominal x-ray films, which might reveal a medially displaced stomach on a flat abdominal film (Frey, 1976). Peritoneal aspiration and lavage positive for blood are characteristics of splenic injuries. Spleen scanning and angiography may be performed.

Nursing Care and Related Interventions
Treatment of hepatic injuries depends on the location of the injury, severity, and whether the bile ducts have been injured. If the ducts have been injured, as evidenced by hemobilia, a cholecystojejunostomy may be performed with T-tube decompression of the bile ducts (Burt and Nelson, 1981). An exploratory laparotomy may be done to repair liver lacerations or for debridement. Treatment also includes intravenous (IV) fluid resuscitation to prevent hypovolemic shock and central venous pressure monitoring. In liver and spleen injuries, similar to other types of abdominal injuries, the pregnant woman may require fluid resuscitation with packed red blood cells or whole blood to improve fetal oxygenation. Constant fetal monitoring is extremely important.

Treatment of splenic injuries may require a splenectomy. Because of the immunologic role of the spleen and the chance of postsplenectomy septicemia, however, medical management of splenic trauma has proven to be effective, especially in children (Kakkasseril et al., 1982). Central venous pressure monitoring and IV fluid resuscitation are important in patient care and treatment.

Kidney, Bladder, Ureter, or Urethra

Pathophysiology
Kidney injuries may be from blunt or penetrating trauma. They usually are caused by motor vehicle accidents or sports injuries resulting in contusions, lacerations, a shattered kidney, or pedicle injuries (Morgensen et al., 1980). The most common cause of *bladder injury* is blunt trauma (Palomar et al., 1980). *Ureteral injuries* most often occur with a fracture of the pubic arch of the pelvis, which in turn penetrates the ureter. Seventy-four percent of bladder injuries are associated with fractures of the pelvis (Palomar et al., 1980).

Clinical Manifestations
With *urinary tract injuries,* hematuria may or may not occur. Usually there is colicky flank pain and, less frequently, abdominal pain. Shock symptomatology depends on blood loss. Extraperitoneal signs, such as swelling of the anterior abdominal wall, scrotum, buttocks, or perineum, may be present (Frey, 1976).

Diagnostic Studies
Diagnostic studies for urinary tract injuries begin with an intravenous pyelogram (IVP). Choices of further radiological studies are based on the results of the initial IVP and may include angiography, a cystourethrogram, or retrograde cystography.

Nursing Care and Related Interventions
The treatment of blunt kidney trauma usually does not require surgery, but the treatment of penetrating trauma does. Kidney surgery includes repair of lacerations, debridement, and possibly a nephrectomy. *Bladder* surgery would be indicated for the repair of lacerations or rupture. Since *ureteral trauma* is most frequently penetrating, surgical intervention is performed, usually involving an end-to-end anastomosis of ureteral tissue. *Urethral injury* repair has not been very satisfactory because

of the high incidence of stricture and incontinence. Suprapubic drainage followed by a two-stage urethroplasty, however, has proven effective (Frey, 1976).

Aorta and Diaphragm

Pathophysiology
Injuries to the aorta and diaphragm are caused by motor vehicle accidents, gun butts, surfboards, motor vehicle steering columns, lap seat belts, and stab wounds. Aorta and diaphragm injuries are almost always associated with other injuries (Ward et al., 1981). Myles and Yellin (1979) reported that patients with injuries of the aorta have a 52 percent mortality rate. Diaphragm injuries usually occur secondary to penetrating trauma and are more frequently on the left side because the left diaphragm lacks the protection of the liver.

Clinical Manifestations
Aorta injuries are characterized by nausea and vomiting, hypotension, rapid respirations, and other signs of hypovolemic shock. Any patient admitted with a penetrating abdominal wound and hemorrhagic shock should be suspected of having an aorta injury (Myles and Yellin, 1979). Ecchymosis of the midline peritoneum area may be present as well as abdominal tenderness. Distal pulses may or may not be present. The hemoglobin and hematocrit may be normal or decreased.

Assessment of *diaphragm injuries* is sometimes difficult due to associated injuries such as pulmonary contusion and hemothorax (Ward et al., 1981). Patients with diaphragm injuries display signs and symptoms of shock. Respiratory difficulty is evident. Chest x-ray film reveals an elevated diaphragm and/or hemothorax. Angiography or lung scan may be performed.

Nursing Care and Related Interventions
Initial treatment of aorta injuries is important for patient survival. One of the most important factors affecting survival is the presence of a means for rapid tamponade of the hemorrhage. External counterpressure from antishock (MAST) trousers may be used initially. A thoracotomy may be performed for manual clamping of the aorta above the injury until a celiotomy for repair can be performed.

The possibility exists for herniation and subsequent bowel strangulation if diaphragm injuries are not rapidly treated. Treatment consists of a thoracotomy or laparotomy to control bleeding and to repair diaphragm tears.

Pancreas, Stomach, and Intestines

Pathophysiology
Injuries to the pancreas, stomach, and intestines may be either blunt or penetrating. Blunt injuries are caused by motor vehicle accidents, such as the deceleration force exerted by a steering wheel resulting in a shearing force to the abdomen. Penetrating injuries are most often caused by gunshot wounds. Such injuries can cause further

complications, such as bacterial peritonitis. Many injuries are associated with each other because injuries usually involve multiple structures.

Pancreatic trauma can be serious, and it is often associated with other abdominal injuries. Such an injury can occur as a result of impact with a steering wheel in a motor vehicle accident. Pancreatic injury has a morbidity rate of 36 percent and a mortality rate of 20 percent (Karl and Chandler, 1977). The single most important factor leading to morbidity and mortality in pancreatic injuries is a delay in diagnosis. Any patient with a retroperitoneal hematoma should be assessed for a pancreatic injury.

Clinical Manifestations
The symptomatology associated with *stomach and intestinal injuries* is usually related to peritoneal irritation, for example, muscle guarding, rebound tenderness, and hypotension. Edema, crepitus, and microscopic hematuria may be evident (Hunt et al., 1980).

The patient experiencing a pancreatic injury may be in shock and exhibit abdominal guarding and tenderness without signs of pneumoperitoneum. The patient may also complain of epigastric and back pain. However, the patient may be asymptomatic unless the injury causes peritoneal irritation. Symptoms may not develop until 12 hours after the injury.

Diagnostic Studies
Peritoneal lavage is a useful procedure in assessing and diagnosing stomach and intestinal injuries, more helpful, in fact, than any x-ray studies (Hunt et al., 1980). The WBC count may be elevated.

Peritoneal lavage is also a useful tool in assessing and diagnosing pancreatic injuries. Peritoneal fluid should be tested for amylase, the level of which would be elevated if injury to the pancreas is present. Abdominal and thoracic x-ray films and angiography are usually not helpful in assessing pancreatic injuries (Majeski and Tyler, 1980). Computerized tomography scanning and cholangiopancreatography, however, may be helpful (Dickerman and Dunn, 1981).

Nursing Care and Related Interventions
Treatment of injuries to the stomach and intestines usually involves surgery. Prevention of further contamination of the peritoneal cavity is particularly important. Surgical intervention, performed for debridement or to repair lacerations and perforations, may require a resection or stoma formation.

Resection of the distal portion of the body and tail of the pancreas may be the required treatment. Surgical intervention is performed via an exploratory laparotomy or a pancreaticojejunostomy. In addition, IV fluid resuscitation, central venous pressure monitoring, and nasogastric decompression are also necessary.

CONCLUSION

Abdominal trauma is an increasingly common occurrence in the United States. Nurses must be prepared to assess correctly and care appropriately for patients experiencing both blunt and penetrating abdominal trauma. This process is best achieved if the emergency department nurse is proficient in triaging such patients, recognizing patterns of injury and clinical manifestations, assisting with diagnostic studies, developing appropriate nursing plans of care, and actively participating in discharge planning. The nursing process is used in formulating a plan of care and in identifying appropriate interventions for patients suffering abdominal trauma.

BIBLIOGRAPHY

Barber, J. M., and S. A. Budassi: *Mosby's Manual of Emergency Care*. St. Louis: Mosby, 1979.

Bouterie, R. L.: The assessment and diagnosis of the patient with abdominal trauma. *Internal Surgery* 66(1):59–61 (1981).

Burt, T., and J. Nelson: Extrahepatic biliary duct trauma. *Western Journal of Medicine* 134(4):238–289 (1981).

Cummings, P. H.: *Quick Reference of Common Emergency Drugs*. New York: John Wiley & Sons, 1983.

Dickerman, R., and E. Dunn: Splenic, pancreatic, and hepatic injuries. *Surgery Clinics of North America* 61(1):3–16 (1981).

DiVicenti, F. C.; J. D. Rivers; E. J. Laborde; I. D. Fleming; and I. Cohn: Blunt abdominal trauma. *Journal of Trauma*. 11(3):207–218 (1971).

Editorials: Diagnosis of management of pancreatic injury. *Annals of Emergency Medicine* 10(3):172 (1981).

Flint, L. M.: Intraperitoneal injuries. *Heart and Lung* 7(2):273–277 (1978).

Frey, C. F.: *Initial Management of the Trauma Patient*. Philadelphia: Lea and Febiger, 1976.

Hunt, K.; R. N. Garrison; and D. Fry: Perforating injuries of the gastrointestinal tract following blunt abdominal trauma. *American Surgery* 46(2):100–104 (1980).

Kakkasseril, J.; D. Stewart; J. Cox; and M. Gelfard: Changing treatment of pediatric splenic trauma. *Archives of Surgery* 117(6):758–759 (1982).

Karl, H., and J. G. Chandler: Mortality and morbidity of pancreatic injury. *American Journal of Surgery* 134:549 (1977).

Luckmann J., and K. C. Sorensen: *Medical-Surgical Nursing: A Psychophysiologic Approach*. Philadelphia: Saunders, 1980.

Majeski, J. A., and G. Tyler: Pancreatic trauma. *American Surgery* 46(10):593–596 (1980).

Moore, E. E.: Evaluating and managing penetrating abdominal injuries. *Emergency Room Reports*. 2(9):85–90 (1981).

Morgensen, P.; P. Agger; and H. Ostergaard: A conservative approach to management of blunt renal trauma: Results of a follow-up study. *British Journal of Urology* 52(5):338–340 (1980).

Myles, R., and A. Yellin: Traumatic injuries of the abdominal aorta. *American Journal of Surgery* 138(2):273–277 (1979).

Palomar, J.; E. Polanco; and G. Frentz: Rupture of the bladder following blunt trauma: A plea for routine peritoneotomy in patients with extraperitoneal rupture. *Journal of Trauma* 20(3):239–241 (1980).

Perdue, P.: Abdominal injuries and dangerous fractures. *RN* (7):35–37, 84 (1981).

Sube, J.; H. H. Siperman; and W. J. McIver: Seat belt trauma to the abdomen. *American Journal of Surgery* 113(3):346–350 (1967).

Ward, R.; T. Flynn; and W. Clark: Diaphragmatic disruption secondary to blunt abdominal trauma. *Journal of Trauma* 21(1):35–38 (1981).

Wilkins, E. W., ed: Abdominal emergencies: *MGH Textbook of Emergency Medicine*. Baltimore: Williams and Wilkins, 1978, pp. 420–436.

Williams, J. S., and J. R. Kirkpatrick: The nature of seat belt injuries. *Journal of Trauma* 11(3):207–218 (1971).

24
Multiple Trauma

Janet Gren Parker

After completing this chapter, the reader will be able to do the following:

1. Triage a patient experiencing multiple trauma.
2. Identify factors influencing the care of the multiple trauma patient.
3. Discuss the diagnostic studies used in the care of the multiple trauma patient.
4. Prioritize the care of the multiple trauma patient.
5. Discuss immediate interventions necessary in the care of the multiple trauma patient.
6. Discuss the emotional impact experienced in multiple trauma situations.

Trauma is the fourth leading cause of death in the United States, and the first cause of death in people under the age of 40. One-half of childhood deaths are the result of major trauma. *Multiple trauma,* or *polytrauma,* is defined as an injury to two or more body systems. Multiple trauma must be approached in an organized, team fashion to prevent confusion and to aid in organizing the delivery of care.

Advancements have been made in the care of trauma victims. Ambulance attendants are trained and licensed by most states. Established radio communication exists between the prehospital personnel and the emergency department staff. Emergency departments are staffed appropriately and equipped with the necessary supplies and machinery to treat the trauma victim. In most hospitals with intensive care units for continual care of the trauma patient, the nurse-to-patient ratio is usually 1 to 2. Some institutions have even developed trauma units to provide care specifically designed for the trauma patient.

Hicks et al. (1982) revealed that the quality of care of the trauma victim, however, could still be improved. Trauma care delivered in rural emergency departments was studied because 70 percent of trauma fatalities occur in rural areas. Care was measured according to standards developed by the American College of Surgeons committee on trauma and the American College of Emergency Physicians. Approximately 100 patients were studied. Overall, for 70 percent of the patients, care departed in some major way from the standards. Airway control was not adequate in

77 percent of the patients. Ninety-one percent lacked adequate intravenous tube size or correct fluid type or amount. The study concluded that emergency department health care providers needed education in every aspect of trauma care.

The emergency department nurse is a vital member of the team necessary to provide quality care for the trauma patient. To maintain quality and minimize the time involved, this care must be organized. The nurse must ensure that the patient receives the necessary care so that optimal life-functioning is achieved.

TRIAGE

An organized and efficient approach to the sorting of trauma vitims is necessary. Four accident victims may present to the emergency department simultaneously in the event of an automobile collision, for example, all having experienced trauma of some type. The triage nurse must collect data, analyze the data, and determine the priority of care needed in this situation. The data provide the framework for the planning and delivery of care.

Subjective Data

The history of the event that resulted in the injury is of prime importance. If conscious, the patient can relate this information, or it may come from the ambulance attendants, police, or witnesses to the event. The mechanism of the injury is also important. If a motor vehicle is involved, ascertain whether the patient was the driver or the passenger. What was the rate of speed involved? Was it a single car or a multicar accident? The more facts that can be determined about the event, the more likely injuries can be suspected and handled appropriately.

Ascertain if the patient ever had a loss of consciousness prior to or after the accident. Did the patient complain of anything immediately prior to the event? Where is the person complaining of pain now? What symptoms does the person currently exhibit in the emergency department?

Past medical history is extremely important because it may alter the prescribed care of the patient. Record current medications, allergies, and tetanus immunization status as well.

Objective Data

The triage nurse must quickly observe for adequate airway maintenance, respiratory effort, and circulatory status. Document vital signs, such as pulse rate, respirations, and blood pressure. Assess skin for pallor, temperature, and the presence of moisture. Document areas of ecchymosis and assess any extremity with obvious deformities for pulses, pallor, paresis, pain, and paralysis. Also assess the patient's back for injury. Note and document sites of bleeding.

Objects embedded anywhere in the body should be immobilized, not removed.

TRIAGE

Objects should be removed only after everything has been set up to handle the consequences—usually in the operating department.

Prehospital care is documented in the objective data. If an airway maintenance mechanism is in place, an intravenous infusing, a leg splinted, or a pressure dressing on an area, this treatment is documented in complete detail. It is extremely important to document prehospital neck and spine stabilization techniques used in the care of the patient.

Assessment and Planning

By analyzing the subjective and objective data collected, the triage nurse makes an assessment of the patient's injuries and initiates a plan of care. This plan of care includes the patient's priority of care and appropriate nursing interventions. (Table 24.1 contains examples of triage notes for patients presenting to the emergency department with multiple trauma.) A thorough discussion of the care of a multiple

TABLE 24.1 Examples of Triage Notes for Patients Experiencing Multiple Trauma

S: 19 yo WM with c/o being in a single-car MVA app. 30 min PTA. Was thrown out of car through windshield and landed on pavement. Pt. was only occupant of the car. PMH: neg., no current drugs, NKA, last tetanus 5 yrs ago. Now c/o diffuse abdominal pain and pain in Ⓡ leg.

O: Airway, breathing, and circulation stable. RR 20, P 100, BP 110/80. Awake, alert and oriented. Skin without pallor, warm to touch, but slightly moist. Abdomen has ecchymosis over entire upper left quadrant. Ⓡ leg over tib/fib area swollen with ecchymosis. Pulses present, pain present, slight pallor of foot.

A: Multiple trauma, R/O abdominal blunt trauma and fractured tib/fib.

P: Surgical evaluation, admit examination room immediately, monitor vital signs for impending shock due to abdominal injury, splint Ⓡ leg, apply ice to leg and continue to assess presence of pulses in Ⓡ foot.

S: 32 yo construction worker who fell five stories at building site app. 20 min PTA. Safety line broke and patient fell to concrete covered ground feet first. PMH: neg., NKA, current drugs and tetanus status unknown.

O: Comatose, on backboard with C-collar applied. Blood coming from mouth and nose with audible respirations of 40. P 140, BP 80/P. Open fractures of both femurs visible. Distended abdomen and unstable chest wall with decreased breath sounds on the right side. Cyanotic.

A: Multiple trauma.

P: Surgical evaluation, admit trauma room immediately, prepare for adequate airway maintenance and resuscitation of circulatory system. Cover open fractures with saline soaked gauze.

trauma patient follows in the next sections. Knowledge of this material will aid the nurse in performing accurate and appropriate triage.

MULTIPLE TRAUMA

Effective intervention for the multiple trauma patient requires simultaneous and multiple assessment and treatment. A general principle to remember in caring for the multiple trauma victim is the following: Assume that everything that could possibly be wrong with the patient *is,* until proven otherwise. Do not assume everything is fine solely because the patient arrives from another hospital with his intravenous (IV) site wrapped in gauze. A dislocated elbow may be hidden under the gauze with a radial artery tear accompanying the injury. Another principle to remember is this: do not be fooled by the obvious. Do not focus on the profusely bleeding extremity wound while the patient's airway is slowly compromised by a laryngeal spasm.

Trauma patients are utterly dependent on others for survival because of the overwhelming injuries they have sustained. Life-saving measures must be instituted immediately. The nurse must assure the coordination of all personnel, all necessary assessment and treatment procedures, and the emotional support for the patient and the patient's family. This difficult task is not easily accomplished, but it is imperative, for the patient's sake, that effective intervention is done through appropriate teamwork and organization.

Diagnostic Studies

Several general diagnostic studies will usually be performed on patients experiencing multiple trauma. These studies serve as baselines in many situations. They are important, because they help provide a measure of the patient's progress.

Blood studies are done for type and crossmatch, hematocrit, hemoglobin, and blood gas values. These studies will help determine the care necessary in the emergency department. Additional studies may be requested, including electrolytes, glucose, blood urea nitrogen, clotting studies, and drug screens.

Urine samples must be obtained from all multiple trauma patients and tested for the presence of blood. It is best to obtain a voided sample, if at all possible. Catheterization may be traumatic and can cause red blood cells to appear in the urine. Nonetheless, catheterization is frequently necessary to help monitor the hemodynamic status of the patient.

Electrocardiograms may be ordered on patients with chest trauma of any type. Radiographic studies provide important information concerning the extent of injury in the patient. Chest, abdominal, cervical spine, skull, and extremity x-ray films are frequently ordered to help assess the extent of injury. Computerized tomography and arteriograms may be necessary to fully assess the extent of injury. Intravenous pylograms, cystograms, and urethrograms are also used to assess the full extent of injury to the genitourinary tract system.

Nasogastric aspirant and samples of stool should be guiaced to assess for the presence of blood. A peritoneal lavage may be done to assess for intra-abdominal bleeding.

Many of these tests may have to be repeated several times. How many times depends on the condition of the patient, the extent of injuries, and the interventions performed in the emergency department.

Priorities of Care

It is difficult to list priorities of care when dealing with a patient who has suffered multiple injuries. Several events must be occurring simultaneously for the patient to receive adequate care. The care of the trauma patient must include the simultaneous assessment of the patient's airway and circulatory status together with the assessment of all of the other injuries, with appropriate actions implemented after the assessment has been completed. This care is best accomplished by using an alphabetical organization method in the care of the trauma victim (Molyneux-Luick, 1977). Someone must assume the responsibility to ensure that all the steps are done in the appropriate order so that quality care is delivered.

Airway

Adequate maintenance of the airway is always the top priority in multiple trauma. (Chapter 5 discusses airway maintenance in detail.) One important fact to remember is that the airway encompasses the area from the nose to the diaphragm. The thoracic cavity must be assessed for injury and appropriate actions taken to stabilize the entire airway.

Upper airway maintenance includes the use of oral airways, esophageal obturator airways (EOAs), cricothyrotomy, endotracheal tubes, and tracheostomy. Whichever mechanism is chosen, be sure not to hyperextend the neck until a cervical spine fracture has been ruled out. The EOA can be effectively used without hyperextending the neck.

Most life-threatening thoracic injuries are diagnosed by physical examination, not x-ray studies. The patient may even expire if x-ray studies are insisted upon prior to treatment. Table 24.2 lists life-threatening thoracic injuries, their clinical manifestations, and appropriate immediate interventions necessary to maintain the patient's airway.

The patient's airway must be assessed continually to ensure its patency and maintenance. Supplemental oxygen must be employed as quickly as possible and suction readied to help maintain airway patency. Arterial blood gas studies are the only reliable measure of the adequacy of the airway. Clinical observations are not reliable measures.

Bleeding and Shock

An arterial bleed can cause shock and death in minutes. An adult's blood volume may be reduced by 10 percent before any clinical signs of shock are observable. In fact, 20 percent of an adult's blood volume may be lost before blood pressure starts to fall. Maintenance of the blood volume in children is just as tenuous. A rule of

TABLE 24.2 Life-Threatening Thoracic Injuries

Type of Injury	Clinical Manifestations	Interventions
Open, sucking chest wound	1. Cyanosis, sound of sucking, wound in chest wall in front, back, or sides 2. Restlessness 3. Subcutaneous emphysema	Cover immediately with hand or Vaseline-impregnated gauze during expiration, if possible. Chest tube to underwater seal for long-term management.
Tension pneumothorax	1. Cyanosis 2. Decreased chest movement on affected side 3. Shifted trachea	Immediately relieve the tension by inserting 18-gauge needle into second intercostal space on the affected side. Chest tube to underwater seal for long-term management.
Flail chest	1. Difficulty breathing 2. Fractured ribs 3. Unstable chest wall with paradoxical respirations	Stabilize the chest by immediately applying external pressure (sandbag) until the patient can be placed on positive pressure ventilation equipment.
Ruptured thoracic aorta	1. Hoarseness 2. Shock 3. Left hemothorax 4. Tearing chest pain 5. Difference in blood pressure between right and left arms 6. Widened mediastinum	Open the chest and clamp the aorta above the tear, if possible. Patient must be transported to the operating room as soon as possible.
Traumatic asphyxia	1. Bleeding from mouth and nose 2. Purple around face and neck 3. Subconjunctival hemorrhages 4. Visual disturbances	Patent upper airway needed immediately with the patient placed on a respirator. The patient may also need chest tube placement if a hemo or pneumothorax is also involved.
Ruptured trachea or bronchus	1. Hemoptysis 2. Mediastinal shift 3. Subcutaneous emphysema 4. Airway obstructed with blood	Stabilize the airway as quickly as possible, usually with a cricothyrotomy. Place chest tubes as needed to manage pneumo/hemothorax.

MULTIPLE TRAUMA

TABLE 24.2 (*continued*)

Type of Injury	Clinical Manifestations	Interventions
Pulmonary contusion	1. Restlessness 2. Tachypnea 3. Hemoptysis 4. Tachycardia 5. Inability to cough 6. Severe chest pain 7. Hypoxia	Stabilize the airway as quickly as possible. The patient may require ventilator assistance.

SOURCE: Perdue, 1981.

thumb for approximating a child's total blood volume is to use the figure 80 cc/kg regardless of the child's age (Lyon, 1981).

The first intervention in this category is to stop the bleeding. Apply direct pressure with pressure dressings and use pressure points to stop the bleeding. Hemostats may be used to occlude arterial bleeds, but they may cause tissue damage if used improperly. Tourniquets should be used only when applying pressure fails or in the case of a total amputation. The time when the tourniquet is applied must be documented.

Observe continually for signs and symptoms of shock. The patient's skin will become cold, clammy, and cyanotic or pale. The pulse rate will increase, while the blood pressure and central venous pressure fall. In fact, the patient's central venous pressure will change before blood pressure changes.

Occult bleeding can also produce shock. Three to eight units of blood can bleed occultly into the abdomen from a pelvic fracture, three units of blood from a femur fracture, one to three units of blood from a tibia or fibula fracture, and one unit of blood from a humeral, radial, ulnar, spine, or shoulder girdle fracture (Perdue, 1981). Double these estimates if the fracture is an open one.

Immediate fluid replacement is essential. A large-bore (16- to 18-gauge) peripheral intravenous line, as well as a central subclavian line, must be started immediately. The preferred fluid is Ringer's lactate because of its isotonic effect. Blood replacement is the optimal treatment. In the patient receiving blood, the nurse must observe closely for any complications. The blood should be warmed, filtered, and replaced as soon as possible—preferably before the blood pressure starts to fall.

Massive transfusions may cause coagulation disturbances, elevated potassium levels, acid-base imbalance, and ammonia intoxication (Turner, 1982). Hypocalcemia can also result because the citrate in banked blood binds calcium, leading to hypocalcemia or citrate intoxification. This condition can be corrected by giving 10 ml of 10 percent calcium gluconate intravenously for each liter of blood given to the patient. Hypothermia is also a complication of massive blood transfusions. Citrate is metabolized in the liver and excreted by the kidneys. Hypothermia slows this mechanism, thus increasing the likelihood of citrate intoxification.

If the patient has experienced penetrating or blunt chest trauma and continues to be hypotensive, the nurse should suspect cardiac tamponade. Cardiac tamponade is another life-threatening condition that requires immediate intervention. The patient may be restless, have a paradoxical pulse, narrow pulse pressure, and a central venous pressure of greater than 12 cm H_2O. Beck's triad—hypotension, neck vein distention, and distant, muffled heart sounds—is indicative of cardiac tamponade. A pericardiocentesis must be performed immediately to relieve the pressure in the pericardial sac and to allow the heart to maintain an adequate cardiac output.

Consciousness

The level of consciousness is the index of brain damage. The neurological assessment in the emergency department must establish a baseline to monitor intracranial pressure. The patient's response to stimuli should be described and documented. Pupillary size, reactivity, and equality should be continually assessed and documented. Bilateral movement and sensation of the extremities should be assessed and documented. Injuries may result in skull fracture, concussion, contusion, cord concussion, cord penetration and transection, cord fracture and compression, and cerebral edema.

Repeat the neurological assessment and observations as often as necessary to monitor the development of increased intracranial pressure. Remember, however, that, in children especially, hypothermia can complicate and confuse the neurological assessment. Clinical manifestations of increased intracranial pressure are contained in Table 24.3.

Artificial hyperventilation is the immediate intervention for increased intracranial pressure. Hyperventilation decreases the CO_2 levels in the brain, causing cerebral vasoconstriction. This vasoconstriction allows the fluid causing the increased pressure more space to expand, thereby actually decreasing the intracranial pressure, at least temporarily. Osmotic diuretics and steroids may also be used to help decrease intracranial pressure. Osmotic diuretics are fast-acting but may cause rebound. The acute effect of steriods is controversial, but they are felt to have some positive long-term effect on intracranial pressure.

Burr holes may be used as an intervention after hyperventilation and medication therapy are prescribed. Holes are drilled (or burred) into the cranium to release the accumulated pressure. Hematomas are frequently evacuated in the emergency department by the use of burr holes to help prevent permanent brain damage.

Digestive Organs

The abdomen must be inspected for signs of injury. Scars, contusions, abrasions, wounds, distention, and rigidity must be documented. Palpation is done with caution because it may aggravate the injury. Bowel sounds are auscultated and girth mea-

TABLE 24.3 Clinical Manifestations of Increased Intracranial Pressure

	Compensated	*Decompensated*
Pulse rate	Decreased	Increased, then nothing
Respiratory rate	Decreased	Increased, then nothing
Blood pressure	Widening pulse pressure	Decreased
Temperature	Elevated	Further elevation
Pupils	Unequal	Fixed and dilated
Level of consciousness	Decreased	Decreased further

TABLE 24.4 Clinical Signs in Abdominal Injuries

Sign	Suspected Injury
Lower rib fracture	Spleen or liver
Kehr's sign—referred pain to left shoulder tip	Spleen, liver, or pancreas
Cullen's sign—purplish discoloration around umbilicus	Dissection of blood from retroperitoneal tissue into the abdominal wall
Turner's sign—purplish discoloration of flank	Extravasation of blood from retroperitoneal tissue to the flank
Ballance's sign—fixed area of dullness in upper left quadrant	Subcapsular or extracapsular hematoma of the spleen

SOURCE: Turner, 1982.

surements made to help establish baseline data. In a motor vehicle injury, the lap seat belt may have caused a contusion if it was worn incorrectly above the iliac crest. If there is a penetrating injury that creates an open abdomen, simply cover the open area with a sterile saline-soaked dressing. The injury will be repaired in the operating department.

A nasogastric tube is inserted to help decompress the stomach, which helps to prevent vomiting and aspiration. Decompression of the stomach is extremely important in children because children commonly hyperventilate in traumatic situations, causing their stomachs to accumulate a large amount of air. Nasogastric aspirant should be guiaced to check for the presence of occult blood. If the patient has ingested red meat recently, the guiac may be falsely positive.

Detection of occult bleeding into the abdominal area is of prime importance. The most commonly injured abdominal organs are the solid organs (liver and spleen). A peritoneal lavage is the most helpful test to indicate the presence or absence of blood in the abdomen, particularly intraperitoneal bleeding. The lavage may be falsely negative in retroperitoneal bleeding or injury. Table 24.4 lists other clinical signs that are helpful in assessing the extent of abdominal injury.

In the emergency department a definitive diagnosis is usually not made, but the decision whether to operate *is* made. Currently, many surgeons feel that spleens should not automatically be removed, particularly in children (Pachter, 1982). Overwhelming infection occurs in less than 1 percent of splenectomized adults; but, when it does, the mortality is in excess of 50 percent and death occurs within 24 to 48 hours (Pachter, 1982, p. 209).

Excretory Organs

All patients experiencing multiple trauma should be catheterized with a Foley catheter except in the presence of a ruptured urethra or a severe pelvic fracture. The patency of the urethra, especially in children, must be documented before a Foley is placed. Children should be bagged for a urine sample and adults asked to void for one, if possible. A Foley catheter aids in evaluating bladder rupture, fluid maintenance, and kidney injury. It must also be in place before a peritoneal lavage can be attempted.

TABLE 24.5 Complications of Musculoskeletal Fractures

Injury	Complication
Humerus	Brachial artery or radial nerve injury
Distal femor shaft	Femoral or popliteal vessel injury
Proximal tibia	Tibial nerve injury
Ankle dislocation	Pedal artery compression
Knee dislocation	Popliteal vessel compression
Elbow dislocation	Brachial artery compression

SOURCE: Perdue, 1981.

Hematuria is present in 85–90 percent of all multiple trauma victims. Intravenous pyelograms are the only way to rule out significant genitourinary tract trauma.

Urinary output must be maintained at a rate of 30 cc/hour in both adults and children. An inadequate urinary output is an early sign of shock. Prolonged inadequate urinary output may lead to acute renal failure.

Fractures
All extremities must be assessed for possible fractures. Any suspected fracture should be splinted and immobilized immediately. Open fractures should be covered with saline or betadine soaked dressings, splinted for immobilization, and eventually repaired in the operating department.

Each extremity should be assessed for pain, pallor, paresis, paralysis, and pulses. Other assessment factors include localized swelling, tenderness, deformity, ecchymosis, crepitation, and muscle spasm. Table 24.5 lists complications that need to be watched for in relation to specific musculoskeletal trauma.

Fat embolism is a common complication seen usually within the first 24 hours after injury in young people with fractures of the femur or humerous. Fractures of the long bones allow fat droplets to be released from the marrow into the general circulation. The patient may become apprehensive, short of breath, diaphoretic, cyanotic, and tachycardic. The development of petechial hemorrhages on the chest, shoulders, axillae, and conjunctiva are indicative of fat emboli. Intervention is supportive in nature.

Pain management may become of prime importance in the management of fractures. Morphine sulfate is the preferred drug given intravenously as long as the respiratory and neurological status of the patient is stable.

Emotional Reactions to Multiple Trauma

Although the trauma patient's family or significant others are frequently the last to be considered in the situation of multiple trauma, their needs are also significant. Resource people to help with the family include the supervisor, chaplain, social worker, psychiatric nurse, or clerical support personnel. The family should be kept informed and updated as much as possible in simple terms. The parents of injured children feel guilt or disbelief coupled with concerns about the care of their other children.

Impact, retreat, acknowledgment, and reconstruction are stages that both the family and patient must pass through successfully to achieve optimal mental health. The family's initial encounter with the critical situation is that of impact. Behavior demonstrated in this stage will include automatic, poorly controlled behavior. The family may appear depersonalized and numb. Be careful not to interpret this behavior as revealing an uncaring or unconcerned attitude. It is simply the best coping mechanism available at first.

The retreat stage is usually manifested by anxiety. The family may be unable to face the trauma, so they may try to retreat to the situation existing prior to the critical event. They may demonstrate behavior ranging from indifference to euphoria.

Realization that the loss has occurred starts the acknowledgment phase. The family enters the grieving process starting with shock and disbelief. Verbalization should be encouraged in this stage. Questions should be answered with short replies that are truthful. False reassurance is improper and may hinder the passage onto the next stage.

Reconstruction occurs when the family reintegrates the altered family member back into the family. The alteration may be as permanent as death or as short-lasting as a week's stay in the hospital.

CONCLUSION

The care of the multiple trauma patient is a complex, multifaceted task. It must be organized to ensure quality patient care. Priorities must be identified and interventions carried out immediately to provide the best opportunity for maintenance of life. Education of emergency department health care providers is imperative to help ensure the high level of care required for the patient experiencing multiple trauma.

BIBLIOGRAPHY

DeMuth, W. E.: The injured, unconscious patient. *Consultant* 20:217–218 (Mar. 1980).

Hicks, T. C.; D. F. Danze; D. M. Thomas; and L. M. Flint: Resuscitation and transfer of trauma patients: A prospective study. *Annals of Emergency Medicine* 11:296–299 (1982).

Lyon, S. H.: Critical care of the child with multi-trauma. *Nursing Clinics of North America* 16:657–70 (1981).

Molyneux-Luick, M.: The ABCs of multiple trauma. *Nursing 77* 7:30–36 (Oct. 1977).

Pachter, H. L.: Some tips on trauma care. *Emergency Medicine* 14:204–206+ (Feb. 15, 1982).

Perdue, P.: Abdominal injuries and dangerous fractures. *RN* 44:34–7+ (July 1981).

———: Life-threatening head and spine injuries. *RN* 44:36–41+ (June 1981).

———: Life-threatening respiratory injuries. *RN* 44:26–33 (Apr. 1981).

———: Stab and crush wounds to the heart. *RN* 44:63–65+ (May 1981).

Turner, P. S.: Test your knowledge of the multiple trauma patient. *Nursing 82* 12:129–133+ (1982).

Witter, M.: Priorities in trauma management. *Occupational Health Nursing* 29:27–29 (Sept. 1981).

25

The Pediatric Patient

Mitzi M. Lamberth

After completing this chapter, the reader will be able to do the following:

1. Triage a pediatric patient experiencing an illness.
2. Describe the pathophysiology of fever.
3. Discuss abdominal pain related to children.
4. Identify signs of dehydration.
5. Describe the stages of Reye's syndrome.
6. Describe the pathophysiology of sickle cell disease.
7. Identify signs and symptoms of a child in sickle cell crisis.
8. Identify signs of child abuse.
9. Identify signs of child neglect.
10. Discuss specific discharge teaching plans for children.

Children are treated in emergency departments for a variety of problems ranging from a sore throat to multiple trauma. Pediatric patients are often among the most perplexing to enter the emergency department. A child's condition can change quite rapidly because of immaturity of the body's systems and functions. Children are not small adults. Some of the common childhood complaints are discussed in this chapter as well as some life-threatening illnesses that require immediate care.

TRIAGE

Subjective Data

The nurse should begin the triage process by obtaining an initial history of the presenting problem from the patient, parents, guardians, or ambulance personnel. Obtain an explanation of the symptom that caused the parents to use the emergency department. Common symptoms for which children are frequently brought to the emergency department include sore throat, fever, vomiting and diarrhea, and seizures. If his condition allows and if he is old enough to describe it, interview the child about the presenting problem. Remember to use terms that the child can understand. Obtain information as detailed as possible about the illness. Most of the information will probably be obtained from the family. A child who presents to the emergency department with vomiting, for example, may be extremely ill. The vomiting could be caused by gastroenteritis or an emergent illness such as Reye's syndrome that is causing the child to vomit from increased intracranial pressure. The triage nurse should determine if the child has had a prodromal illness or any other symptoms associated with this illness. Find out how quickly the child became ill. It is also important to determine if the child has been under more physical or emotional stress than usual.

If a child is brought to the emergency department because of unexplained lethargy, ask the accompanying parent whether the child could possibly have ingested any medications or poisons; also ask for other symptoms and about recent illnesses. Inquire whether any trauma has occurred recently.

If there is pain, document when it began, what type of pain it is, and whether it has changed since it first began. Note whether the pain is relieved by anything (e.g., different positions, eating, moving about). Inquire about the patient being exposed to any illnesses. Always obtain a past medical history after completing the history of the present illness. Document any allergies or any medications the patient is taking.

Objective Data

The patient exhibits many signs about his present health status and underlying problem when entering the emergency department. Observe the mode of entry, skin color, facial expressions, actions, level of consciousness, and orientation. These facts must be considered by the triage nurse when assessing and planning the patient's care. The triage nurse should do a brief physical assessment of the patient as quickly as possible. The patient who has a decreased level of consciousness or confusion or is having respiratory difficulty must be taken to a treatment room immediately for further evaluation. Examine the skin to determine whether the child is hot, cold, warm, moist, or dry. Take the temperature of any child complaining of fever, before sending the child to the waiting area. An antipyretic may be needed if the child is febrile.

Assessment and Planning

A nursing diagnosis is made and a plan of care initiated by the triage nurse after obtaining the subjective and objective data. Determine first if the child is in distress and if an immediate plan of action is indicated. In the treatment room, the nurse assuming care of the child should obtain an initial set of vital signs including blood pressure. (Table 25.1 lists normal pulse, respiration, and blood pressure values for children.)

TRIAGE

TABLE 25.1 Normal Pediatric Vital Signs

Age	BP	P	RR
Newborn–6 wks	70/40	140 ± 50	30–50
6 wks–6 months	80/50	130 ± 45	20–30
6 months–1 yr	80/60	120 ± 40	20–30
1–3 yrs	95–100/60	100–120	18–30
4–8 yrs	100/60	100	12–20
10–14 yrs	115/60	80	12–20

SOURCE: Lyon, 1981, p. 658.

The parents of most children entering the emergency department should be given teaching instructions for fever control, clear liquids, and other nonemergent problems while waiting for the physician. If the wait will be long, the parents should be told that the child needs medical care, but that there will be a delay and that they are advised not to leave.

A thorough discussion of pediatric problems, such as fever, abdominal pain, vomiting and diarrhea, Reye's syndrome, meningitis, sickle cell disease, and child abuse, is presented in the balance of this chapter. Knowledge of this material will aid the nurse in performing accurate and appropriate triage. (Two examples of triage notes for children are contained in Table 25.2.)

TABLE 25.2 Examples of Triage Notes for Pediatric Patients

S: 9 month-old WF brought to E.D. by mother with c/o 2 d hx of vomiting and diarrhea, fever for 6 hrs. Unable to tolerate liquids for 8 hrs. Sleeping continuously. PMH: neg., NKA, no current meds.

O: Carried in mother's arms. Sleeping, pale, skin hot and dry, mucous membranes dry. Drowsy but alert when aroused with no tearing. Eyes dull and sunken, anterior fontanelle sunken. T 101°F rectal, P 162 regular, RR 42.

A: Vomiting and diarrhea with dehydration.

P: Pediatric evaluation, to treatment room immediately, mother with pt., mother reassured.

S: 10 yo BM brought to ED by parents with c/o abdominal pain and bilateral knee pain for 4 hrs. No nausea, vomiting, constipation, or diarrhea. Denies fever. PMH: sickle cell disease, NKA, no current meds.

O: Ambulatory with limp, leaning forward with hands holding abdomen, skin warm, no cyanosis noted. T 99°F oral.

A: Abdominal and joint pain. Possible sickle cell crisis.

P: Pediatric evaluation, to treatment room as soon as possible.

FEVER

Pathophysiology

Fever is one of the most common pediatric complaints seen in the emergency department. Parents become alarmed when their child develops a fever. The child may not have any other signs of illness or may exhibit symptoms that are clues to why there is a fever. Infection, dehydration, and an inflammatory process are three of the most common causes of a fever. Drugs, tumors, or an impaired hypothalamus are less frequent causes of fever.

The body temperature is regulated by the hypothalamus. The hypothalamus works as a thermostat and has a set level. It is believed that the hypothalamus is stimulated by pyrogens from bacteria or deteriorating tissues of the body during various diseases (Guyton, 1981). The pyrogens cause the hypothalamus to raise its thermostat, which causes an elevation of body temperature. Dehydration also causes the thermostat to become elevated.

A person has chills when the hypothalamic thermostat is at a temperature higher than the body temperature. An elevated hypothalamic thermostat causes vasoconstriction; the skin is cool, and the person begins to shiver until the body temperature is as high as the hypothalamic setting (Guyton, 1981). A fever lasts until the factor causing the increasd hypothalamic setting is removed. Then the hypothalamic setting decreases until it returns to a normal level. At this time, the body begins to sweat and the skin feels hot due to vasodilation (Guyton, 1981). This phenomenon occurs when the body temperature is higher than the hypothalamic setting and ends when both the body temperature and hypothalamic setting return to normal.

Clinical Manifestations

The child presenting to the emergency department with fever may have flushed skin, tachycardia, restlessness, and irritability. Some children with fever present to the emergency department with a *seizure,* usually of the generalized tonic-clonic type, which occurs most often in children under age five. Unless the family lives close to the hospital, the seizure will probably be over and the child will be postictal when he arrives for treatment.

Dehydration may occur when a child has a fever of prolonged duration, especially if it is associated with vomiting and diarrhea. The dehydrated child usually has pale, dry skin with poor turgor and dull, sunken eyes. The infant may have a sunken anterior fontanelle. This child usually has a decreased urine output and fluid intake.

Diagnostic Studies

A history should first be obtained including other signs and symptoms. Inquire about recent immunizations and exposure to illnesses. Next, a complete physical examination should be done. A diagnosis may be made without any laboratory data. The examination may reveal the cause of fever, such as otitis media. A urinalysis should be done if no causes for the fever are found on examination or if the child has suprapubic tenderness. A complete blood cell count may be done to rule out infection. An x-ray film of the chest may be ordered to rule out pneumonia.

A neurological examination should also be performed for the child with a seizure. A lumbar puncture is usually done to rule out meningitis. The cerebrospinal fluid should be cultured. Cultures of the blood, nasopharynx, and urine may be done to determine the cause of the fever. A complete blood count and urinalysis should be done and electrolyte levels should be checked. Measuring the glucose level is important because hypoglycemia may cause a seizure. A skull x-ray study should be done if there is a history or evidence of head trauma.

Nursing Care and Related Interventions

The child who is having a seizure or is postictal should be taken to the treatment room immediately. Assess the airway for obstruction. Suctioning may be required to prevent aspiration of secretions. Always protect the child from injury during a seizure. Inserting a padded tongue depressor between the teeth will prevent injury to the tongue and cheeks unless the teeth are clamped shut. Forcing the teeth apart could cause injury and should not be done. Vital signs, including a blood pressure and rectal temperature, should be measured as soon as possible in all children with a fever. Weigh the child so that the correct dosage of antipyretics can be administered. The goal is to reduce the fever that may have caused the seizure. Reducing fever may be accomplished by antipyretics such as aspirin or acetaminophen and by sponging with tepid water. Alcohol should not be added to the water because its fumes can be toxic and it cools the skin too quickly. Neither ice water sponging nor enemas are recommended because they cool the body too rapidly, causing the child to begin to shiver, which in turn causes the body temperature to rise even higher. Antipyretics should be given because they act on the pyrogens that cause the hypothalamic setting to rise.

Be sure to explain the procedures to the child and parents to reduce their anxiety. Explain what the physical examination will consist of, telling them, for example, that you will be looking at the child's ears, eyes, nose, and throat. If specific diagnostic studies are requested, explain how they are done.

The parents of a child who had a seizure will need reassurance. They should be told that a seizure does not mean the child has a serious illness or has suffered brain damage. Also tell the parents that a febrile seizure does not indicate that the child is an epileptic. These points should be reinforced even if the parents do not ask any questions. Many parents are afraid to ask because they are afraid of the answers.

Discharge Planning

The parents should be given careful written instructions concerning fever control. Many times the parents are so upset that they have forgotten what they were told by the time they arrive home. Encourage parents to give acetaminophen instead of aspirin to their children during outbreaks of influenza and varicella because aspirin may be a precipitating factor for Reye's syndrome. The amount of aspirin or acetaminophen to give the child should be specified. Also remind them to store the medications securely out of reach after they have given them to the child. They should be taught how to give a sponge bath and never to add alcohol to the water. Instruct them about the hazards of adding ice to the water or giving enemas to reduce the fever. It is imperative that the parents have a thermometer and know how to use it. Always inquire about this before they leave the emergency department.

Most children do not feel like eating when they have a fever. Parents should be instructed to encourage fluid intake to prevent dehydration. Clear liquid diet instructions are important so that they will know what fluids are best tolerated when the child is ill.

The same discharge instructions apply to the child who had a febrile seizure. Such a child is not always admitted to the hospital for further evaluation if the cause of the fever is determined and is not serious. The child's parents need reassurance and instructions on seizure precautions. Reinforce fever control and explain that they must check the temperature frequently while the child is ill. It is important that they keep the fever under control. The child who has had one febrile seizure is more likely to have another.

ABDOMINAL PAIN

Pathophysiology

Abdominal pain occurs frequently in children. Parents usually bring a child to the emergency department with abdominal pain because they suspect acute appendicitis, but a child may have abdominal pain for a wide variety of reasons. Otitis media, gastroenteritis, and pneumonia are frequent causes of abdominal pain. Urinary tract infections are quite common in children and usually cause abdominal pain.

Clinical Manifestations

The child with abdominal pain may present to the emergency department with no physical signs of illness. Others may have a clinical presentation of fever, vomiting and diarrhea, or cold symptoms. The child may be seen holding a hand over the area that is painful. The infant may be seen crying and drawing his legs up toward the abdomen when pain occurs.

Diagnostic Studies

A history of the illness and a complete physical examination may be all that is required to diagnose the cause of abdominal pain. The abdomen should be inspected for contour, and any abnormalities such as distention should be documented. Next, the abdomen should be auscultated for bowel sounds. Percussion and palpation should never be done until auscultation is completed because they may stimulate the bowel and cause an increase in bowel sounds that could be misleading. The child who is old enough to point to where the pain is should not have that area palpated first. The palpation could cause pain that would distract the child from feeling pain in another area, thereby masking the findings.

Laboratory information may not be required if the history and physical examination reveal a cause of illness such as otitis media or gastroenteritis. Most children with abdominal pain, however, should have a urinalysis to rule out a possible urinary tract infection. A complete blood count may be requested to rule out infection and anemia. Stool may be examined for blood or ova and parasites. Pinworms can be a cause of abdominal pain, especially in the school age child.

A chest x-ray film is required to rule out pneumonia if there is evidence of a respiratory tract infection. An x-ray film of the abdomen is usually not required, but may be ordered to rule out or to confirm a diagnosis of intestinal obstruction. A child under one year of age who seems to have abdominal pain should be examined carefully for intussusception. The diagnosis can be confirmed with a barium enema.

The age of the child should always be considered. Psychological aspects should be considered when there are no physical causes for the pain. The young school age child, for example, may be experiencing abdominal pain because of the stress caused by being separated from the family. This reaction is most likely to occur when the child has not been away from the family before and is attending school for the first time. Age is also an important factor in a female with abdominal pain. The female who has reached the age of puberty may experience abdominal pain prior to the onset of menses.

Nursing Care and Related Interventions

A complete set of vital signs including blood pressure should be done. An accurate temperature is extremely important. A rectal temperature is the most accurate when the patient has abdominal pain. A rectal temperature will usually be elevated before an oral temperature if there is an inflammation in the abdomen, especially if the inflammation is recent. The nurse should explain this fact to the older child, especially one who is going through the stage of shyness and does not want anyone to see his naked body. The blood pressure, pulse, and respiratory rate should be evaluated before the rectal temperature, since the latter upsets many children and may cause an increase in the other measurements.

The nurse should explain to the patient and family information about the examination. It is important that the child remain as calm as possible during the abdominal examination so that any abnormalities can be detected. The child who is aware of what will be done will probably be more cooperative.

The infant and toddler who are not toilet trained should be bagged for a urine specimen before the examination is started. It is important to clean the perineal area before the bag is placed on the child. All children should have a midstream urine specimen obtained if possible. The child should be informed before any blood is drawn. A simple explanation that the needle stick will hurt for only a minute can be helpful.

Discharge Planning

Many parents believe that a child must eat solid food or they will not get well. Explain that the child will begin to eat normally when he feels better, but he should be encouraged to drink plenty of fluids. If the child has had vomiting or diarrhea, the parents should be given a list of clear liquids to give the child for approximately 24 hours. Stress the importance of taking fluids to prevent dehydration.

Fever control instructions should be explained. Parents should be told the importance of checking the child's temperature. Many adults do not know how to read a thermometer and should be taught how to do this before they leave the emergency department.

Parents should be told about medications prescribed for the child and how they should be given. Emphasize the importance of taking all of an antibiotic as directed and not to stop the medicine because the child seems well. They should be told not to give laxatives or enemas unless the health care provider directs them to do so.

Instructions should be given to call or to return to the emergency department, clinic, or their private physician if the pain becomes worse, fever increases, or any other symptoms develop. Discuss other symptoms the child may develop if an illness such as otitis media or gastroenteritis is diagnosed.

VOMITING AND DIARRHEA

Pathophysiology

Vomiting and diarrhea are quite common occurrences in infants and children. They may be the first signs of illnesses such as otitis media, meningitis, or diseases of the gastrointestinal tract. The most common cause of vomiting and diarrhea is nonspecific gastroenteritis. Another frequent cause, especially in infants, is improper feeding.

Diarrhea and vomiting may also be caused by bacterial infections, viruses, and intestinal obstruction. Both may be caused by parasites. Milk allergy may be a cause of diarrhea, especially in infants.

The body weight of an infant or young child is comprised of considerably more fluid than an adult's. Vomiting and diarrhea, therefore, can easily become a serious condition in this age group. Because their body functions are immature and occur at a higher metabolic rate, dehydration and electrolyte imbalances can occur quickly.

Clinical Manifestations

The child who presents to the emergency department with vomiting and diarrhea may exhibit no signs of dehydration. Others may present with dry mucous membranes and no tearing; this indicates that there is approximately five percent dehydration (Chow et al., 1979). Tachycardia, poor skin turgor, and sunken eyes or fontanelle are indicative of 7–10 percent dehydration (Chow et al., 1979). A child with greater than

10 percent dehydration may be hypotensive and show signs of listlessness, stupor, and seizures.

Diagnostic Studies

The history should include the length of time the child has been ill and how frequently the vomiting and diarrhea have occurred. It is important to inquire about the amount of emesis or stool the child expels and when it occurs. The health care provider should attempt to determine whether the vomiting has been projectile or nonprojectile. Projectile vomiting may be indicative of increased intracranial pressure or pyloric stenosis. Any other symptoms regarding the illness, such as fever or abdominal pain, should be documented.

The physical examination will provide most of the data needed to determine how the illness should be treated. Although the examination may not reveal any physical cause for the illness, it will help determine the degree of dehydration, a factor that is extremely important. Data can be acquired by examining the skin, mucous membranes, and the fontanelle of an infant.

Blood tests may not be necessary unless the child has signs of dehydration. Then tests should be ordered to rule out an electrolyte imbalance. A complete blood count may be done to rule out infection. A urinalysis should be ordered to determine whether the vomiting and diarrhea are caused by a urinary tract infection. Stool cultures are usually not ordered unless the diarrhea has been present for several days. The stool may be tested for ova and parasites depending on the findings of the history and physical examination. The emesis and stool should be tested for the presence of blood.

Nursing Care and Related Interventions

Initially, vital signs, including a blood pressure, should be checked and a weight taken. Always explain to the child and family what is being done. Often, children are administered intravenous fluids while in the emergency department and then are sent home if they are less than 5–7 percent dehydrated. Dehydration of more than 7 percent usually requires admission to the hospital. Most infants are admitted to the hospital if they have any signs of dehydration. Explain the venipuncture procedure for the intravenous fluids and try to obtain blood samples with only the single venipuncture. The intravenous fluid rate must be monitored carefully to prevent overloading the patient.

Record the frequency and amount of stool and emesis. Document any abnormal characteristics such as a foul odor. Urine output should be measured and recorded. Proper handwashing techniques should always be practiced, but take even more care after caring for a child with vomiting and diarrhea. Assume that the vomiting and diarrhea are infectious until proven otherwise.

The child should be made as physically comfortable as possible. It is frightening for a child to have to go to the hospital. Try reducing the child's anxiety by reading to him or by providing some toys for him to play with or hold. Once the child is more comfortable and the vomiting has ceased, he can start taking ice chips. If this is tolerated, progress to clear liquids or an oral electrolyte solution.

Discharge Planning

Parents must be instructed not to give their child antiemetics or antidiarrheal agents. Explain that these medicines often cause drowsiness and could possibly mask any other signs and symptoms that could develop. Clear liquid diet instructions should be written down and given to the parents. It is important that they understand to keep the child on clear liquids for a least 24 hours or the vomiting and diarrhea may get worse. Instruct them to start the child on small frequent feedings such as one-half tablespoon of liquid every 15 to 30 minutes until it is well tolerated. At this time, the amount of liquids may be increased. After 24 hours, they may begin full liquids or a bland diet. Other discharge teaching may include abdominal pain instructions and fever control.

REYE'S SYNDROME

Pathophysiology

Reye's syndrome was first described in 1963 as acute encephalopathy with fatty infiltration of the viscera. There is a rapid development of hepatic dysfunction and various degrees of central nervous system disturbance. The syndrome is a disease entity that is life-threatening and often fatal. It occurs from infancy to young adulthood, but is most commonly found in children between the ages of five to fifteen. The disease has occurred worldwide, but is apparently more prevalent in the United States, with a higher incidence in the suburban areas.

The cause of Reye's syndrome is unknown. Studies have shown that it usually occurs after a viral illness such as varicella, influenza type B, or upper respiratory infections. Other viruses associated with Reye's include echovirus, adenovirus, and herpes. A high percentage of children with Reye's syndrome received salicylates during their preceding viral illness. Evidence suggests that salicylates may interfere with the mitochondria; therefore, the Center for Disease Control has recommended that salicylates not be given to children during influenza or varicella outbreaks because this might be a factor precipitating Reye's syndrome. Researchers also suggest that the genetic makeup of an individual child may be a factor in Reye's. Although there is evidence that this is doubtful due to the small number of cases developing in one family, it cannot be excluded.

There is change and injury to the mitochondria affecting all tissues in Reye's syndrome. During the initial phase of the illness, the size of the liver may be normal, but as the liver cells become infiltrated with small droplets of fat the liver becomes enlarged. As the disease progresses, the liver may also appear yellow or white in color. Once the mitochondria become damaged, there is a breakdown in the urea cycle and ammonia is no longer changed to urea for excretion from the body. Consequently, a decrease occurs in nitrogen output in the urine because the ammonia is not being converted, which leads in turn to an elevation in the serum ammonia level, and ammonia begins to flood the body.

The serum transaminase levels, SGOT and SGPT, become elevated and may be as high as double the normal levels early in the disease. They may increase even more as the disease progresses. The transaminases must be synthesized for protein formation to proceed normally. Patients may also become hypoglycemic as the disease advances into later stages. Glucose is normally stored in the cells as glycogen, with the largest portion being stored in the liver cells. The cells require glycogen as their source of energy, but the glycogen stores are rapidly depleted in Reye's. After the glycogen stores are depleted, the cells begin to malfunction and die. Although many functions of the liver are interrupted, there are usually no signs of jaundice, and the bilirubin levels also remain normal. The prothrombin time may be prolonged.

The brain cells lose their store of glycogen and become watery and distorted. As the disease progresses, there is marked cerebral edema with increased intracranial pressure, which is partially due to the cell's retention of sodium and the increasing ammonia levels. As the brain becomes flooded with ammonia, it tries to buffer the ammonia with cerebrospinal fluid (CSF) glutamine, but eventually the buffering becomes overloaded. The ammonia then has a profound effect on the brain. The cerebral edema and intracranial pressure increase even more. The opening pressure for a lumbar puncture is increased, but the CSF values are essentially normal. The glucose level may be low if the child is in a state of hypoglycemia.

The heart and kidneys may also be affected. The fatty infiltration of the heart may lead to myocardial damage; in the kidneys it may cause uremia.

Clinical Manifestations

Many children are brought to the emergency department because of an acute onset of vomiting that is probably due to the encephalopathy. Taking a good history is most important. The data will most likely show that there was a prodromal illness three to seven days prior to the onset of vomiting. The child seemed almost completely well, the fever probably had subsided, and the child had returned to a normal routine when the vomiting began. Parents often assume their child has another virus when vomiting starts again and may not bring the child in for treatment until there is a change in his neurological status. It may be difficult to assess clear signs of neurologic changes in the infant, but the parents may describe vomiting and refusal to eat. In addition, the infant may be stuporous or unresponsive. Infants are more likely to have seizures than older children. The seizures may be due to anoxia or hypoglycemia. The older child may be brought to the emergency department because of irritability, listlessness, or agitated delirium.

As the disease progresses, the child becomes tachypneic, hyperventilates, and becomes tachycardic. This phase is possibly due to the cerebral edema and brainstem compression. Respirations increase because of the increased ammonia levels in the body. The liver may or may not be enlarged initially but becomes enlarged during the progression of the illness. (Five progressive stages seen in Reye's syndrome are listed in Table 25.3.)

TABLE 25.3 Stages of Reye's Syndrome

Stage I	Lethargic but able to follow verbal commands. Posture normal, response to pain is purposeful. Pupils are brisk with normal reflex.
Stage II	Combative or stuporous. Normal posture, may or may not respond purposefully to pain. Pupils are sluggish with conjugate deviation.
Stage III	Comatose. Decorticate posturing and decorticate response to pain. Pupils sluggish with conjugate deviation.
Stage IV	Comatose with decerebrate posturing with response to pain. Pupils sluggish and reflex may be absent.
Stage V	Comatose. Flaccid posture with no response to pain. Pupillary reaction and reflex are both absent.

SOURCE: National Institute of Health, 1981.

Nursing Care and Related Interventions

Reye's syndrome is a disease that involves many systems. All functions of the body must be monitored closely. Most important is support of the brain during the illness. Injury to other organs in the body, however, has been found to be almost completely reversible. Although Reye's is well known for its hepatic dysfunction, it is the injury to the brain that is fatal. The neurologic function and status, therefore, must be carefully observed.

After the child enters the emergency department, obtain a complete set of vital signs including blood pressure. Always explain to the patient and family what is going to be done, in order to reduce their anxiety as much as possible. Be prepared to start an intravenous line of 10 percent dextrose and draw blood for laboratory tests. If possible, try to do this with only one venipuncture to prevent upsetting the child. If the child is already comatose, be prepared for a respiratory arrest. Always have intubation and suction equipment nearby and ready for use. Measure the vital signs and assess the neurological status frequently, while documenting all findings. The patient should be placed on a cardiac monitor so that any dysrhythmias can be noted immediately. Elevate the head of the bed to decrease intracranial pressure. If the child is extremely anxious or combative, sedation may be necessary to help prevent an increase in intracranial pressure.

After the child has been stabilized, he should be transported to the intensive care unit for careful monitoring. If the hospital is not equipped to handle this type of patient, transfer him to the nearest hospital with the needed capabilities. If transport to another hospital is necessary, a physician or nurse should accompany the patient in the ambulance to assist the emergency medical technician (EMT) or paramedic in monitoring the patient and handling any problem that could develop.

The various types of monitors and equipment used should be discussed in detail with the patient and family. This information will help alleviate their fears concerning any devices that they are not familiar with. Explain to the family the condition of the child and be prepared to answer their questions.

MENINGITIS

Pathophysiology

Meningitis is an inflammation of the covering of the brain and upper spinal cord known as the meninges. It is caused by bacteria, viruses, and other organisms that spread to the meninges. Bacterial meningitis usually develops after an upper respiratory tract infection near the meninges such as otitis media.

Organisms that cause meningitis in children vary from year to year and may vary from one geographic location to another. The most common organisms that cause bacterial meningitis are *Hemophilus influenzae, Neisseria meningitidis,* and *Diplococcus pneumoniae* (Barltrop and Brimblecombe, 1978). *Escherichia coli, streptococci,* and *staphylococci* are less frequent causal agents. The bacteria that is in the blood circulates and invades the spinal fluid. The bacteria may enter the meninges directly by penetrating wounds or lumbar punctures. Once the bacteria enters the spinal fluid, the meninges become inflamed and exudation occurs. There may be brain injury due to tissue damage.

Clinical Manifestations

The onset of symptoms in bacterial meningitis is usually sudden and includes vomiting, headache, fever, and photophobia. Stiffness of the neck occurs and causes pain when the neck is flexed. Infants up to the age of two will most likely have a bulging anterior fontanelle due to increased intracranial pressure (Barltrop and Brimblecombe, 1978). Infants may have a high-pitched cry and vacant stare. Positive Kernig's and Brudzinski's signs signify meningeal irritation.

Meningococcus is caused by *Neisseria meningitidis* and can cause upper respiratory infections, septicemia, and meningitis (Barltrop and Brimblecombe, 1978). It may start as an infection of the tonsils or nasopharynx and then is followed by meningococcal septicemia. This infection extends to the meninges of the brain and spinal cord.

One of the first symptoms of meningococcus is fever due to the infection. Next, nausea and vomiting, severe headache, irritability, confusion, and convulsions may occur as a result of increased intracranial pressure. Neck and shoulder stiffness is due to meningeal irritation. Kernig's and Brudzinski's signs are both positive. Petechiae may be present and progress to purpuric lesions due to septicemia. The diagnosis of meningococcus is almost always correct if the child presents with petechiae or purpura, fever, and meningismus. The onset of meningococcus is sudden and usually severe. Death may occur within a few hours because the septicemia causes total peripheral vascular collapse (Barltrop and Brimblecombe, 1978).

Diagnostic Studies

The diagnosis of meningitis or meningococcus should be suspected by the history obtained and the patient's clinical presentation. To confirm the diagnosis, a lumbar puncture is performed in order to obtain cerebrospinal fluid. The cerebrospinal fluid pressure will be elevated due to increased intracranial pressure. The white blood cell count of the fluid will be high and these cells will be mostly polymorphonuclear cells. The glucose level will be low, and the protein level is usually elevated but may be normal. The spinal fluid should be cultured to determine the causative organism.

Blood testing should include a complete blood cell count, platelet count, PT-PTT, electrolyte values, and glucose levels. Measures of creatinine and blood urea nitrogen levels should also be ordered. Blood, nasopharynx, and urine cultures should be done. A chest x-ray film and a skull x-ray film should be obtained to help establish baseline data.

Nursing Care and Related Interventions

The child should be taken to a private treatment area immediately if meningitis or meningococcus are suspected. A complete set of vital signs including blood pressure and weight should be recorded. Measuring weight is important so that the dosages of drugs can be calculated and the proper amount of the drugs given. Neurologic status at time of arrival in the emergency department should be documented and monitored frequently along with vital signs and blood pressure. Observe the child closely and document any change in physical findings such as petechiae developing. The child with meningococcus may soon become unconscious and develop respiratory difficulties and deteriorate rapidly. Intubation equipment should be nearby and ready for use. Arterial blood gas values should be measured if respiratory problems develop.

Intravenous fluids should be started immediately to give intravenous antibiotics and other drugs such as Valium if seizures begin. Intravenous chloramphenicol and ampicillin are the preferred drugs with meningococcal septicemia. The antibiotics for bacterial meningitis may vary depending on the causative organism, but ampicillin intravenously is usually the initial drug of choice.

Hydration of the patient may be necessary if there is evidence of dehydration due to vomiting and fever. Intake and output must be accurately recorded. Give antipyretics to lower a high fever; tepid water sponging may be necessary.

The nurse should be supportive of both the child and the family. They will both be frightened. Explain procedures before they are carried out. Answer any questions that the child or family may have. Before the lumbar puncture is done, discuss it with the parents and the child. The parents may have many questions about stories they have heard regarding lumbar punctures. Assure them that it is a relatively safe procedure and that few complications occur. The parents would probably prefer to wait out of the room while the procedure is done, but they may not leave voluntarily. Always ask them if they would like to wait outside the room and assure them they will be called back in when the procedure is completed. Explain to the child that the parents will return soon.

After the lumbar puncture is done, blood drawn, and intravenous fluids started, the antibiotics should be given. Never give the antibiotics before the culture samples have been obtained. After all of these initial procedures are completed, including x-ray examination, the child should be transported to his room in the hospital where he

SICKLE CELL DISEASE

and the family can be together. If the child has meningococcus, he should be admitted to the intensive care unit for close observation and monitoring of cardiac and respiratory status.

Meningococcus is transmitted by contact and droplet infection. If petechiae develop or are present at the onset of care, respiratory isolation precautions must be taken. All care givers should wear masks at all times. Any person having close contact with meningococcus may need antimicrobial prophylaxis such as rifampin.

SICKLE CELL DISEASE

Pathophysiology

Sickle cell disease is an inherited chronic hemolytic anemia that is found primarily in black Americans. It is the most common form of inherited anemia and occurs in persons with identical hemoglobin genes. The person with sickle cell disease is homozygous and has an abnormal hemoglobin in the red blood cells called hemoglobin S. The person with sickle cell trait is heterozygous, does not have anemia, and is asymptomatic. Approximately 8 percent of black Americans have the sickle cell trait and 1 of every 600 has the disease.

The function of hemoglobin is to carry oxygen from the lungs to the tissues. In persons with sickle cell anemia, the abnormal hemoglobin S molecules make up a large portion of the red blood cell. The abnormal hemoglobin molecule carries the normal oxygen capacity, but once the molecule releases the oxygen, it creates a deoxygenated state that causes the red blood cell membrane to become distorted and assume a sickle shape. Once the red blood cells sickle, they become entangled, leading to an increase in the viscosity of the blood. Circulation is either partially or completely blocked in the capillaries, arterioles, and veins by the entangled cells. This causes venostasis and hypoxia, which leads to venospasm, ischemia, and damage to many organs. Eventually the damage to the tissues and organs becomes permanent.

The sickled red cells are fragile and are destroyed rapidly during circulation. Sickled red cells have a life expectancy of only 15–30 days, whereas normal red cells have a life expectancy of 120 days. The destruction of these abnormal red cells is the cause of the anemia. The cells are destroyed faster than they are produced. Normal hemoglobin levels usually range from 12 to 16 g per 100 ml, but in sickle cell anemia the hemoglobin level usually ranges from 6 to 9 g per 100 ml.

Clinical Manifestations

The symptoms of sickle cell disease usually do not occur until a child is about six months of age. By then, the fetal hemoglobin level has fallen and the hemoglobin S is present. A sickle cell crisis can occur sporadically and may be precipitated by hypoxia, infection, dehydration, fatigue, or trauma. Physical or mental stress may also cause a crisis to occur.

Three forms of sickle cell crisis may occur. These are aplastic, sequestration, and painful (Linehan, 1978). Infection is the most common cause of an *aplastic crisis,* although it may also be due to a folic acid insufficiency. The bone marrow has temporarily stopped production of red blood cells and the hemoglobin level falls. Therefore, the parents may bring the child to the emergency department because of an increase in pallor and the child may be more tired than usual.

A *sequestration crisis* develops when large amounts of blood pool in the spleen and liver causing them to become enlarged. This may cause circulatory failure and death. In the child, the spleen may be hyperactive, which in turn causes the red cells to be destroyed even faster. The liver continues to enlarge as the child grows older, but the spleen may become fibrous and smaller due to multiple infarcts (Jolly, 1981).

The most common crisis seen is the *painful crisis*. This is caused by the small blood vessels becoming occluded with sickled cells. The blood flow is reduced or blocked to various organs and tissues, causing ischemia and infarction. Hematuria may be present with renal infarction, and pulmonary infarcts may occur. The patient may develop a fever and have pain in the abdomen, back, joints, and extremities. Cerebral vascular accidents, hemiplegia, and blindness may result from cerebral occlusion. Liver function is impaired and the abdomen may be enlarged. Jaundice is common. Abdominal pain may result from vaso-occlusion in the abdominal viscera.

Chronic problems exist with sickle cell disease such as osteomyelitis and septicemia. There is a high incidence of cholelithiasis in adolescents and young adults. The spleen becomes fibrotic and renal function is impaired as multiple infarcts occur. Most patients die before the age of 40, and 50 percent die before the age of 20 as a result of cerebral vascular accidents, splenic sequestrations, and bacterial infections (Linehan, 1978).

Diagnostic Studies

A careful history and examination should be done to help determine what diagnostic tests are necessary. The findings will differentiate the type of crisis that is occurring and will influence the need for further diagnostic studies. If pain and fever are present, the patient is probably in metabolic acidosis; therefore, arterial blood gas studies should reveal a decrease in the bicarbonate and pH of the blood. Many health care providers prefer drawing a venous blood sample to assess pH, to prevent further anxiety and trauma to the child. This blood may be obtained at the same time blood is drawn for other samples.

A complete blood count should be done to determine if there is a fall in the hemoglobin. During a painful crisis, the hemoglobin will remain at its normal 6 to 9 g, but it will drop during an aplastic or sequestration crisis. The white blood cell count usually is elevated in sickle cell crises as a result of the red blood cell destruction.

The unconjugated bilirubin level will usually be elevated in a child with sickle cell anemia. However, the conjugated bilirubin level should be normal. An elevated conjugated bilirubin level is indicative of a biliary obstruction and requires further evaluation.

Urine should be tested for blood and a culture and sensitivity to rule out a urinary tract infection. Other cultures should be considered because infection may be the primary cause of the crisis.

SICKLE CELL DISEASE

Radiologic studies may be helpful in determining if there is any necrosis or deformities from bone infarcts. A flat plate x-ray film of the abdomen can help determine the presence of gallstones.

Nursing Care and Related Interventions

The nursing care for the patient with sickle cell crisis consists of hydration, reducing emotional stress, and treating the pain. Because there is no cure for sickle cell disease, care of its victims is aimed at symptomatic relief.

Hydration of the patient in sickle cell crisis is most important to combat the effects of the sickled red cells. Intravenous fluids of 5 percent dextrose in water or 5 percent dextrose with half normal saline are the fluids of choice. Sodium bicarbonate may be given or added to the fluids if the patient is acidotic. After any nausea and vomiting subsides, the child should be encouraged to take small frequent amounts of fluids orally. Keep an accurate record of intake and output. Offer the bedpan or urinal frequently.

Relief of pain may be accomplished by a combination of measures. Medications for milder pain may include oral analgesics such as aspirin, acetaminophen, or codeine. Meperidine or codeine may be given intramuscularly or intravenously for pain not relieved by the oral analgesics. Although morphine can be given, it should be avoided if at all possible because it depresses respirations. The patient should be instructed to remain on a stretcher with the bedrails raised while receiving narcotics. Observe and document the results of the medication. The pain may also be reduced with proper positioning of the patient and supporting the extremities with pillows. Distracting the patient with toys or reading books may help. Allowing the parents to stay with the child may alleviate anxieties and fears of the child that might cause the pain to seem worse.

Oxygen may be ordered for the patient, although there is no documented evidence that it is beneficial in the treatment or relief of pain in sickle cell crisis. (Linehan, 1978). Nonetheless, because many young sickle cell sufferers feel that it is helpful, some physicians give them low flow oxygen through nasal prongs to help them psychologically.

Antipyretics are given to reduce fever because fever increases dehydration. The patient's temperature should be checked frequently and recorded.

Support must be given to the child and parents. Talk with them about their fears and answer any questions honestly. Always explain procedures before they are done and tell them what is to be done next. Offer toys and books to distract children from their illness. Parents may vent feelings of guilt, frustration, and resentment. Provide counseling and information for the parents. They will then be able to answer questions their child may have.

Discharge Planning

Discharge planning and teaching is important for the patient with sickle cell disease. The parents should be counseled on what activities are best for the child in order to prevent a crisis from occurring. Strenuous sports should be avoided. Parents should be instructed in recognizing signs of dehydration and the importance of maintaining adequate fluid intake. The child should also be taught to avoid excessive emotional stress. Teach the parents and the child the signs of a mild crisis, such as fever, pallor, and pain in the back, abdomen, and extremities, so that the family can seek treatment *before* a severe crisis occurs.

CHILD ABUSE

Child abuse is a problem that existed for centuries but was rarely discussed or reported. In times past, abuse was regarded as overpunishment for something the child had done wrong. As a consequence, no one became involved. People felt it was none of their business what parents did to their children and they did not want to interfere. Today, child abuse is publicized more and people are becoming more aware of the problem. It occurs in all levels of society, regardless of race, religion, level of intelligence, or socioeconomic status.

Often thought of only as physical trauma, child abuse also occurs as emotional and sexual abuse. Often the term *child abuse* is used to describe child neglect. *Child neglect* means the child has not been given enough attention for the basic needs of survival, either physical or emotional survival. Child abuse thus refers to a physical, emotional, or sexual injury that is nonaccidental to any child under the age of 18.

In 1977, the U.S. Department of Health, Education and Welfare conducted a nationwide analysis that estimated that one million children in the United States are abused or neglected each year. It also estimated that annually a minimum of 2,000 children die as a result of the abuse or neglect. Many children will have permanent physical or emotional problems as a result of abuse.

Physical Abuse

Physical abuse can occur at any age but usually occurs to a child under age three. Many times the injury is a result of severe punishment for a behavior that is appropriate for the age of the child such as diaper wetting in the infant. The older child may be severely beaten for poor grades or for not behaving properly. Mothers usually abuse infants, whereas fathers are more likely to abuse older children (Jolly, 1981). The mother often feels the baby cries because she is unable to make the baby happy, so she strikes the baby to stop the crying.

There are many physical characteristics of child abuse. Burns in an unusual area are frequently a result of abuse. Cigarette burns are often on the palms of the hands, soles of the feet, and buttocks. A child usually will not burn himself repeatedly. In addition, infected cigarette burns may resemble impetigo or ringworm. Children often burn themselves accidentally on an appliance, but they may also be burned intentionally with these appliances. The location of the burn is often the key indicator of accident or abuse. An example would be a burn in the shape of an iron on a child's back.

CHILD ABUSE 485

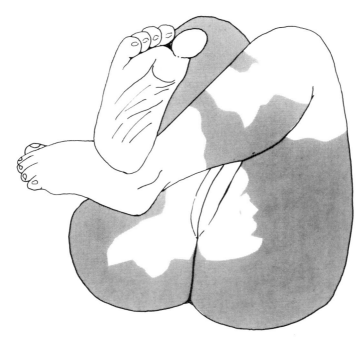

Figure 25.1 A scald burn of the perineum, feet, and legs resulting from physical child abuse.

Another type of burn related to abuse occurs by scalding. The child is lowered into a tub of hot water often as a means of punishment for diaper wetting. The child will be burned on the perineum, feet, and legs (see Fig. 25.1). Although a toddler might accidentally step into a tub of hot water, such an accident victim would likely fall forward and have burns on his hands, forearms, feet, and lower legs, rather than on the buttocks or feet.

Another indication of abuse is clusters of bruises or welts on the face, back, buttocks, thighs, chest, and abdomen. They may form patterns that reflect the type of object used to inflict them, such as a handprint, belt buckle, or a looped electrical cord as illustrated in Figure 25.2. There may be bruises over several areas of the body that are in various stages of healing. They may not be compatible with the history of the injury in respect to what caused the injury and when it occurred.

Child abuse should be suspected in children with fractures and dislocations that are inconsistent with the age of the child. Abused children often have spiral fractures as a result of twisting of the extremities. They commonly have facial and skull fractures. If multiple fractures in different stages of healing are present, child abuse should be suspected.

All children are likely to have lacerations and abrasions at some time in their life, but the key to suspected abuse is the location of the wound. Lacerations and abrasions to the external genitalia, torso, or the backs of arms and legs are probably not

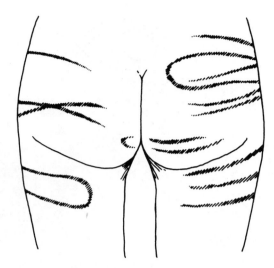

Figure 25.2 Looped electrical cord bruises.

accidental. Human bite marks of adult size are indicators of abuse. In addition, bald areas on a scalp with normal hair growth is an indication that hair has been pulled out.

Behavioral signs of abuse may not be as easy to detect as physical signs. The child may show a wide range of reactions and appear afraid of any adult approaching, and avoid any physical contact by backing away. Or the opposite may happen, and the child may show an unusual affection for strangers. The child may stare and show no reaction when approached by the nurse or physician and may not turn to the parents for protection. Another indication of abuse is a fear of going home.

Child Neglect

Neglect is the lack of attention for the basic needs of the child, such as food, clothing, medical care, and supervision. Weight loss, failure to thrive, and abdominal distention may be signs that the child is not receiving proper nourishment. These problems may be a sign of constant hunger.

Poor hygiene and inappropriate clothing for the type of weather may mean the child is neglected. The child may not have a coat for the winter and may wear long-sleeved clothes in the summer possibly to hide bruises. A neglected infant may have bald patches on one side of the scalp due to being left in one position for a long time.

Behavioral signs of neglect are often a result of the physical indicators. A child steals food because of improper feeding at home. The child may skip school or may arrive early and stay late to get away from home. The neglected infant may appear gloomy and be inactive.

Sexual Abuse

Sexual abuse is described as any sexual activity between an adult and a child. This type of abuse affects both boys and girls but most commonly affects girls. Signs of physical injury may not be apparent, and the abuse may not be discovered until the child confides in someone. Sexual abuse is often not reported because there are no signs of physical injury or because only a family member knows and he does not want anyone else to know. He thinks it will not happen again.

Physical signs of sexual abuse include bruises and lacerations of the external genitalia, vagina, and anal area. There may be bruises and lacerations of the mouth and throat if the child is forced to perform oral sex. A child may complain of dysuria or genital itching. A penile or vaginal discharge and poor anal sphincter tone may be indications of sexual abuse. Any girl under the age of 13 who becomes pregnant or has a venereal disease may be a victim of sexual abuse.

Children who have been sexually abused often demonstrate an unusual amount of sexual knowledge. They may be withdrawn and have poor relationships with peers. They also may show a decrease in performance at school or refuse to participate in physical activities.

Emotional Abuse and Neglect

The signs of emotional abuse and neglect are very difficult to identify. The child is often rejected and threatened. The child may show signs of failure to thrive or difficulty learning. Frequently the child is hyperactive or displays some form of disruptive behavior.

Although physically abused children are frequently emotionally affected, not all emotionally abused children are physically abused. Emotionally abused children may have feeding problems or habits such as biting, rocking, or improper toilet habits. They are sometimes withdrawn and exhibit unacceptable behavior such as cruelty to others. Their emotional and intellectual development may be retarded and they may seem to be emotionally disturbed. However, parents of an emotionally abused child avoid seeking help and blame the child for the behavior.

Diagnostic Studies

History and physical examination of the child are the most useful diagnostic tools in determining whether a child has been abused. A careful history from the parents or guardians must be obtained to help determine how and when the child was injured or became ill. A history should be obtained from the child in private. The history may be inconsistent with the illness or injury. The attitude, appearance, and behavior of the child and parents should be noted. Document the history and physical findings in detail.

A complete physical examination must be done. The head should be examined for hematomas, bald areas of the scalp, and other injuries. A fundoscopic examination of the eyes may reveal retinal detachment due to blunt trauma, retinal hemorrhages as a result of a subdural hematoma, or papilledema due to increased intracranial pressure. The abdomen should be palpated for tenderness and enlargement of organs. Observe for symmetrical movement of extremities and normal range of motion of joints. Examine the genital area for any evidence of sexual abuse.

Findings of the physical examination determine what other diagnostic studies should be done. When child abuse is suspected, a series of x-ray films including skull, chest, abdomen, and extremities should be requested. Many health care providers order full body x-ray films. A complete blood count, platelet count, and PT-PTT should be ordered if the child has multiple bruises. (The parents may claim that the child bruises easily.) Urine should be checked for blood if there is trauma to the back or abdomen. A toxicology screen should be ordered if the child exhibits an altered level of consciousness or any bizarre behavior. (Parents have drugged infants so that they would sleep and not cry.) Further diagnostic studies may be necessary such as a computerized tomographic scan of the head if there is evidence of a subdural hematoma or increased intracranial pressure. The x-ray films may show fractures that are in different stages of healing.

When sexual abuse is suspected, the penis or vagina and anal area should be examined. The external genitalia should be examined for blood, hair, or discharge. A Wood's light will fluoresce any seminal fluid that may be present on the perineum. Any discharge should be cultured for gonorrhea and examined under the microscope for the presence of sperm. A rectal examination should be done to reveal any tears or poor sphincter tone, and a culture for gonorrhea should be obtained. A Venereal Disease Research Laboratories (VDRL) test should be ordered to rule out syphilis.

An extremely gentle vaginal examination must be done to check for the presence of a hymen. A child-sized speculum can be inserted to examine for tears, bruising, or a discharge. Any discharge should be examined for sperm and cultured for gonorrhea. If the girl has reached the age of menarche, the physician may elect to give her some form of estrogen such as diethylstilbesterol to prevent pregnancy if rape or incest has occurred.

Nursing Care and Related Interventions

In most emergency departments the nurse is the first person who sees a patient who comes in for care. Therefore, nurses are in a primary position to recognize indications of child abuse or neglect. If child abuse is suspected, never accuse the parents of causing the injury. Try to remain emotionally uninvolved and remember that the parents may be seeking help for themselves as abusers by bringing the child in for medical care.

The nurse should try to develop a trusting relationship with the child. The child may be hysterical or calm. After the child is in a treatment room, a complete set of vital signs, including blood pressure, should be obtained. Explain to the child and family what is to be done next. This will help reduce their anxiety. A weight should be obtained when possible. The child should be undressed for a thorough examination. An older child may be reluctant to undress because of shyness or because he has injuries that have been hidden by the clothing. Respect the rights of the child and allow him to undress in private.

Support must be given to the child and the family. If abuse is suspected, the child should be admitted to the hospital for further evaluation and protection. The appropriate agency should be notified immediately in cases of suspected abuse or neglect. The physician may elect to communicate to the parents that abuse is suspected and that the appropriate agency has been notified. The agency will help them receive counseling.

Child abuse and neglect must be reported even if only suspected and not proven. The community agency will have the responsibility of determining whether abuse or neglect has occurred. Nurses who suspect child abuse or neglect and fail to report it may be held liable. Learn about the laws of the state where you practice.

CONCLUSION

Children can become ill very quickly. Their body systems are immature and their condition can change rapidly. Health care providers must remember that children are not adults in small packages. The nurse must make a thorough and accurate assessment of the patient presenting to the emergency department to provide optimum care. A thorough understanding of the psychological, physiological, and educational needs of the patient and parents is imperative in order for the emergency department nurse to provide the highest possible quality of care.

BIBLIOGRAPHY

Barltrop, D., and F. Brimblecombe: *Children in Health and Disease*. London: Balliere Tindall, 1978.

Chow, M.; B. Durand; M. Feldman; and M. Mills: The gastrointestinal system. *Handbook of Pediatric Primary Care*. New York: Wiley, 1979, pp. 625–650.

Guyton, A. C.: *Textbook of Medical Physiology*. Philadelphia: Saunders, 1981.

Jolly, H.: *Diseases of Children*. Boston: Blackwell Scientific Publications, 1981.

Linehan, M.: Sickle cell anemia—the painful crisis. *The Journal of Emergency Nursing* 4:12–19 (1978).

Lyon, S. H.: Critical care of the child with multi-trauma: *Nursing Clinics of North America* 16:657–670 (Dec. 1981).

Stages of Reye's Syndrome. National Institute of Health, Washington, D.C., 1981.

26
An Overdose or Poisoning

Pamela W. Bourg
Denise A. Gornick

After completing this chapter, the reader will be able to do the following:

1. Triage a patient experiencing an overdose or poisoning.
2. Discuss the priorities of appropriate and accurate triage.
3. Identify broad classifications and clinical manifestations of each classification (e.g., barbiturates, acids/alkalies, street drugs).
4. Discuss different modes of poisonings, i.e., oral ingestion, injection or surface contamination, and the effects of each.
5. Describe potential life-threatening complications of poisonings.
6. Identify the pathophysiology related to poisonings.
7. List and describe nursing interventions indicated for poisonings.
8. Discuss antidotes commonly used in poisonings in the emergency department.

Care of the poisoned patient has markedly improved during the last decade as a result of sophisticated advances in poison centers, emergency departments, and prehospital care. With the proliferation of available chemicals and drugs, however, the potential increases for poisoning by both intentional and accidental means. In 1978 alone, there were 12,171 deaths due to poisonings in the United States. One-half of those deaths were due to carbon monoxide poisonings (*Clearinghouse Bulletin,* 1981). No end is in sight. In fact, the advent of new pharmaceutical agents (such as verapamil and the tricyclic antidepressants) promises to test further toxicologists' ingenuity in discovering how best to manage overdoses of new drugs (Kulig and Rumack, 1982).

Emergency nursing will need to develop further expertise in poison management. The toxic emergency may range from the life-threatening crisis that demands immediate resuscitative care to stable clinical conditions that may become unstable in time (Rumack et al., 1981). It is essential, therefore, that the emergency nurse be knowledgeable about the clinical manifestations associated with the commonly abused drugs and the methods by which these drugs can be counteracted or removed from the body.

TRIAGE

The victim of a reported or suspected overdose requires prompt management and should *never* be relegated to the waiting area in the emergency department (Budassi and Barber, 1981). Several clinical manifestations that can alert the triage nurse to the possibility of a drug overdose when it is not immediately apparent include a change in a state of consciousness, a fairly abrupt change in behavior or personality, lethargy, stupor, and coma. Other potential signs that may indicate overdose include unexplained cyanosis, seizures, and vascular collapse (Fauman and Fauman, 1978).

A poisoned patient must be cared for similar to any other critically ill patient. Initial observation of airway, breathing, and circulation are of primary importance. Often the ABCs are overlooked by the emergency department staff more concerned with learning the specific treatment for the poison than with the vital signs of the patient. The ambulatory, stable patient must be differentiated from the comatose patient. The emergency nurse must consider associated injuries and illness in a patient who is comatose from a drug ingestion. Almost all patients in a toxic condition have the potential for seizures and thus must be observed for seizure activity.

For the patient with toxic exposure to the skin or eye, immediate consideration must be given during the initial triage period to prevent any further absorption. Before any further assessment, therefore, the patient may have to be taken to an area where he can receive decontamination: for example, in the event of organophosphate exposure, removal of the contaminated clothes and decontamination of the skin can be life-saving.

The patient's presenting behavior is a significant observation to make before triage is completed. The poisoned patient may present as controlled, withdrawn, agitated, or combative. The patient out of control must be placed in an appropriate area to provide safety for himself as well as for the care providers. It is appropriate at the time of triage to assess the need for physical restraint in the intentionally overdosed patient. Restraints may have to be applied immediately to prevent the patient from further harming himself.

After it has been ascertained that the patient's vital functions are intact, more detailed subjective and objective data can be collected.

Subjective Data

Obtaining subjective data on a poisoned patient in the emergency setting may be difficult because many patients who take an overdose present with coma, seizures, or delirium (Bayer and Rumack, 1979). The emergency nurse should conduct a focused interview, if possible, to obtain the information contained in Table 26.1. Often the depressed patient who ingests an intentional overdose is reluctant to reveal the

TABLE 26.1 Subjective Data Base for the Poisoned Patient

1. What type of medication (poison) was taken?
2. How much of the particular substance was taken?
3. How long ago was it taken?
4. Was anything else taken, i.e., alcohol, other drugs?
5. Why did you take the medication?
6. Were you attempting to commit suicide?
7. Have you ever attempted suicide in the past?
8. Have you ever been treated for this problem?
9. If so, what type of treatment did you receive?
10. When were you last treated?
11. Were any antidotes given prior to arrival in the emergency department?
12. Has there been any vomiting or attempts to remove the poison?
13. When was your last meal? What did it consist of?
14. If the patient is unconscious, question significant others regarding when the patient was last seen in a normal state.
15. If the patient is unconscious, question significant others regarding events leading to the poisoning.
16. Is there a history of drug abuse? What types of drugs?
17. Any allergy history?
18. Are there any routine medications?

substance taken. In a study of drug-abuse patients in 1980, emergency department histories of 150 patients were compared with toxicology analysis; in only 20 percent of the cases was the history confirmed by the results. Furthermore in one out of four cases, a drug was found unsuspected from the history (*Analytical Toxicology,* 1980). Nevertheless, it is necessary to obtain a reliable estimate of the type and amount ingested because this is the first step in assessing the severity of the ingestion. Knowing the time of ingestion assists the nurse in determining when peak effects might be expected and whether preventing absorption would be useful.

In some cases, prior medical conditions, allergies, and administration of routine medications may influence the severity of the toxicity as well as the treatment. If no history is available, it is always advisable to focus on the patient's presenting symptoms. (For the subjective data collection relating to the substance abuser, see Chapter 27.)

When the overdose is intentional, it is important to try to ascertain what event actually precipitated the overdose. Family members and significant others should be interviewed. In interviewing the family, the emergency nurse should look for suicide attempts by other family members and other significant family pathology, such as divorce or death of a loved one. Families tend to offer independent verification of the patient's situation (Bayer and Rumack, 1979).

To complete the subjective history, the emergency nurse must interview prehospital personnel for any further information that may be pertinent, such as the patient's condition on his arrival or suggestive evidence of any other injury. Did the patient fall and strike his head after ingesting the poison? What field treatment, if any was done? It is especially important to have the poison container brought to the hospital.

Objective Data

Measuring vital signs is imperative upon the poison victim's arrival at the emergency department. Obtain vital signs repeatedly at regular intervals, the frequency to be determined by how critically ill the patient is. A head-to-toe assessment should be carried out, concentrating on the neurological and cardiopulmonary status.

Respiratory rate and rhythm are essential; do not use guesswork. Check for the presence of the gag reflex; however, in the assessment of obtundation, the presence of the gag reflex can be misleading and should not be relied on as an isolated diagnostic tool (Kulig et al., 1982). Measure blood pressure and pulse. Note any irregularities that will determine the type of monitoring required.

During the assessment of neurological status, concentrate on the level of consciousness (use of the Glasgow Coma Scale is a reliable objective assessment), pupil size and responses, deep-tendon reflexes, and the detection of any seizure activity. Any comatose patient should be investigated for potentially associated head or neck injuries or other medical problems. The mental status examination should include orientation, hallucinosis, memory, agitation, confusion, and suicidal ideation.

Additional assessments for ocular exposure include visual acuity, photophobia, spasm of the eyelid, and tearing. For skin exposures, assess the area of contamination, degree of absorption, and degree of burn. In caustic ingestions, assess the oral mucosa.

The objective data are useful not only for establishing a baseline but also in monitoring whether the patient is improving or deteriorating. The data collected will guide the emergency nurse in the assessment phase.

Assessment and Planning

Each poisoned patient should be assessed and planned for on an individual basis. It is important to assess the clinical manifestations, not the poison. Table 26.2 lists common presentations by poison classification. In addition, Table 26.3 lists pupillary changes and cites poisons that could possibly cause those changes.

Several common poisoning syndromes can guide the emergency nurse to a possible assessment. Patients with narcotic and sedative hypnotic poisonings may present as comatose, hypotensive, hypothermic, and with cardiorespiratory depression and hyporeflexia. Lomotil toxicity can be delayed for up to 12 hours or more and can be associated with anticholinergic activity because it contains atropine.

Anticholinergic drugs will cause patients to have warm, dry skin, dilated pupils, tachycardia and other dysrhythmias, hypertension, delirium, and hallucinations.

TABLE 26.2 Substance Manifestations

Specific Substance	Clinical Manifestations
Acids/alkalies	1. Respiratory distress due to edema. 2. Burning pain from mouth to stomach. 3. Oral burns: mucous membranes soapy and white initially, may become brown, edematous, and ulcerated. Absence of oral burns does not rule out esophageal burns. 4. Bloody vomitus that may contain shreds of mucous membrane. 5. Drooling due to inability to swallow. 6. Signs of esophageal or gastric perforation include subcutaneous air, rales, Hamman's crunch.
Barbiturates	1. Respiratory depression, pulmonary edema. 2. Decreased level of consciousness, may be stuporous to comatose. 3. Hypotension: BP typically reduced to levels less than 80 mm HG. 4. Absence of corneal and deep-tendon reflexes. 5. Rectal temperature reduced to levels averaging 35°C.
Salicylates	
Mild or early	Burning in the mouth, throat or abdomen; slight to moderate hyperpnea; lethargy, vomiting, tinnitus, hearing loss or dizziness.
Moderate	Severe hyperpnea, marked lethargy, delirium, fever, sweating, dehydration, incoordination, restlessness, ecchymosis.
Severe	Hyperpnea, convulsions, cyanosis, anuria, uremia, coma, pulmonary edema, respiratory failure, hypoglycemia.
Chronic	Tinnitus, abnormal bleeding, gastric ulceration, weight loss, rash, mental deterioration.
Acetaminophen	1. Nausea, vomiting, anorexia, abdominal pain; may be asymptomatic. 2. If untreated, may develop signs of hepatic failure.

TABLE 26.2 *(continued)*

Specific Substance	Clinical Manifestations
Opiates	1. Symmetrical pinpoint pupils (do not have pinpoint pupils with mephridine); dilated pupils do not rule out opioid ingestion. Mydriasis can result if asphyxia has occurred or may be due to concurrently ingested nonnarcotic drugs. 2. Depressed respiratory rate; rate is slow and shallow, decreasing at times to 2–6/min; may see Cheyne-Stokes respirations. 3. May present with convulsions, general excitement, and tremors. 4. Cardiovascular deterioration may occur as a result of respiratory depression and is usually manifested initially with hypotension.
Amphetamines	
Mild	Restlessness, tremors, insomnia, irritability, tachycardia, flushing of skin, increased sweating, dilatation of pupils, dry mouth, glycosuria, hyperactive reflexes, fever.
Moderate	Confusion, delirium, hallucinations, panic states, profuse sweating, tachypnea, hypertension, extrasystoles, dyskinesia.
Severe	Convulsions, circulatory collapse, hyperpyrexia, chest pain, subarachnoid hemorrhage, coma.
Tricyclics	Hypotension, seizures, lethargy, ECG abnormalities, supraventricular tachycardia, multifocal PVC, ventricular dysrhythmia, heart block, widening QRS, dysrhythmias, tachycardia, abnormal reflexes, coma, mydriasis, myoclonus, respiratory depression, delirium and hallucinations, hypo- or hyperthermia, dry mouth, absence of bowel sounds, blurred vision.
Cyanides	
Early	Resembles an anxiety state with headache, giddiness, excitement and tachycardia, dyspnea.

TABLE 26.2 *(continued)*

Specific Substance	Clinical Manifestations
Severe/late	Drowsiness, coma, seizures, cyanosis. If ingestion, gastric mucosal damage: blood-stained gastric aspirate, palpitations, hypotension, hypoxic ECG changes including atrial fibrillation, ectopic ventricular beats, abnormal QRS with the T wave originating high on the R wave.
Food poisoning *Salmonella* *Staphylococcus* *Clostridium botulinum* *Clostridium perfringens*	Nausea, vomiting, diarrhea, fever, and abdominal pain are the most common manifestations with botulism. (See the above symptoms and include the following: dysphagia, dysarthria, muscle weakness, urinary retention and respiratory paralysis, descending paralysis.)
Alcohol Methanol	Slight CNS depression, may be asymptomatic for up to a day before the onset of headache, nausea, and vomiting, severe abdominal pain; visual disturbances ranging from diminished vision to total blindness; may be accompanied by photophobia, pain, or conjunctival changes; coma and respiratory failure take place late in the course.
Ethylene glycol	1. May present as acute ethanol intoxication with mild to marked inebriation and GI distress. 2. During first 12 hrs, hypertension and leukocytosis frequently encountered; may progress to pulmonary edema, respiratory failure, convulsions, coma, CNS depression, cardiovascular collapse. 3. Twenty-four to 48 hrs after ingestion, may present with acute oliguric renal failure.
Isopropyl alcohol	Acetone breath, dizziness, headache, confusion, a flushing sensation, ataxia, stupor, hypothermia, hypotension, nausea, vomiting and diarrhea, severe gastritis occasionally accompanied by GI bleeding; acetonuria and acetonemia in

TABLE 26.2 (continued)

Specific Substance	Clinical Manifestations
	the absence of glucosuria, hyperglycemia or acidemia should arouse suspicion in patients with altered states of consciousness.
Iron	Vomiting, hemorrhagic gastroenteritis, lethargy, rapid and weak pulse, hypotension, pallor, cyanosis, ataxia; coma may appear ½–1 hr after ingestion. These symptoms may disappear after 4–6 hrs followed by 6–24 hrs asymptomatic period. A second crisis occurs with cyanosis, vasomotor collapse, pulmonary edema, hepatic and renal failure, coma.
House plants (Calcium oxalate)	Nausea, vomiting, diarrhea, fever, flushed face, dilated pupils, depressed respiratory status, hypotension/shock, drowsiness, stupor, convulsions, bradycardia, dizziness, dyspnea, respiratory or circulatory collapse, severe burning of mucous membranes with swelling of tongue and throat.
Sedatives/hypnotics	Nausea, vomiting, dry mouth, drowsiness, motor excitation followed by deep coma, rapid variations in pupillary width and reaction to light, hyperreflexia, hypotension, hypothermia, stupor to coma, slow, shallow respirations, seizures, bradycardia, cardiac dysrhythmias (A-V conduction disturbances).
Street drugs Phencyclidine (PCP)	1. Abdominal cramping, nausea, vomiting, muscle rigidity, head and neck posturing, increased deep-tendon reflexes, ataxia, very unsteady, staggering, swaying, and in need of support to stand; slurred, incoherent speech; eyes appear blank and glassy with an intense, piercing gaze; may be catatonic, stuporous, or extremely agitated; visual or auditory hallucinations (auditory predominant); muscle rigidity. 2. When hypertension and nystagmus, both vertical and horizontal, present

TABLE 26.2 *(continued)*

Specific Substance	Clinical Manifestations
Street drugs	
Phencyclidine (PCP)	together, usually indicates PCP abuse, as this is only abused drug that produces the two signs at the same time.
	3. Hypertensive crisis, seizures, renal failure, respiratory and cardiovascular collapse, and prolonged psychosis occur with high doses.
	4. PCP-induced coma will typically possess marked muscle rigidity—most other causes of drug-induced coma produce flaccid paralysis.
Cocaine	
Phase I	Early stimulation: nausea, vomiting, vertigo, headache, cold sweats, twitching of small muscles, especially of face, fingers, and feet; tics; tonic, clonic movements; rise in core temperature; elevated BP, pallor, PVCs; increased respiratory rate and depth.
Phase II	Decreased responsiveness, increased deep-tendon reflexes, generalized hyperflexia, seizures; increase in pulse and blood pressure; gasping, rapid or irregular respirations; peripheral, then central cyanosis.
Phase III	Flaccid paralysis; coma; fixed, dilated pupils; loss of reflexes; circulatory failure, ventricular fibrillation, pulmonary edema, respiratory failure.
Lysergic acid Diethylamide (LSD)	Bizarre visual experiences; heightening of brightness and color perception; distortion in perception of real objects; visual delusions or hallucinations; apprehension, panic, elation, or depression; may have "flashbacks" up to 1 yr after ingestion of drugs.

TABLE 26.3 Pupillary Changes in the Poisoned Patient

No change
  Acid/alkali
  ± barbiturates
  Demerol
  Salicylates
  Acetaminophens
  Cyanides
  Heavy metal (e.g., arsenic, lead)
  House plants (calcium oxalate)
  Sedatives/hypnotics/benzodiazepines

Unequal
  Anisicoria normal in 10% of all people
  Doriden

Mydriasis (dilatation)
  A. Anticholinergics (e.g., Atropine, Sominex)
      Phenothyazines (e.g., Haldol, Prolixen, Thorazine)
      Antihistamine
      Atropine/scopolamine
      Mushrooms
      Some house plants (e.g., Jimson Weed)
      ± Marijuana
  B. Sympathoimetics
      Speed
      Epinephrine/neosynephrine
      Thyroid medication

Miosis (constriction)
  Opiates (except Demerol)
  PCP
  Topical miotic drops
  Insecticides
  Organophosphates
  Carbamates: Tensilon, Physostigmine

Vertical nystagmus
  Sedatives
  PCP
  Dilantin
  Barbiturates (after ruling out brainstem lesions)
  Alcohol

NURSING CARE AND RELATED INTERVENTIONS 501

Commonly ingested anticholinergics include tricyclic antidepressants, antihistamines, phenothiazines, and over-the-counter sleep preparations.

Organophosphate and carbamate insecticide poisonings may present with cholinergic signs and symptoms such as increased salivation, lacrimation, and sweating. Frequently these types of poisoning mimic asthma, respiratory tract infection, and gastroenteritis.

Salicylate poisoning can cause hyperpnea, fever, vomiting, and hyperthermia. Other causes of hyperpnea may be metabolic acidosis as a result of methanol, ethylene glycol, isoniazid, and iron intoxication.

Hypotension and cyanosis that is unresponsive to oxygen therapy may be secondary to methemoglobinemia caused by ingestion of nitrates, nitrites, benzocaine, or a phenacetin compound.

Delirium and psychosis can be caused by phencyclidine (PCP). Chronic heavy metal poisoning may manifest as toxic psychosis (Gerstner and Huff, 1977).

The initial assessment should focus on vital functions. Next, the effects of the poison on body systems can be determined using the material thus far presented. Complications to watch for include central nervous system depression, respiratory depression or airway occlusion, seizures, cardiovascular compromise, temperature changes, cerebral edema, and pulmonary edema. (Table 26.4 outlines several sample triage notes for the poison patient.)

PATHOPHYSIOLOGY

The fundamental pharmacologic properties of a drug, such as rate of absorption, distribution in the body, and rate of elimination, provide valuable information regarding the degree of severity and length of the clinical course of a poisoned patient and determine methods that may be effective in eliminating the drug.

Knowledge of drug absorption after oral ingestion helps predict potential toxicity and helps determine if the use of absorbents such as activated charcoal will be effective in preventing absorption of the drug. A drug that is rapidly absorbed and reaches a plasma peak in one hour will not be effectively absorbed by charcoal administered two hours after ingestion. However, gastric emptying may be delayed in a mixed-drug ingestion, and the use of activated charcoal may be effective even several hours after the overdose occurs.

Some drugs have a low absorption constant. This may affect the ability to diagnose toxicity based on a plasma level obtained too early. This is the case with phenytoin, salicylates, and tricyclics, which are usually not well absorbed until many hours after the toxic ingestion. Absorption of most drugs occurs in the small intestines, and therefore drugs or conditions that delay gastric emptying will result in delayed absorption of the drug (Rumack et al., 1981).

NURSING CARE AND RELATED INTERVENTIONS

The major thrust of nursing intervention is to terminate the exposure of the patient to the poison, after life-threatening problems are dealt with. Any patient in coma also

TABLE 26.4 Examples of Triage Notes for Patients Experiencing Overdose or Poisoning

S: 25 yo M found comatose in bathroom. Multiple "track marks" present on both arms. PMH: history of IV drug use "on occasion," according to friend. Allergies unknown.
O: BP 100/p, P 92, RR 8. Responds only to noxious stimuli. No evidence of trauma on physical exam. Pupils pinpoint. Skin pale.
A: Possible drug overdose through IV injection.
P: Rapid medical evaluation, airway, O_2.

S: 19 yo F with reported ingestion of 50 tablets Triavil approximately ½ hr prior to arrival in emergency department. PMH: suicide attempt, with overdose, two times in past. History of severe depression in recent weeks. NKA, according to parents.
O: BP 84/48, P 120 irregular, RR 16. Becomes extremely agitated with attempts to arouse. Skin pale and cool to touch.
A: Suicidal attempt with tricyclic overdose.
P: Rapid medical evaluation, airway, O_2, cardiac monitoring.

S: 16 yo M found crawling and rolling in street and brought to emergency department by police. Became extremely combative and abusive while en route to emergency department. PMH: unable to obtain due to agitation.
O: BP 168/98, P 110, RR 28. Incoherent, slurred speech. Vertical nystagmus noted. Noxious body odor, unkept appearance.
A: Possible drug reaction or psychotic reaction.
P: Medical evaluation, quiet room to minimize agitation, restrain if necessary.

S: 45 yo F with chief complaint of nausea, vomiting, abdominal pain, and generalized muscle weakness. Also complains of difficulty focusing on near objects. Husband also complaining of some nausea and abdominal pain. PMH: no history of disease or illness; history of consumption of home-canned foods 24 hrs prior to onset.
O: BP 130/76, P 92, RR 20. Skin warm and dry. Oriented ×3.
A: Possible food poisoning.
P: Medical evaluation, admit examination room as soon as possible.

deserves to receive oxygen, glucose, and naloxone. This treatment is warranted and will certainly not be harmful.

A number of interventions can be used for care of the poisoned patient. The selection depends on the drug taken, the time elapsed since ingestion, and the presenting condition of the patient.

First-line intervention should include an intravenous line of normal saline or Ringer's lactate with a large-bore catheter (16 or 18 gauge) on any comatose or somno-

TABLE 26.5 Specific Diagnostic Studies

Substance	Lab Studies or Specific Tests
Acetaminophen	Blood level 4 hrs or more after ingestion—levels obtained before 4 hrs may not represent peak plasma levels; SGOT, SGPT, bilirubin levels, PT, PTT—see elevation in all of these 24–48 hrs after ingestion due to hepatotoxic reaction.
Caustic ingestion	CBC, T & C × 4, chest x-ray exam/abdominal x-ray exam, KUB x-ray exam.
Cyanide	Methemoglobin levels, ABGs.
Ethylene glycol	ABGs—see metabolic acidosis, look for increased anion gap, U/A—calciumoxalate cystalluria.
Lead	Lead concentration of blood, urine lead concentrations.
Hydrocarbon	WBC—see increase, ABGs, methemoglobin level, chest x-ray exam.
Iron	Serum iron concentration; abdominal x-ray if suspected ingestion of iron tablets; blood glucose—increase; increased WBC.

lent patient. Baseline blood samples for glucose, complete blood count, electrolyte values, and toxicology screens should be obtained prior to initiation of the intravenous fluids. (Table 26.5 specifies which tests are necessary for certain substances.) The general toxicology screen is probably overused. The care of the poisoned patient should be based on clinical status and not on drug levels. There are two cases in which drug levels are important for prognostic reasons: salicylate poisoning and acetaminophen poisoning. (Bayer and Rumack, 1979).

All comatose patients and patients with cardiac irregularities should have electrocardiogram monitoring. Baseline arterial blood gas studies should be obtained to monitor potential acidosis where applicable. A chest x-ray film should be obtained to determine if there has been any aspiration due to the poisoning.

Removal of the substance can be accomplished in one of two ways: gastric lavage or ipecac-induced emesis. Emesis is contraindicated in any patient who is comatose, seizing, or has ingested a caustic substance. Ipecac syrup is administered in doses of 30 cc for the adult and 15 cc for the child orally. It should be followed with one or two glasses of water. Sometimes walking the patient may help to induce emesis. Ipecac should be repeated only once because it may create cardiac dysrhythmias.

For the patient who is lavaged, there should be a cuffed endotracheal tube in place to provide airway protection. The size of the orogastric tube varies between 28 and 40 on the French scale. The patient should be placed in a left-lateral, head-down position and his stomach irrigated with an isotonic or half-normal saline up to 2,000 cc or until clear. The large-bore orogastric tube (Lavacuator) is also being used with increased frequency. Whole pills and pill fragments are being retrieved with good results with this type of tube.

Activated charcoal absorbs most drugs. It should be administered either orally or via an orogastric tube. The dose is 50–100 g for adults and 20–50 g in a child. Use of multiple doses of charcoal may be warranted in tricyclic antidepressant overdoses. Charcoal will also act as a marker of intestinal transit time so that when it appears in the stool it will be unlikely that any more absorption of the drug from the gastrointestinal (GI) tract will occur. Cathartics are another mechanism to decrease potential drug toxicity. They move the drug rapidly through the GI tract so that absorption will be decreased. The adult dosage of magnesium sulfate is 15 to 30 g; for children, it is 250 mg/kg.

An antidote is a physiologic antagonist that may reverse the signs and symptoms of the poisoning. Table 26.6 outlines the available antidotes. Other specific treatments to reverse signs and symptoms are listed in Table 26.7.

Ocular decontamination can be accomplished by flushing the eyes with plain tap water as soon as possible. Eyes should be irrigated for at least 20 minutes for acids, alkalies, and hydrocarbons. Ophthalmologic consultation should be obtained for corneal injuries.

External decontamination includes removal of clothes and cleansing of the skin. Organophosphates and carbamate insecticides may contaminate medical personnel.

TABLE 26.6 Antidotes

Poison or Agent	Symptoms Requiring Treatment	Antidote
Narcotic Analgesics or Related Agents Sedatives/hypnotics	CNS depression Respiratory depression	Naloxone (Narcan): Adult and pediatric dose, 0.8–2 mg IV. May need to repeat frequently due to short half-life (30 min).
Anticholinergic Agents Antihistamines Belladonna alkaloids Tricyclic antidepressants Over-the-counter sleep preparations	Central and/or peripheral symptoms accompanied by one or more of the following: hypertension, hallucinations, coma, convulsions, dysrhythmias	Physostigmine: Adult, 1–2 mg IV; children, 0.5 mg IV. Give slowly as it may precipitate seizures and brady dysrhythmias.
Cholinergic Agents Organophosphate Pesticides Carbamate pesticides Physostigmine Neostigmine Tensilon	Cholinergic crises: diaphoresis, lacrimation, bronchial secretions, excessive urination/defecation, convulsions, fasciculations	Atropine Sulfate: Adult: 2 mg IV; children, 0.05 mg/kg IV. Repeat every 10–30 min until cessation of secretions. Pralidoxime (After Atropine): Adult, 1 g IV over 2 min; children, 25–50 mg/kg IV. Repeat × 3 at 8–12 hr intervals if muscle weakness not relieved.

TABLE 26.6 (continued)

Poison or Agent	Symptoms Requiring Treatment	Antidote

Cyanide
  Potassium cyanide
  Hydrocyanic acid
  Laetril
  Nitroprusside sodium
	Cyanosis
	Convulsions
	Coma
		Amylnitrite: Inhaled 30 sec of each 60 sec.
		Sodium Nitrite: Adult, 300 mg IV (10 ml of 3% solution); children, 10 mg/kg STAT and 5 mg/kg in 30 min.
		Sodium Thiosulfate: Adult, 12.5 g (50 ml of 25% solution); children, 1.65 ml/kg of 25% solution. If child weighs 25 kg or more, give adult dose.

Iron Salts
  Ferrous sulfate
  Ferrous gluconate
	Hypotension, shock, coma, free serum iron present	Deteroxamine: shock and/or coma, 15 mg/kg/hr, IV infusion for 8 hr. If no shock or coma, but SI > TIBC, 90 mg/kg IM q 8 hrs.

Methemoglobin-producing Agents
  Nitrates
  Nitrites
  Phenazopyridine
	Methemoglobinemia	Methylene Blue: 1–2 mg/kg or 0.2 ml/kg of 1% solution IV. NOTE: Contraindicated if methemoglobinemia secondary to sodium nitrite in cyanide poisoning.

Acetaminophen
  Tylenol
  Nebs
	Hepatotoxicity, hepatocellularnecrosis	N-Acetylcysteine (Mucomyst):[a] 140 mg/kg PO of 20% solution loading dose. Maintenance dose, 70 mg/kg PO q 4 hrs for 17 doses.

Beta Blockers	Bradycardia, shock	Glucagon: 50 μg/kg IV bolus followed by 0.1 mg/kg/hr.[b]

[a] Investigational.
[b] Salzberg and Gallagher, 1980.

TABLE 26.7 Specific Treatments for Poisoning

Enhancement of Excretion

Alkaline diuresis: effective with salicylates, phenobarbital, and herbicides mecoprop and 2,4D (dichlorophenoxyacetic acid)

1. Administer IV fluids at rate required to keep output at 3–6 ml/kg/hr.
2. Add 2–3 ampules of sodium bicarbonate to each liter of D_5W (88–132 mEq/L).
3. Keep urine pH at 7.5 or greater.
4. Monitor hourly fluid intake and output and urine pH.
5. Monitor serum electrolytes.
6. Diuretics may be indicated.

Chelate Poisons to Form a Nontoxic Compound

1. EDTA (calcium disodium edetate) used in lead toxicity. Dose: 50 mg/kg/24 hrs IV or IV in three divided doses for 5 days. Course may be repeated as needed, being sure to allow two days between courses.
2. BAL (dimercaprol) used with mercury, arsenic toxicity. Dose: 3–5 mg/kg IV q 4 hrs for 2 days; 3 mg/kg/dose IV q 8 hrs for 2 days, 3 mg/kg/dose q 12 hrs for a week.
3. D-penicillamine used with mercury, arsenic, lead toxicity. Dose: 25 mg/kg up to 1 g PO QID.

Acid Diuresis

1. Ascorbic acid may be given in doses of 500 mg to 2 g orally or IV to obtain acid urine—pH 4.5–5.5.
2. Ammonium chloride may be used at a total dose of 2–6 g/day or 75 mg/kg/dose in four divided doses.
3. Many times mannitol diuresis will accomplish an acid urine alone without any additional measures.

Therefore, personnel should protect themselves with rubber gloves, masks, and rubber aprons. Whenever possible, the decontamination should occur outside the medical facility.

Serial vital signs and mental status evaluations must be continued. Follow-up should be made on any physical or somatic complaints. Maintain the patient's cleanliness after substance removal. (See Chapter 27 for a detailed discussion of psychological intervention with regard to the suicidal patient.)

DISCHARGE PLANNING

The decision to admit or discharge a poisoned patient from the emergency department is based on initial clinical condition, continued assessment, or the predicted severity of the poisoning. Several different types of poisonings require reevaluation hours after ingestion (e.g., tricyclic antidepressants). Observation units in emergency departments may obviate the need for these patients' admission to the hospital.

Psychiatric evaluation is another important aspect. It should be obtained before an overdose patient is discharged.

If the poisoning is accidental, appropriate family teaching regarding safety in the home should occur. Community health nurse referrals may be indicated in selected instances of repeated ingestions within the same household. Multiple ingestions may be a form of child abuse (Budassi and Barber, 1981).

Poison control systems evolved out of the need to regionalize linkages of the poison center to the Emergency Medical Service. The goal of such systems in the United States is to provide information and consultation, professional education, data collection, public education and prevention, research and evaluation, and further development of the system.

The Poisindex is a computer-generated microfiche system of specific and detailed emergency poison treatment protocols. It is published on a quarterly basis. Access to this system takes less than a minute and treatment can be instituted promptly.

CONCLUSION

The goal for the emergency nurse in the care of patients experiencing overdose or poisoning is to care for the patient, not the poison. In general, good supportive care followed by general poison management will contribute to a successful patient outcome. The nurse's efforts may take the form of early crisis management and patient family teaching.

BIBLIOGRAPHY

Arena, J.: *Poisoning: Toxicology Symptoms and Treatment.* 3rd ed. Springfield, IL: Thomas, 1976.

Bayer, M., and B. Rumack: Poisoning and overdose. *Topics in Emergency Medicine* 1(3): entire volume (Oct. 1979).

Budassi, S., and J. Barber: *Emergency Nursing Principles and Practices.* St. Louis, MO: Mosby, 1981, pp. 617–740.

Clearinghouse Bulletin for Poison Centers 35 (6) (Aug. 1981).

Cyanide poisoning: Medical emergency. *New York State Journal of Medicine,* 69:10–12 (June 1969).

Doull, J., C. Klaassen; and M. Amdur: *Toxicology: Basic Science of Poisons.* New York: Macmillan, 1975, pp. 677–698.

Drug abuse patients. *Journal of Analytical Toxicology* 1:6 (1980).

Elenbass, R., ed.: Poisonings and overdose. *Critical Care Quarterly* 4 (4): entire volume (Mar. 1982).

Fauman, B., and M. Fauman: Recognition and management of drug abuse emergencies. *Comprehensive Therapy* 4:38–43 (1978).

Gerace, R. V.: Near fatal intoxication by 1,1,1-trichlirethane. *Annals of Emergency Medicine* 10(10):533–534 (1981).

Gerstner, H. B., and J. E. Huff: Selected case histories and epidemiologic examples of human mercury poisoning. *Clinical Toxicology* 11(2):131–150 (1977).

Goldfrank, L., and R. Weisman: Bacterial food poisoning—what to do if prevention fails. *Postgraduate Medicine:* 72:171–179 (1982).

Greenland, P., and T. Howe: Cardiac monitoring in tricyclic antidepressant overdose. *Heart and Lung* 10(5):856–859 (1978).

Kulig, K., and B. Rumack: Update on overdose management. *The Digest of Emergency Medical Care* 2(4):1–3 (April 1982).

Kulig, K.; B. Rumack; and P. Rosen: Gag reflex in assessing level of consciousness. *Lancet,* 6 March 1982, p. 565.

Riegel, J., and C. Becker: Use of cathartics in toxic ingestions. *Annals of Emergency Medicine* 10(5):254–258 (1981).

Rumack, B.; J. Sullivan; and R. Peterson: Management of acute poisoning and overdose. *Rocky Mountain Poison Center Syllabus,* 1981, p. 23.

Salzberg, M., and E. Gallagher: Propranolol overdose: A case report. *Annals of Emergency Medicine* 9(1):26–27 (1980).

27
Drug or Alcohol Dependency

Pamela W. Bourg
Marilyn K. Bourn

After completing this chapter, the reader will be able to do the following:

1. Define *substance abuse* and relate the scope of the problem to emergency nursing.
2. Triage a patient with a drug or alcohol dependency.
3. Examine potential life-threatening complications of substance abuse.
4. Identify the pathophysiology relating to the substance abuser.
5. Identify noncritical pathology associated with substance abuse.
6. List and describe nursing interventions indicated for the abusing patient.
7. Discuss appropriate psychological interventions.
8. Describe alternative potential modes of discharge and followup care.

Alcoholism and drug abuse are recognized as two of contemporary society's most widespread and devastating problems. The many advances in pharmacology since World War II have provided extensive health benefits to patients today. Unfortunately, the advances have also engendered a belief that chemicals can solve our problems in these stressful and hectic times. Most health care providers know the many negative and harmful effects of substance abuse; patients, however, frequently ignore the warning signs of the serious side effects.

The incidence of drug and alcohol abuse is extensive throughout society. Alcoholism, for example, is the third-ranking major disease in this country and is considered a widely neglected medical problem (Bluhm, 1981). Heart disease and cancer are the only two disease entities that produce a higher mortality rate. Approximately 95 million adults consume alcohol; of those, it is estimated that 10 million could be classified as either abusers or alcoholics. In the adult population, 4 to 8 percent are suffering from some form of chemical dependency. In addition, studies indicate there is a cross-tolerance between drug and alcohol abuse. The terms *substance abuse* or *substance dependency* refer to these two combined disease entities.

TABLE 27.1 Commonly Abused Substances

Class	Examples
General CNS depressants (represents large group of drugs whose abuse brings patients to hospitals)	Alcohol, hypnotics, barbiturates, tranquilizers
CNS sympathomimetic or stimulants	Amphetamine, cocaine
Narcotic analgesics (opiates)	Heroin, morphine, methadone, propaxyphene, and synthetic drugs with similar actions
Cannabinols	Marijuana, hashish
Psychedelics or hallucinogens	LSD, mescaline, psilocybin
Solvents	Aerosol sprays, glue, toluene, gasoline, paint thinner
Over-the-counter drugs	Contain atropine, scopolamine, antihistamines
Others	Phencyclidine (PCP), bromides

The problem of substance abuse is becoming so prevalent that emergency nurses must deal with it frequently. In one major city emergency department, for instance, it was found that 25 to 50 percent of all ambulatory patients were significantly influenced (either mentally or physically) by large quantities of alcohol (Dilts et al., 1978). Patients involved in some form of substance abuse also manifest a 20 percent incidence of associated medical complications. Finally, statistics indicate that more than half of all motor vehicle fatalities are a result of alcohol intoxication (McElroy, 1981). (Table 27.1 describes commonly abused substances seen in the emergency setting.)

The emergency department presents a unique opportunity to intervene with substance abusers. Their presentation to the emergency department may be varied and confusing. The emergency nurse should recognize signs that signal a potential drug or alcohol problem. The abusers may be the great deceivers. They may present as ill-kempt or disheveled people—or as finely tailored, meticulously groomed executives.

Their presentation to the emergency medical system may include acute intoxication, withdrawal symptoms, syncope, seizures, hepatitis, gastrointestinal bleeding, trauma, and bizarre or suicidal behavior. Most frequently, substance abusers present with a variety of somatic complaints (Westie and McBride, 1979).

Problems resulting from substance abuse appear more extensive in modern society because of the increased availability and number of substances that are subject to experimentation and use. Drug and alcohol problems cross all socioeconomic lines and age groups, with adolescents and young adults particularly prone to involvement and experimentation. Several factors, however, have emerged as predisposing an individual to dependency.

In general, more men than women have substance dependency problems, often in the range of 3 or 4 to 1. This ratio varies considerably with the social and cultural group, the patient's age, and the type of substance. Changing social conditions that prevail in modern society have increased the number of women who abuse substances (Liban and Smart, 1980).

A common misconception is that impoverishment causes dependency. Studies indicate that alcoholism exists to about the same extent in both elite and nonelite groups. The overall rate of substance dependence tends to rise as disposable income increases. An example of this theory can be noted among adolescents in the United States. As a group, they have enjoyed affluence and have been associated with increasing rates of substance dependency.

Availability appears to play a major role in the genesis of substance abuse epidemics. Heroin usage increases in the United States after wars because of the soldier's international travel (as during and after the Vietnam War). It increases as well during good economic times. America's heroin usage decreases during bad economic times and after increased pressure from police and immigration officials. Emergency nurses may predict trends of other substance abuse that may affect the patients for whom they care. For example, an increase in the use of phencyclydine (PCP) among adolescents may be seen during appearances of well-known rock bands in a particular geographic area.

Learned behaviors also predispose individuals to develop substance dependency. Children are apt to emulate behaviors of parents when they reach adulthood. If one or both parents respond to problems with excessive use of alcohol or drugs, children may subsequently do the same.

Another interesting phenomenon reported in recent literature has suggested that "last borns" are more likely to develop substance dependence because they are at risk at an early age to experience parental loss. Loss of a parent disturbs family dynamics and the child's sense of security is often affected, therefore causing dependency on drugs or alcohol as a coping mechanism (Westermeyer, 1974).

Experimentation with alcohol and drugs is a phenomenon of contemporary society. The patterns described previously, however, do predispose individuals to abuse leading to dependency.

TRIAGE

The obvious substance abuser represents a minority of all patients seen in emergency departments. Commonly the patient presents with a variety of complaints. Since the prevalence of substance abuse is widespread, the nurse should consider the possibility of substance involvement whenever an emergency patient shows puzzling signs and symptoms.

The stereotypic motions surrounding the intoxicated patient sometimes cloud accurate assessment and triage. The emergency nurse, therefore, must be especially diligent when triaging. Initial observation of airway, breathing, and circulation is most important. The alert, ambulatory, stable patient must be differentiated from the comatose patient with an unprotected airway. Concomitant life-threatening illnesses or injury must be ruled out.

The patient's general behavior is an extremely important observation to make before triage is completed. The substance abuser may appear to have a normal mental status, be withdrawn, agitated, controlled, combative, or passive. The person's overall behavior can vary from stable to erratic. Emphasis must be placed on the importance of safety for the health care providers and other patients. The agitated or combative patient must be triaged to the appropriate area to provide proper care and safety for those involved.

Hygiene can be used as a guide to appropriate triage. Personal hygiene can distinguish between an acute or chronic problem. It can also indicate changes in mental status and/or coping mechanisms.

Using the three basic assessment tools, the ABCs, and judging by the patient's general behavior and personal hygiene, the emergency nurse can make a rapid and generally accurate initial triage decision. After assessment of more detailed subjective and objective data, the nurse can institute appropriate triage action.

Subjective Data

The basis of an emergency department nurse's subjective data gathering is the patient history. The major purpose of the subjective (history) data collection is to obtain as much information as possible, organize it into categories, develop patterns, and identify medical and nursing needs.

Frequently, the importance of this nursing process is underestimated. An incomplete data base may prevent adequate planning and intervention. A profile of medical, psychological, sociological, and environmental histories is essential. The goal of subjective data collection is to collect information that relates to the patient's current health problems; in this case, the substance abuse patient. In general, the patient's data base consists of three basic elements: (1) the patient's presenting problem(s); (2) the relationship between symptoms and relevant physiological manifestations; and (3) the patient's health state as it relates to the person's history and current health practices (Thompson, 1979). After establishing this basic approach, the emergency nurse can begin to develop an insightful and more complete data base for the substance abuser.

The patient entering the emergency department with a possible drug or alcohol problem may not voluntarily offer this information. Skill and tact are often the keys to accurate history-taking. Beginning the subjective data collection with general, nonthreatening components may help to establish a trusting environment so that more intimate information may be obtained. A firm, but kind and compassionate approach may be useful. It is important not to appear judgmental or disapproving (Bluhm, 1981). Begin the patient's history by asking the person why he came to the emergency department. Allow the patient to explain the various symptoms that have caused concern. The substance abuser often presents with traumatic concerns (fall, auto accident, assault) as well as nontraumatic ones (tremors, abdominal pain, insomnia). Attempt to determine the duration of the presenting complaint as well as the possible underlying abusive pattern. Allow the patient, using his own words, to describe the "quantity" and "quality" of the complaint. Such terms as "squeezing," "stabbing," "frightening," "uncontrollable" may help to describe the chief complaint. Discuss with the patient his concept of the precipitating factors. The patient may be unable to recall the onset of the abuse problem, but may be capable of competently discussing the onset of the current complaint. Time of onset is not considered a high priority in the emergency setting.

Patterns of past physical, medical, or mental conditions are important. Examine with the patient previous modalities of medical intervention (Antabuse, Methadone, counseling). Were these successful or unsuccessful? Has the patient received outpatient or inpatient care? In addition, assess what types of nonmedical interventions (home remedies, more drinking) made the problem better or worse. It is also imperative to look for other acute or chronic health problems that may influence the patient's condition. Myocardial infarctions, angina pectoris, chronic obstructive pulmonary disease (COPD), seizure disorders, pregnancy, diabetes, infection, and other complicating medical problems may significantly influence the medical intervention. In addition, the emergency nurse should assess for acute/chronic health problems that may be directly related to the patient's substance abuse. Delirium tremens, withdrawal symptoms or seizures, hallucinations, depression, hyperactivity, or suicidal gestures may also have an influence on the planning of treatment modalities. Concomitant use of prescribed medications or possible allergies to medications must be assessed before treatment is initiated. Devastating and potentially fatal results, including anaphylaxsis, may occur as a result of combining medications (prescribed or not).

After obtaining the history of a physical complaint, assessment of psychosocial factors can then be completed. Discuss with the patient the presence of support systems such as family, friends, or clergy. Does the patient have a significant other? An understanding of how the patient has influenced those around him provides further insight into the problem. How has the presenting problem interfered with the person's activities of daily living (job, family, home responsibilities) (Thompson, 1979)? During these initial phases, it is also helpful to determine if support systems will be available upon discharge of the patient. Alternate support mechanisms may be required; early planning for these can be beneficial in rapid and definitive treatment of the patient (see Table 27.2).

Finally, the comments of associated health professionals and medical records may help to complete a subjective history. Assessments made by emergency medical technicians and paramedics in the field (at home or work) may provide a missing link to a patient's history. Emergency departments and drug and alcohol services and clinics frequently keep unofficial logs or card files on chronic abusers. It is not unusual for the chronic abusers to be recognized immediately by one or more health professionals working in a system. These logs and experienced health professionals may serve as untapped resources for the chronic abuser. When information is unobtainable because the patient is in coma or uncooperative for some reason, previous medical records are invaluable.

Family, friends, and significant others may possess a wealth of information. Their presence during history-taking may or may not be advantageous. If their presence interferes with the collection of information, tactful diversion may be required. On the other hand, their companionship may be the support needed for the patient to discuss personal or embarrassing information openly. The emergency nurse may also

TABLE 27.2 Subjective Data Base for the Substance Abuser

1. Have alcohol or drugs ever been a problem in your life?
2. How much do you usually drink or take in a day?
3. What do you drink or take?
4. When was your last drink or drug?
5. Have friends or family ever been concerned about the amount of alcohol or drugs you take?
6. At what age did you first become high?
7. How would you describe your drinking/drug patterns?
8. Do you ever use alcohol/drugs to help you get through the day?
9. Have you ever missed work or lost jobs because of your habits?
10. Have you had any of the following problems: ulcers, hepatitis, neuritis, gastritis, pancreatitis, pneumonia, D.T.s?
11. When you drink or use drugs, do you feel happy, depressed, relieved, unchanged?
12. Do you have a significant other?
13. Have you ever had treatment?
14. What kind of treatment?
15. When was your last treatment?

find it helpful to speak with the family or friends on a private basis. Their input and insight may provide an added dimension to the data base. Closely examine any areas of discrepancy.

Objective Data

The objective baseline assessment often provides a clue to the presence of chemical dependency. Objective findings are often nonspecific. The emergency nurse must pay special attention to physical signs when considering substance dependence. General characteristics to assess include multiple odors of alcohol, paint, glue, almonds, ketosis; poor grooming; a demanding attitude; obstreperousness; behavior inappropriate to the setting; poor eye contact; facial tics; or tremors.

Vital signs may assist the nurse in determining the severity of the chemical dependence. Temperature may be elevated due to toxic effects or withdrawal from sedatives and narcotics. The patient who blacks out from drug use may be hypothermic. Careful assessment of the respiratory rate and effort is important. Tachycardia in the absence of infection may be an additional indication of substance abuse. Hypertension or a fluctuating blood pressure may also be present. Determine orthostatic pulse and blood pressure, which may indicate fluid loss caused by dehydration or occult bleeds.

Examination of the neurological system should include the following: deep-tendon reflexes, pupil size and responses (see the pupil chart in Chapter 26), presence of nystagmus, level of consciousness, and gait. The mental status survey should include orientation, hallucinosis, memory, agitation, confusion, and suicidal ideation. The Glasgow Coma Scale is an excellent quantitative tool for the objective assessment of level of consciousness. The objectivity it affords may be particularly helpful when a variety of emergency clinicians are assessing the acutely or chronically intoxicated patient.

Assessment and Planning

Collective consideration of the subjective and objective data is required when planning nursing care and assisting with the medical intervention for the substance abuser. Providing holistic care that encompasses emergent needs and basic needs requires skillful priority setting by the emergency nurse. Many authorities attempt to categorize patients according to signs and symptoms. Although categories may assist in organizing, they may also create tunnel vision in one's approach to the patient and may actually hinder priority setting. Each patient should be assessed and planned for on an individual basis. Two functions are used in assessing the substance abuse patient. (1) Determine whether the patient is acutely intoxicated or is withdrawing; then assess the degree. (2) Identify any conditions that will affect the care to be provided, such as mental status depression, seizures, dysrhythmias, unstable or abnormal vital signs, concomitant injury, occult bleeds, metabolic disturbances, and delerium tremens.

Alcohol, hypnotics, barbiturates, and tranquilizers are the most commonly abused central nervous system depressants, whose abuse brings patients to the hospital. The presence of these substances may cause a variety of neurological signs and symptoms. The degree of neurological deficit will be directly related to the type and quantity of substance abused.

A head-to-toe surface examination should be conducted for signs of abrasions, bruises, old scars, infections, and infestations. Be on the lookout for intravenous track marks.

Slow or stertorous respirations in the absence of an adequate gag reflex may require immediate suctioning, positioning, or intubation. The acutely intoxicated patient may experience respiratory depression or compromise at much lower levels than the chronic abuser. Alcohol levels of 300–400 mg percent may be associated with hypoventilation, and levels of 500 mg percent may be lethal.

Drug and alcohol withdrawal are common seizure etiologies. Focal seizures are rarely a result of withdrawal syndromes unless there is an underlying physiologic basis. Withdrawal seizures seldom result in status, and further assessments may be required (Bourn and Driscoll, 1982). Approximately 1–3 percent of the patients experiencing alcohol withdrawal will suffer a major motor or grand mal seizure. Of these, 90 percent will occur from 7 to 48 hours after the beginning of abstinence. Severe tremors may be mistakenly labeled as grand mal seizures. Differentiation is necessary to ensure appropriate emergency treatment and avoidance of overtreatment for the patient in simple withdrawal.

The presence of cardiac dysrhythmias, regardless of the underlying etiology, is potentially dangerous. Sinus tachycardia may be present during intoxication or withdrawal. Stimulants that produce tachycardia may exacerbate underlying cardiac anomalies. Depressants that produce bradycardia causing decreased myocardial function may result in inadequate cardiac output and poor cerebral perfusion. When abused, cocaine, phenytoin, tricyclic antidepressants, and numerous other substances may cause a variety of dysrhythmias. The underlying etiology of any dysrhythmia must be researched. In addition to the presence of an abused substance, underlying hypotension, hypoxia, and myocardial infarction must be considered.

Abnormalities in vital signs may exist. In the presence of poor nutrition and dehydration, the patient may experience postural hypotension and suffer syncope or near syncopal episodes. These periods of syncope may in turn result in trauma secondary to the fall. Because of overall poor health and hygiene and consequent underlying infection, the abusing patient often suffers also from fever of low or high grade. A progression of such infections as pneumonia, upper respiratory illness, cystitis, and meningitis may eventually lead to sepsis and a fatal outcome. Hypothermia is as serious a concern as hyperthermia. As a result of poor living conditions or decreased mental comprehension, many abusing patients suffer from mild to severe hypothermia. Certain toxins, LSD or phenothiazines, for example, are causal in hypothermia despite ambient temperature.

Mild hypothermia (35°C) is frequently treated in the emergency department with discharge to follow. Profound hypothermia (32°C or below), however, may produce more serious complications. Hypothermia is associated with such complications as cardiac dysrhythmias, aspiration, and damage to the central nervous system as well as death. Underlying respiratory manifestations are a result of an unprotected airway due to intoxication. Pneumonia, COPD, emphysema, bronchitis, tuberculosis, and other respiratory diseases are repeatedly seen in the abusing patient.

The potential for unstable or abnormal vital signs, then, may result from a number of sources. It is important that the emergency nurse recognize abnormal vital signs and complete a thorough assessment looking for each potential problem.

Concomitant injury is possibly the most common associated complication seen. Falls, automobile accidents, and assaults occur frequently during intoxication and withdrawal. In many cases the injury is minor and requires only a few stitches or orthopedic support. However, serious injuries, such as femur fractures, penetrating wounds, and skull fractures, often do occur. The determination of head injury versus intoxication is both complicated and confusing. The signs and symptoms of both may have a similar appearance and may mimic or mask each other. Careful observation of vital signs, level of consciousness, pupillary reaction, reflexes, vomiting, and drainage from the ears or nose is helpful (Budassi and Barber, 1981). Overlooking an intracranial bleed may be devastating and potentially lethal to the patient.

Certain metabolic disturbances are restricted to, and are much more likely to be seen, in the alcohol abuser. Alcoholic ketoacidosis typically occurs following a prolonged binge in the malnourished individual. The patient usually presents with protracted vomiting and moderate to severe ketoacidosis following several days of abstinence. The diagnosis is determined from the history, findings of metabolic acidosis, and, generally, a normal serum glucose level.

Alcohol-induced hypoglycemia may mimic acute ethanol intoxication. Hypoglycemia may occur in a wide variety of clinical settings, but it is especially likely to occur in the malnourished alcoholic, or in young children and adolescents during alcohol use or up to one day following alcohol use. The appropriate use of the Dextrostix or a serum glucose level will aid in the diagnosis.

Practitioners often fail to recognize Wernicke-Korsakoff syndrome as a result of its variable clinical presentation. Thiamine deficiency in some patients predispose them to develop structural neurologic pathologies. This leads to distinctive features, including nystagmus, gaze palsy, ataxia, confusion, hypothermia, hypotension, and possibly coma. More than 50 percent of the patients show ataxic changes and 90 percent have abnormal mentation (Marx and Rosen, 1981). Consequently, this symptomatology is frequently mislabeled as solely intoxication. The greatest degree of morbidity occurs with the sustained mental changes and residual memory impairment suffered.

Delirium tremens is a withdrawal state. It is the most severe withdrawal state and is manifested by excessive sympathetic discharge. The patient is delirious and has gross tremors, marked agitation, and auditory and visual hallucinations that prevail about 72 hours after withdrawal and may continue for several days (McElroy, 1981). Shock and hyperthermia are associated with a 10 to 20 percent mortality rate. Seizures occur in approximately 30 percent of these cases and may compromise the airway and be a major complication.

Disulfiram (Antabuse) and dolaphine (Methadone) are two commonly used medications for the treatment of alcohol and heroin addition, respectively. Complications may arise, however, as a result of these drugs. Withdrawal from Methadone may ensue in a fashion similar to withdrawal from heroin itself. Methadone remains in the body approximately 48 hours; 24 to 36 hours after this level falls, withdrawal symptoms become evident. Pupil dilation and increased blood pressure, pulse, and respirations, along with abdominal cramps, nausea, vomiting, restlessness, and diaphoresis may be experienced (Budassi and Barber, 1981). Although the patient experiencing Methadone withdrawal may wish to die, withdrawal is seldom fatal. Antabuse reactions, on the other hand, *are* potentially fatal. The effectiveness of this medication is due to behavioral modification as a result of its unpleasant side effects. Antabuse, when combined with alcohol, causes nausea, vomiting, and headache. In extremely sensitive patients or when mixed with larger quantities of alcohol, Antabuse may cause a bright red flushing of the face, neck, and upper thorax; hypotension, hyperventilation, tachycardia, decreased level of consciousness, nausea and vomiting, or coma. Recognition of this possibility is essential.

In addition to serious withdrawal complications, a continuum of noncritical withdrawal symptoms exists. As blood levels of the abused substance decline, metabolic changes occur, resulting in such general syndromes as tremors, nausea, vomiting, and headache. Mild withdrawal, popularly called *the morning after syndrome,* is the most commonly observed side effect of acute alcohol intoxication. The symptomatology occurs within several hours of cessation of intake and is characterized by headache, mild tremors, nausea, vomiting, irritability, and malaise (Budassi and Barber, 1981). Although mild withdrawal is experienced by a large number of the drinking population at one time or another, it is usually seen in the emergency department only as a result of the frightened amateur who has experienced acute intoxication the night before.

As the substance abuse becomes more chronic, the degree of withdrawal experienced proportionally increases. Depending on the particular substance of abuse, its half-life, and the duration of chronicity, severe withdrawal may occur from 7 to 24 hours after the substance has been stopped. It should be emphasized that the substance blood levels do not have to be completely depleted for withdrawal to occur. The chronic alcoholic who normally functions with a blood level of 300 mg percent may experience withdrawal when levels drop to 100 mg percent (legally intoxicated in many states). General physical condition and ability to cope may also influence the onset of severe withdrawal. Patients with diabetes, pancreatitis, infection, or cirrhosis may be more vulnerable to withdrawal. These patients may also experience increased symptomatology such as insomnia, diaphoresis, confusion, tremors, body aches, abdominal cramping, and the onset of auditory or visual hallucinations. The progress of severe withdrawal to the more serious delirium tremens must also be considered. (Table 27.3 outlines several sample triage notes on substance abuse patients.)

PATHOPHYSIOLOGY

Considerable variability exists in the presenting signs and symptoms of chemical dependency. The characteristics, of course, differ according to the type of drug, the person using the drugs, the various situations and environmental contexts, and the economic, social, and cultural milieu. A fairly consistent presentation can be discerned in all types of abuse, however. (Table 27.4 details the various stages.)

The early stage is problematic heavy usage. During the early phase, usage attains an increasingly important role in the individual's life-style. Decisions are made and behaviors chosen to include more frequent usage and higher doses. For example, an individual may gradually begin to avoid acquaintances or family members who do not use drugs or who use them infrequently and may increase contact with people whose usage is heavy and frequent. The chemically dependent individual begins to rationalize regular drug use. Drug effect is sought during unpleasant states such as anger, sadness, or anxiety, whereas previously it had been used only for social events or for celebrations.

The middle phase of chronic addiction is the stage of increased tolerance. In order to duplicate the desired drug effect, higher doses become necessary. This leads to greater expenditures for the drug and more prolonged periods of intoxication. With some addicting substances (e.g., alcohol, opiates, and sedatives), the person requires the drug to avoid withdrawal illness. The person's thoughts and behavior revolve around obtaining and using drugs. Usually at this time, the individual is unable to keep drug usage within normal limits. Personality changes may lead to solitary drinking or fights. The individual develops withdrawal effects. There is a tendency during this stage to develop respiratory, urogenital, or skin infections. Accidental overdose and suicide attempts occur because of poor judgment while under the influence, which causes decreased self-esteem and hopelessness about the future.

In the advanced stages, severe physical problems or incapacitating psychologic symptoms predominate. Loss of control occurs more than half and eventually 90 to 100 percent of the time. Thinking is distorted or confused for long periods of time. Cheap drugs or any substance that may be available (e.g., rubbing alcohol, glue) are used in a crisis when drugs of choice cannot be obtained. By this stage, chemically

TABLE 27.3 Examples of Triage Notes for Patients With a Drug/Alcohol Dependency

S: 27 yo M with chief complaint of severe abdominal "burning," c/o nausea, no emesis, SOB, or diaphoresis. PMH: none, NKA.
O: BP 114/72, P 98, R 24 shallow while lying; BP 98/P, P 122, R 28 shallow while sitting. Skin pale and warm. Abdomen tender to palpation. ETOH on breath.
A: Abdominal pain, R/O GI bleed, pancreatitis, gastritis.
P: Medical evaluation, admit examination room.

S: 64 yo F apparently has fallen several times with multiple contusions and abrasions. Verbally abusive and appears intoxicated. PMH: unknown, allergies/tetanus unknown.
O: BP 164/82, P 82, RR 18 uncompromised. Awake and alert but not oriented. 2 cm lac. to forehead, with minimal bleeding. No apparent LOC, PERRLA.
A: Possible intoxication, with suturable laceration.
P: Evaluate for head injury, medical evaluation for detoxification, admit examination room now.

S: 16 yo F found comatose in bathroom with numerous superficial self-inflicted lacerations to forearms. PMH: depression, according to boyfriend. Allergies/tetanus unknown.
O: BP 98/P, P 72, RR 10 shallow. Responds slightly to noxious stimuli. Minimal bleeding from arms. Incontinent of urine, rare unifocal PVC noted on monitor.
A: Possible suicide attempt with suturable lacerations and possible substance ingestion.
P: Rapid medical evaluation, airway, O_2.

S: 45 yo well-dressed man complaining of long-term cocaine abuse and requesting assistance. Staggering gait, cooperative with no other complaints. PMH: none, NKA.
O: BP 142/88, P 104, RR 18. Skin warm and dry. Patient is tearful and emotional.
A: Possible chronic drug abuse.
P: Medical evaluation with drug treatment referral, to waiting room.

dependent persons become increasingly dependent on others to manage their lives, solve problems, and provide sustenance and shelter.

It is important for the emergency nurse to try to ascertain what phase the patient is in. Care in the early phase is easier. As the course progresses, the patient becomes less cooperative and may not be amenable to therapy. Understanding these phases may assist in appropriate patient care interventions (Westermeyer, 1974).

TABLE 27.4 **Phases of Chemical Dependency**

Acute	Chronic	Deterioration
1. Increased amounts and frequency.	1. "Titer" or "binge" usage.	1. Continuous usage.
2. Seeks occasion to use.	2. Loses control.	2. Loses control most of the time.
3. Episodic intoxication.	3. Develops ingenuity for obtaining, paying for, hiding, and using the drug.	3. Plans daily activity around usage.
4. Emotional lability.		4. Poor grooming; unconcern with opinions of others.
5. Begins to exercise poor judgment.	4. Impairment between intoxication episodes.	5. Enjoys less but cannot stop.
6. Tolerance increases.	5. Decreased productivity.	6. Erratic, unable to conceptualize current status, poor judgment.
7. May incur vehicular or industrial accidents, falls, burns.	6. Uses to feel normal, personality changes, deterioration of self-image, cannot solve problems.	7. Manipulates others.
8. Somatic complaints may include insomnia, headache, palpitation, cramps, episodic distress, irritability, puffy face or extremities.		8. Alienated.
	7. Alienates others, abuses family.	9. Decreased tolerance, withdrawal seizures.
	8. Infections: respiratory, skin, accidental overdose, suicide attempts.	10. Parenteral users: septicemia, pulmonary edema, endocarditis, cirrhosis, homicide, vitamin deficiency.
	9. Withdrawal, apprehension, visual disturbances, malaise, weight change, depression.	

The acutely intoxicated adolescent presents a special problem to the emergency department nurse. When dealing with the young adult or child experiencing some form of substance abuse, it is important to realize the significance of such a problem. Early intoxication may be a result of experimentation, anxiety, peer pressure, rebellion, or imitation. Although it is important to question the underlying etiology of drug or alcohol abuse, it is imperative to recognize the significance of the medical situation. Blood levels of hallucinogens, sedatives, alcohols, or amphetamines need not be high in the young person to cause serious exacerbated signs and symptoms. Airway complications, cardiac dysrhythmias, and organ dysfunctions should be monitored with caution in the young adult. Appropriate assessment distinguishes those experimenting with substances and who need only observation versus those who are, in fact, dependent and may need detoxification.

The substance abusing patient may suffer a wide variety of concurrent medical problems. Gastric ulcers, hepatomegaly, systolic hypertension, cardiomegaly, anemia, thrombocytopenia, pancreatitis, coagulation disorders, and myopathies are not uncommon complications.

NURSING CARE AND RELATED INTERVENTIONS

The goal of this section is to teach nursing interventions for substance abuse emergencies. The emergency nurse must first address life-threatening problems to all who warrant it. This priority overrides all other considerations. Level of consciousness can be used as a guide to nursing interventions.

Priority in the comatose patient is to maintain an adequate airway, which may include straightening the head, removing any obstructions from the throat, and endotracheal intubation, if necessary. Simultaneously, intravenous fluids with a large-bore needle (16 or 18 gauge) should be started. Use physical restraint, if necessary, to make sure that the catheter will stay in place. Maintain adequate circulation. Use fluid challenges whenever appropriate. The ECG should be monitored because toxic agents may affect cardiac rhythm. Use side rails and restraints to prevent falls.

Baseline blood samples should be obtained for sugar, complete blood cell count (CBC), blood urea nitrogen (BUN), electrolyte values, and toxicology screens, including alcohol (see Table 27.5 for clinical significance of laboratory data). Initial management should never be delayed for toxicology determinations. After the blood has been drawn, unconscious patients should have boluses of two ampules (0.8 mg) of Narcan and 50 cc of 50 percent dextrose to treat possible hypoglycemia or narcotic-related causes of coma (see Table 27.6 for therapeutic drugs). If there is minimal or no response, a second 50 cc of 50 percent dextrose may be indicated and up to five ampules of Narcan may be necessary for deep coma or suspected Darvon abuse. A partial response may indicate that the patient may have taken a combination of drugs or has profound hypoglycemia or may have concomitant medical problems.

A Foley catheter is placed to monitor urine output and pH. Dip stick the urine specimen for ketones. An electrocardiogram is obtained to observe any dysrhythmias and to detect any calcium and potassium abnormalities. Arterial blood gas levels are also measured.

Emptying the stomach in the unconscious patient is a dangerous procedure even when a cuffed, inflated endotracheal tube is in place to prevent aspiration. The large-bore tube necessary for adequate lavage can perforate the esophagus while being positioned in the unconscious patient. Care must be taken during its insertion to prevent this complication. Sufficient fluid should be used until gastric return is clear. Then instill 30–50 g activated charcoal, which absorbs drugs so they are no longer available for absorption into the blood.

The somnolent patient is less of an immediate problem but can become worse if his condition is underestimated and not managed appropriately. Because the patient may still be absorbing the drug, attention should be paid to techniques that decrease further absorption (see Chapter 26 for specific information). If the somnolent patient becomes worse in the initial period, particularly with decreased respirations, the same nursing interventions should be used as for the comatose patient.

If the somnolent patient is easily arousable and breathing is adequate, oxygen

TABLE 27.5 Laboratory Studies and Clinical Significance in the Substance Abuse Patient

Test	Purpose
Dextrostix	Provides a quick determination for presence of low blood glucose and helps determine need for administration of dextrose, which may be the cause of coma.
Blood glucose	Hypoglycemia may be secondary to glycogen depletion in the liver as well as inhibition of gluconeogenesis from lactic, pyruvate, and amino acids.
Urine	Checks for presence of ketones.
CBC	Rules out infection. Checks for elevated WBC. Rules out occult bleed. Checks for decreased HCT.
Electrolytes	Rules out any metabolic problems (hyponatremia, hypocalcemia). Magnesium levels may help in clinically treating Wernicke-Korsakoff's syndrome.
Arterial blood gas	Helpful in ruling out metabolic problems such as DKA or hypoxia as a cause of coma.
Blood alcohol level/Toxicology screen	Provides baseline for determining intoxication vs. withdrawal. (Alcohol levels of 100 mg percent are considered legally intoxicated.)
Coagulation studies	Abnormal values can be found with advanced liver disease of alcoholism.
Amylase	Abnormal values can be found in patients with pancreatitis.
BUN	Can assist in ruling out renal failure as a cause for coma and/or seizure.

should be administered via nasal cannula, 2–5 l/minute. Simultaneous with history-taking, nursing interventions (e.g., IV, laboratory studies) as described for comatose patients should be carried out.

Emesis or lavage should be used in this group of patients. If the somnolent patient recovers in the emergency department and maintains normal vital signs, the person should be observed until alert enough to be evaluated by a psychiatrist or a drug/alcohol counselor. In the conscious patient, the emergency nurse must be careful not

TABLE 27.6 Medications in Patients with Drug/Alcohol Dependency

Medication	Action in Drug/Alcohol Dependent Patients	Dosage and Route	Administration Pearls for Drug/Alcohol Dependent Patients
Narcan (Naloxone)	Antidote for narcotics, Darvon, and Lomotil. Differentiates coma caused by drugs from other cause.	0.8 mg or more, usually given IV. Pediatric dose is the same.	Will precipitate narcotic withdrawal in drug-abusing patient. Be prepared to deal with a combative patient after administration.
Dextrose 50%	Reverses hypoglycemia. Can assist in the differentiation of unconsciousness and unknown illness.	$D_{50}W$ solution 50 ml IV bolus. Pediatric dose: $D_{50}W$ solution 1 ml/kg IV bolus	Draw serum glucose before administration.
Thiamine/ Multivitamins	Prophylaxis of thiamine/vitamin deficiency. Usually seen in alcoholics.	50–100 mg IV added to glucose solution or IM	
Valium (Diazepam)	Acute alcohol withdrawal; status seizures	2–10 mg IV titrated over 3–4 min (half-life is short, only 7 min)	Do not mix with any other injectable. DO NOT add to IV solution. Be prepared to deal with adverse reaction, including apnea and cardiac arrest.
Tranxene (Chloraxepate)	To relieve mild tremulousness in withdrawal patients.	15–30 mg P/O	Peak effects within 60 min.
Librium (Chlordiazepoxide hydrochloride)	To relieve acute tremulousness in the alcoholic patient or in those patients who are unable to take P/O preparations.	50–100 mg IM or IV	Use cautiously until patient is calm. Absorption is erratic by intramuscular route.
Haldol (Haloperidol)	To treat hallucinosis. Can be used in addition to benzodiazepines.	1–5 mg IM, P/O, or IV	IV use is still in research phase but has been found to be effective.

to underestimate the seriousness of substance abuse. Blood should be drawn for the same laboratory determinations. Emesis should be induced as well. Toxicological laboratory studies are usually not indicated for the conscious patient who does not have a concomitant medical problem.

The alcohol withdrawal patient should be treated symptomatically, depending on the stage of withdrawal. In the mild state, hydration, rest, buffered aspirin or acetaminophen and time are usually the only interventions necessary. The serious withdrawal patient may need a large-bore IV for volume restoration; thiamine is added to the dextrose solution or administered intramuscularly. Laboratory studies should include CBC, electrolyte values, levels of glucose, creatinine, and BUN. Benzodiazepines may be used to relieve tremulousness (Tranxene, 30 mg by mouth every four to six hours.) Librium may be used if nausea or vomiting is present. If psychosis is present, parenteral haloperidol (Haldol) is indicated.

Delirium tremens is an uncommon but serious syndrome of alcohol withdrawal. Nursing interventions include ensuring adequate airway, establishing an intravenous line (usually 5 percent dextrose with 0.45 percent normal saline is preferred), and obtaining laboratory studies as indicated previously. Parenteral diazepams are administered. Since hypoglycemia often accompanies delirium tremens, supplemental glucose may be administered. Fluid administration is vitally important in the management of delirium tremens because extreme dehydration may require up to 6 l for correction over 24 hours. At least one-quarter of the solution should consist of normal saline. An ECG should be obtained for a baseline, and monitoring should be continued. Temperature must be followed carefully since hyperthermia is a lethal complication of delirium tremens. If seizures occur, they should be managed with diazepam (Valium).

Discontinuance of drugs such as Methadone, morphine, Demerol, codeine and Darvon also produces varying degrees of withdrawal. Withdrawal treatment for narcotic addiction is not indicated in the absence of withdrawal signs. Always ensure the ABCs. In the presence of mild withdrawal, relieve the accompanying gastrointestinal symptoms, and manage with chlorazepate (Tranxene). In the presence of severe withdrawal symptoms, treat symptomatically. After withdrawal is complete, treatment with most medications is avoided, except for disulfiram (Antabuse) and Methadone.

Other groups of drugs such as CNS stimulants, psychedelics, and psychotomimetics may present emergency problems. Nursing interventions for these drugs are described in Chapter 26.

Inspect the skin for evidence of old trauma, pressure sores, infestation, and infection. Serial recording of vital signs and mental status must be continued. If there is not an altered level of consciousness, repeat the diazepam administration. A decreasing level of consciousness may signal intracranial pathology.

Follow up on any physical or somatic complaints, such as back pain. Administer fluids and assure the patient's comfort and personal rights.

Psychological Intervention

After the substance abuse patient has been stabilized for the medical emergency, the emergency nurse is responsible for ensuring that he is not left alone. Often these patients have expressed either suicidal or homicidal ideas. The intoxicated patient may refuse to stay in the emergency department before or after he sobers up. Two points are important:

1. The patient is emotionally needy and vulnerable, and he feels he deserves help.
2. The patient may evoke mixed feelings from emergency department staff due to manipulative and emotionally draining behavior (Budassi and Barber, 1981).

The substance abuse patient's right to refuse medical treatment should be carefully evaluated with injuries threatening to life or limb. A holding procedure should be instituted to restrain the patient and keep him from leaving the department until the patient is able to make an informed decision. Patients too intoxicated to walk should be detained until ambulatory to prevent injury.

The initial confrontation with substance abuse patients may be extremely difficult, especially if the encounter in the emergency department is the first time the patient faces his addiction problem. It is not unusual for the patient to continue his habit for months before receiving treatment.

The families of substance abuse patients require information. They need to know they are not alone and that there are millions of people who have loved ones suffering from substance abuse. The emergency nurse's role is to provide a supportive environment for both the patient and his loved one. Allow an appropriate amount of time for interaction with both the patient and family. This may be extremely difficult in a busy emergency department. The emergency nurse must effectively use available time for this to occur. Using time during serial monitoring can often be quite effective. Provision for counseling services for families should be arranged, if appropriate.

Disposition

After medical stabilization of the substance abuse patient, there are usually two alternatives to care in the inpatient hospital setting. The choice is usually made by a physician, depending on the severity of the illness. The patient may be admitted to a medical unit or to a detoxification unit. Some of the criteria used to determine whether a patient should be admitted to an inpatient medical unit versus a detoxification unit are as follows (adapted from "Standard Policies and Procedures," 1979):

A. First documented seizure.
B. Need for continued suctioning.
C. State of unconsciousness.
D. Need for continuous oxygen.
E. Need for intravenous therapy for longer than 24 hours.
F. Skull fracture.
G. Laboratory analysis values:
   1. BUN—40+.
   2. K—2.5.

3. Na—120.
   4. Po$_2$—50.
   5. pH—7.35+.
   6. Amylase elevated with fever and abdominal pain.
   7. Methanol—40+.
   8. HCT—less than 30 percent, acute or chronic bleeding.
H. Vital signs
   1. Temperature 38°C or greater.
   2. Pulse
      a. Irregular.
      b. Pulse rate of 140 to 160 and/or blood pressure systolic below 90.
      c. Rate of 160 will need to be evaluated before considered for inpatient detoxification admission.
   3. Blood pressure 250/160.

Before the patient is transported out of the emergency department, a verbal report is usually given to the nurse on the inpatient unit. Essentials of the report should include the following:

1. Synopsis of patient's emergency department course.
2. Patient's current vital signs.
3. Level of consciousness.
4. Report of any laboratory values.
5. Report of laboratory specimens sent.
6. Whether the patient has relatives accompanying him.
7. Any special problems (e.g., current behavior and/or mental status).

Discharge Planning

Virtually all treatment programs educate the patient and the family regarding the substance abuse syndrome. Families should be taught early warning signs of dependency, its effect on the family, and the usual outcomes of abuse if interventions are not instituted. Although the importance of education has not been tested formally, most individuals active in the field of substance abuse believe that patients and family gain considerably from learning about their disorder.

A variety of resources exist within the community that can benefit the substance abuse patient. These resources often go hand in hand with institutional treatment. Alcoholics Anonymous (AA), for instance, is an excellent resource for treatment. This best known self-help group, composed of individuals who are themselves recovering alcoholics, establishes a milieu where help is available 24 hours a day. AA also offers groups that discuss special problems of children of alcoholics (Alateen) and of spouses (Alanon). AA can be used as a referral source where no other outpatient service is either available or acceptable to the patient. Halfway houses and outpatient counseling are other alternatives when available in the community.

Disulfiram (Antabuse) is a drug useful to patients who want to attempt sobriety but have episodic motivations to return to alcohol. Antabuse interferes with the metabolism of alcohol in such a way that increased amounts of plasma acetaldehyde build up. This, in turn, produces flushing, throbbing in the head and neck, headache, and nausea and vomiting.

The opiate abuser does tend to differ from the alcoholic. He tends to be younger and has more antisocial problems. There is a documented level of crime associated with illicit use of opiates. Dolaphine (Methadone) does not cure opiate addiction. Methadone maintenance is used to help the addict develop a life-style free of street drugs.

Basic rules of rehabilitation for all substance abusers are as follows: (1) detoxify the abuser; (2) encourage the patient to reach out to family and significant others; (3) evaluate the patient's efforts; (4) help the patient establish goals; and (5) offer a program of counseling. In order to continue and reinforce the need for referrals to rehabilitation agencies, emergency department personnel require feedback regarding referral outcomes. Some type of follow-up system should be initiated and maintained.

CONCLUSION

The emergency nurse's role with a substance abuse patient can be pivotal. The nurse may be the first knowledgeable person an abuse patient encounters who can help him identify his illness and assist him on the road to recovery (McElroy, 1981). Although the nurse may experience rebuffs, it is still important to try to assist a chronic substance abuser to a rehabilitation program.

The goal for the nurse should be to interact with the patient nonjudgmentally. It is not enough to know the treatment regimen and pathophysiology of substance abuse; the nurse must also understand the roots of the abuser's behavior.

BIBLIOGRAPHY

Anderson, D., and J. Cosgriff: *The Practice of Emergency Nursing*. Philadelphia: Lippincott, 1975, pp. 71–89.

Anderson, R.: Recognition of drug and alcohol use and abuse. *Occupational Health Nursing* pp. 25–26 (Sept. 1981).

Berdie, M. A.: An evaluation of services provided drug abusers in an emergency room. *International Journal of the Addictions* 13(5):695–707 (1978).

Bluhm, J.: When you face the alcoholic patient. *Nursing 81* pp. 71–73 (Feb. 1981).

Bourn, S., and M. Driscoll: Understanding and managing the seizure patient. *Emergency Nursing Update Series* 2:19 (1982).

Briggs, T.: General management guidelines for the alcoholic and other chemically dependent. *Minnesota Medicine* 3:176–177 (1979).

Budassi, S., and J. Barber: *Emergency Nursing: Principles and Practice*. St. Louis, Mo: Mosby, 1981.

Chambers, C. D.; D. M. Peterson; and S. C. Newman: The acute drug reaction in a hospital emergency room: a demographic and social assessment. *Journal of the Florida Medical Association* 60:40 (1972).

Danis, J.: Stigma management with the alcoholic patient. *Journal of Emergency Nursing* 7:204–208 (Sept./Oct. 1981).

Dilts, S. L.; B. R. Berns; and E. Casper: The alcohol emergency room in a general hospital: A model for crisis intervention. *Hospital Community Psychiatry* 29:795–796 (1978).

Fauman, B., and M. Fauman: Recognition and management of drug abuse emergencies. *Comprehensive Therapy* 4:38–43 (1978).

Ficarra, B.: Toxicologic states treated in an emergency department. *Clinical Toxicology* 17:143 (1980).

Goodman, A., and A. Gilman: *The Pharmacological Basis of Therapeutics*. 6th ed. New York: Macmillan, 1980.

Khantzian, E. J., and G. J. McKenna: Acute toxic and withdrawal reactions associated with drug use and abuse. *Annals of Internal Medicine* 90:361–372 (1979).

Levy, L.; J. Duga; M. Girgis; et al.: Ketoacidosis associated with alcoholism in nondiabetic subjects. *Annals of Internal Medicine* 78:213–219 (1973).

Liban, C., and R. G. Smart: Generational and other differences between males and females in problem drinking and its treatment. *Drug and Alcohol Dependence* 5:207–221 (1980).

Marx, J., and P. Rosen: Increasing detection of Wernicke-Korsakoff syndrome. *Emergency Room Reports* 2:121–126 (1981).

McElroy, C.: Alcohol withdrawal syndromes. *Journal of Emergency Nursing* 7:195–198 (1981).

Shuckit, M.: *Drug and Alcohol Abuse—A Clinical Guide to Diagnosis and Treatment*. New York: Plenum, 1979.

Standard Policy and Procedures. Department of Health and Hospitals, Division of Psychiatric Services, Denver, Colo., #2028179 (1979).

Svitlik, B.: Helping the alcoholic patient on the road to recovery. *Journal of Emergency Nursing* 7:199–202 (Sept./Oct. 1981).

Thompson, J.: Subjective data collection in the emergency department. *Emergency Nursing Update Series* 1:2 (1979).

Valle, S.: A model for alcoholism treatment in general hospitals. *Maryland State Medical Journal* 3:77–79 (1980).

Westermeyer, J.: Alcoholism from the cross cultural perspective: A review and critique of clinical studies. *American Journal of Drug and Alcohol Abuse* 1(1):89–105 (1974).

Westie, K., and D. McBride: The effects of ethnicity, age and sex upon processing through an emergency alcoholic health care system. *British Journal of Addiction* 74:21–29 (1979).

28
A Psychiatric Emergency

Janet Gren Parker

After completing this chapter, the reader will be able to do the following:

1. Triage a patient experiencing a psychiatric emergency.
2. Categorize such a patient according to exhibited behaviors.
3. Discuss the nursing care of a patient experiencing a psychiatric emergency, describing how to use therapeutic communication, restraints, and medications.
4. List common medications used in the care of such patients.
5. Discuss the discharge planning necessary for patients experiencing a psychiatric emergency.

One of the more anxiety-provoking situations in the emergency department is the arrival of a patient in need of emergency psychiatric care. A psychiatric-mental health emergency is a sudden change in behavior or an unforeseen, isolated incident that, if ignored, may result in life-threatening or psychologically damaging consequences. The following elements are included in the patient's behavior:

1. The change is sudden, occurring within days, not months of time.
2. The behavior is unusual for that patient.
3. The behavior is disordered, lacking a pattern or purpose.
4. The behavior is inappropriate, not fitting the circumstances or situation in which the patient finds himself (Sclar, 1981).

As the emphasis of care has shifted from state hospital-based care to community-based care, the number of people using the emergency department for psychiatric care has increased. The need for emergency care can be defined by the patient, family, or agents of society. Depression and suicide attempts are the primary reasons people seek care; in addition, other reasons include anxiety, intoxification, aggressive behavior, psychosis, confusion, excitement, bizarre behavior, and hysteria (Sclar, 1981).

The goal in an emergency psychiatric situation is to reduce stress and the emotional distress of the patient and family and to alleviate the immediate crisis (Sclar, 1981). This chapter discusses the categories of patient behaviors that present in the emergency department, specific nursing care interventions, and discharge planning necessary in the care of the patient experiencing a psychiatric emergency.

TRIAGE

Triage is extremely important to help differentiate psychiatric and organic origins of the patient's behavior and to establish priorities of care. The patient should be triaged to the medical service whenever there is a doubt about a possible organic cause. Medical causes should always be ruled out before psychiatric evaluation is attempted. Table 28.1 lists common medical disorders with their psychiatric symptoms that often confuse the diagnosis.

Subjective Data

The triage nurse must obtain as much data as possible from the patient, family, or significant other. Obtaining data is sometimes difficult, particularly when the patient will not speak or responds only with inappropriate comments. The triage nurse must ascertain the immediate concerns of the patient and the patient's family or significant others. What recent events happened in the patient's life to precipitate the present behavior? What is the patient's usual mode of behavior? Has the patient's usual behavior changed? How has the patient been interacting at work, with his family, and with his peers?

Organic indicators must also be considered. Is there a history of an abrupt personality change without an identifiable precipitant? Is there a history of central nervous system trauma or disease or a history of drug or alcohol abuse? Does the patient have any past medical history that might indicate an organic origin to the problem? Is the patient currently taking any medications?

Every patient presenting to the emergency department with altered behavior must be evaluated for possible suicidal or homicidal ideation. The patient, even if a child or an adolescent, should be asked directly whether he has ever contemplated harming himself or others. This question does not give a person the idea of suicide, but instead suggests to him that it is appropriate to talk about such thoughts and actions. It is usually reassuring to the patient.

Objective Data

Describe the patient's behavior as much as possible rather than labeling it. Observe the interaction between the patient and any family member or significant other. Vital signs should be recorded to help rule out organic causes.

TABLE 28.1 Medical Disorders With Psychiatric Symptoms

Disorder	Psychiatric Symptoms
Cushing's syndrome	Anxiety, thought disorder, delusions
Addison's disease	Depression, apathy, thought disorder, confusion, agitation
Hyper- and hypoparathyroidism	Anxiety, hyperactivity or depression, confusion, disorientation, thought disorder, somatic delusions
Hyperthyroidism	Anxiety, depression, hyperactive or grandiose behavior
Hypothyroidism	Clear mental status with anxiety, irritability, thought disorder, and hallucinations
Thiamine deficiency	Confusion, decreased memory, auditory and visual hallucinations
Vitamin B_{12} deficiency	Apathy, irritability, depression, mood swings, delusions, hallucinations
Pernicious anemia	Depression, feelings of guilt or worthlessness, confusion
Huntington's chorea	Mood swings, delusions, auditory hallucinations
Alzheimer's disease	Dementia, aphasia, decreased cognition, depression, paranoid delusions
Encephalitis	Stupor, coma
Epilepsy	Impulsive violent behavior
Lupus	Thought disorder, depression, confusion
Meningitis	Agitation, confusion, disorientation, hallucinations, stupor
Porphyria	Anxiety, severe mood swings, excitement or withdrawal, angry outbursts
Multiple sclerosis	Personality change, inappropriate behavior, mood swings, depression
Intracranial tumor	Depression, anxiety, decreased memory, agitation
Pancreatic carcinoma	Depression, imminent sense of doom, decreased drive and motivation

SOURCE: Casadonte et al., 1980.

A brief mental status examination is helpful in documenting the patient's present condition. The elements of a mental status examination include the following (Cohen and Harris, 1981):

Physical appearance—clothing, hygiene, odor, use of cosmetics, physical health, appearance in relation to age.
Psychomotor behavior—gait, handshake, posture, abnormal movements, pace and energy of movements.
Mood and affect—attitude toward the nurse, appropriateness of affect, range of affect, specific feelings and moods.
Intellectual performance—attention and concentration, insight, orientation, short-term memory, social judgment.
Speech—amount, clarity, liveliness, rate, rhythm, volume.
Thought—clarity, content, flow.
Level of consciousness.

Assessment and Planning

By analyzing the subjective and objective data collected, the triage nurse makes an assessment and develops a plan of care. The plan of care should include the patient's priority of care and appropriate nursing actions such as restraints, close observation, or suicidal precautions. The assessment is usually more meaningful if it can be in the form of exhibited behavior, rather than disease oriented. (Table 28.2 contains two examples of triage notes for patients experiencing a psychiatric emergency.)

CATEGORIES OF PATIENT BEHAVIOR

Psychiatric emergencies are best understood by classifying them according to categories of patient behavior rather than the more traditional diagnostic categories because emergencies often require decisions and actions before a diagnosis is determined. Behavior classification includes behavior that is threatening to others, behavior that is self-destructive, disruptive behavior, and behavior that immobilizes the patient so that it is impossible for the person to negotiate life demands (Sclar, 1981).

Behavior That Is Threatening to Others

Violent patients pose a genuine danger for all personnel in the emergency department. Unfortunately, it is difficult to predict violence with certainty. Eighty percent of violent acts are performed by people under the age of 50 (Slaby, 1981). Violence may be anticipated in patients with a history of unprovoked, unexplained acts of violence prior to their arrival at the emergency department, impulsive and aggressive behavior, previous arrests or juvenile records, alcohol or drug toxicity, organic disturbances, or acute paranoia. Violent behavior is usually due to social maladjust-

TABLE 28.2 Examples of Triage Notes for Patients Experiencing Psychiatric Emergencies

S: 19 yo WF with c/o not eating or sleeping the last 3 days. "My boyfriend left me and I can't handle it anymore." Unable to work last 2 days because "I can't concentrate." No sign of drug or alcohol abuse. Patient denies suicidal or homicidal thoughts. PMH: none, no current meds, NKA.
O: Well-dressed, clean woman, energy of movements decreased, flat affect, thought processes and LOC normal, speech slowed and soft; BP 110/70, P 80 regular.
A: Depression.
P: Psychiatric evaluation, waiting room.

S: 25 yo WM found in tree by police with butcher knife to his throat. Neighbors say he has been in the tree for 3 days. They called the police when they saw the knife. He has been "talking out of his head" in the tree. PMH: unknown, current meds unknown.
O: Disheveled, head shaved, feces and urine all over body, will not speak, handcuffed, gait shuffling, no eye contact, spits occasionally at policemen.
A: Disruptive behavior, R/O acute psychosis.
P: Psychiatric evaluation, admit to examination room now with handcuffs in place with policemen.

ments without manifested psychotic disorders (Slaby, 1981; Sclar, 1981). Violent behavior can also be seen as a defense mechanism that protects the patient from unbearable and overwhelming feelings of helplessness (Pisarcik, 1981).

Behavior That Is Self-Destructive

Suicidal behavior is also difficult to predict. Kaplan et al (1982) found that among mental health professionals the accuracy with which suicide can be predicted is limited. In fact, in most mental health settings, the management of suicide risk is based on only two clinical observations: the imminence of suicidal feelings and the severity of past suicide history.

Previous suicidal attempts are helpful indicators of the development of potentially self-destructive behavior. Women attempt suicide more frequently, whereas men succeed more often. This pattern is changing, however, because of the changing role of women in society. Adolescent suicide is on the increase, with suicide being reported in children as young as five and six years of age (Herman and Schowalter, 1981). The widowed and the divorced, as well as the single person, have a higher incidence of suicide compared to married people.

Emergency department health care providers should investigate all single-car accidents to identify accidents that the patient could have initiated himself. When the account of the accident does not add up to a true picture, questioning the patient may help identify behavior problems that should be addressed. Impulsive, independent, and action-oriented people will initiate a single-car accident on the spur of the moment as the result of a recent stress that was embarrassing or humiliating (*Emergency Medicine,* 1981).

Depression is the major predisposing factor for suicide, with psychosis and drug abuse closely related to self-destructive behavior. Fifty percent of depressed patients present with physical complaints, such as headaches, insomnia, anorexia, constipation, and fatigue (Guze, 1981). Feelings of sadness, hopelessness, and apathy are frequently present. Children who have suffered chronic illness, severe trauma, several hospitalizations, deprivation, losses or separations, or abuse are at high risk for developing depression. Depression can be manifested by despondency, psychomotor retardation, agitation, sleep disturbances, changes in eating and bowel habits, and sexual dysfunction (Guze, 1981).

Disruptive Behavior

Patients who exhibit disruptive behavior can be a major problem in the emergency department. They are not violent or suicidal, yet they are often disruptive and difficult to handle effectively. Patients with disruptive behavior usually are psychotic, depressed, anxious, or have a psychosomatic disorder, a grief reaction, or a reaction to physical or sexual trauma.

A true psychosis is due to a functional disorder manifested by disturbances in speech, delusions, and/or hallucinations. The health care provider must differentiate between a functional and organic psychosis. The following findings would support an organic cause for the psychosis:

1. Rapid onset of symptoms with no past medical history of emotional problems.
2. Symptoms developing after the age of 40.
3. Changes in vital signs or abnormal pupils.
4. Tumors, diaphoresis, or disorientation.
5. Impaired recent memory, ataxia.

Manic-depressive states are manifested by a wide variety of behaviors. The patient's speech pattern may be slow, soft, and monotone or fast, racing, and high-pitched. The patient's thoughts may race or be apathetic and disinterested. Behavior may be agitated or slow in movement. The patient may complain of sleeping all the time or of insomnia. His affect may be flat, sad and tearful, or excited and animated.

Anxiety is an emotional response to a perceived danger. The patient may complain of headaches, dizziness, fainting, body aches and pains, hyperventilation, severe agitation, fear, panic, phobias, or hysteria.

Immobilizing Behavior

Behavior that immobilizes the patient so that it is impossible for the person to negotiate life demands can be confused with many psychiatric disorders. This category, however, refers to behavioral changes that are the result of some type of biological dysfunction. Elderly patients with organic brain syndrome and patients with drug overdoses are examples of patients with immobilizing behavior that is due to biological dysfunctions. Patients suspected of suffering from biological dysfunction require complete medical, neurological, and psychiatric evaluations. Even then, the diagnosis may be difficult to determine and the patient may be referred from one service back to another in an apparently endless cycle.

NURSING CARE AND RELATED INTERVENTIONS

Caring for the patient with a psychiatric emergency is a challenge that is often rewarding and satisfying for the nurse as well as for the patient and family. Many such patients simply need someone to talk with and to listen to their problems. Crisis intervention techniques are extremely helpful in most situations.

Therapeutic communication is the goal in talking with psychiatric patients. The nurse should be honest, open, and show genuine interest in the patient. The nurse should acknowledge the feelings and behaviors the patient is exhibiting and also validate and recognize the person's positive qualities. To assist in developing an understanding of what the problem is, encourage ventilation and exploration of feelings and thoughts. Listen attentively, reflect back feelings, and state and restate the patient's feelings when the person is unable to express them (Sclar, 1981). Offer reassurance by providing clear, concise information and by answering questions honestly and directly. All activities should be directed toward facilitating a problem-solving process.

Touch is an effective means of nonverbal communication that can convey caring and concern. It should not be used with patients who are paranoid, in panic, or assaultive because they may misconceive any bodily contact as a threat, an intrusion, or a violation.

If the patient is a child, observe the family interaction carefully. Try to see the problems through the child's eyes, speaking with the child separately from the family. A sudden change in a child's behavior may indicate that the entire family has problems that should be addressed.

Restraints

When a patient is unable or unwilling to control his behavior or is harmful to himself or others, restraints may be necessary. The patient actually may feel relieved when someone else takes charge and provides him with the necessary controls he is unable to impose on himself. The nurse should assess the need for the restraints and obtain authorized consent for their use, if possible. The time and the reason for the restraints must be documented. Describe the patient's activities and behaviors that necessitated the restraints. The patient must be closely monitored and observed to prevent any anxiety complications. The restraints should be removed immediately if there are any signs of physical distress or an alteration in the condition of the patient.

Mechanical restraints are the most common type used, usually leather straps and/or a posey belt. Sheets and bandages may also be used. Whatever is chosen, the patient's circulation must be checked below the site of each restraint to ensure that circulation to the distal extremity is not being compromised. People restraints may also be used. Five people (one for each extremity and one for the trunk) physically restrain the patient until mechanical restraints are applied. Restricting the patient to a particular examination room is another technique that is sometimes helpful in keeping a patient in a confined area, not totally restrained.

Medication Therapy

Another form of restraint that is commonly used in the emergency department is chemical—specific drugs to calm the patient. These drugs are often referred to as *major tranquilizers, neuroleptics,* or *antipsychotic* medications. Some sources classify these drugs according to chemical structure, but it seems to be more convenient to classify them into high- and low-potency categories. Low-potency drugs tend to cause orthostatic hypotension and sedation, but they have less extrapyramidal side effects. High-potency drugs have less of an effect on the blood pressure and cause less sedation, but they have increased extrapyramidal side effects. Both categories of drugs exert their effects by blocking the dopamine receptors in the brain. They also have anticholinergic properties. Table 23.3 contains common antipsychotic drugs used in the emergency department.

Antipsychotic medications are contraindicated in patients in coma as a result of alcohol, barbiturate, or narcotic use and in patients with severe central nervous system depression, allergies to the drug, blood dyscrasias, liver disease, Parkinson's disease, or increased intraocular pressure, and in pregnant women.

The dosage depends on the patient's size, age, weight, past response to drugs, severity of illness, degree of sedation required, and risk of side effects. The dosage for children is usually 20–50 percent less than the adult dosage. In children, it is usually recommended that drugs not be used unless the patient is behaviorally out of control.

Rapid neuroleptization may be tried to calm a violent patient. A physical examination should be done initially to rule out intracranial tumors, hypertension, head injury, hypotension, and toxic delerium. One to ten milligrams of Haldol intramuscu-

TABLE 28.3 Emergency Department Antipsychotic Drugs

Trade Name	Generic Name	Common Dosage (IM)
Haldol	Haloperidol	2–5 mg
Thorazine	Chlorpromazine	25–50 mg
Navane	Thiothixene	4 mg (not recommended for children under 12)
Stelazine	Trifluoperazine	1–2 mg
Prolixin	Fluphenazine	1.25 mg
Compazine	Prochlorperazine	5–20 mg

larly or 25–100 mg of Thorazine intramuscularly is given initially. This is repeated every 30–60 minutes until the patient is calm. Check and document the patient's blood pressure and pulse before each dose of medication.

Common side effects associated with antipsychotic medications include a decreased tolerance to alcohol, decreased seizure threshold, orthostatic hypotension, sedation, alterations in sexual function, nasal congestion, dry mouth, blurred vision, increased appetite, phototoxicity, and constipation. Thorazine can also cause electrocardiogram (ECG) changes with QRS prolongation and ST and T wave depression and blood dyscrasias.

Extrapyramidal Side Effects

It is estimated that approximately 33 percent of the patients taking antipsychotic drugs experience some form of extrapyramidal side effects from the drugs (Harris, 1981). Parkinsonism, dyskinesias and dystonias, akathisia, and tardive dyskinesia are four classes of side effects that may be seen in patients presenting to the emergency department.

With Parkinsonism side effects, the patient presents with Parkinson disease symptoms. These symptoms usually clear if the dosage of the drug is decreased. The temporary use of antiparkinsonism agents, such as Cogentin or Symmetral, may be necessary in some cases.

Dyskinesias and dystonias are more common side effects seen frequently in young people in their upper teens and twenties. These side effects usually appear dramatically and suddenly. The patient is frightened and usually afraid that he is desperately ill. The use of 25–100 mg of Benadryl intravenously or intramuscularly will convert the dyskinesias and dystonias. Cogentin may also be used.

If akathisia develops, the patient may present with feelings of restlessness and agitation. The drug dosage should initially be reduced. If the side effect remains, the use of another antipsychotic agent may be necessary. Antiparkinsonism agents may also be helpful. Valium is recommended only as a last resort.

Tardive dyskinesia is a long-term side effect. There is currently no treatment recommended to help handle it except discontinuance of the drug. Electric conversion therapy may be used in some situations.

The Violent Patient

The goal in caring for the violent patient is to establish control of the patient and the situation in order to create a safe environment for the patient, other patients, and the staff. It is not wise to be passive and reflective with the violent patient. Firm limits must be established and the patient treated with honesty, dignity, and respect. Offer reassurance, explaining where the patient is, what is being done, and why it is being done. Answer questions directly and honestly.

The patient's behavior often must be controlled immediately through force, verbal communication, physical restraints, and drugs. Enlist the support of other team members, including security officers, in the emergency department. Haldol is the preferred drug, 5–10 mg intramuscularly or 5–20 mg orally. The examination area for the violent patient must be large enough to provide the patient a feeling of private space. It should be well lit with no dangerous furnishings, readily accessible to security officers, and have multiple exits. The health care provider should always be between the patient and an exit so that escape is possible, if necessary.

After treating a violent patient, the nurse may feel overwhelmed. Thoughts may need to be ventilated and feelings and experiences shared with peers.

The Suicidal Patient

Goals in caring for the suicidal patient include opening lines of communication, identifying and exploring resources and options, establishing or renewing social supports, and beginning some type of therapeutic intervention. Evaluation of the suicidal potential is extremely important because outpatient versus inpatient treatment must be decided. Hospitalization is recommended if the patient is dangerous to himself or others, social support systems are nonexistent or ineffectual, or medication is ineffective.

The patient should be cared for in a safe, comfortable, and quiet environment. Security should be notified for backup and the patient checked for possession of weapons. Reassure the patient that he is safe in the emergency department and that the staff will not allow him to harm himself. Therapeutic communication is used to help diffuse the crisis and to plan adequate long-term interventions.

DISCHARGE PLANNING

Often the patient experiencing a psychiatric emergency will be discharged from the emergency department into the care of police officers to be transferred to the local psychiatric hospital for further care. Signed commitment papers enable the police to transport the patient. The nurse must prepare the patient for such a disposition, reassuring him that the police will not harm him and that he is being transported to a hospital for further care, not to jail. This is often a traumatic time for the patient and his family. They must be prepared for what is happening, told why it is happening, and be given an idea of what the immediate future will be for the patient.

If the patient is discharged and referred for continued outpatient therapy, the nurse must be sure that the patient understands when and where he should return. The family must also be aware of the planned follow-up care. Everyone involved in the situation, including the patient, must be cognizant of the fact that the emergency department is always available if the patient feels his behavior is becoming a concern or if he feels the need to discuss his feelings with someone. All prescribed medications and their potential side effects must be explained to the patient and family.

Referrals for follow-up care may include actual outpatient psychiatric follow-up in a local mental health clinic or nonpsychiatric follow-up. Social and residential issues may be the cause of the problems, or medical and legal issues may have to be addressed. Public health nurses, social workers, and chaplains may have to be contacted to help in discharge planning.

CONCLUSION

Patients requiring emergency psychiatric care usually create anxiety and disruption in the emergency department. The nurse must realize, even though the disruption is not appreciated, that the patient requires quality care to help reduce his stress and anxiety. A therapeutic climate that facilitates resolving problems must be created. All members of the health care team must be included in the care of a patient experiencing a psychiatric emergency. Group intervention guarantees that such a patient will receive the best care available within the emergency department and the local community.

BIBLIOGRAPHY

Casadonte, P. P.; D. E. McPherson; B. Z. Paulshock; E. D. Peselow; and C. Rohrs: Psychiatric emergencies in primary care. *Patient Care* 14:14–17+ (Nov. 30, 1980).

Cohen, S., and E. Harris: Mental status assessment. *AJN* 81:1493–1518 (1981).

Cordoba, O. A.: Antipsychotic medications: Clinical use and effectiveness. *Hospital Practices* 16:99–100+ (Dec. 1981).

Guze, S. B.: Early recognition of depression. *Hospital Practices* 18:87–89+ (Sept. 1981).

Harris, E.: Antipsychotic medications. *AJN* 81:1316–1323 (1981).

———: Extrapyramidal side effects of antipsychotic medications. *AJN* 81:1324–1328 (1981).

Herman, S. P., and J. E. Schowalter: Depression, suicide, and the young child. *Emergency Medicine* 13:60–62+ (Sept. 30, 1981).

Kaplan, R. D.; D. B. Kottler; and A. J. Francis: Reliability and rationality in the prediction of suicide. *Hospital Community Psychology* 33:212–215 (1982).

Pisarcik, G. K.: Psychiatric emergencies and crisis intervention. *Nursing Clinics of North America* 16:85–94 (Mar. 1981).

Sclar, B.: Psychiatric Emergencies. In A. W. Burgess (ed.): *Psychiatric Nursing in the Hospital and the Community*. Englewood Cliffs, NJ: Prentice-Hall, 1981, pp. 471–486.

Slaby, A. E.: Emergency psychiatry: An update. *Hospital Community Psychology* 32:687–98 (1981).

Suicide by accident. *Emergency Medicine* 13:128–130 (Apr. 15, 1981).

29

Heat Disorders and Cold Disorders

Margaret E. Moser

After completing this chapter, the reader will be able to do the following:

1. Triage patients experiencing heat disorders and cold disorders.
2. Explain body heat production and dissipation mechanisms.
3. Describe causes of hyperthermia, hypothermia, and frostbite.
4. Recognize symptoms and signs relating to heat disorders and cold disorders.
5. Evaluate laboratory data relating to heat stroke.
6. Develop nursing interventions for the treatment of patients with disorders due to temperature extremes.
7. Recognize and interpret symptoms of frostbite.
8. Identify dangers of treatment in the hypothermic rewarming process.
9. Develop discharge planning for patients with disorders due to temperature extremes.

Hyperthermia and hypothermia are complex medical disorders that are directly related to environmental temperatures. The disorder may be deemed a true emergency, requiring immediate intervention. The nurse must be able to perform a rapid, adequate, well-organized assessment and develop an appropriate plan of care. Nursing intervention must be effective in order to assist the patient in restoration and maintenance of normothermia in relationship to environmental factors that may influence the patient's situation and life-style.

TRIAGE

Subjective Data

Collection of the history from the patient, family, ambulance personnel, or others is the first step in the triage process. Patients having heat disorders or cold disorders will usually present with temperature changes and associated symptoms. To what depth the triage nurse explores the chief complaint will, of course, depend on the severity of the patient's condition. If the patient appears stable, collect the data by asking, "What is the complaint?" and "What is it like?" The *quantity* of the problem is conceived by questions such as "How severe is the problem?"; "How often does it occur?"; and "How long does it last?" *Chronology* is obtained by questions such as "When did it start?" and "How has it progressed?" The *setting* is established by such questions as "Where was the patient when it started?" and "What was he doing at that time?" The nurse continues with factors that *aggravate* or *alleviate* the problem by asking, "What makes it better or worse?" *Associated manifestations* of the problem are approached by asking, "What other signs or symptoms is the patient experiencing with this problem?"

A pertinent past history assists the nurse in evaluating the patient's complaint. This history includes the patient's age, history of cardiovascular problems, cerebral or pulmonary problems, skin disorders, chronic diseases, recent illnesses, past heat- or cold-related problems, hyperthyroidism or other metabolic disturbances, what medications are currently being taken, use of alcohol or amphetamines, any known allergies and history of tetanus toxoid immunization.

Objective Data

The triage nurse collects objective data from the patient by means of the general survey immediately on the patient's arrival in the emergency department. Simple, close observation reveals whether the patient is seriously ill; signs of respiratory distress, extreme pain and pronounced changes in the level of consciousness will be readily observed. In the less acutely ill patient, skin color, diaphoresis, shivering, posture, irritability, edema, and facial expressions (denoting apprehension or malaise) may be present and will assist the nurse in making a rapid assessment.

After the patient is made comfortable, a complete set of vital signs are taken. Temperatures above 103°F (39°C) or below 97°F (36°C) should be taken again at a different anatomical site, preferably a rectal measurement. If extremes exist, a thermocoupler should be used.

Neurological symptoms are noted early in both hyperthermia and hypothermia, ranging from confusion and disorientation to delirium and frank coma.

Assessment and Planning

After obtaining subjective and objective data, the nurse integrates the findings and makes an initial assessment. This assessment is accomplished by identifying one or more nursing diagnoses and preparing a related plan of care. The plan must include priority of care for the patient, indicating whether the patient should be placed in an examining room or be retained in another area where appropriate nursing intervention may be initiated. (Table 29.1 contains examples of triage notes for patients experiencing heat or cold disorders.)

HYPERTHERMIA 543

TABLE 29.1 Examples of Triage Notes for Patients Experiencing Heat and Cold Disorders

S: 50 yo WM c/o headache, fatigue, dizziness, nausea, with vomiting, leg cramps (severe pain Achilles area both legs). Onset this p.m. while playing baseball at local church. PMH: negative, no allergies, and taking no meds.
O: Skin pale, warm, profuse diaphoresis. T 104°F oral, P 100, RR 28, BP 100/72. Mental status: anxious and irritable.
A: Heat exhaustion, R/O heat stroke.
P: Admit to examining room, medical evaluation immediately.

S: 64 yo BF admitted per ambulance stretcher. Family states found mother in BR 30 min ago (where she lives alone). PMH: high blood pressure for 2 yrs. Takes (1) BP tablet each a.m.
O: Patient unconscious. Extremities rigid, skin cold, dry, cyanotic, BP 70/40, P 32 weak, RR 8–10 shallow. Receiving O_2 per mask at 10 L/min.
A: Hypothermia, R/O CVA.
P: Admit to examining room, medical evaluation immediately.

HYPERTHERMIA

Hyperthermia is a complex medical disorder that refers to an increase in deep body heat (core temperature) due to the environment, exercise, or a defective thermoregulatory system. The amount of heat necessary to affect change of the human body's heat balance structure is dependent on a number of precipitating factors that include hyperthyroidism, amphetamine use, alcohol use, and fever. Chronic heart disease, old age, prematurity, obesity, and abnormalities of skin and sweat glands are other factors that increase susceptibility to heat.

The heat-regulating center in the hypothalamus is the body's thermostat, measuring core and peripheral blood temperatures and initiating cardiovascular and sweating reflexes to dissipate heat. Callaham (1979) relates that 97 percent of cooling takes place at the interface between skin and air. Cutaneous vessels dilate dramatically, increasing blood flow and maximizing the cooling of blood circulating at the surface.

Ambient heat or environmental temperatures of 90°F (30°C) account for heat disorders in 90 percent of individuals who seek medical treatment, according to Callaham. In temperatures above 99°F (37°C), conductive and radiant mechanisms of heat loss are hindered. These mechanisms account for more than 60 percent of regulatory heat loss; therefore, only evaporation remains to cool the body. Doris and Baker (1981) discuss in detail experimental measurements of evaporative water loss in high ambient temperatures.

Humidity affects performance ability and may be quantitated by a psychrometer. This instrument is composed of three thermometers and measures effects of ambient, radiant, and evaporative heat (a regular thermometer measures dry/air temperature). The wet bulb globe temperature reading (WBGT) is a good figure for assessing humidity. This device is used to plan activities for athletic practice and military training.

Acclimatization, or body adjustment to activity in high temperatures, occurs via two processes. First, sweat production increases (2.5 times normal); and second, sodium content in sweat decreases. When maximal acclimatization occurs, the individual begins to perspire earlier and 2–3 times the normal amount of sweat will be produced. This sweat contains less sodium than normal. Maximal cardiac output and stroke-volume will be attained. This acclimatization process takes several weeks to develop usually occurring with gradual increases or exercise in a hot climate. (Goldfrank et al., 1980).

The disturbances resulting from direct effects of environmental heat on body tissues include changes in mental status, cardiovascular and renal function, and electrolyte balance.

Mental status changes occur due to vascular shunting for peripheral dilatation. Cerebral ischemia may develop, especially in patients with already decreased vascular volume, such as those on diuretics, fasting, or with history of congestive heart failure (CHF) or alcohol abuse. These changes present clinically as confusion, abnormal behavior (combativeness, irritability), cerebellar ataxia, delirium, and frank coma. Seizures are inconsistent but may occur in patients with heat stroke.

Cardiovascular changes are the earliest symptoms noted. As the anterior hypothalamus senses the rise in temperature, reflex mechanisms cause splanchnic vasoconstriction and peripheral vasodilatation. The central regulating mechanism normally maintains the core temperature approximately 3° to 5°F higher than the temperature at the surface. Surface vasodilatation may shunt as much as 4 l of circulating blood per minute, resulting in core heat loss and increased cardiac output. The net result is an increased heart rate and a decreased blood pressure. As the core temperature continues to rise, cardiac output may double and then drop suddenly at temperatures above 108°F (42°C). Oxygen consumption follows a similar pattern. Anemia may occur due to heat-induced destruction of red blood cells, further increasing circulatory flow. Renal failure may develop due to the decreased renal blood flow resulting from cardiovascular shunting.

Changes in the electrolyte values of sodium, potassium, calcium, and serum phosphate occur. Sweat losses are great (often 1.5 l per hour), and losses of sodium and potassium occur. Calcium losses occur during the second or third day, possibly due to deposits of calcium phosphate and calcium carbonate into skeletal muscles that occurs with rhabdomyolysis.

Callaham (1980) refers to rhabdomyolysis in patients with exertional heat stroke who will have muscle tenderness, myoglobinuria, and ischemic compartment syndrome. They also have dangerously elevated potassium levels and plummeting serum calcium because a considerable amount of plasma will leak into damaged tissue. High temperatures may damage body cells in many different ways, resulting in widespread pathology.

Bleeding diathesis is one of the most feared consequences of extreme hyperthermia. Clinically, it presents with massive ecchymosis, hematemesis, and epistaxis. Direct thermal injury to the endothelial vascular lining results in clinical signs of disseminated intravascular coagulation (DIC). Alterations of all clotting factors in the direction of hypocoagulability may be caused even by normal exercise in heat.

Other pathophysiological occurrences may be noted in gastrointestinal dysfunction, ulceration, or massive bleeding. Respiratory problems of pulmonary edema, vascular thrombosis, and concomitant systemic acidosis may occur with hypoxemia and hypercapnia. Hepatocellular dysfunction will result in jaundice.

LESS COMMON HEAT ILLNESSES

Pathophysiology

Heat edema is the result of exposure to a hot environment. *Prickly heat* develops primarily in humid climates where sweating is ineffective; thus, the skin is kept wet for longer periods of time. *Heat tetany* is probably related to the hyperventilation that develops in people suffering from heat exposure. *Heat syncope* is postural hypotension caused by heat exposure. It is probably related to vascular shunting through dilated cutaneous vessels. *Anhidrotic heat exhaustion* is preceded by prickly heat in 80 percent of the cases. *Malignant hyperthermia* is a rare, genetically determined condition precipitated by inhalants and neuromuscular blocking agents that are used during general anesthesia.

Clinical Manifestations

Heat edema is clinically manifested by mild swelling of the extremities, with occasional pitting edema of the ankles. The patient with ankle edema from heat presents with complaints of (1) tightness of the extremities; (2) swelling; and (3) possibly itching. This disorder occurs in any age group. The history should note exposure such as lying in the sun, walking on the beach, or working in a hot environment. Objectively, the nurse notes a slightly elevated pulse rate, reddened and warm skin (which may be sunburned), and a slightly elevated temperature.

A patient with prickly heat presents with an erythematous, fine papular rash that may cause a prickly, itching sensation. The patient states that the rash appeared suddenly and that he feels hot. He may also complain of nausea, malaise, and irritability. The patient's temperature may be slightly elevated (99°–104°F) and the pulse rate increased. The blood pressure is usually within normal limits.

Heat tetany presents with carpopedal spasms occurring during exposure to heat.

Anhidrotic heat exhaustion is manifested clinically by symptoms of weakness, failure of normal sweating, and vasopressin-resistant polyuria and it occurs particularly in people who are acclimatized.

Primary signs of malignant hyperthermia include tachycardia, tachypnea, hypoxia, hypercarbia, and metabolic acidosis. Other signs sometimes present include cardiac dysrhythmias, cyanosis, skin mottling, rigidity, and profuse sweating.

Nursing Care and Related Interventions

For a patient experiencing heat edema, the nurse must formulate the plan of care that relates to the patient's symptoms, which would include cold wet dressings to the affected area and elevation of the affected part. Discharge planning includes teaching the patient avoidance of hot or humid environments until the swelling is reduced.

Treatment for prickly heat is symptomatic; discharge planning includes teaching proper skin cleansing techniques and providing an environment for good air movement to assist in the healing process.

Heat tetany resolves itself promptly when the patient is removed from a hot environment to a cool environment.

For a patient experiencing heat syncope, the avoidance of any quick movements and sudden or prolonged standing positions are adequate preventative measures.

For anhidrotic heat exhaustion, intervention is symptomatic and begins with creating environmental changes—that is, placing the patient in a cool climate. A potassium supplement may be useful for replacement. Burch et al. (1979) have shown that a total body potassium depletion of approximately 517 mEq (20 percent) occurs in about the third week of acclimatization, a condition that may be the cause of anhidrotic heat exhaustion.

For a patient experiencing malignant hyperthermia, Dantrium may be effective in some situations.

HEAT CRAMPS

Pathophysiology

Heat cramps occur most frequently in healthy people who perspire freely and replace fluid losses with large amounts of water, which causes rapid changes in extracellular fluid osmolarity. It is believed that the serum sodium level decreases because of hypotonic dilutions resulting in heat cramps.

Clinical Manifestations

The pain is generally moderate to severe and located in the most worked muscles; the extremities, shoulders, or dorsal buttocks. The patient may have a slightly elevated temperature, pulse rate, and respiratory rate, but the blood pressure is usually within normal limits. The patient may also complain of weakness, headache, and nausea.

Diagnostic Studies

The history and physical examination are usually sufficient for diagnosis, but measurement of arterial blood gas levels may be ordered to assist in a differential diagnosis for ruling out hyperventilation and alkalosis from muscle fatigue. Hyperventilation is virtually universal at respiratory rates up to 60, which may be common in heat stress. Heat loss is thereby increased, and respiratory alkalosis is often present.

Nursing Care and Related Interventions

The goal in the care of the patient with heat cramps is to relieve the cramps by replacing the sodium the patient has lost.

Place the patient in a cool environment to rest. Administer a sodium chloride solution, prepared by adding 1 teaspoon of salt or two 10-grain salt tablets to 1 quart of water. The patient drinks three to four glasses of this solution. Intravenous fluids may be needed and normal saline (0.9 percent sodium chloride) or a hypertonic saline solution (23.5 percent sodium chloride, 10–20 ml) may be used (Callaham, 1979; Rosen, 1983).

HEAT EXHAUSTION

Pathophysiology

Heat exhaustion tends to develop throughout a period of several days. This syndrome is primarily a manifestation of the strain being placed on the cardiovascular system in its attempt to maintain normothermia. Heat exhaustion may be due to either water depletion or salt depletion, or both.

Clinical Manifestations

The symptoms of heat exhaustion include headache, giddiness, anorexia, malaise, thirst, vomiting, and muscle cramps. The patient's temperature may be moderately elevated, up to 104°F (40°C), with increased pulse and respiratory rates. Orthostatic blood pressure changes and syncope may be present; even though the mental status remains intact, the patient may be anxious and irritable.

Diagnostic Studies

An absolute criterion for distinguishing heat exhaustion from heat stroke is that no significant changes are noted in the laboratory values of serum glutemic pyruvic transaminase (SGPT) in the patient experiencing heat exhaustion. Sodium, protein, blood urea nitrogen (BUN), and hematocrit studies are performed to help establish the degree of dehydration.

Nursing Care and Related Interventions

The goal in the care of the patient with heat exhaustion is the adequate replacement of water and salt and the restoration of the body to normothermia. Place the patient in a cool environment dressed in minimal clothing, such as a hospital gown. Assess the degree of dehydration and start fluid replacement. Three to four glasses of an oral electrolyte solution of 0.5 percent sodium chloride or a commercial drink, like Gator Ade, is given to the patient. Intravenous solutions are titrated by the patient's cardiovascular status; a solution of 5 percent dextrose in 0.9 percent sodium chloride (normal saline) or 5 percent dextrose in 0.45 percent sodium chloride (half normal saline) solution are the fluids of choice. Fit young athletes may require as many as 4 l of fluid during a period of six to eight hours.

Discharge Planning

Discharge planning for patients with all of the previously mentioned heat disorders must include several factors. Assessment of the patient's readiness to learn is the initial step. Next, the patient and any significant other responsible individual must understand what caused the problem and how to prevent a future occurrence.

Factors that may increase the patient's susceptibility to a heat disorder should be stressed. The patient must understand what signs and symptoms to watch for that would signal a need to return to the emergency department. The nurse should also explain that aspirin may not be effective in the treatment of heat disorders because its action is related to fever that is caused by infection, not by fevers due to heat disorders. (Table 29.2 contains an example of written instructions that should be provided to the patient upon discharge.)

TABLE 29.2 Discharge Planning/Heat Disorders

1. While exercising, working, or performing other activity in a hot or humid environment:
  (a) Dress minimally.
  (b) Drink one or two glasses of water every 1–2 hrs.
  (c) Take frequent rest periods.
2. Watch for symptoms of heat disorders such as:
  (a) headache   (b) weakness   (c) rapid pulse
  (d) rapid breathing (e) muscle cramps   (f) restlessness
  (g) excessive perspiring (h) elevated temperatures (i) nausea/vomiting
3. If the above symptoms occur:
  (a) Lie down and rest in a cool area
  (b) Circulate air with a fan
  (c) Bathe in cool water
  (d) Avoid coffee, alcohol, or stimulants
  (e) Do not take salt tablets undiluted—rapid absorption causes gastrointestinal (stomach) problems
  (f) Drink fluids such as water with ¼ teaspoon salt added to 1 qt of water or Gator Ade mixed half and half with water.
4. Acclimatization is a slow, gradual experience that builds body resistance to heat exposure.
5. Heat exposure can threaten your life. Call your physician if symptoms persist or you feel worse.

HEAT STROKE

Pathophysiology

Heat stroke is a life-threatening, emergency situation requiring immediate intervention. It is the second must common cause of death in athletes. Two types of heat stroke exist, nonexercise and exercise-induced. The *nonexercise* heat stroke occurs in the elderly who have degenerative vascular disease, obese people with cardiovascular disease, and people on medications with side effects causing increased temperatures (thyroid compounds, amphetamines), decreased thirst, and sweating (antihistamines). *Exercise-induced* heat stroke occurs in athletes, soldiers, or anyone who is unable to dissipate body heat after strenuous exercise.

The basic pathology of heat stroke is total failure of the sweating mechanism. It is believed that when a person's core temperature reaches 106°F (41°C), the central regulating mechanism fails and sweat production ceases. Studies have shown the mortality rate of heat stroke to range between 30 and 80 percent. Eighty percent of these deaths occur in people who are more than 50 years old (Goldfrank et al., 1980).

Clinical Manifestations

Characteristic signs of heat stroke include hyperpyrexia with temperatures above 106°F (41°C); altered levels of consciousness; hot, dry skin; rapid respirations; tachycardia; abrupt decrease in urine output; and electrocardiogram changes that include ST depressions, T wave changes, bundle branch blocks, and/or ventricular fibrillation. Seizures may occur, and the patient may go into deep coma. If coma persists longer than ten hours, prognosis is poor.

Diagnostic Studies

Blood values should be determined as soon as possible and include complete blood count (CBC) and platelets, electrolyte values, levels of BUN, glucose, creatinine, phosphokinase (CPK), SGOT, LDH, SGPT, uric acid, lactate acid, calcium, prothrombin time (PT), and partial prothrombin time (PTT). Arterial blood gas (ABG) studies reveal the level of acidosis. Lactate levels are usually elevated, reflecting anaerobic metabolism. The CBC may be elevated, and serum sodium and osmolarity will vary depending on the degree of dehydration.

Nursing Care and Related Interventions

The nursing goal in the care of the patient experiencing heat stroke is to restore and maintain normothermia and treat underlying pathophysiological complications. Treatment consists of rapid cooling of the body temperature by using the most effective means available. Therapy begins in the field by placing iced water or saline towels or sheets over the patient, immersing the patient in a stream, or spraying him with a hose. In the emergency department, an iced bath, hypothermia blanket, and fanning may be used to reduce surface temperature.

Core temperature cooling methods include gastric lavage with iced saline, cooled intravenous (IV) fluids, cooled oxygen mist under pressure with a flow high enough to maintain perfusion, and cold saline enemas. Constant monitoring of the temperature during cooling is necessary. Cooling should be halted when the patient's temperature reaches 102°F (38.9°C) because he may continue to drift downward to dangerously low temperature levels. If this happens, shivering may begin and produce heat; and violent shivering may lead to convulsions.

Maintenance of the airway is a top priority because coma, seizures, and vomiting are not uncommon occurrences. An intravenous infusion of Ringer's lactate, 5 percent dextrose in 0.45 percent sodium chloride solution or normal saline solution should be started, and the patient observed for signs of fluid overload, for example, restlessness, productive cough, cold and clammy skin, neck vein distention, cyanosis, and shock. A central venous pressure (CVP) line and Foley catheter are placed in order to monitor both vascular volume and urine output (specific gravity should be measured every two hours). Careful monitoring of vital signs and the level of consciousness must be continued until the patient is stable. An Isuprel or dopamine IV drip may be considered for shock, titrated with blood pressure readings.

Thorazine 10 to 20 mg IV may be given to control delirium and shivering, and Valium 2.5–20 mg may be needed for seizures (see Fig. 29.1). The patient with heat stroke is admitted to the hospital for continual observation.

Children under 12 years old experiencing hyperthermia may require many of the same core cooling treatments used for adults; however, due to the smaller body size, a child may easily be placed in a tub of ice cold water for surface cooling. Caution should be used in administration of drugs to children. Thorazine 0.1 mg/kg may be used for shivering and delirium, and Valium 0.05 mg/kg up to a maximum of 10 mg may be needed for seizures. Intravenous Ringer's lactate, 5 percent dextrose in one-half normal saline, or 2.5 percent dextrose in one-quarter normal saline solution (10–20 ml/kg/hour) are used for the smaller child. Children should be admitted to the hospital for observation and further treatment if symptoms of heat stroke exist.

HYPOTHERMIA

Hypothermia is a state of reduced surface and core temperature to less than 95°F (35°C) that can be attributed to either an increase in heat loss or a decrease in heat production, or both. Heat production results from increased metabolism (thermogenesis), exercise, acclimatization, and cold weather shivering. Heat loss results from exposure to wet, cold, or windy environments with prolonged exposure ending in dangerous fluid and electrolyte imbalances.

A number of predisposing factors exist that place a greater risk on the individual who is exposed; therefore, one may become extremely hypothermic in relatively warm climates of 50°F to 60°F. A person with a lowered metabolic rate or a central nervous system disorder is at high risk. Drug abusers, the elderly, and neonates (particularly premature infants) are also at a high risk because of heat energy loss by radiation (Marks et al., 1981).

HYPOTHERMIA

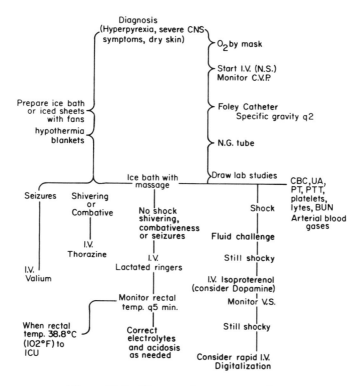

Figure 29.1 Heat stroke treatment chart.

Pathophysiology

Systemic effects of hypothermia begin with peripheral vasoconstriction as the body attempts to conserve its core heat. Shivering and increased muscle metabolism are major factors in heat production; however, shivering will cease as the body's core temperature drops to 86°F (30°C) or insulin is no longer available for glucose transfer. If either happens, physiologic responses lead to a decline in respiration, pulse, blood pressure, pH, and oxygen saturation. A rapid onset of electrolyte imbalances occurs. The heart becomes an ineffective pump, and a diffuse decrease in voltage is noted on the electrocardiogram. Increased sodium and potassium, decreased temperature, low pH, and a low Po_2 are probably key factors in predisposing the patient to ventricular fibrillation (see Fig. 29.2).

Clinical Manifestations

A healthy, unintoxicated individual who undergoes an increase in shivering and vasoconstriction due to a cold environment may appear well oriented and have only minor complaints; but he may progressively show increased signs of apathy, poor

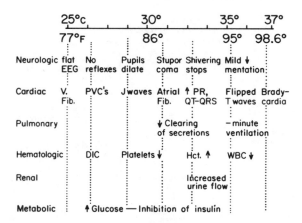

Figure 29.2 Accidental hypothermia—systemic effects.

judgment, dysphasia, dysarthria, and ataxia. As the shivering decreases, it is replaced by marked skeletal rigidity. Breathing becomes shallow and irregular. Blood pressure may not be detectable, but a carotid pulse is usually present. The electrocardiogram shows a gamut of dysrhythmias including bradycardia, tachycardia, and/or ventricular extrasystoles. The skin appears bluish, and the hands, face, and feet may be swollen.

Diagnostic Studies

The complete blood cell count (CBC) will reveal volume depletion and hemoconcentration. Hemoglobin and hematocrit levels may be elevated. The platelet count may be depressed; however, all of these may return to normal after rewarming. The white blood cell count (WBC) is variable but usually elevated, and blood viscosity will be elevated.

BUN rises slowly, indicating a mild azotemia due to tissue destruction (Speich, 1977). Potassium levels are normal at onset, and hypokalemia secondary to therapeutic measures may occur later in the course of treatment. Glucose is frequently elevated as a direct result of the inability of insulin to function properly; however, hypoglycemia is occasionally present due to glycogen depletion. Serum enzymes, SGOT, and CPK may be elevated, particularly if there is tissue damage.

ABG studies are ordered to help follow and treat predictable acidosis. ECG changes reveal prolonged PR, QRS, and QT intervals, nonspecific ST segment and T wave changes and bradycardia. Atrial fibrillation, atrial flutter, idioventricular rhythms, J waves and muscle artifact, ventricular fibrillation, or asystole may be present. Hypothermia creates myocardial irritability that hinders attempts to restore normal sinus rhythm; thus medication, countershock, or pacing may be ineffective until the core temperature is close to normal.

Nursing Care and Related Interventions

The goals in the care of the patient experiencing hypothermia are to restore and maintain normothermia and to prevent the development of complications during therapeutic procedures.

Handle the patient gently because the hypothermic heart can be made to fibrillate by rough handling (Bangs and Hamlet, 1980). Oxygen is administered to support decreased respiratory intake and to provide more oxygen during rewarming. Removing the patient's clothing and replacing it with a dry, warm covering is a necessary part of the nursing care. The patient should not be left uncovered or exposed while therapeutic procedures are instituted. Vital signs are taken upon the patient's arrival and every five to ten minutes during the rewarming procedures. The patient must be placed on a cardiac monitor to ensure that cardiac function is adequate. The correction of hypovolemia using glucose and water solutions or physiological saline, after baseline blood gas studies and electrolyte values are obtained, is necessary. However, because hypothermia patients are susceptible to electrolyte and fluid imbalances, it is important to keep an accurate account of fluid intake and output. Cardiopulmonary resuscitation (CPR) must be initiated when necessary and maintained, even if pupils are fixed and dilated and the body is cold. Prolonged CPR may be effective after two or more hours.

Rewarming methods include both surface and core rewarming. Surface rewarming begins with warm, dry clothing, hot blankets, or the use of the hyperthermia blanket. Hot wet sheets or towels may be applied to the skin surfaces. A Hubbard tub or other device for a hot bath is considered for rewarming with water temperature settings at 98° to 100°F. This technique is especially useful with children.

Core rewarming methods are used for moderate and severe hypothermia. The core rewarming methods that are used include the following:

1. Warmed humidified intermittent positive pressure breathing accomplished by using warm distilled water.
2. Warmed IV fluids using either a blood warmer or immersing the IV tubing in warmed water.
3. Gastric lavage using warm fluids (water or normal saline solution).
4. Irrigation of the bladder and/or colon with warm fluids.
5. Peritoneal dialysis with warm normal saline or Ringer's lactate.

More invasive techniques, such as use of the cardiopulmonary bypass or thoracotomy with lavage of the mediastinum using warm normal saline, are considered in extreme cases. All fluids used in the rewarming processes should be at temperatures of 98°–100°F (37°C).

The rewarming procedure must be done with strict monitoring of vital signs and cardiac monitoring in order to recognize and treat potential complications and to evaluate the degree of rewarming. Temperatures are raised cautiously, 1°F to 2°F per hour, ensuring that surface rewarming does not occur much faster than core rewarming.

Complications that may arise as a direct result of the rewarming procedure include dilatation of the peripheral vessels, causing hypotension due to lowered cardiac output and blood entering the heart that contains high concentrations of metabolites. The minimal use of drugs during the hypothermic state is essential. Decreased cellular metabolism causes a build up of drugs resulting in excessive accumulation. Diazepam 5–10 mg may be used to treat seizures. Chlorpromazine 10–25 mg is used for shivering or combativeness. Sodium bicarbonate (dosage titrated or 44.2 mEq) is used to treat acidosis.

The primary cause of hypothermia in children is accidental immersion in cold water, but environmental hypothermia is not an uncommon occurrence. Children's young, healthy bodies resist effects of hypothermia; however, the smaller body surface cools faster. Treatment may range from simply holding a baby close to one's warm body (which is an excellent source of heat) to any of the methods previously explained. Pediatric drug doses will be used, and such drugs as whiskey balls (cotton balls saturated with whiskey), Tylenol and Benadryl may be considered.

Marks et al. (1981) refer to the susceptibility of the premature infant to hypothermia within the hospital setting and proper handling of the premature infant in order to prevent the occurrence of hypothermia.

Discharge Planning

Prevention of hypothermia is the main goal in discharge teaching. Patients should be instructed in the importance of wearing warm clothing during exposure, preferably in layers starting with long underwear and adding loose-fitting additional garments. Mittens are preferable because they lock air in and the fingers warm each other. A pulldown cap covering the face, ears, and neck and two pairs of socks with waterproof shoes or boots should be worn. The patient should be instructed to avoid nicotine because of its vasopressive action, as well as alcohol, which may hasten heat loss and increase chances of frostbite. The patient should avoid being cold in bed because the metabolic rate may drop 10–15 percent below normal during sleep. The patient should also eat more because for every 10°F colder it gets, the body uses approximately 150 extra calories.

FROSTBITE

The exposure of peripheral tissue to the extremes of cold, either wet or dry, are manifested by three different modes: (1) frostbite—a chilling and ischemic insult to the tissue, either from exposure to low atmospheric temperature or freezing by contact exposure; (2) immersion injury—an ischemic insult to the tissue due to localized immersion into water of temperatures less than 50°F (10°C); and (3) chilblains—a chronic, subcutaneous vasculitis, usually at the pretibial area, hands, or feet due to chronic or recurrent exposure to cold.

FROSTBITE

Pathophysiology

Freezing damages the tissue by disrupting enzyme function, denaturing proteins, and dessicating the cell with ice crystal formation, which becomes hyperosmotic in respect to the intracellular fluid. There may also be cell wall damage in nerves, muscles, and arteries; however, the skin may be able to recover unharmed as long as its neurovascular blood supply remains intact. Freezing below 21°F (5°C) is irreparable. Prolonged cold exposure causes ischemic injury due to arteriospasm and microvascular stasis. Rapid rewarming minimizes this discrepancy.

Clinical Manifestations

Frostbite begins with paresthesia and numbness. Freezing that reaches into the epidermis appears as a shallow, blanched wheal. This formation is known as *frostnip* and is easily treated by passive rewarming with the hands. A full-thickness injury of the tissues appears usually on the extremities as a pale, waxy area with a doughy consistency, a mottled cyanotic symblance, and some swelling and erythema. A dark eschar may form and appear necrotic. Deeper injury involves the bone. When this injury occurs, the affected part appears pale, lifeless, hardened, and devoid of movement or sensation. A thick, gangrenous eschar may develop, and the entire thickness of distal portions of the extremities may be devitalized.

Nursing Care and Related Interventions

The nursing goal in the care of the patient with frostbite is to intervene effectively to counteract the dessicating effects of freezing of localized tissues and reestablish homeostasis.

The patient may present with symptoms of hypothermia, and restoration of core temperatures must be accomplished before treating the frostbite. Airway maintenance, ventilation, and cardiovascular status should be evaluated, and necessary emergency measures initiated immediately.

Rapid rewarming of superficial or deep frostbite is a highly effective measure for preservation and recoverability of damaged tissues. The injured part should be immersed gently into a well-agitated bath at 104°–108°F (40°–42°C) for 20 to 30 minutes or until erythematous flushing appears. Pain may be excruciating, requiring the use of analgesics. The frostbitten area should never be rubbed because the tissue is particularly sensitive to trauma (Goldfrank and Kirsten, 1979).

The rapid rewarming procedure should not be attempted when there is any danger of refreezing. An extremity once thawed and refrozen almost certainly results in total tissue destruction.

Another treatment, employed primarily to enhance microvascular perfusion, is administration of intravenous heparin. This drug is given for its antisludging and anticlotting properties at a rate to maintain a PT level of 2.0 to 2.5 times more than normal.

Systemic vasodilators such as alcohol may be used. Enzymes may be used in the form of a topical ointment for debridment. Extreme invasive measures, such as sympathectomy, faciotomy, and amputation, are delayed as long as possible to avoid removal of viable tissue.

Discharge Planning

Discharge planning for the patient with frostbite includes several factors. The patient or significant other should understand the cause of the problem, measures to prevent further occurrences, and what to do if there is a recurrence. Because the hands and feet are most susceptible, tell patients to wear protective clothing—mittens, insulated waterproof boots, and layers of socks. Stress the importance of avoiding alcohol, which hastens heat loss and increases chances of frostbite, and nicotine, which causes peripheral vascular constriction. Increasing calorie intake should be advised because it increases metabolism and internal heat. In case of recurrence, the patient should be instructed to cover the affected part with extra clothing or blankets; come indoors; handle the part gently, not rubbing it; and contact a physician. Further instructions regarding antibiotic use, physical therapy, and return follow-up visits should be given to the patient both verbally and in writing.

CONCLUSION

The patient with a heat disorder or cold disorder requires an adequate and rapid assessment followed by the development of a plan of care that will help restore the patient to an optimal level of functioning. The emergency department nurse must initiate this type of care and include adequate discharge planning to help prevent a recurrence of a similar situation. Preventative health maintenance is a primary goal to help improve the quality of life of every person.

BIBLIOGRAPHY

Bangs, C., and M. Hamlet: Out in the cold. *Topics in Emergency Medicine* 2(3):19–36 (1980).

Buckingham, L. L.: Environmental medicine. *Family Medicine: Principles and Practice*. New York: Spinger-Verlag, 1978, p. 606.

Budassi, S., and J. Barber: Hyperthermia. *Emergency Nursing: Principles and Practice*, St. Louis, MO: Mosby, 1981, pp. 581–587.

Burch, G.; J. Knochel; and R. Murphy: Stay on guard against heat syndromes. *Patient Care* 13(12):67–80 (1979).

Callaham, M. L.: *Emergency Management of Heat Illness*. Emergency Physician Series. Chicago: Abbott Laboratories, 1979.

Callaham, M. L.: When it gets too hot, cool it. *Consultant* 20(8):59–63 (1980).

Chaim, B.; T. Haygai; K. Gad; E. Yoram; and S. Yair: Heat tolerance in patients with extensive healed burns. *Plastic Reconstructive Surgery* 67(4):499–504 (1981).

BIBLIOGRAPHY

Conn, H. F.: *Current Therapy.* Philadelphia: Saunders, 1982, pp. 952–955.

Costrini, A.; H. Pitt; A. Gustafson; et al.: Cardiovascular and metabolic manifestations of heat stroke and severe heat exhaustion. *American Journal of Medicine* 66:296 (1979).

Doris, P., and M. Baker: Effects of dehydration of normoregulation in cats exposed to high ambient temperatures. *Journal of Applied Physiology* 51(1):46–54 (1981).

Ebertowski, S. K.: Heat stroke vs. heat exhaustion. *Emergency Nursing Update Series.* Biomedia, 1979, pp. 3–6.

Goldfrank, L., and R. Kirsten: Emergency management of hypothermia. *Hospital Physician* 15:12–15(1979).

———.; H. Osborn; and R. Wiesman: Heat stroke. *Hospital Physician* 16:24–36 (1980).

Gunby, P.: Cold facts concerning hypothermia. Medical News *JAMA* 243(14):1403–1409 (1980).

Hayward, J.; J. Erickson; and J. Ballis: Thermal balance and survival time prediction of man in cold H_2O. *Journal of Physiological Pharmacology* 53:21–32 (1981).

Heimler, R., et al.: Effects of thermal environmental change in premature infants. *Pediatrics* 68(1):82–98 (1981).

Lloyd, E. L. I.: Accidental hypothermia treated by central rewarming through the airway. *British Journal of Anaesthesiology* 45:41–47 (1981).

McElroy, C. R.: Update on heat illness. *Topics in Emergency Medicine* 2(3):1–18 (1980).

Marcus, P.: Laboratory comparison of technics for rewarming hypothermic casualties. *Aviation Space Environmental Medicine* 49(5):692–697 (1978).

Marks, K. H., et al.: Oxygen consumption and temperature control of premature infants in double wide incubators. *Pediatrics* 68(1):93–98 (1981).

Morrison, J.; M. Conn; and J. Hayward: Thermal increment provided by inhalation rewarming from hypothermia. *Journal of Applied Physiology* 46(6):1061–1065 (1979).

Proppe, D. W.: Influence of skin temperature on thermoregulatory control of leg blood flow. *Journal of Applied Physiology* 50(5):975–978 (1981).

Proulx, R.: Heat stress disease. *Principles and Practice of Emergency Medicine.* Philadelphia: Saunders, 1978, pp. 815–822.

Rolnick, M.; T. Stair; and E. Silfen: Hypothermia—Cold weather is only one cause. *Consultant* 20(3):132–138 (1980).

Rosen, P., et al.: *Emergency Medicine Concepts and Clinical Practice.* St. Louis, MO: Mosby, 1983, pp. 477–519.

Rund, D., and T. Rausch: *Triage.* St. Louis, MO: Mosby, 1981.

Ryan, J. F.: High fever. In S. S. Gellis and B. M. Dayun (eds.): *Current Pediatric Therapy,* vol. 9. Philadelphia: Saunders, 1980, pp. 767–768.

Shapiro, Y.; A. Magazanik; R. Udassin; et al.: Heat intolerance in former heat stroke patients. *Annals of Internal Medicine* 90:913–916 (1979).

Speich, P.: Brought back to life. *Journal of Emergency Nursing* 3(2):9–12 (1977).

Sturyenberger, A. J.: Differentiating among heat syndromes. *Journal of Emergency Nursing* 4:24–28 (1978).

Surpure, J. S.: Hyperpyrexia in children. *JACEP* 8:130–133 (1979).

30
Obstetrical and Gynecological Problems

Mary Ann Brown

After completing this chapter, the reader will be able to do the following:

1. Triage a patient experiencing obstetrical and gynecological problems.
2. Discuss pathophysiology, clinical manifestations, nursing care, and discharge planning for selected obstetrical and gynecological patients.
3. List steps in the management of an emergency delivery.
4. Identify assessment guidelines and discuss management of the rape victim.

Many changes occurring in the health care system affect which types of patients and problems are encountered in the emergency department. A major trend in obstetrical care is regionalization of hospitals into a trilevel system with high-risk patients being cared for in tertiary centers, secondary centers providing care for about 80 percent of the obstetrical population, and primary centers caring only for low-risk patients. Because of fewer patients, many primary hospitals may close their obstetrical departments, necessitating a redistribution of patients to other centers. The redistribution will lead to increased travel time for patients and greater use of the local emergency department for stabilization and transfer.

Birth patterns are constantly changing, and more infants today are being born to mothers who are 16 or under and 35 or older. These population groups tend to have a higher rate of complications. Increasing costs of care, coupled with fewer federally funded programs, may increase the number of patients receiving no prenatal care. Many mothers are choosing to have their infants at home or in alternative birthing centers. These factors may affect the emergency department by making it the initial contact center for prenatal patients; thus, the emergency department will treat more patients with obstetrical and gynecological complications and will receive more transfers from home or other health care systems.

TRIAGE

The purpose of the triage system is to direct the patient to the appropriate level of care. Most triage areas do provide an area for the nurse to obtain a history, establish a chief complaint, and obtain vital signs. Further assessments may be done depending on facilities, personnel, and established protocols.

Subjective Data

Subjective data obtained from the patient should include age, previous pregnancies using the FPAL system (the letters stand for *full term, premature, abortions,* and *living children*), last normal menstrual period, and estimated data of confinement.

Obtain the first day of the last normal menstrual period (LNMP), noting the number of days of flow and the normal amount of flow. It is important to *establish the date of the LNMP* because 25 percent of women who are pregnant will continue to have some vaginal bleeding at the time of the expected period.

The estimated date of confinement (EDC) can be established using Nagele's rule. This estimate is calculated by taking the first day of the LNMP, adding seven days, and subtracting three months. It is vital to establish the week of gestation at the time the patient presents in the emergency department. Key events that may assist in establishing the EDC include *quickening* (the first fetal movement perceived by the expectant mother) at 16 to 18 weeks in a multigravida, 18 to 20 weeks for a primigravida, and fetal heart tones (present with a fetascope by the twentieth week).

The *chief complaint* should be described in the patient's own words including the onset, previous episodes, associated symptoms, and pertinent negatives, such as the presence of vaginal bleeding (character, amount), vaginal discharge (consistency, color, odor), pain (location, duration), and urinary symptoms (frequency, urgency, burning).

Objective Data

The objective data collection should include the patient's general appearance, mental status, and vital signs. Hemodynamic changes of pregnancy may result in a slightly elevated pulse rate (five beats per minute) and a lowered blood pressure. It is important to take the blood pressure with the patient sitting or lying on the left side, and in between contractions if in active labor, because back-lying positions and uterine contractions produce blood pressure elevations. Temperature and respiration are unchanged by pregnancy.

Further assessment of the obstetrical patient would include measurement of the fundal height. The fundal height will be halfway to the umbilicus at 16 weeks, slightly below at 20 weeks, and should correspond with centimeters (measured from the top of the symphysis pubis to the top of the uterus) after 20 weeks.

Leopold maneuvers are done to determine the lie of the fetus—the presentation, location of small parts, and degree of engagement. The maneuvers are as follows:

First maneuver. Presenting part, lie, and engagement. Stand at the patient's side and grasp between thumb and fingers the lower uterine segment just above the symphysis. The head will feel hard and round and will swing from side to side if engagement has not taken place.

Second maneuver. Location of back and small parts. Stand at the patient's side facing her head and place hands on either side of the uterus, using one hand to exert pressure and the other to palpate. The back will feel firmer and smoother. It may help to compare findings with the mother's impression of the area of greatest or strongest fetal movement.

Third maneuver. Still facing the patient to determine the location of a breech, move the hands from the sides of the uterus to the fundus. The breech will fill the fundal area and is therefore less movable.

The fetal heart tones are best heard on the side of the baby's back and below the umbilicus if the baby is in a vertex presentation or above the umbilicus in a breach presentation. The rate should be between 120 and 160 beats per minute. The patient's extremities should be examined for edema, presence of varicosities, and reflexes.

It is important to note the color, odor, and amount of vaginal discharge and any associated symptoms such as itching, swelling, or pain.

Assessment and Planning

Once this initial triage assessment is completed, the nurse develops a plan of management that includes the priority of treatment, further assessment needed, possible transfer to another department or hospital, or referral to another appropriate agency. (Examples of triage notes using the subjective data, objective data, assessment, and plan of management (SOAP) format with the obstetrical and gynecological patient are presented in Table 30.1.)

THE PELVIC EXAMINATION

Who will perform the pelvic examination and the extent of the examination will depend on hospital protocols and the type of health care provider available in the hospital system. Speculum examinations might be performed by the physician, certified nurse midwife, or nurse practitioner with pelvic assessment for labor being done by the emergency department nurse. The complete pelvic examination includes a speculum examination as well as the bimanual examination.

Speculum Examination

The patient should empty her bladder to make the examination more comfortable and to facilitate palpation of pelvic organs. She should be assisted to the examining table and properly draped. Selection of an appropriate speculum is based on size and parity. Obese patients may require a large speculum, nuliparas a speculum with a narrow blade, and an infant speculum is available for examining children. A sterile speculum is necessary if there is a history of ruptured membranes. A light, gloves, lubricant, microscope slides, swabs, and various culture media should be readily

TABLE 30.1 Examples of Triage Notes for Patients Experiencing Obstetrical and Gynecological Problems

S: 21 yo WF p0010 with LNMP July 1, EDC April 8 and EGA 16 wks, followed in county clinic, c/o intermittent lower abd. pain and cramping × 3 hr ∅ N/V, D, UTI symptoms or vaginal bleeding. PMH: diabetic on 32 u NPH insulin qd. NKA.
O: BP 110/60, P 82, RR 18, FH halfway to umbilicus FHTs ∅ with fetascope, 146 doptone, pelvic: deferred, extremities: neg.
A: Lower abd. pain, R/O threatened AB, ectop. pg.
P: OB-Gyn evaluation, admit examination room ASAP.

S: 29 yo WF p0000 with LNMP 26 days ago for 4 days, normal flow. On OCP × 4 yrs without problems ∅ missed pills. PMH: negative. c/o painful blister rt. labia × 3 days, sl. watery discharge with odor or itching, dysuria. Last intercourse 10 days. NKA.
O: BP 110/70, P 86, RR 20, T 38°C, 1 × 1 cm vesicle rt. labia.
A: Vaginal lesion, R/O herpes.
P: OB-Gyn evaluation, waiting room.

S: 28 yo BF p4004 with LNMP Nov. 1, EDC Aug. 8, EGA 41 wks, c/o lower abd. pain associated with backache, rectal pressure q 2 min ∅ bleeding, rupture of membranes. NKA. PMH: ∅.
O: FHTs 140, cervix complete/complete + 3.
A: Labor second stage.
P: OB evaluation, admit to examination room, prepare for imminent delivery.

available. Patients with a history of third trimester bleeding should be examined only by a physician after placenta previa has been ruled out (with ultrasound if available). The examination might be deferred until the patient is transferred to labor and delivery and type specific blood is available. The speculum examination helps the health care provider assess the presence of vaginal discharge, site of origin of the discharge, amount of the discharge, the color and size of the cervix, and the condition of the vaginal vault.

Bimanual Examination

Bimanual examination is performed to determine the size and position of the pelvic organs and any abnormal findings such as areas of pain or pelvic masses. An evaluation of possible labor would consist of positioning the patient on the examining table with her knees flexed and her feet together, allowing the knees to fall apart. The perineum is sprayed with an antiseptic solution, and, with a sterile gloved hand, the labia are separated using the thumb and ring finger. The index and middle finger are inserted using a down and backward motion. The examiner then locates the cervix and determines its position (anterior, posterior), consistency (soft, hard), and dilation in centimeters. Next, the examiner should palpate the presenting part (vertex or breech) and locate the ischial spines on the mother's pelvis. One should determine if the presenting part is above ($-1-2-3$ station) or below ($+1+2+3$ station) the spines. This procedure helps determine how close the presenting part is to the vaginal opening.

BLEEDING IN PREGNANCY

Clinically evident vaginal bleeding occurs in 22 percent of normal pregnancies. Other causes of vaginal bleeding during pregnancy include abortion, ectopic pregnancy, and gestational trophoblastic disease.

Abortion

Pathophysiology
Abortion is defined as the termination of pregnancy prior to the twentieth week. The incidence of spontaneous abortion is 15 to 20 percent and of these 62 percent are associated with abnormal embryonic development. Maternal structure abnormalities, hormone deficiencies (diabetes), and external trauma account for the remainder (Quilligan, 1980).

Clinical Manifestations
Threatened. Only slight vaginal bleeding and pain are present. The cervix is closed and the size of the uterus corresponds to the weeks of gestation.
Imminent. Cervical dilatation is present.
Inevitable. An imminent abortion with the added sign of rupture of the membranes is termed inevitable.
Incomplete. Some of the products of conception are passed, pain is present, and bleeding is usually profuse.
Complete. All products of conception are passed. Bleeding and pain are minimal.
Missed. The uterus retains the dead fetus. Bleeding is usually dark brown, the urine pregnancy test negative, and the uterine size less then the dates would indicate.
Habitual. A label applied when a woman experiences three or more consecutive abortions.

Nursing Care and Related Interventions
The goal of care for the patient with a threatened abortion is rest, adequate hydration, and treatment of any underlying conditions. After the cervix has dilated and the abortion is inevitable, the objective is to empty the uterus enabling it to contract and prevent hemorrhage. If 12 weeks of gestation or less, dilation and curettage (usually suction curettage) may be performed in the emergency department using paracervical block anesthesia. Analgesics (usually Demerol and/or Valium) may be given intravenously, but recovery from sedation requires more time and closer observation than with local anesthesia. Orders might include an intravenous line of 5 percent dextrose

with Ringer's lactate with Pitocin added and a type and cross for two units whole blood. Pitocin is used to contract the uterine muscle. After the procedure, the vital signs, the consistency of the uterus, and the amount and color of vaginal bleeding should be noted every 15 minutes for one hour. The nurse should assess the emotional state of the patient and provide appropriate support. Patients can be expected to exhibit a wide range of emotions. Patients may be discharged within four to six hours.

Patients who are more than 12 weeks of gestation are usually admitted for dilatation and curettage (D&C) or evacuation of the uterus through the use of intravenous oxytocin or prostaglandin vaginal suppositories. Patients with missed abortions will usually abort spontaneously within three weeks after fetal death. Those undelivered after five weeks are at risk for disseminated intravascular coagulation as a result of repeated small infusions into the maternal circulation of thromboplastic material from the degenerating placenta. Weekly fibrinogen levels are obtained. If the fibrinogen level drops below 150 mg/100 ml or the patient notices easy bruising of the skin, nose bleeds, or bleeding gums, she should be admitted for heparin therapy to normalize the clotting factors and for emptying of the uterus.

Rh negative mothers whose pregnancies have been terminated for whatever reason should receive antiRHo (D) immunoglobulin to prevent sensitization and protect future pregnancies.

Discharge Planning
Patients with a threatened abortion are usually discharged with instructions for bed rest. They may be given a mild sedative. If uterine contractions and bleeding increase or if tissue is passed, they should return to the emergency department for evaluation. The tissue specimen should be brought to the hospital for inspection. Patients undergoing a D&C should be discharged with a companion and be provided with a written explanation regarding the need for taking Methergine (which is to stop the vaginal bleeding) and the schedule (one tablet every four hours for six doses). Bed rest is usually recommended for 24 hours with gradual resumption of normal activity during the next week. Signs such as chills, fever, lower abdominal pain, abnormal bleeding, foul smelling discharge, or scant, dark urine should be reported immediately. Intercourse should be avoided until bleeding has stopped. A follow-up evaluation should be done in three weeks. Patients should be provided with information about local support groups and Planned Parenthood.

Ectopic Pregnancy

Pathophysiology
The incidence of ectopic pregnancy has doubled in the last ten years accounting for 12 percent of all maternal mortality (Quilligan, 1980). According to some experts, the rising incidence of sexually transmitted diseases coupled with the success of antibiotic therapy in the treatment of pelvic inflammatory disease (PID) may have contributed to this increased incidence of ectopic pregnancy. It is the leading cause of mortality during the first trimester. Tubal physiology is impaired because pelvic inflammatory disease causes an agglutination of the tubal cilia and narrowing of the

tubal lumen. Antibiotic treatment prevents complete closure, so the patient remains fertile, but the ovum cannot be carried into the uterus for implantation. Ninety percent will implant in the tube, the other 10 percent in the peritoneal cavity, uterine cornua, ovary, or cervix.

Clinical Manifestations
Ectopic pregnancy should always be suspected in a woman of childbearing age who has some disturbance of menses and abdominal pain. The onset may be gradual with intermittent, diffuse abdominal pain and slight to absent bleeding, or it may be acute with severe pain and shock. If there is bleeding into the peritoneal cavity, the patient may complain of referred shoulder pain when placed in a recumbent position due to irritation of the diaphragm by blood. Seventy-five percent of the patients will have a mass on the adnexa uteri on pelvic examination.

Nursing Care and Related Interventions
Ultrasound can be used to rule out intrauterine pregnancy. Patients should be instructed regarding the need for a full bladder. If the ultrasound is performed in another department, a nurse should accompany the patient. Constant observation is necessary because rupture of the ectopic pregnancy followed by hemorrhage and shock can occur suddenly.

Culdocentesis is performed by passing a long spinal needle attached to a 20 cc syringe into the culdosac during a speculum examination. A ruptured ectopic pregnancy will cause intraperitoneal bleeding and pooling of dark nonclotting blood in this area. Laparoscopic examination under general anesthesia can be done to visualize the pelvic organs. Urine pregnancy tests are unreliable in ruling out ectopic pregnancy. Blood tests, though more sensitive, can be falsely negative. Patients exhibiting signs of shock must be prepared for immediate surgery. An intravenous line of 5 percent dextrose with Ringer's lactate is started and a complete blood cell count (CBC) and blood type and cross are obtained. The patient might need to be placed in the shock position and given oxygen.

Discharge Planning
Patients discharged without a clear diagnosis are cautioned to observe for signs of bleeding, increasing pain, or signs of shock, such as dizziness, fainting, weakness, cold clammy skin, and pallor. They should be cautioned about taking medication for pain because the medication may mask symptoms. Aspirin should be avoided because it may affect bleeding. Patients should be discharged in the company of another person. Bed rest should be encouraged for 24 hours. The patient should remain on a full liquid diet for 24 hours since admission for exacerbation of symptoms and surgical intervention is more common during this time period.

Gestational Trophoblastic Disease

Pathophysiology
Gestational trophoblastic disease develops from a degeneration of the chorionic villi that are converted into clear vesicles resembling grapes. This tissue can develop into

choriocarcinoma with metastasis to the lungs, liver, and brain. Usually there is no fetus present. The mass may grow to fill the uterus to resemble a four-month to six-month gestation size.

Clinical Manifestations
Patients may experience normal signs of pregnancy, but nausea is usually more severe and prolonged. The size of the uterus does not correspond to the weeks of gestation. Fifty percent will be sized greater than dates and 20 percent sized smaller than dates. There is an absence of fetal heart tones. As the pregnancy progresses, the patient exhibits signs and symptoms of preeclampsia, such as elevated blood pressure, edema, and proteinuria. It is usually bleeding and/or passage of tissue from the vagina that causes the patient to seek emergency treatment.

Nursing Care and Related Interventions
Diagnosis can be confirmed by the identification of grapelike vesicles on ultrasound. The patient is admitted for treatment including evacuation of the uterus.

BLEEDING IN LATE PREGNANCY

The most common cause of bleeding in late pregnancy is a bloody show. Nevertheless, two conditions—placenta abruption and placenta previa—pose a considerable threat to the mother and infant and must be differentiated from a simple bloody show.

Placenta Abruption and Placenta Previa

Pathophysiology
Placenta abruption is defined as a premature separation of the placenta, either partially or totally. The incidence is 1 in 100 deliveries and it is associated with hypertension, multiparity, previous abruption, precipitous delivery, trauma, and a short umbilical cord.

Placenta previa exists when the placenta is abnormally implanted in the lower uterine segment and is either partially or totally covering the cervical os. The incidence is 1 in 200 deliveries and is associated with multiparity, advanced maternal age, multiple pregnancy, and breech presentation.

Clinical Manifestations
The patient experiencing placenta abruption presents with pain and signs of labor, such as contractions and cervical dilatation. The uterus is firm and tender to touch. Bleeding is usually dark red and may be profuse or hidden. Fetal heart tones may be present if the abruption is incomplete. Signs of shock may be out of proportion to the amount of bleeding noted.

The patient experiencing placenta previa presents with a sudden onset of bright red vaginal bleeding usually not accompanied by signs of labor or complaints of pain. The fetal heart tones are usually present.

PREGNANCY-INDUCED HYPERTENSION (TOXEMIA)

Nursing Care and Related Interventions
Particular attention must be paid to the patient's vital signs and the character and amount of vaginal bleeding. Any tissue passed should be saved. The abdomen is carefully examined for the presence or absence of uterine contractions noting frequency, duration, quality of the contraction, and uterine tone. The fundal height should be measured and marked (concealed intrauterine hemorrhage may be detected by a rising fundal height). Blood is drawn for a CBC, type and cross, and clotting studies. An intravenous infusion of 5 percent dextrose with Ringer's lactate is started. Ultrasound can be used for placental localization and also to determine the degree of abruption. Patients with partial abruption, provided the fetal heart tones are stable, may be allowed to labor with continuous internal fetal monitoring in labor and delivery. They are usually made ready for an immediate cesarean section (shave, prep, and Foley catheter), if it becomes necessary. Only patients with a small degree of placenta previa are allowed to labor. Most patients must have a cesarean section in labor and delivery. Most patients fear for their own safety and their baby's. In most hospitals, the father of the baby is encouraged to remain with his partner in labor, and if regional anesthesia is used, accompany her to delivery.

Discharge Planning
Although it is advisable to keep the patient who is not at term in the hospital until delivery, financial reasons and patient's requests may necessitate discharge. If this situation arises, instructions must include the importance of inserting nothing in the vagina and no sexual stimulation to orgasm (this may cause uterine contractions). The patient must always have a companion with her and transportation to the hospital available immediately. The nurse may need to arrange suitable accommodation for the patient, especially for a single woman or for one whose significant other is not available.

PREGNANCY-INDUCED HYPERTENSION (TOXEMIA)

Pregnancy-induced hypertension is the third leading cause of maternal mortality. Because of its insidious onset, the patient presenting in the emergency department will probably be acutely ill. This disease is characterized by the classic triad of edema, hypertension, and albuminuria after the twenty-fourth week of pregnancy. The etiology is unknown.

Pathophysiology

Plasma levels of renin and angiotensin are elevated during pregnancy. These increased levels may be necessary to counterbalance the salt-losing action of progesterone and enable the maternal system's blood volume to expand by the end of the first trimester. In a normal pregnancy, a hypertensive response to these strong pressor agents is prevented by some unknown mechanism.

In pregnancy-induced hypertension, there is an altered reactivity in the arterial wall to angiotension II and renin, leading to arterial spasm and increased blood pressure. Intravascular blood volume progressively decreases leading to a rising hematocrit, decreased urinary output, altered placental circulation, and fetal compromise. Progressive central nervous system irritability as evidenced by hyperreflexia may lead to convulsions.

Clinical Manifestations

Women at risk are the extremely young and considerably older primigravidae, those receiving no prenatal care, those from a low socioeconomic level, those of multiple gestation, and those with polyhydramnios, diabetes, and hypertension.

Preeclampsia
Mild. The blood pressure is 140/90 mm Hg, or there is an elevation of 30/15 mm Hg over a previous reading. There is 1−2+ edema, 1−2+ proteinuria, and an occasional headache.
Severe. The blood pressure is 160/100 mm Hg, with 3−4+ proteinuria and 3−4+ edema. Other signs and symptoms include hyperreflexia, persistent headaches, scotoma, blurred vision, and/or epigastric pain.

Eclampsia
The patient has experienced a seizure.

Nursing Care and Related Interventions

Controversy exists concerning whether the mildly preeclamptic woman can be treated at home with bed rest and a diet high in protein and fluids. Women with severe preeclampsia are admitted. In the emergency department, the nurse must be prepared to deal with potential seizures. The patient should be admitted to a quiet, darkened room under constant observation with oxygen, suction, side rails, magnesium sulfate, and Apresoline readily available.

Apresoline is the preferred drug to effect a rapid decrease in the blood pressure because it does not affect uterine blood flow. It is used with patients whose diastolic pressure exceeds 110 mm Hg. Doses of 5 mg are given intravenously every 20 minutes until the diastolic pressure reaches the 90–100 mm Hg range.

Magnesium sulfate is the preferred drug for the treatment and prevention of seizures. It acts directly on the neuromuscular junction and is excreted by the kidney. It should be administered as soon as the diagnosis of preeclampsia is made. Intravenous magnesium sulfate, 4 g of a 50 percent solution mixed in 150 cc of 5 percent dextrose in water is given initially for 20 minutes, followed by 1–2 g per hour. The dosage may be decreased or stopped if the urinary output is less than 50 cc in one hour, the reflexes are less than 1+, and the respirations are less than 10 in one minute. Magnesium sulfate may be given intramuscularly. The Z-tract method should be used to keep the medication deep in the muscle. Leakage into fatty tissue causes pain. One milliliter of 1 percent xylocaine can be added to the intramuscular medica-

EMERGENCY DELIVERY

tion to reduce the discomfort. Respiratory depression from overdose of magnesium sulfate can be reversed by the administration of 1 g calcium gluconate. The patient should assume a left lateral position to improve placental circulation. A Foley catheter is inserted to enable accurate measurement of urinary output and to obtain a urine sample for protein content. Vital signs, FHTs, reflexes, and signs of labor should be documented every 15 to 30 minutes. Sibai (1981) reported in a study of 67 eclamptic patients that 30 percent had no signs of edema, 20 percent had normal blood pressure, one patient convulsed with a systolic blood pressure of 130, and one patient convulsed with a diastolic pressure of 80.

If the woman is indeed sent home with mild preeclampsia, the nurse must be sure the patient understands to watch for increased swelling of the face or fingers, a sudden weight gain of more than 2 pounds in one week, headaches, visual disturbances, or epigastric pain. She should return to the emergency department promptly if necessary.

EMERGENCY DELIVERY

The main goal in managing an emergency delivery is to provide a controlled delivery in as safe an environment as possible. To assess the immediacy of delivery, it is necessary to recognize the stage and phase of labor (see Table 30.2) and the appropriate time frame for the primiparous and the multiparous patient.

The primiparous patient will normally dilate 1.0 to 2.0 cm per hour in the active phase of labor, and the transition phase may last from 45 minutes to one hour. It usually requires one hour for expulsion to take place. The multiparous patient can be expected to dilate 1.5 to 2.0 cm per hour in the active phase, and the transition phase may last 5 to 10 minutes. Expulsion takes place within a few minutes. In an emergency situation, the normal process of labor may be altered, becoming either more rapid or prolonged.

Nursing Care and Related Interventions

The nurse must prepare for imminent delivery if the fetal head is visible at the introitus or if the patient is multigravida and is completely dilated with sudden rupture of the membranes and complaints of rectal pressure. The patient who is completely dilated may be transferred to labor and delivery if her membranes are intact, contractions five minutes or longer apart, and a precip basin is readily available. Patients who are not in the second stage of labor may be transferred directly to labor and delivery regardless of parity or rupture of membranes. The management of the laboring patient may vary with individual hospital policies and procedures.

Delivery Procedure
The primary focus is to gain confidence and control of the patient and the delivery. Cleanliness is a secondary consideration. The patient is never left alone; equipment is obtained by another person and consists of two Kelly clamps, scissors, cord clamps, bulb suction, towels and blankets, and a basin for the placenta. (The step-by-

TABLE 30.2 Stages and Phases of Labor

Stages	Contractions	Dilation	Reaction
Stage I Early phase	5–20 min intervals 30–40 sec duration	0–3 cm	Excited, talkative
Stage I Active phase	3–5 min intervals 40–60 sec duration	3–8 cm	Serious, answers questions with difficulty, fearful, contraction painful
Stage I Transition phase	2–3 min intervals 60–90 sec duration	8–10 cm	Introverted, restless, loss of control, c/o nausea and vomiting, rectal pressure
Stage II Pushing phase	2–4 min intervals 40–50 sec duration	Complete	More calm, rectal pressure, involuntary pushing
Stage III Placenta	Signals beginning of separation, may see cord lengthening and gush of blood from vagina, change in uterine shape (becomes firm)		c/o cramping, nausea, and vomiting

step process of conducting an emergency delivery is shown in Table 30.3. Table 30.4 contains the Apgar scoring system.)

Managing the Third Stage
Observe for the signs of the placenta separation, such as the uterus becoming firm and globular, a sudden gush of blood from the vagina, and the lengthening of the cord. When these signs occur, ask the mother to push to expel the placenta. Control the bleeding after delivery of the placenta by fundal massage and/or an intravenous infusion of 20 units of Pitocin in 5 percent dextrose with Ringer's lactate or 10 mg Pitocin IM. Breastfeeding stimulates the release of oxytocin and may be the most effective way to control bleeding.

It is important to conceptualize the delivery as a normal event rather than a medical emergency. Including the patient's significant other helps the woman to focus on the experience as that of giving birth rather than focusing on the place or the circumstance of the experience.

Patients who are hemorrhaging during the third stage because of retained placenta or lacerations of the cervix and/or vagina should be transferred to the delivery room or operating room where manual removal of the placenta and inspection and repair of

TABLE 30.3 Conducting an Emergency Delivery

Signs	Activity	Rationale
Gain eye contact	Ask specific questions, name, FPAL, medical problems, allergies.	Assists in focusing attention, calming the patient.
Breathing instructions	Demonstrate and breath with the patient, pant or push to assist in gradual expulsion of the head.	Easier to learn by observation. Helps control delivery and prevention of lacerations.
Comfortable position	Side lying or lounge chair, avoid stirrups.	Facilitates placental circulation and pushing efforts. Placing in stirrups may increase stretching and tearing of perineum. Easier to deliver slippery baby on a flat surface.
As head becomes visible	Gently place fingertips on vertex. As head continues to emerge, spread fingers and allow more of the hand to be in contact with the head. Fingers should be directed toward the rectum with elbow up. Apply gentle downward restraining pressure.	Helps to control delivery. Keep the head flexed, allowing gradual delivery of the head.
Head delivery	The patient should be instructed to stop pushing and use a panting breathing technique. Support the head with one hand, using the other hand to slide down the back of the head to the neck for the cord. If the cord is loose, slip it over the shoulders as the delivery proceeds. If it is tight around the neck, clamp it in two places, cut it in between, and unwrap the cord. Clean the infant's airway with a bulb sy-	Facilitates circulation and prevents trauma to the cord. A tight cord prevents delivery.

TABLE 30.3 (*continued*)

Signs	Activity	Rationale
	ringe. If meconium is present use Delee mucus trap to suction deeply down each nare.	To prevent aspiration of meconium.
Delivery of shoulders	As external rotation of the head occurs, place one hand on either side of the head with fingers pointing toward the infant's face. Deliver the anterior shoulder by exerting downward and outward pressure with the top hand until the anterior shoulder impinges under the symphysis. Deliver the posterior shoulder by exerting upward and outward pressure with the lower hand.	Head will rotate to right or left as shoulders engage. Proper hand placement will assist in "catching."
Complete delivery	Clean the infant's airway again with the bulb syringe, clamp the cord in two places, and cut between the clamps. Note the delivery time. Dry the infant and place against mother's skin. Do 1- and 5-min Apgar scores. (See Table 30.4.)	To clear amniotic fluid. Assists in preventing heat loss.

lacerations can be accomplished. If the patient presents with signs of hemorrhage after the placenta has been expressed, administration of 10 mg Pitocin IM, fundal massage, or bimanual compression of the uterus will usually terminate the bleeding. Bimanual compression of the uterus can be accomplished by placing the gloved left hand in a fist position into the anterior fornix of the vagina and the right hand on the abdomen. The fundus of the uterus is compressed between the two hands. The abdominal hand applies vigorous massage until the uterus contracts. Compression should be maintained for at least five minutes.

Malpresentations of the fetus such as breech, face, and brow will usually result in a longer labor so that there is ample time to transfer these patients to the delivery

TABLE 30.4 Apgar Scoring System

Signs	0 Points	1 Point	2 Points
Heart rate	Absent	<100	>100
Respiratory effort	Absent	Slow, irregular	Good cry
Muscle tone	Limp	Some flexing of extremities	Active motion
Reflex irritability	No response	Grimace	Cough, cry, and sneeze
Color	Blue-white	Body pink, extremities blue	Body and extremities pink

Apgars > 6
1. Keep baby warm and dry off immediately.
2. Clear airway using bulb syringe.
3. Provide gentle stimulation by rubbing back. (Strong stimulation may cause breath holding.)
4. Give the infant some oxygen via mask.

Apgars < 6
Do the proceeding steps and provide oxygen by positive pressure using a bag and mask. Heart rate 110–120/min.

Apgars < 3
Use positive pressure for oxygen delivery and obtain assistance for intubation and ventilation.

---

room. No attempt should be made to perform a breech delivery in the emergency department unless trained obstetrical and neonatal personnel and equipment are available.

SEXUALLY TRANSMITTED DISEASES

There are 14 sexually transmitted diseases listed by the Center for Disease Control. Although cases of syphilis and gonorrhea are required to be reported to public health authorities, many are not. It is estimated that there are between 2 and 2.5 million cases of gonorrhea each year. Chlamydia trachomatis is probably the second most frequent infection with an estimated incidence of 4–5 million cases per year. Herpes genitalis may approach 400,000–600,000 cases per year. Factors contributing to this growing public health problem include changing sexual practices (more nonmarital sex with more partners), contraceptive methods (nonuse of barrier methods), and the problem of subclinical infections in women that may go untreated.

Sexually transmitted diseases pose grave problems for the pregnant woman and her infant. PID increases the risk of sterility and ectopic pregnancy, while other infections increase the risk of spontaneous abortion, premature rupture of the membranes, and preterm delivery. Approximately 1 million neonates will become infected each year, and neonatal herpes has an estimated mortality rate of 50 percent.

Sexually transmitted diseases can be classified according to the disease syndrome, such as cervicitis or vaginitis, or the causative organism. The following six organisms are responsible for 95 percent of all vaginal infections.

Chlamydia Trachomatis

Pathophysiology
Chlamydia trachomatis is an intracellular bacterial pathogen sexually acquired. It causes a purulent discharge and urethritis in the male and cervicitis in the female.

Clinical Manifestations
Cervicitis is characterized by a cloudy, thick discharge emanating from the external os. The cervix may appear swollen and bleed easily. Vaginal symptoms such as itching and odor are usually absent. Urinary symptoms such as frequency, urgency, and burning are present.

Diagnostic Studies
Culture techniques are not readily available so the diagnosis is made by excluding other causes of cervicitis such as gonorrhea and *Trichomonas vaginalis*. A patient with a negative Thayer-Martin culture, a negative gram stain, and the absence of *Trichomonas vaginalis* on a wet saline slide should be treated for Chlamydia.

Nursing Care and Related Interventions
The patient and her sexual partner should receive tetracycline 500 mg four times a day (QID) for seven days or erythromycin 500 mg QID for seven days.

Neisseria Gonorrhea

Pathophysiology
Neisseria gonorrhea is a gram-negative diplococci, sexually contracted, causing symptoms of purulent discharge and urethritis in the male.

Clinical Manifestations
Cervicitis and urinary symptoms are common in the female, although some women may be asymptomatic. The diagnosis is confirmed by a positive gram stain and positive culture on Thayer-Martin media.

Nursing Care and Related Interventions
The patient and her sexual partner should be treated with procaine penicillin G 4.8 million units given intramuscularly (IM) in two divided doses. Probenecid, which maintains an elevated blood level of penicillin, is given orally in a 1 g dose 30 minutes prior to the injection. Patients should remain in the emergency department 20–30 minutes after receiving penicillin to be observed for an anaphylactic reaction. Patients who are allergic to penicillin may receive tetracycline 250 mg by mouth QID for

10 days. Penicillinase-producing *Neisseria gonorrhea* should be treated with spectinomycin 2 g IM.

Herpes Simplex Virus (HSV)

Pathophysiology
There are two types of Herpes simplex virus: HSV-Type I is associated with lesions above the waist, and HSV-Type II is associated with genital lesions. Cross-infection does occur. Infection is sexually contacted, and there may be transfer of infection to the genitals by hand contact with an oral lesion or oral genital sex.

Clinical Manifestations
The initial infection usually takes place three to seven days after exposure and is characterized by irritation, pain, watery discharge, and multiple vesicles that may appear on the cervix, vulva, and/or perianal skin. These vesicles rupture within 24–48 hours, leaving extremely painful ulcers. Systemic symptoms include fever, headaches, and anorexia. The lesions usually subside within three to six weeks. Recurrent infections have mild to absent systemic symptoms. Diagnosis is made on pap smear or viral culture.

Nursing Care and Related Interventions
Acyclovir is useful in lessening the course of the primary infection, but it has no value in treating recurrences. Treatment concentrates on the relief of symptoms and the prevention of secondary infections. Patients may be admitted for cleansing of the painful ulcers. They are given sedation to help them rest. An indwelling Foley catheter may be necessary if the patient is unable to void. Hot sitz baths are soothing and may be used to help the patient empty the bladder.

Gardnerella Vaginitis (*Hemophilus Vaginalis,* Nonspecific)

Clinical Manifestations
Gardnerella is one of the most common sexually contracted vaginal infections but may not cause symptoms severe enough for the patient to seek treatment. It is not a tissue irritant so complaints of redness, burning, or itching are rare. Vaginal symptoms include a thin, watery, profuse discharge with odor. There is little or no itching.

Diagnostic Studies
The infection is suspected when a gray-white discharge is noted. It may be frothy with a pH of 5.0–5.5. A fishy odor is emitted when a 10 percent solution of potassium hydroxide (KOH) is added to a slide smear. Diagnosis is confirmed by the microscopic identification of "clue cells," which are speckled vaginal epithelial cells with obscure cell borders.

Nursing Care and Related Interventions
The patient and her sexual partner should be treated with metronidazole 250 mg eight tablets immediately or ampicillin 500 mg once every six hours for five days.

Trichomonas Vaginalis

Pathophysiology
Trichomonas vaginalis is caused by a protozoa and is sexually contracted. Its prevalence is declining because of effective treatment. Cervicitis and urinary symptoms are common.

Clinical Manifestations
The patient complains of slight to profuse yellow or greenish discharge that is usually frothy. There is an inflammatory skin response or soreness, postcoital bleeding, and strawberry marks on the cervix or vaginal mucosa. Diagnosis is confirmed by the presence of mobile, flagellated, pear-shaped organisms on a wet saline slide.

Nursing Care and Related Interventions
The patient and her partner should each be treated with metronidazole 250 mg eight tablets immediately or 250 mg three times a day for seven days.

Candida Vulvovaginitis

Clinical Manifestations
Candida vulvovaginitis occurs more commonly in diabetes, oral contraceptive users, and those who are pregnant. Patients complain of a thick discharge, pruritus, and dyspareunia. The vulva may appear red and swollen. The discharge has a yeastlike odor.

Diagnostic Studies
Diagnosis is made by identification of pseudomycelia and buds on a microscopic smear with a 10 percent KOH solution added or via culture on Nicherson's medium.

Nursing Care and Related Interventions
The infection is treated with nystatin vaginal suppositories twice a day for 7 to 14 days or miconazole nitrate cream, applied vaginally at bedtime for seven nights.

Pelvic Inflammatory Disease

Pathophysiology
Pelvic inflammatory disease is a symptom complex characterized by lower abdominal pain, mild to severe tenderness of the adnexa uteri, and cervicitis. Nausea and vomiting and fever are common symptoms. The most frequent causative organisms

are *Neisseria gonorrhoeea, Chlamydia trachomatis, Mycoplasma hominis,* and *Bacteroides fragilis.*

Nursing Care and Related Interventions
The Center for Disease Control's recommendations include ampicillin or tetracycline 500 mg QID for 10 days preceded by a loading dose of procaine penicillin G 4.8 million units IM or ampicillin 3.5 g by mouth accompanied by 1 g of probenecid. Patients with a high fever, severe abdominal pain with rebound tenderness, and nausea and vomiting should be admitted for intravenous antibiotic therapy.

Assisting the Patient with a Vaginal Infection

The emergency department nurse must become comfortable in obtaining the sexual history, describing the signs and symptoms of present and past infections, and noting the type of sexual contact. Be supportive and nonjudgmental during the examination and praise the patient for obtaining treatment.

The following equipment is helpful to have readily available during the examination: saline and KOH solution, cotton-tipped applicators, slides, Thayer-Martin media, LEM culture, speculum, and sponge forceps.

Use the saline solution to prepare slides for trichomonas and gardnerella, and the KOH solution to diagnose candida. Thayer-Martin media is used to culture secretions for gonorrhea and the LEM culture for herpes.

Discharge Planning

Patients should be instructed to take medication as directed until it is totally finished. Those taking Flagyl (metronidazol) should be cautioned against mixing this drug with alcohol because it causes an Antabuse-like reaction. It should be taken after meals to reduce stomach irritation; the patient might notice a metallic taste in the mouth. Systemic antibiotics may lead to an increased incidence of candida. Plain yogurt inserted vaginally may prevent this from happening by maintaining the acidity of the vagina. Plain boric acid powder in a number 2 sized gelatin capsule inserted vaginally is also effective. Patients should refrain from intercourse for one week or use a combination of foam and condoms to prevent cross-infections.

The patient should be made aware of several things that may help relieve symptoms and prevent further infections. Avoiding soap, vaginal sprays, or perfumed bath oils on mucous membranes, and using a hair dryer to dry the vaginal hair after a bath or shower are helpful. Wearing cotton underpants, avoiding many layers of clothing, and taking warm sitz baths also help.

Patients who are unable to obtain immediate medical care and whose main symptoms are a foul-smelling discharge and/or itching may use a mild vinegar douche (1 tablespoon vinegar per 1 l of water) or plain yogurt vaginally to reduce symptoms until medical attention can be obtained. A hanging douche bag is less traumatic than a squeeze bag. Patients should be semireclining in a bathtub and should hang the bag not more than 14–16 inches above the hips. This home treatment may make the patient more comfortable, but it will also make identification of the causative agent more difficult.

TOXIC SHOCK SYNDROME

Toxic shock syndrome has received wide attention from the news media since it was first described by a pediatrician in 1978. Dr. James Todd recognized the syndrome in seven children, three boys and four girls. He established the causative agent as *Staphylococcus aureus*. The Center for Disease Control reported 299 cases in the first nine months of 1980 with 29 fatalities. It was noted that 100 percent of the women affected used tampons and the onset of symptoms occurred during the menses. The syndrome is characterized by rapid onset of fever, nausea, vomiting, and diarrhea. There is a rapid decrease of the blood pressure and shock. The patient often has an erythematous macular sunburnlike rash with marked peeling of the hands and feet ten days later.

Nursing Care and Related Interventions

Nursing care is supportive with observation of vital signs, intake and output, character of skin lesions, and condition of joints.

Laboratory tests include blood, throat, urine, cerebral spinal fluid, and vaginal cultures. Tests may be obtained to rule out Rocky Mountain spotted fever, leptospirosis, or measles. Tests to evaluate renal and hepatic function may be ordered. Antibiotic therapy has little value in treating the acute episode, but may be useful in preventing recurrences.

Women can reduce the risk of toxic shock syndrome by avoiding the use of superabsorbent tampons, alternating tampons with pads, and changing tampons frequently. Toxic shock syndrome has also been linked with the prolonged wearing of a diaphragm.

RAPE

Rape is considered a crime of violence. It is the fastest growing crime in the United States. The rape victim may be young or old, male or female. Male rape has been associated with homosexuals, but a recent study reported several cases of men who have been sexually assaulted by women (Masters and Sarrel, 1982).

Confidential and empathetic care of the rape victim in the emergency department can profoundly affect the recovery process. Patients may actually benefit from seeing a caring male figure (Hicks, 1980).

The role of the nurse in the emergency department is to obtain and document evidence of support for the patient, not to establish a crime. In some states, it is mandatory to report rape to the authorities. Well-documented medical records are essential.

Clinical Manifestations

Most rape victims experience a sense of humiliation, loss of control, and violation of self. The emotional response may range from supreme control to hysteria. The process of adjustment is not unlike a grief reaction, with the patient passing through periods of fear, denial, guilt, depression, and an organizational period in which the victim comes to terms with the event and herself (Freeman, 1980).

Nursing Care and Related Interventions

It is helpful to assign the patient to one nurse who will be able to care for her throughout the entire emergency department visit. A careful history of the assault, including a description of the assailant, any threats, the use of weapons, and the type of physical and sexual contact attempted or completed, is important to document. A description of the patient's emotional state and general appearance should also be included. The entire body should be examined for any signs of trauma, especially around the head and neck. Scrapings are taken from the fingernails. By placing the patient's buttocks on a paper towel and combing the pubic hair, specimens of foreign hair can be obtained. A pap smear, sample of vaginal secretions for an acid phosphatase test, and a gonorrhea culture are made.

Medications for preventing pregnancy, such as conjugated estrogens 25 mg QID for five days or ethinyl estradiol 0.5 mg BID for five days may be prescribed. These medications usually are accompanied by severe side effects such as nausea and vomiting. Patients may be given follow-up appointments for pregnancy testing and, if the tests are positive, may undergo induced abortion if they do not desire completion of the pregnancy.

Preventative treatment for gonorrhea consists of 4.8 million units of procaine penicillin G IM plus 1 g probenecid orally or, if the patient is allergic to penicillin, 1.5 g oral tetracycline immediately, followed by 500 mg QID for 15 days.

Discharge Planning

Plans should be made to discharge the patient in the company of a friend, and a change of clothing should be obtained. Written instructions regarding the use of medication, possible side effects and follow-up appointments should be given. If the incident will be reported to the police, the patient should be provided with information about the investigation process, including the types of questions usually asked. This information may be given by a counselor, nurse, physician, or police officer. If no rape counselor is available, the nurse should explore with the patient the support options (such as the local crisis center) available to her for follow-up within 48 hours. Additional information for the patient and the staff may be obtained from the National Center for Prevention and Control of Rape, 5600 Fishers Lane, Rockville, Maryland.

CONCLUSION

Changing birth patterns, increasing costs of medical care, and reorganization of obstetrical care are factors that will contribute to more obstetrical and gynecological patients seeking treatment in the emergency department. Consequently, it is necessary that the emergency department nurse be familiar with these major problems. The process of assessment is essential and must focus on either noting or ruling out pregnancy.

Since obstetrical and gynecological emergencies concern the female's reproductive function, there is usually a concern about reproductive ability, a fear of pregnancy, or a fear of losing a pregnancy. In any case, emotional reactions should be expected. Sometimes in an emergency situation, the emotions are forgotten. To provide support, it is important to allow the patient privacy, an opportunity to express feelings, and the support of significant others whenever possible.

BIBLIOGRAPHY

Bolton, G., and E. Cohen: Detecting and treating ectopic pregnancy. *Contemporary Obstetrical Gynecology* 18:101–104 (1981).

Cavanagh, D.; R. Woods; and T. O'Connor: *Obstetrical Emergencies*. 2nd ed. Hagerstown, MD: Harper & Row, 1982.

Cotton, D.; R. Paul; J. Read; and E. Quilligan: The conservative aggressive management of placenta previa. *American Journal of Obstetrical Gynecology* 137:687–695 (1980).

Fleury, F.: Adult vaginitis. *Clinical Obstetrical Gynecology* 24:407–438 (1981).

Freeman, M.: Sexual assault: A discussion. *American Journal of Obstetrical Gynecology* 137:933–935 (1980).

Freeman, P.: Gonorrhea. *Journal of Emergency Nursing* 6:16–22 (1980).

Handsfield, H.: Sexually transmitted disease. *Hospital Practices* 17:99–116 (1982).

Hicks, D.: Sexual assault. *American Journal of Obstetrical Gynecology* 137:931–933 (1980).

Jennings, B.: Emergency delivery: How to attend one safely. *MCN* 4:148–153 (1979).

Kaufman, R.: How to diagnose infectious vaginitis. *Contemporary Obstetrical Gynecology* 11:61–64 (1978).

McGovern, C.: Recognizing a tubal pregnancy. *MCN* 6:303–305 (1978).

Masters, W., and Sarrel, P.: When men are raped by women. *Sexual Medicine Today* 6(7):14–20 (1982).

Miles, P.: Sexually transmissible disease. *Journal of Emergency Nursing* 6:6–12 (1980).

Oill, P.: Herpes virus type 2 infection of the genital tract. *Journal of Emergency Nursing* 6:13–16 (1980).

Ostheimer, G.: Resuscitating the depressed neonate. *Contemporary Obstetrical Gynecology* 15:27–41 (1980).

Quilligan, E.: *Current Therapy in Obstetrics and Gynecology*. Philadelphia: Saunders, 1980.

Sibai, B., et al.: Reassessment of intravenous $MgSO_4$ therapy in preeclampsia-eclampsia. *Obstetrical Gynecology* 57:199–202 (1981).

Varney, H.: *Nurse Midwifery*. Oxford, England: Blackwell Scientific, 1980.

Wheeler, H.: Pregnancy induced hypertension. *JOGN* 10(13):212–231 (1981).

Williams, P., and M. Joseph: *Differential Diagnosis in Obstetrics*. New York: Arco, 1978.

Wroblewski, S.: Toxic shock syndrome. *American Journal of Nursing* 81:82–25 (1981).

Zuspan, F.: Problems encountered in treatment of pregnancy induced hypertension. *American Journal of Obstetrical Gynecology* 131:591–597 (1978).

———., and K. Zuspan: Strategies for controlling eclampsia. *Contemporary Obstetrical Gynecology* 18:135–141 (1981).

EMERGENCY NURSING AND COMMUNITY RESOURCES

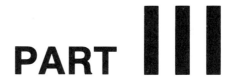

PART III

31

Disaster Planning

Janet Gren Parker

After completing this chapter, the reader will be able to do the following:

1. Define a disaster situation.
2. Discuss the stages of a disaster.
3. Discuss federal, state, and local plans that help coordinate activities during a disaster.
4. Discuss disaster triage.
5. Discuss the role of the emergency department as it relates to the hospital disaster plan.
6. Define a radiation disaster.
7. Discuss psychological reactions that may be exhibited during and after a disaster.

Disaster planning encompasses all personnel affiliated with the hospital, the community, and the state and the federal government. The emergency department nurse, of course, is directly involved in most disaster situations. Consequently, the emergency department nurse must be active in disaster planning at all levels.

By definition, a disaster is any patient-generating incident that overloads either existing personnel or existing supplies and equipment, or a disaster is any patient-generating incident in which backup supplies and personnel are not available in a reasonable amount of time (Simoneau and McCall, 1981). Disasters may be external or internal in nature. External disasters occur outside of the hospital (e.g., an airplane crash), while internal disasters occur within the institution (e.g., a hospital fire or bomb threat). External disasters can also be labeled natural or manmade disasters. Examples of natural disasters include tornadoes, earthquakes, tidal waves, and volcanic eruptions. Manmade disasters include fires, airplane crashes, collapses of buildings, and train wrecks.

Regardless of the type or the cause of the disaster, delineating specific situations according to expected patient volume is instrumental in developing a thorough disaster plan.

Multiple Patient Incident—The multiple patient incident occurs daily in emergency departments throughout the country. An incident that generates at least two, but fewer than ten, patients is self-limiting and can usually be handled effectively without requiring aid from resources outside of the community. Most emergency departments have some type of plan for recalling additional personnel, if needed, in a limited situation. Typical incidents that generate multiple patients are automobile accidents, house fires, and bus accidents.

Multiple Casualty Incident—A multiple casualty incident generates at least ten, but fewer than 100, casualties and necessitates total community and perhaps state involvement. Airplane crashes, snow storms, and floods are examples of multiple casualty incidents. The community-wide disaster plan must be established and functional to adequately coordinate this type of situation.

Mass Casualty Incident—A mass casualty incident generates more than 100 victims. Because a mass casualty overwhelms the local community and local health care professionals, additional aid and assistance is required from the state and the federal government. Although these incidents occur infrequently, they must be anticipated in any disaster planning activity. Examples include wars, major hurricanes, and earthquakes in which thousands of casualties may be generated on a continuing basis.

STAGES OF A DISASTER

Seigler-Shelton and Marks (1980) identified several stages of a disaster. Regardless of the origin, type, or extent of the disaster, the stages are identical. Although the time involved in each stage will vary depending on the type of the disaster, each situation will progress through the following stages:

1. *Warning stage*—In every situation a warning period exists. The warning stage can extend from two seconds to days in length. This stage may provide sufficient time for preparing to handle the potential event.
2. *Impact*—During the impact stage, the primary objective is staying alive. The event occurs that produces the disaster situation and everyone involved attempts to survive the event.
3. *Inventory*—After the impact stage, survivors first assess the effects of the event, and then they identify what must be done next. During the inventory stage, people assess or inventory personal injuries and/or family involvement.
4. *Rescue*—During the rescue stage, help arrives to rescue survivors and to help the injured casualties. This stage requires help from members of the community.
5. *Remedy*—Recovery activities are initiated during the remedy stage. Utilities are reconnected, clothing is found, and temporary food and shelter are identified and used. This stage may last from days to weeks or even months before normal activities are resumed.
6. *Recovery*—The recovery stage encompasses total recovery from the impact and the resulting situation. This stage includes psychological recovery as well as phys-

COMMUNITY PLANNING

ical recovery from the event. It also involves the development of adaptive behavior required to produce lasting changes.

All six stages must be remembered and integrated into any disaster plan, whether it is the federal, state, local, or hospital plan. This chapter will discuss in detail the community plan and the hospital plan that help the emergency department nurse to function as well as possible in any disaster situation.

COMMUNITY PLANNING

Community disaster planning involves, in fact, federal plans, state plans, and local community plans. All three plans are integrated and coordinated to avoid duplicating activities and services.

The Federal Disaster Relief Act specifying *federal* response to disasters is initiated by and administered through the President of the United States. Implementation begins after the President decides an event has depleted the resources from either a state or from several neighboring states. The governor of the state requests assistance directly from the President. Military resources are used to help the affected state or states to recover from the disaster situation.

The *state* plan is developed in cooperation with the federal plan and local area disaster coordinators. Most state plans, implemented when the disaster constitutes several local areas, requires regional coordination within the state. Emergency department nurses, therefore, should understand the fundamental aspects of the disaster plan in their particular states.

Local Community Planning

The local community disaster plan may vary considerably, depending on the specific resources available within the community. The community committee should include representatives from all agencies within the community that would be involved in handling a disaster situation. (Table 31.1 contains many agencies that probably should be represented, if they are functional within the community.)

The plan developed and established by this committee must address several areas of concern (Simoneau, 1981):

1. Actual declaration of the disaster.
2. Communication pathways and links.
3. Record-keeping.
4. Establishment of triage teams and command posts in the field.
5. Identification of disaster workers and medical personnel.
6. Patient transportation activities.
7. Public utility restoration.
8. Procurement of additional supplies and equipment.

TABLE 31.1 Composition of Local Disaster Planning Committees

Public utilities
Fire department
Police department
Civil defense
Mayor's office
Each local hospital
American Red Cross
Mental health centers
Funeral director association
Medical association
Emergency medical services
Highway patrol or state police
National Guard
Any other agency directly involved in disaster relief

9. Review and update of plan.
10. Periodic drills using the plan.
11. Public education regarding the plan.

This list, though not all-inclusive, provides an excellent starting point for further discussion and planning. Although preplanning is necessary to enable everyone to function well during a disaster, the established plan should be as simple as possible. The more complicated the plan, the harder it will be to implement. If the plan closely resembles day-to-day activity, it will be easier to remember and to implement when necessary.

Disaster Triage

During a disaster, triage activities in the field are different from triage activities in an emergency department. The goal in field triage is saving the greatest number of lives while using the simplest measures possible. The hopelessly injured are made as comfortable as possible, while efforts are directed toward treating the many who may respond quickly to lifesaving treatment and intervention.

Four categories of field, military, or disaster triage have been identified (Mahoney, 1969). *Minimal treatment* includes the injured who either treat themselves or are handled by paraprofessionals, and then begin helping other casualties. *Immediate treatment* includes casualties who have a reasonable chance of surviving, with minimal time required to provide lifesaving interventions. *Delayed treatment* includes casualties who can wait for extensive treatment after they receive initial first aid. *Expectant treatment* includes critically injured casualties. Younger people in this

TABLE 31.2 Examples of Disaster Triage

Category	Example
Minimal	Sprained extremities
	Simple extremity fractures
	Minor lacerations and abrasions
	Dislocations
Immediate	Accessible respiratory obstruction
	Accessible hemorrhage
	Sucking chest wounds
	Tension pneumothorax
	Shock
	Readily correctable major medical problems
Delayed	Major fractures
	Closed cerebral injuries
	Spinal cord injuries
	Eye injuries
	Complicated major medical problems
	Genitourinary tract injuries
Expectant	Major multiple trauma
	Victims with little hope of survival

category are treated first, and then older people. The casualties in the expectant category may be reclassified at a later time. (Table 31.2 contains examples of disaster casualties classified according to the four major categories.)

HOSPITAL PLANNING

The emergency department nurse must have direct input into the development, testing, and revision of the hospital disaster plan. The emergency department is probably the first area of the hospital that will receive word from the community about the occurrence of a disaster. The Joint Commission on Accreditation of Hospitals requires that hospitals devise, implement, and practice (twice a year) a hospital-wide disaster plan. The plan should be simple enough to be implemented easily and require minimal staff education. The closer the plan emulates normal, everyday activity, the higher the probability that it will be implemented without excessive anxiety, indecision, and stress.

The hospital plan should be established by a hospital committee including the following members:

1. Emergency department nurse and physician.
2. Hospital administration.
3. Public affairs office.

4. Security department.
5. Pharmacy.
6. Social work department.
7. Surgical department.
8. Nursing department.
9. Medical department.
10. Volunteer associations.

This list, used as a starting point, can be expanded to accommodate the needs of each individual hospital organization. The committee ensures that each hospital department develops its own specific plan that is included within the overall plan of action. The disaster plan, which is published and updated in manual form, should be located for easy reference in every department of the hospital and on each patient care division. The hospital disaster committee is also responsible for educating hospital employees about the plan, coordinating hospital disaster drills, evaluating the drills, and revising the plan appropriately. Inservice education programs are necessary to update all hospital personnel regarding the revisions made in the plan.

The Emergency Department Plan

The emergency department is usually the first area of the hospital to be notified that a disaster situation either potentially exists or has already occurred. The emergency department must be prepared to receive multiple casualties within a short period of time and to provide the optimal care these patients require. The emergency department is the hub of activity in the hospital. After incoming victims arrive at the emergency department, they are dispersed throughout the hospital according to the established plan. All emergency department personnel should know the fundamental plan of action. The following discussion examines specific areas in the emergency department plan.

Implementation
The physician and nurse in charge at the time of the incident must decide when to implement the disaster plan. Most hospital plans have several phases that depend on the number of expected casualties. Obtaining data concerning the disaster and verifying the data collected from the community agencies involved are required before a decision is made based on the data. Different phases of the plan may be implemented, ranging from increased involvement in the emergency department to a hospital-wide effort affecting all hospital departments.

Command Post
In the command post, decisions made and implemented reflect major administrative functions, such as staff call back, obtaining needed supplies and equipment, assign-

ing staff, identifying staff members, and delegating certain hospital responsibilities. Moreover, central communications are also maintained in this area.

After the nurse in charge of the emergency department identifies staff required, the command center should be directed to contact the appropriate staff. A current list of staff and their telephone numbers should be maintained in the department and average response time noted so that staff who can respond faster can be called first. Furthermore, the nurse coordinator must also assign the staff to specific areas of responsibility. Areas of responsibility might include triage action, treatment, and delayed treatment areas.

Triage Action
Triage action provides a rapid assessment of each incoming casualty and assigns the patient to the appropriate area for treatment. Most hospital plans permit the triage of victims to all areas within the hospital, rather than confining patients to areas just within the emergency department. The triage area also provides a barrier to the influx of relatives, news media personnel, curious onlookers, and other unauthorized individuals.

Personnel in the triage area must include at least one physician, one nurse, clerical support, and transporters. The physician and nurse must understand disaster and emergency department triage, assessing each incoming victim according to the care required to ensure the patient's survival.

The clerical personnel must generate the paper work at triage, tagging the patient according to hospital policy and maintaining a list of all patients received. The hospital tagging system should include a packet with appropriate laboratory, radiology, and treatment record sheets necessary to care for the victim. All paper work generated for each patient should be affixed with the same number that was assigned to the patient upon arrival. This number is affixed to the patient, not to the person's clothing, preferably tied to an extremity where it will not be removed.

The triage area must be stocked with required supplies. A triage cart should be ready at all times with supplies available to maintain airways, stop bleeding, provide first-aid measures, support the clerical tasks, and to communicate effectively in case of telephone failure. Furthermore, a mechanism should also be established for immediate receipt of additional stretchers, wheelchairs, sheets, and other supplies required to help support the triage area.

Critical Care Teams
Staff should be immediately assigned to critical care teams that minimally include a physician, a nurse, and a clerk. A transporter and an aide are also beneficial, if they are available. The staff functions as a team to care for victims triaged to care areas within the emergency department. The team approach must be used to provide quality patient care. The physician in charge should assign the team to a patient. The team should remain with the patient until the person is transported to another area within the hospital to receive continual care. The team is responsible for the following: continuous assessment of the patient; emergency interventions for the patient (stabilization); documentation of the care provided; and transportation to other areas within the hospital for continuing care.

Supplies and Ancillary Services

Arrangements must be made for ready access to at least a 30-day supply of backup materials and drugs. Local supply houses must be ready and willing to cooperate in this area. A mass casualty incident generating more than 100 seriously injured patients can quickly deplete supplies.

Furthermore, ancillary services must also be available to support both the emergency department and other patient care areas within the hospital. Laboratory and radiological support, of course, is mandatory. Special services can be provided by departments not directly involved in patient care activities, including the following departments: public affairs, security, housekeeping, and social services. Public affairs and social services can handle the news media as well as the families and relatives of victims. Security must ensure that patient flow patterns remain uncongested while securing the hospital itself from outside intruders. Housekeeping can help transport patients, direct visitors from the triage area, obtain required supplies and equipment, and clean the treatment areas after a patient is transported to another department.

Evaluation of the Plan

After the disaster is over and everyone has adjusted to its impact, the disaster plan itself must be reevaluated and revised. The literature describing personal accounts of disasters identifies numerous problem areas that developed in existing plans. Establishing adequate communication mechanisms often is a major problem. Proper staff identification is another problem. Furthermore, adequate psychological intervention for staff, as well as for disaster victims, has also been identified as a problematical area.

Radiation Disasters

With the number of nuclear power plant increases and the concomitant increase in the amount of radioactive supplies and chemicals transported, the emergency department must be capable of treating victims of a potential radiation exposure.

People arriving at the scene of a radiation disaster should approach the scene from an upwind direction, and they should be equipped with basic radiation survey meters to measure the amount of existing radiation. The maximum exposure for anyone dealing with a radiation victim should be 100 Rem. Health care providers and ambulance personnel should wear gloves, boots, overalls, caps, and masks, if time permits (Richter et al., 1980). Life-threatening emergencies should be treated before any decontamination is attempted. The patient's clothing should be removed, and then the patient should be washed with soap and water.

After the patient arrives at the hospital, a control area should be established to treat and decontaminate the patient. The floor should be covered with paper, the area isolated with ropes, and the health care providers should wear protective clothing.

The radiation disaster plan should be coordinated with a radiation safety specialist, if possible.

PSYCHOLOGICAL REACTIONS

In considering the aftereffects of a disaster situation, one must consider the effects on the victim, on the victim's significant others, and on the health care providers and other disaster workers. Hargreaves (1980) identifies three stages of disaster coping mechanisms.

Stage I (Impact)—The person is dazed, stunned, and apathetic. The person's behavior may be so disorganized that he responds minimally to directions.

Stage II (Recoil)—The person exhibits extreme suggestibility, altruism, and gratitude for help. The person minimizes personal injuries and is extremely compliant. The person is grateful to be alive and is quiet about anyone who has died.

Stage III (Posttrauma)—After the person's spirits lift, he experiences a feeling of euphoria and a sense of brotherhood within the community. The person actively participates in plans for reconstruction.

Although panic is not a common response, it is more prevalent if the following limitations exist: the disaster occurs with only minimal warning, limited escape routes exist, and insufficient or inadequate leadership and information are available.

Harrison (1981) identified five acute reactions that may occur during a disaster. Overwhelmed by stressful external stimuli, a person may use defense mechanisms necessary for maintaining homeostasis. The *normal* or expected reaction is calmness and an ability to function appropriately. The person may be *depressed* because a major effect of the disaster is loss, particularly for the person who is elderly. An *overreactive* or hysterical reaction is demonstrated through purposeless motor behavior and unrealistic beliefs. A *somatic* reaction is a physiological reaction that originates from an emotional or nonemotional source. *Panic* is uncontrollable and hysterical behavior that may require gentle restraints.

The elderly, children, psychiatric patients, disaster workers, and people who have experienced a recent loss are at high risk for developing psychological problems after a disaster situation. A flexible, pragmatic, immediate crisis intervention response is the best approach to the emergency phase of disaster intervention (Fraser and Spicka, 1981). The American Red Cross and the community mental health center can provide emotional support training for potential disaster workers. Mental health services should be directed toward prevention. Crisis intervention techniques seem to be the most appropriate during the disaster and immediately after during the recovery phase.

CONCLUSION

The emergency health care provider must be prepared to handle any potential disaster situation to ensure saving as many lives as possible in a minimal amount of time. To accomplish this goal, the nurse must be aware of federal, state, local, and hospital disaster plans. The emergency department plays an integral role in the management of a disaster. The staff of the department must be organized and efficient to provide the best care possible to the victims of a disaster situation.

BIBLIOGRAPHY

Berren, M. R.; A. Beigel; and S. Ghertner: A typology for the classification of disasters. *Community Mental Health Journal* 16:103–111 (Summer 1980).

Campbell, P. M., and C. A. Pribyl: The Hyatt disaster: Two nurses' perspectives. *Journal of Emergency Nursing* 8:12 (1982).

Fraser, J. R. P.; and D. A. Spicka: Handling the emotional response to disaster: The case for American Red Cross/community mental health collaboration. *Community Mental Health Journal* 17:255–264 (Winter 1981).

Hargreaves, A. G.: Coping with disaster. *American Journal of Nursing* 80:683 (1980).

Harrison, D. F.: Nurses and disasters. *Journal of Psychosocial Nursing* 19:34–6 (Dec. 1981).

Mahoney, R. F.: *Emergency and Disaster Nursing.* New York: MacMillan and Company, 1969.

Melton, R. J., and R. M. Riner: Revising the rural hospital disaster plan: A role for the EMS system in managing the multiple casualty incident. *Annals of Emergency Medicine* 10:39–44 (1981).

Orr, S. M., and W. A. Robinson: The Hyatt disaster: Two physicians' perspectives. *Journal of Emergency Nursing* 8:6–11 (1982).

Seigler-Shelton, C., and L. N. Marks: The Wichita Falls experience. *Supervisor Nurse* 11:28–30+ (April 1980).

Simoneau, J. K.: Disaster Aspects in Emergency Nursing. In S. A. Budassi and J. M. Barber (ed.): *Emergency Nursing Principles and Practice.* St. Louis: Mosby, 1981, pp. 641–679.

———, and P. McCall: Disaster! prepare for the possibility. *Critical Care Update* 8:35+ (Dec. 1981).

32
Evolving Trends in Emergency Nursing

June D. Thompson

After completing this chapter, the reader will be able to do the following:

1. Describe the history and development of the emergency medical services in the United States.
2. List the 15 components of a functional Emergency Medical Services System (EMSS).
3. Summarize the current situation of emergency care in the United States.
4. List nine selected consumer needs and discuss the extent to which their needs are being met by nursing.
5. Discuss characteristics of at least three types of specialists in emergency nursing.
6. Describe the challenge of the future for emergency nursing.

Emergency Nursing: Where did it start? How and why is it developing? This chapter explores selected issues pertaining to American health care, the response of the emergency care system, and the future responsibilities of emergency nursing to respond to and affect the delivery of health care services.

The last half of the twentieth century may someday be remembered as the age of depersonalization—the era in which people were computerized, numbered, herded into mass-education, mass-transit, and mass-health care systems. Technology is increasing at an astounding rate, and young professionals are specializing, experimenting, testing, and individually enhancing their professions. Toffler (1970) has termed this the era of "Future Shock." Because the technological world is expanding so rapidly, people often feel either trapped by or excluded from the systems.

A proportional dissonance exists among the technological advances in this country, the development of professional specialities and the subspecialities, and the health care needs of the public. After technology advanced to produce high-speed motor vehicles, motor vehicle related deaths significantly increased. Health care professionals have subspecialized, for example, to produce experts in the field of pediatric cardiovascular surgery and neonatology, but the general practitioner is slowly disappearing. Finally, almost all health professionals are working diligently to expand the body of scientific knowledge in their specialty; but some professionals may have neglected learning how to care for people and how to analyze the public's health care needs. The professionals, however, are not solely responsible for enhancing the depersonalization and inadequacy of health care. Economics, politics, and fundamental professional availability are other equally important variables.

In 1966, the National Academy of Science published a research paper entitled, "Accidental Death and Disability: The Neglected Disease of Modern Society." This study highlighted the type of emergency care that was being delivered in this country and exposed the ways in which the health care needs of the public were being neglected. The study labeled this "neglected epidemic" the leading cause of death in children and in young adults and identified it as the nation's most important environmental health problem.

This paper was produced simultaneously with two other types of research. The first type of research examined improved methods for delivering emergency care. The studies were based on war experiences in VietNam, as well as on primarily prehospital management of cardiac emergencies (Heaton, 1966; Cobb, 1976; Lund and Skulberg, 1976). The second type of research analyzed the patterns and trends in the use of emergency services in the United States. Extensive research by Gibson (1978), for example, documented that there was a continuing increase in the use of hospital emergency departments as primary health care centers. Consequently, the development of emergency care services became quite complex. On one hand, researchers and health care professionals focused extensively on the components of trauma, critical care stabilization, and management; and, on the other hand, the number of people using emergency departments for primary care or for nonemergency care increased. Inconsistencies existed within the prehospital ambulance systems. Moreover, inconsistencies existed in both the preparation of and type of health care professionals available to care for the ambulatory or nonemergency care patients after they arrived at the emergency facilities. Emergency care was primitive and basically disorganized.

Finally, in 1973, Public Law 93-154, the Emergency Medical Services Systems (EMSS) Act, was passed. This law authorized $185 million for a three-year program to plan, implement, improve, and expand comprehensive regional systems for emergency medical services. The work accomplished from the pilot program was so successful that in 1976 the law was slightly amended, and an additional $200 million was authorized for three more years (Montgomery, 1980). This federal legislation has significantly helped identify and develop the initial steps for operating an efficient EMS System in this country. (Table 32.1 identifies the fifteen major components of a comprehensive and functioning EMS System.)

The emergency care group that became most clearly developed and standardized throughout the 1970s included emergency medical technicians (EMTs) and paramedics who provided prehospital care and transportation. Standards of education and practice were developed, and research clearly documents that organized prehospital

TABLE 32.1 Components of a Functioning Emergency Medical Services System

Provision of manpower
Training of personnel
Communications
Transportation facilities
Critical-care work
Use of public safety agencies
Consumer participation
Accessibility to care
Transfer of patients
Standard record keeping
Consumer information and education
Independent review and evaluation
Disaster linkage
Mutual-aid agreements

SOURCE: Public Law 93-154, Emergency Medical Services Systems Act, 1973.

care made a significant difference in mortality rates (Emergency Medical Services, 1980).

By the early 1980s, the picture of emergency services began to emerge. Although some components of the 1973 proposed EMS System have been addressed and significant strides have been made, other areas either have been ignored or have become entangled in the interprofessional and intraprofessional territorial disputes (Gann, 1981; Leitzell and Riggs, 1981).

The current situation of emergency care may be summarized as follows:

1. Significant improvements have occurred since the 1960s.
2. The emergency care system is disorganized and fragmented.
3. The prehospital care of emergency victims in some parts of the country is both advanced and standardized.
4. Prehospital emergency care in other parts of the country, however, barely exists.
5. Hospital administration and physician groups are disputing the cost as well as the effectiveness of various services (e.g., categorizing the capabilities of hospital emergency services, free-standing emergency centers, hospital-based ambulance services, and helicopter rescue services).
6. Hospital administrators, physicians, and nurses are debating the following topics: employing paramedics, physician assistants, and nurse practitioners in the emergency department; using advertising to increase business and to improve revenue for the hospital; expanding the emergency center services versus trying to find alternative care services for patients who require less expensive, nonemergency care; and encouraging the use of board-certified emergency care

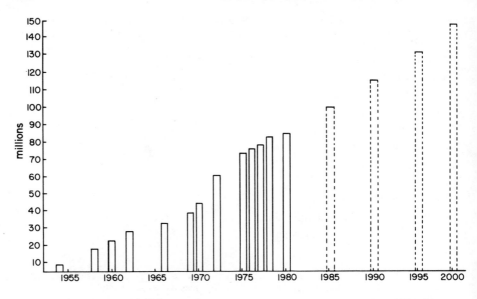

Figure 32.1 The total number of emergency department visits 1954–1980 with projections for 1985–2000.

professionals in emergency nursing and medicine versus either increasing nonprofessional emergency care staff or using trauma surgeons and family practice physicians.

7. The public is affected by this "future shock" situation. Throughout the years, the American health care system has encouraged the dependency of the "patient" on the "doctor." Emergency care centers are witnessing the results of this "dependency education," because many people now are dependent on physicians and the health care system. Since 1954, the emergency departments have witnessed a 760 percent increase in emergency department use. Emergency department usage skyrocketed from 9.7 million in 1954 to 83.5 million in 1979. The increase in emergency department use, as illustrated in Figures 32.1 and 32.2, is dependent on concomitant increases in population (American Hospital Association, 1955, 1967, 1970, 1971, 1976, 1978, and 1979).

8. Many patients should be treated by the emergency department. According to a study determining the urgency of patients' problems (Gifford et al., 1980), of the 10,253 patients who arrived at 24 different hospital emergency departments, only 12 percent of the patients had life-threatening disorders requiring emergency intervention within 20 minutes. Fifty-five percent of the patients were described as urgent cases requiring intervention within 12 hours. The remaining 33 percent of the study population were categorized as nonemergent. These individuals could easily have received care someplace else. Although many studies indicate the abuse and misuse of the emergency facility, the study by the American

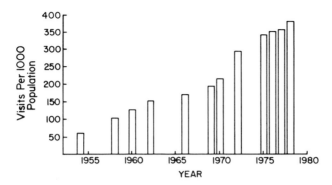

Figure 32.2 The number of emergency department visits per 1000 population, 1954–1978.

College of Emergency Physicians (ACEP) suggests that in two-thirds of the cases the public correctly uses the emergency department for care (Gifford et al., 1980).

9. Although emergency care technology has increased significantly, it appears to be primitive compared to the technology available in other health care specialities.
10. Emergency care education is not standardized for health care professionals. In some universities, medicine and nursing have been aggressive in their approach to establish emergency care curricula for students and to establish emergency medicine residency programs. In other universities, however, emergency care education is either disorganized or even ignored.
11. Emergency care research is minimal among all disciplines.
12. In general, great strides have been made, but the development of a specialized profession is just beginning. Emergency care is still in its infantile stage.

Before predicting future events, however, one must systematically consider the past, the players, the professions, the politics, the turfs, and the actual needs of the consumers. Emergency care entered the health care scene at a time when the nation began to focus on the quality and delivery of all health care in this country. Because of its nature and its revenue-generating potential, emergency care became a focus for many groups. Emergency service extends beyond merely stabilizing and treating the critically ill or injured patient. It is, in fact, a philosophy extending from an earlier definition proposed by the American College of Surgeons (ACS): in essence, the purpose of an emergency department is to provide adequate appraisal and initial treatment or advice to every person who considers himself or herself acutely ill or injured and presents himself or herself to the emergency department. Consequently, emergency care services, as defined by the ACS and in accordance with the standards defined by the EMSS, still require development and implementation.

In the balance of this chapter we examine the needs of the consumer and the potential of nursing either to meet or to assist in meeting those needs.

CONSUMER NEEDS

Several types of consumer needs can be easily identified. The critically ill or injured patient, for example, requires physiological stabilization and continued assessment and care. Furthermore, the patient also needs information about his status, in addition to nurturing kindness and support. The family of the critically ill patient needs support through crisis intervention, in addition to information and education about the patient's situation.

The needs of all other emergency care patients are numerous. Most patients will require some type of physiological assessment, intervention, continued monitoring, support, reassurance, and education. Many patients using the emergency facilities require extensive education on the following topics: self-assessment, self-care, and the availability of community resources. The families of these patients will also require reassurance and education. Other patients such as "repeaters" need support and reassurance, as well as referrals to supporting services.

Although this list is incomplete, it provides a tentative profile of the needs of patients who enter the emergency center. Table 32.2 uses a Likert scale analysis as a model for portraying patients' needs. The placement of the "*" on each line of the scale indicates the extent to which nursing is attempting to meet the patient's designated need. If the "*" is toward the left end of the scale, the need is not being met. As the "*" moves along the scale to the right, it indicates the extent of emergency nursing's attempt to meet the patient's specific need.

After identifying the patient's needs, one can define the scope of emergency nursing practice.

EMERGENCY NURSING—THE PRESENT

Current emergency nursing practice often appears reactive and mechanical. Because of the infancy status of emergency care throughout the United States, only the most basic issues have been addressed. Systems previously developed usually addressed the care of the critically ill and injured. Consequently, most advances in emergency nursing, as illustrated in Table 32.2, affect only the physiological aspects of emergency care. Although physiological care is crucial for the patient, it is also the aspect of nursing practice that is most dependent on or interdependent on the practice of medicine. Thus, the physiological aspects of emergency nursing are the dependent components of practice. Nurses are restricted in their ability to determine their own scope of practice in providing care. Nursing practice frequently is restricted by the limitations of the nursing and medical practice act, which often prohibits the nurse from making diagnoses or from initiating independent interventions that may be interpreted as medicine. Consequently, the nurse depends on or is interdependent on the physician for direction of practice.

Emergency nursing's efforts to expand and to standardize practice relating to the care of the critically ill or injured patient has resulted in several types of subspeciality roles, including the following: emergency rescue flight nursing; mobile intensive care unit nursing; paramedic or prehospital nurse coordinator; and, trauma nursing (Various Roles of EDNA Nurses, 1980). Although these roles have indeed enhanced the

EMERGENCY NURSING—THE PRESENT

TABLE 32.2 Patient and Family Needs Overview and Emergency Nursing Efforts to Meet Those Needs

	Patient Needs Not Met		Patient Needs Met
Physiological care of critically ill or injured patients		———————————————	*
Psychological and supportive care of critically ill or injured patient		* ——————————————	
Psychological and supportive care of family of critically ill or injured patient		* ——————————————	
Average E.D. patient physiological assessment, intervention, and continual monitoring		———————————————	*
Average E.D. patient support, reassurance, and education		* ——————————————	
Family of average E.D. patient reassurance and education		* ——————————————	
Education for all patients regarding self-assessment, self-care, and availability of community resources		*————————————	
Education, support, and referral for repeaters		* ——————————————	
Public education regarding accident prevention, selected first-aid techniques and purpose and use of emergency care facilities		* ——————————————	

practice of emergency nursing and have improved the care patients receive, the roles still are primarily geared toward the physiological needs of the patient.

In addition to the specialists in trauma and critical care, two other major types of specific emergency nursing roles have evolved. The first type is the emergency nurse practitioner. The nurse practitioner, educated primarily in certificate programs (Various Roles of EDNA Nurses, 1980), provides care in select emergency departments and in associated walk-in clinics. The role was justified because of the tremendous increase in emergency department use, especially by patients with minor problems. The potential role of the nurse practitioner in emergency care has not been fully explored. Most of the current programs focus on the physiological assessment and management of patient complaints, but place minimal focus on other areas of patient care. Consequently, many aspects of patient and family needs are not met even by the emergency nurse practitioner.

The other type of emergency nursing specialist is the masters-prepared clinical specialist. The functions of the clinical specialists are diverse. Some nurses focus on the physiological aspects of trauma care, while others are involved in such nursing aspects as family and patient crisis intervention, psychiatric assessment and support, rape crisis care, and public and staff education (Various Roles of EDNA Nurses, 1980). The role of the clinical specialist emphasizes in particular the nursing aspects of emergency care.

The predominant issue regarding emergency nursing today concerns the lack of a standardized emergency nursing role. In most centers, the level, scope, roles, and standards of the nursing department in the facility are determined by the nurse director in the emergency care center, or, in some cases, by the medical director of the emergency department. Many nurses, when asked about their scope of practice, reply: "I do whatever they let me do." Many emergency nurses apparently allow others to specify the current scope of practice and to determine its future. If this practice continues, however, nursing will fail to meet the patient's needs, and perhaps many of the components of the EMSS standards will not be met.

EMERGENCY NURSING—THE FUTURE

Nursing, particularly emergency nursing, can dramatically influence the delivery and scope of services provided to emergency care patients (*Standards of Emergency Nursing Practice,* 1983). To have a significant impact, however, nurses must have a collective vision of the needs of the patients and the scope of care. This vision will provide the power to shape and to influence the current systems. Nevertheless, nurses have not yet developed a collective vision (Rodgers, 1981) because of various factors, including differences in background and educational preparation of the nurses, as well as differences in the reward structures in employment settings (Welch, 1980; Millar, 1981).

Emergency nursing as a specialty is at an advantage because it is a focused area of practice. Nonetheless, emergency nurses must also cope with many of the same problems that face all nurses.

To impact emergency care effectively, emergency nurses require a focus that will enable them to develop unified efforts directed toward achieving their goal. In determining the focus, nurses must examine the current status of emergency care, current standards of health, and current standards of health care. The professionals who are available to provide comprehensive care must be examined to identify the complementary skills among all types of care givers. Furthermore nurses must analyze the fiscal impact of providing comprehensive care. Moreover, emergency nurses must expand their analysis to include not only nursing questions, but also social work, medical, political, and economic questions. Agreeing to use or not to use paramedics in the emergency department, for example, may be easier than agreeing to use licensed vocational nurses. Emergency nurses must study the issues, before determining the most appropriate course of action.

Nurses are responsible for becoming educated because education not only will increase their freedom and autonomy, but it will assist nurses in their ability to analyze the patients' needs and to identify appropriate care required.

Emergency nursing, which will continue to require the expertise of trauma nurse specialists and clinical specialists interested in crisis intervention, should determine future roles intelligently and consciously. Emergency nursing is a young and informed speciality. If emergency nurses cooperate in developing a collective vision, they will then be able to develop innumerable emergency nursing roles to meet all patient needs.

Emergency nursing resembles an evolving society. The process of becoming developed, however, is not smooth. It is a cycle of fits, starts, pitfalls, and an unending sequence of steps forward and backward. Nevertheless, nursing has a great deal to offer. Emergency nursing must outgrow its medical model prototype to address all emergency care issues. Although the analysis in Table 32.2 demonstrates that many areas of patient needs are still unmet, we must remember the process is just starting. By the year 2000, if deliberate efforts are initiated, emergency nursing can dramatically impact the type and quality of health care services.

Although the issues remain, emergency nurses must become aware, must educate themselves, must be willing to risk, and must believe in their own potential.

The rung of a ladder was never meant to rest upon, but only to hold a man's foot long enough to enable him to put the other somewhat higher. (T. H. Huxley)

BIBLIOGRAPHY

American Hospital Association: *Hospitals, guide, issue.* 29(15), part 2 (Aug. 1, 1955).

American Hospital Association: *Hospitals, guide, issue.* 41(15), part 2 (Aug. 1, 1967).

American Hospital Association: *Hospitals, guide, issue.* 44(15), part 2 (Aug. 1, 1970).

American Hospital Association: *Hospitals, guide, issue.* 45(15), part 2 (Aug. 1, 1971).

American Hospital Association: *Hospital statistics.* Chicago: American Hospital Association, 1976, 1978, 1979.

Cobb, L. A.; H. Alvarez, III; and M. K. Kopas: A rapid response system for out-of-hospital cardiac emergencies. *Medical Clinics of North America* 60:238–290 (1976).

Emergency medical services—A new phase of development: *JAMA* 243(10):1017–1021 (Mar. 14, 1980).

Gann, D. S., et al.: Panel: Current status of emergency medical services. *Journal of Trauma* 21(3):196–203 (Mar. 1981).

Geyman, J. P.: Trends and concerns in emergency room utilization. *Journal of Family Practice* 11(1):23–24 (July 1980).

Gibson, G.: Patterns and trends of utilization of emergency medical services. In G. R. Schwartz; P. Safar; L. H. Stone; et al. (eds.): *Principles and Practice of Emergency Medicine.* Philadelphia: Saunders, 1978, p. 1513.

Gifford, M. J.; J. B. Franaszek; and G. Gibson: Emergency physicians and patients assessments: Urgency of need for medical care. *Annals of Emergency Medicine* 9:502–507 (Oct. 1980).

Heaton, L. D.: Army medical services in Viet Nam. *Military Medicine* 131:646–647 (1966).

Leitzell, J., and L. Riggs: Sounding boards—emergency medicine: Two points of view. *New England Journal of Medicine* 304(8):477–483 (Feb. 19, 1981).

Lund, I., and A. Skulberg: Cardiopulmonary resuscitation by lay people. *Lancet* 2:702–704 (1976).

Millar, S.: Our power to become. *Heart and Lung* 10(3):423–430 (May–June, 1981).

Montgomery, B. A capsule history of U.S. emergency medical care. *JAMA* 243(10):1019 (Mar. 14, 1980.)

National Academy of Science, National Research Council.: *Accidental death and disability: The neglected disease of modern society.* Washington, DC: National Academy of Sciences, 1966.

Standards of Emergency Nursing Practice. St. Louis, MO: Mosby, 1983.

Rodgers, J.: Toward professional adulthood. *Nursing Outlook* 29(8):478–481 (Aug. 1981).

The various roles of EDNA nurses. *Journal of Emergency Nursing:* 6:40–61 (Sept./Oct. 1980).

Toffler, A.: *Future shock.* New York: Random House, 1970.

Welch, M.: Dysfunctional parenting of a profession. *Nursing Outlook* 28(12):727 (Dec. 1980).

Index

"ABC" rule, in cardiopulmonary arrest, 178-179
Abdominal pain:
  areas of, and related illnesses, 237t
  causes of, 235
  in children, 472-474
  triage for, 236-238, 239t
Abdominal trauma:
  blunt, 439-440, 445f
  clinical signs in, 463t
  discharge planning for, 446-448
  laboratory studies in, 442
  and local wound exploration, 443, 444f, 445f
  nursing care and related interventions for, 443-446
  other studies in, 443
  penetrating, 438-439, 444f
  peritoneal lavage in, 441, 442f
  radiography in, 441-442
  triage for, 436-437, 438t
Abortion, 564-565
Abrasion, nursing care for, 284-285
Abscess, peritonsillar, 129
Accelerated hypertension, 219
Acetabular fracture, of pelvis, 318
Acetaminophen:
  for fever in children, 471-472
  poisoning by, 495t
  for thrombus, 216
Achilles tendon rupture, 325, 326
Acid, poisoning by, 495t
Acute back pain, 392-393
Acute patients, 40
  conditions of, 48t
Acute renal failure, burn injury and, 350
Acute rhinitis, 127-128
Acyclovir, for herpes simplex virus infections, 575
Adaptive behavior, and crisis intervention, 18

Adenoids, infection of, 136
Adrenocorticotropic hormone (ACTH), chlorine gas inhalation and, 93
Advanced nurse triage system, 41-42
Against medical advice (AMA):
  patient transfer and, 35
  signed statement by patient, 28
Airway maintenance, 55-56
  in cardiogenic shock, 161-163
  in children, 57
  first steps in, 56
  in multiple trauma, 459, 460t-461t
  and nasopharyngeal airway, 57
  and oropharyngeal airway, 56-57
  oxygen use in, 65-67
  in pulmonary edema, 113
  types of, 57-61
Airway obstruction:
  choking phases in, 61
  clinical manifestations of, 61
  nursing care and related interventions in, 62-65
Airway problems, triage for, 53-55
Akathisia, 537
Alcaine, *see* Proparacaine, for ocular trauma
Alcohol abuse, 509-511
  coma and, 78
  discharge planning and, 80
  and hypoglycemia, 516-517
  poisoning by, 497t-498t
Alcoholic ketosis, as cause of coma, 78
Alcoholics Anonymous (AA), 80, 526
Alignment, in spinal cord injury, 391
Alkalies, poisoning by, 495t
Allergic rhinitis, 128
Allergy:
  to Hymenoptera venoms, 291
  to local anesthetics, 277

605

INDEX

Alpha adrenergic drugs, for spinal shock, 390
Alupent, and IPPB therapy, 86
Amantadine hydrochloride, for parkinsonism, 537
American College of Emergency Physicans, 4
American College of Surgeons, and emergency care, 599
American Diabetes Association, 79
Amikacin, in septic shock, 412t
Amikar, see Amikacin, septic shock
Aminoglycosides, in abdominal trauma, 446
Aminophylline:
　for asthmatic patients, 86
　for pulmonary edema, 115
Amphetamines, poisoning by, 496t
Ampicillin, for pelvic inflammatory disease, 577
Anaphylactic shock, following insect stings, 292
Anesthesia, for minor wounds, 276-278
Aneurysm:
　acute dissecting aortic, 228
　aortic and abdominal pain, 250-251
Angina pectoris, stable and unstable, 147.
　See also Stable angina pectoris; Unstable angina pectoris
Angiography:
　celiac, in abdominal trauma, 443
　pulmonary, 120
Anhidrotic heat exhaustion, 545-546
Anisocoria, 367
Ankle, injuries to, 322
Antabuse, see Disulfiram, and alcohol abuse
Anterior cord syndrome, 387
Anterior tibial compartment syndrome, 321
Antianxiety drugs, 18
Antibiotics:
　for pharyngitis, 131
　for septic shock, 411, 412t
　topical, in burn wound management, 356t
　see also individual drug names
Antidepressant drugs, 18
Antidiarrheal agents for children, 476
Antidotes, for poisons, 504t-505t
Antidysrhythmic drugs, for heart blocks, 207
Antiemetics, for children, 476
Antihypertensive medications, 222t-225t
Antimanic drugs, 18
Antipsychotic drugs, 18, 536-537, 536t
　extrapyramidal side effects to, 537
Antiseptic preparations, for wound cleansing, 276
Antivenin, for snakebites, 290-291
Anxiety, in patient, 12-14
Aorta, injuries to, 450
Aortic aneurysm, classification of, 251t

Apgar scoring system, 573t
Aphasia, and level of consciousness, 366
Appendicitis, 245-246
Apresoline, see Hydralazine hydrochloride
Aquatic organisms, care of bite and stings from, 294-296
Aramine, see Metaraminol
Arfonad, see Trimethaphan
Arterial blood gases (ABG):
　in asthmatic patient, 86
　in bronchitis, 133
　in cardiogenic shock, 162t
　in cardiopulmonary arrest, 177
　in pulmonary edema, 113
　in pulmonary embolus, 119
Arterial lactic acid, in cardiogenic shock, 162t
Arthropod infestation and bites, care of, 292-294
Aspirin, Reye's syndrome and, 471-472
Assault, 26
Asthma, 84-85
　clinical manifestations of, 86
　diagnostic studies of, 86
　discharge planning and, 87
　etiology of, 85
　nursing care and related interventions for, 86-87
　pathophysiology of, 85-86
Atrial dysrhythmias, see Dysrhythmias, atrial
Atrial fibrillation (A-fib), 200
Atrial flutter, 199-200
Atropine, 157
　for atrioventricular junctional dysrhythmias, 202
　in cardiopulmonary arrest, 180t
　in heart blocks, 209
　for sinus dysrhythmias, 194, 196
　for spinal shock, 390
Automaticity, 192
Autonomic nervous system abnormalities, 175-176
Avulsions, nursing care for, 285

Babinski's reflex, 369
Baby:
　emergency delivery of, 569-571, 572t-573t
　intestinal obstructions in, 249
Bacitracin, for ocular trauma, 343
Back pain, acute, 392-393
Bag-mask, as oxygen delivery system, 66t
Bandage, see Dressing
Barbiturate, poisoning by, 495t
Barium studies, for lower GI bleeding, 261
Battery, 26

Baxter formula, *see* Ringer's lactate
Beck's triad, 462
Benadryl, *see* Diphenhydramine hydrochloride
Berkow burn chart, 351, 353f
Bicarbonate, for diabetic ketoacidosis, 77
Bigeminy, in PVB, 204
Bilirubin levels, in cholecystitis, 268
Bimanual examination, of pelvis, 562-563
Bites:
　by animals, 289
　　discharge instruction form, 282f
　from aquatic organisms, 294-296
　arthropod infestations, 292-294
　by humans, 288-289
　from insects, 291-292. *See also individual insects*
　from snakes, *see* Snake bites
　triage for, 271-273, 274t
Black widow spider, care of bite from, 294
Bladder, injuries to, 449-450
Bleeding, *see* Gastrointestinal bleeding; Hemorrhage; Vaginal bleeding
Blood alcohol level tests, consent for, 31-32
Blood brain barrier (BBB), coma and, 72
Blood component therapy, for hypovolemic shock, 404, 405t, 406t, 407t
Blood gases, *see* Arterial blood gases (ABG)
Blood supply, arterial, to lower extremities, 316, 317t
Blood type and crossmatch, in abdominal aneurysm, 251
Blunt abdominal trauma, 439-440
　algorithm for, 445f
Bone structure and healing, 308-309
Bordetella pertussis, 136-137
Bowel obstruction, 248-250
Box theory, 377
Bradycardia, in cardiogenic shock, 163
Brain, decompression of, 382-385
Brain computerized tomography scan (CT), in hypertensive encephalopathy, 226
Bretylium:
　in cardiopulmonary arrest, 180t
　for ventricular dysrhythmias, 206-207
Bretylol, *see* Bretylium
Bronchitis, acute and chronic:
　clinical manifestations of, 133
　diagnostic studies in, 133
　discharge planning for, 134
　nursing care and related interventions, 133-134
　pathophysiology of, 132-133
Brooke formula, in burn injury, 354f
Brown recluse spider, care of bite from, 294

Brown-Sequard syndrome, 387
Burns:
　body surface area, 351
　chemical, 358-359
　classification of, 352t
　clinical manifestations of, 350-351
　diagnostic studies for, 351, 352
　electrical, 358
　pathophysiology of, 349-350
　triage for, 347-349, 349f
Burn injury:
　discharge planning for, 359
　fluid replacement formulas in, 354-355, 354t
　medications for, 357
　minor, care of, 357
　wound care in, 355-357
Burn shock, 349-350
Butazoladin, *see* Phenylbutazone, for thrombus

Calcium chloride, in cardiopulmonary arrest, 180t
Candida vulvovaginitis, in sexually transmitted disease, 576
Carbon dioxide, rebreathing of, and hyperventilation syndrome, 96
Carbon monoxide poisoning, burn injury and, 350. *See also* Status asthmaticus
Cardiac chest pain:
　differentiation of, 146t
　pathophysiology of, 148-152
　triage for, 144-148
Cardiac contusions, 428-429
Cardiac dysrhythmias, *see* Dysrhythmias cardiac
Cardiac monitoring, 192-193
Cardiac tamponade, in multiple trauma, 462
Cardiac workload, reduction of, 108-109
Cardiogenic shock, 159
　airway maintenance in, 161-163
　clinical manifestations of, 160-161
　diagnostic studies in, 161, 162t
　establishing assessment parameters for, 163
　pathophysiology of, 159-160
　vital organ perfusion in, 163, 166
Cardiopulmonary arrest:
　"ABC" rule in, 178-179
　conduction system instability and, 176-177
　diagnostic studies in, 177
　ECG monitoring in, 179, 184, 184t
　medications for, 179, 180t-184t
　myocardial infarction and, 176
　pathophysiology of, 174-176
　patients at risk for, 172
　triage for, 172-174, 174t

Cardiopulmonary arrest *(Continued)*
  ventricular fibrillation history and, 177
Cardiopulmonary resuscitation (CPR):
  in near drowning, 99
  status asthmaticus and, 90
Cardiovascular function, and status asthmaticus, 91
Cardioversion, emergency use of, 184t
  for ventricular dysrhythmias, 206
Caring attitude, in crisis intervention, 18
Case law, 25-26
  emergency care provision, 24-25
Cast, care of, 328-329
Catapres, *see* Clonidine, for hypertensive crisis
Catecholamine stimulation, etiology of, 191
Cedilanid-D, in CHF, 109
Centipede bites, care of, 293
Central cord injury, 387
Central nervous system (CNS)
  dysfunction, following status asthmaticus, 91
  stimulation of, 277
Cephalosporins, in abdominal trauma, 446
Cephalothin, in septic shock, 412t
Cerebral autoregulation, in neurologically injured patient, 381-382
Cerebral edema:
  coma and, 72-73
    psychogenic disorders and, 74
    structural disorders and, 73-74
    toxic/metabolic disorders and, 74
  secondary to hypoxia, 91
Cerebral embolus, 231
Cerebral hemorrhage, 231-232
Cerebral thrombosis, 231
Cerebrospinal fluid leaks, 372, 386
Cerebrovascular accident, 229-230
  cerebral embolus in, 231
  cerebral hemorrhage in, 231-232
  cerebral thrombosis in, 231
  diagnostic studies in, 232
  nursing care and related interventions in, 232-233
  transient ischemic attack in, 230
  triage for, 212-213
Cerium nitrate, *see* Silver nitrate chlorhexidine digluconate 0.2%
Cervicitis, and sexually transmitted disease, 573-578
Chemical burns, 358-359
Chemical dependency:
  medications in patients with, 523t
  pathophysiology of, 518-521
  phases of, 520t

Chemotheraphy, in crisis intervention, 18
Chest trauma:
  cardiac contusions in, 428-429
  and esophageal injuries, 426-427
  flail chest in, 424-425
  and fractured ribs, 420-421
  hemothorax in, 423-424
  myocardial or major vessel rupture in, 430-431
  penetrating cardiac or great vessel trauma in, 431-432
  pericardial tamponade in, 429-430
  pneumothorax and tension pneumothorax in, 422-423
  pulmonary contusions in, 427-428
  and sternal fractures, 421
  and tracheobronchial injuries, 426
  triage for, 418-419, 419t
Child abuse, 30-31
  diagnostic studies in, 487-488
  emotional, 487
  nursing care and related interventions in, 488-489
  physical, 484-486, 485f, 486f
  sexual, 487
Child neglect, 486
Children:
  abdominal pain in, 472-474
  abuse of, *see* Child abuse
  airway maintenance for, 57
  airway obstruction in, 65
  fever in, 470-472
  fluid replacement following burn injury in, 355
  meningitis in, 479-481
  neglect of, 486
  Reye's syndrome in, *see* Reye's syndrome
  Sickle cell disease in, *see* Sickle cell disease
  triage and, 457-459, 459
  and urinary tract infection, 242
  vomiting and diarrhea in, 474-476
Chlamydia trachomatis, in sexually transmitted disease, 573, 574
Chlordiazepoxide hydrochloride, in chemical dependency, 523t, 524
Chlorine gas inhalation, 91
  clinical manifestations of, 92-93
  diagnostic studies in, 93
  discharge planning following, 93-94
  nursing care and related interventions for, 93
  pathophysiology of, 91-92
Chlorpromazine:
  for heat stroke, 550
  for pediatric use, 336
  in psychiatric emergency, 536t, 537

INDEX

Choking, *see* Airway obstruction, choking phases in
Cholecystitis, 267-268
Cholecystography, 268
Cholecystojejunostomy, 449
Cimetidine, for gastritis, 257
Circulatory status, in neurovascular alterations, 307
Clavicular fractures, 309-310
Cleocin, *see* Clindamycin, in septic shock
Clindamycin, in septic shock, 412t
Clonidine, for hypertensive crisis, 221
Clonus, in head and spinal trauma, 370
Clorazepate, in chemical dependency, 523t, 524
Clostridium botulism, and wound infection, 297
Clostridium perfringens, and wound infection, 297
Clostridium tetani, and wound infection, 297-298. *See also* Tetanus, *clostridium tetani*
Cocaine, poisoning by, 499t
Cold, common, 127-128
Cold disorder:
  frostbite as, 554-556
  hypothermia as, *see* Hypothermia
  triage for, 541-542, 543t
Colles' fracture, of wrist, 314, 315f
Coma, 69
  clinical manifestations of, 74, 75t
  diagnostic studies for, 74, 76
  discharge planning for, 79-80
  Glasgow Scale for, 71, 71t
  nursing care and related interventions for, 76
  pathophysiology of, 72-74
  specific causes of, 76-79
  triage for, 70-72, 73t
Comminuted neck fracture, of hip, 319
Commitment, forms of, 36
Common cold, 127-128
Community planning, for disaster, 587-588, 588t
Compartment syndrome, 286
Compazine, *see* Prochlorperazine, in psychiatric emergency
Complete heat block (CHB), 209
Computerized axial tomography (CAT) scan, for coma patients, 74
Computerized tomography (CT) scan:
  of abdomen, in pheochromocytoma, 227
  of brain:
    in cerebrovascular accident, 232
    in hypertensive encephalopathy, 226

Concussion:
  head trauma and, 373-374
  of spinal cord, 386-387
Conductive system, interruption of, 191
Conductivity, 192
Confidentiality, 34
Congentin, for parkinsonism, 537
Congestive heart failure (CHF), 106
  clinical manifestations of, 106-107, 107f
    left-sided heart failure, 107-108
    right-sided heart failure, 108
  control of excessive fluid retention in, 109-111
  diagnostic studies in, 108
  discharge planning for, 111-112
  enhancing myocardial contractility in, 109
  pathophysiology of, 106
  pulmonary edema as complication in, *see* Pulmonary edema
  and reduction of cardiac workload, 108-109
  triage for, 104-105, 105t
  venous/arterial vasodilators for, 111
Conjugated estrogens, use with rape victims, 579
Consciousness, level of:
  in head and spine trauma, 365-367
    and increased intracranial pressure, 378
  in multiple trauma, 462
Consent:
  for blood alcohol level, 31-32
  confidentiality and, 34
  for organ donation, 31
  and psychiatric patient, 35-36
  to treat, 26-28
Constitutional law, 26
Contusions:
  cardiac, 428-429
  in head and spine trauma, 374
  nursing care for, 285-286
  pulmonary, 427-428
Convalescence, following chlorine gas inhalation, 93-94
Coral snake, bites from, 290
Coronary atherosclerotic heart disease (CAHD), 148-149
Corynebacterium diphtheriae, 136
Coumadin, for pulmery embolus, 121
Cramp, heat, 546-547
Cranial nerves, in head and spine trauma, 371-372
Cricothyrotomy, 60
Crisis:
  multiple components in, 18
  psychological, 14
    reaction to, 16
    see also Crisis intervention

Crisis intervention:
  assessment in, 16-17
  evaluation of, 19-20
  priorities in, 16
  resolution of, 19
  safety in, 16
  types of, 17-19
"Crisis rounds," 19-20
Critical care teams, in disaster planning, 591
Croup:
  subglottic:
    diagnostic studies in, 137
    differences between epiglottitis and, 140t
    discharge planning for, 138-139
    nursing care and related interventions for, 138
    pathophysiology and clinical manifestations of, 137
    triage for, 126-127
  supraglottic, see Epiglottitis
Crutches, technique for use of, 328
Crystalloid solution, blood loss and, 261
Culdocentesis, in abdominal trauma, 443
Cyanides, poisoning by, 496t-497t
Cystinuria, 243
Cystitis, 240
Cystoscopy, in urinary tract infection, 242
Cystourethrogram, in abdominal trauma, 443

Dantrium, see Dantrolene sodium, for malignant hyperthermia
Dantrolene sodium, for malignant hyperthermia, 546
Darvon, see Propoxyphene, for thrombus
Dead on arrival (DOA), 32
Death, emotional support following, 185-187
Debridement:
  and wet saline dressings, 279-280
  in wound management, 278
Decadron, see Dexamethasone
Decerebration, 369
Decompression, of brain, 382-385
Decortication, 369
Defibrillation:
  emergency use of, 184t
  for ventricular dysrhythmias, 206
Dehydration, in children, 474-475
Delirium tremens, in substance abuse, 517
Delivery of baby, in emergency, 569-571, 572t-573t
Demerol, see Meperidine hydrochloride
Dental trauma, 340-341
Dependency, drug or alcohol, see Alcohol abuse; Chemical dependency; Drug abuse; Substance abuse
Depression, 534
Dermatones, location of, 389f
Deslanoside, in CHF, 109
Detoxification unit, vs. medical unit, criteria for, 525-526
Dexamethasone:
  for brain decompression, 383
  for croup, 138
Dextrose 50%:
  in chemical dependency, 523t
  in sinus bradycardia, 194
  for stabilization in cardiac chest pain, 156
Diabetes, discharge planning and, 79-80
Diabetic ketoacidosis (DKA), as cause of coma, 77, 77f
Diaphragm, injuries to, 449-450
Diarrhea, in children, 474-476
Diazepam:
  for akathisia, 537
  for atrial dysrhythmias, 199
  in chemical dependency, 523t
  in CNS stimulation, 277
  for facial lacerations, 336
  for seizures, 79, 385
Diazoxide:
  for hypertensive crisis, 221, 222t
  for hypertensive encephalopathy, 226
Dibenzyline, see Phenoxybenzamine, for pheochromocytoma
Diethylstilbesterol, sexual abuse of child and, 488
Digestive organs, in multiple trauma, 462-463
Digitalis:
  for atrial dysrhythmias, 198, 199, 199t, 200
  for atrioventricular dysrhythmias, 203
  in CHF, 109
  for pulmonary edema, 113, 114-115
  for sinus tachycardia, 195-196
Digitalis toxicity, 109
  in nonparoxysmal junctional tachycardia, 203
  signs and symptoms of, 110t
Digoxin:
  pediatric use of, 109, 109t
  in septic shock, 411
Dilantin, see Phenytoin, and seizures
Diphenhydramine hydrochloride:
  for dystonic reaction, 537
  for insect stings, 292
  for minor wounds, 277
Diphtheria, 136
Diplococcus pneumoniae, and meningitis, 479

INDEX

Disaster, 585-586
  hospital planning for, 589-592
  local community planning for, 587-588, 588t
  psychological reactions to, 593
  stages of, 586-587
  triage in, 588-589, 589t
Discharge instruction form, 281f, 282f
Dislocation, of temporal mandibular joint, 338. *See also* Orthopedic trauma
Displaced fracture, of hip, 319
Disruptive patient, 534
Disseminated intravascular coagulopathy (DIC), 411-412
  clinical manifestations of, 413
  diagnostic studies in, 413-414
  nursing care and related interventions for, 414
  pathophysiology of, 412, 413f
  triage for, 396-397, 398t
Disulfiram, and alcohol abuse, 517, 527
Diuretics:
  for cardiogenic shock, 165t
  complications of, 110-111
  osmotic, for brain decompression, 384-385
  see also individual drug names
Dobutamine:
  in cardiogenic shock, 165t
  for hypovolemic shock, 409t
Dobutrex, *see* Dobutamine
Documentation, of nursing care, 47
Doll's eyes maneuver, 370
Dolophine, *see* Methadone
Dopamine:
  in cardiogenic shock, 163, 164t, 166
  in cardiopulmonary arrest, 181t
  for hypovolemic shock, 409t
  for pulmonary embolus, 120
  in septic shock, 411
Doppler ultrasound, 215
Drainage, *see* Postural drainage and percussion
Dressing:
  semipermeable membrane, 280
  three-layed approach to, 279, 279f
  wet saline, 279-280
Drowning, near, 96-99
Drug abuse, 509-511
  triage for, 511
  see also Chemical dependency; Substance abuse
Drug ingestion, pathophysiology of, 501
Duodenal ulcer, 255. *See also* Gastric ulcer
Dyskinesia, 537
Dysphasia, and level of consciousness, 366

Dysrhythmias:
  atrial, 197f, 197-200
    discharge planning for, 201
  atrioventricular junctional, 201-203, 201f
    discharge planning for, 203
  cardiac, 191-193
  sinus, 193f, 194-196
    discharge planning for, 196-197
  triage for, 189-190, 191t
  types of, 194
  ventricular, 203-207, 204f
    discharge planning for, 207
Dystonic reaction, 537
Dysuria, 239

Ear:
  discharge from, 372
  inflammation of, 134-136
Eclampsia, 568-569
Ectopic pregnancy, 564-565
Edecrin, *see* Ethacrynic acid
Edema:
  cerebral, *see* Cerebral edema
  heat, 545-546
  pulmonary, *see* Pulmonary edema
Elbow, injuries to, 312-313
Electrical burns, 358
Electrical cell involvement, in cardiac chest pain, 151
Electrocardiogram:
  in cardiogenic shock, 162t
  in cerebrovascular accident, 232
  for coma patients, 74
  congestive heart failure and, 108
  in embolus, 217
  in hypertensive crisis, 221
  status asthmaticus and, 90
Electroencephalogram (EEG):
  in cerebrovascular accident, 232
  for coma patients, 76
Electrolyte imbalance, etiology of, 191
Electrophysiology, of heart's conduction system, 191-192, 192f
Embolectomy, 217
Embolus, 216
  cerebral, 231
  clinical manifestations of, 217
  diagnostic studies in, 217
  discharge planning for, 218
  nursing care and related interventions for, 217-218
  pathophysiology of, 216-217
  triage for, 212-213
Emergency, defined, 4

INDEX

Emergency care:
  consumer needs for, 600, 601t
  hospital's duty to provide, 24-25
  research studies into, 596
Emergency delivery of baby, 569-571, 572t-573t
Emergency department:
  actual and projected number of visits to, 598t, 599t
  consumer relations and, 6-7
  disaster plan for, 590-592
  and emergency nursing, see Emergency nursing
  health care, role of, 4-5
  hospital and, 4
  patient's perception of, 12-14
  psychological crises in, 14
  record-keeping in, 33-34
  sociological factors in use of, 5-6
  staff and equipment standards for, 36
  triage in, see Triage
Emergency Department Nurses Association, 4
  emergency nursing, 7-8
Emergency Medical Service (EMS), 4
Emergency medical services system, 596-597, 597t
  current state of, 597-599
Emergency Medical Services Systems (EMSS) Act 1973, 596
Emergency medical technician (EMT), 478
  Good Samaritan laws, 27-28
Emergency nursing:
  current practice in, 600-602
  consumer needs, 600, 601t
  documentation in, 47
  in future, 602-603
  review of, 595-599
  role and scope of, 7-8
Emergency pacing, in cardiopulmonary arrest, 184
Emergency room, see Emergency department
Emergent patients, 40
  conditions of, 48t
Emotional abuse and neglect, of children, 487
Emotional support, for relatives of cardiopulmonary arrest patient, 185
  following unsuccessful resuscitation, 185-187
Endoscopy, for GI bleeding, 261
Endotracheal intubation, 59-60, 59f
Epigastric pain, triage for, 253-254, 255t
Epiglottitis:
  clinical manifestations of, 139-140
  diagnostic studies for, 140
  nursing care and related interventions for, 140-141
  pathophysiology of, 139, 139f
  triage for, 126-127
Epinephrine:
  aqueous, for insect stings, 292
  for asthmatic patients, 87
  in cardiopulmonary arrest, 181t
  and facial lacerations, 335-336
  nebulized racemic, for croup, 138
  sympathetic nervous system involvement and, 152
  for ventricular dysrhythmias, 206
Epiphyseal injuries, 309, 310f
Equine antirabies serum (ARS), 300
Erythromycin, for *chlamydia trachomatis* infection, 573
Escharotomy, 356-357
Escherichia coli, in urinary tract infections, 240
Esophageal obturator airway (EOA), 58-59, 58f
Esophagus, injuries to, 426-427
Ethacrynic acid:
  for brain decompression, 385
  for cardiogenic shock, 162, 165t
Ethinyl estradiol, use with rape victims, 579
Ethylene glycol, poisoning by, 497t
Evans formula, in brain injury, 354f
Excitability, 192
Excretory organs, in multiple trauma, 463-464
Exhaustion, heat, 545-546
External otitis, 135-136
Extrapyramidal side effects, to antipsychotic drugs, 537
Eye, trauma to, see Ocular trauma

Face mask, as oxygen delivery system, 66t
Facial fracture:
  discharge planning for, 340
  mandibular, 338
  maxillary, 339-340
  nasal, 337-338
  orbital blow out, 339
  zygomatic, 339
Facial lacerations, 333-335
Facial trauma, triage for, 322-333, 333t
Family, in crisis intervention, 18
Family practice, percent of physicians in, 6
Federal Privacy Act 1974, 34
Femur, fracture of, 319-320
Fever, in children, 470-472
Fiberoptic gastroscope, and upper GI bleeding, 261
Fibula, injuries of, 321-322
First degree AV block, 207
Flaccidity, 369

INDEX

Flagyl, see Metronidazol, for vaginal infection
Flail chest, 424-425
Fluid challenge, in cardiogenic shock, 166
Fluid replacement, in burn injury, 354-355, 354t
Fluid retention, control in CHF, 109-111
Fluphenazine, in psychiatric emergency, 536
Food poisoning, 497t
Foot, fractures to, 322-323
Foreign bodies, nursing care and, 286-287
Four-vessel arteriogram, in cerebrovascular accident, 232
Fractures:
 clavicular, 309-310
 Colles', 314, 315f
 of face, see Facial fracture
 of femur, 319-320
 of foot, 322-323
 in head and spine trauma, 376-377
 of hip, 318-319
 humeral, 311-312
 in multiple trauma, 464
 musculoskeletal, complications of, 464t
 of pelvis, 316-318
 of radius and ulna, 314
 of ribs, 420-421
 of skull, 376-377
 of sternum, 421
 types of, 308
Fribrinoid necrosis, 219
Frostbite, 554-556
Furosemide:
 for brain decompression, 385
 for cardiogenic shock, 162, 165t
 for heart failure, 158, 228
 for hypertensive crisis, 225t
 in pulmonary contusions, 428
Fusion beat, 204
"Future shock," 595
 and emergency care, 598

Gamma benzene hexachloride, for arthropod infestations, 292
Gantrisin, see Sulfisoxazole, for urinary tract infection
Garamycin, see Gentamicin, in septic shock
Gardnerella vaginitis, in sexually transmitted disease, 575-576
Gas gangrene, 297
Gastric ulcer, 255, 256-257
 bland diet for, 258, 258t
Gastritis, 254-255, 256-258
Gastrointestinal bleeding, 259-261
 sources of, 259t
Gastroscopy, 257

Gegenhalten, 368-369
Gentamicin, in septic shock, 412t
Gestational trophoblastic disease, 565-566
Gila monster, 289
Glasgow Coma Scale (GCS), 71, 71t
Glucose:
 for alcoholic ketosis, 78
 for coma patients, 76
Good Samaritan laws, 27-28
Grieving, 185-187
G-strophanthin, in CHF, 109
Gunshot wounds, care of, 287
Gynecological problems, triage for, 560-561, 562t

Haldol, see Haloperidol
Haloperidol:
 in chemical dependency, 523t, 524
 in psychiatric emergency, 536t, 537-538
Hands, sensory nerve patterns of, 314, 316, 316f
Hare traction splint, 319
Head and spine trauma:
 brain decompression in, 382-385
 cerebrospinal leaks, 386
 control of seizures, 385-386
 fractures and, 376-377
 hemorrhages in, 374-376
 hypercarbia prevention, 381
 hypoxia prevention, 380-381
 increased intracranial pressure in, see Intracranial pressure, increase in
 neurological assessment in, 363-372
 normotension maintenance in, 381-382
 normothermia maintenance in, 382
 parenchymal injuries in, 373-374
 triage for, 362-363, 364t
 see also Spinal cord injuries
Heart blocks, 207, 208-209, 208f
Heart failure, hypertensive crisis and, 228. See also Cardiopulmonary arrest; Congestive heart failure (CHF)
Heart sounds, see Dysrhythmias
Heat syndromes:
 discharge planning in, 548, 548t
 forms of, 543-550, 551f
 triage for, 541-542, 543t
Heimlich maneuver, 62
 for children, 65
 complications following, 64-65
 in standing patient, 63, 64f
 in supine patient, 63, 63f
Hematoma, in head and spine trauma, 374-376
Hemophilus influenzae, and meningitis, 479

614

Hemophilus vaginalis, in sexually transmitted disease, 575-576
Hemorrhage:
  gastrointestinal, *see* Gastrointestinal bleeding
  in head and spine trauma, 374-376
  in multiple trauma, 459, 461
  in pregnancy, *see* Vaginal bleeding
Hemothorax, 423-424
Herpes simplex virus (HSV), in sexually transmitted disease, 575
Heparin:
  for disseminated intravascular coagulopathy, 414
  for embolus, 217
  for frostbite, 555
  for pulmonary embolus, 121
  for thrombus, 216
Herniation, in head and spine trauma, 378f, 380
Hill-Burton Act, 24
Hip, injuries to, 318-319
Hippocratic method, for glenohumoral joint reduction, 311
House plants, poisoning by, 498t
Human diploid cell rabies vaccine (HDCV), 300
Human rabies immune globulin (RIG), 300
Human tetanus immune globulin (TIG), 299-300
Humerus, fracture of, 311-312
Hydralazine hydrochloride:
  for CHF, 111
  for hypertensive crisis, 225t
  renal function deterioration and, 229
Hydrocortisone sodium succinate, for insect stings, 292
Hydrophobia, 300
Hyperbaric oxygen therapy (HBO), 90
Hypercarbia, prevention of, 381
Hyperemia, coma and, 72
Hyperglycemic-hyperosmolar nonketotic coma (HHNC), 77-78, 78f
Hyperstat, *see* Diazoxide
Hypertension, *see* Hypertensive crisis
Hypertensive crisis, 218-219
  accelerated and malignant, 219, 220f
  clinical manifestations of, 219
  diagnostic studies in, 219, 221
  discharge planning for, 221, 226
  pathophysiology of, 219
  nursing care and related interventions, 221
  and acute dissecting aortic aneurysm, 228
  and heart failure, 228
  and hypertensive encephalopathy, 226-227
  and myocardial infarction, 229
  and pheochromocytoma, 227-228

INDEX

  pregnancy induced, 228-229, 567-569
  and primary renal disease, 229
  and stroke, 229
  triage for, 212-213, 213t
Hypertensive encephalopathy, 226-227
Hypertensive retinopathy, 219, 220f
Hyperthermia, 543-545
Hypertonic resuscitation formula, in burn injury, 354f
Hyperventilation, for decompression of brain, 383
Hyperventilation syndrome, 94-96
Hypnotics, poisoning by, 498t
Hypoglycemia:
  alcohol-induced, 516
  as cause of coma, 76
Hypokalemia, following diuretic therapy, 110-111, 110t
Hyponatremia, following diuretic therapy, 110t
Hypotension, treatment for, in neurologically injured patient, 381-382
Hypothermia, 550-554, 552f
  substance abuse and, 516
Hypovolemic shock, 397
  blood component therapy in, 404, 405t, 406t, 407t
  circulatory system access in, 402-403
  clinical manifestations of, 400-401
  diagnostic studies in, 401-402
  medications for, 408, 409t
  pathophysiology of, 397-400
  pneumatic or MAS trousers in, 402, 403f
  triage for, 396-397, 398t
  volume expanders in, 403
Hypoxia:
  in near drowning, 97, 99
  prevention of, 380-381
  statis asthmaticus and, 89, 90
  cerebral edema secondary to, 91

^{125}I fibrinogen test, 215
IgE reaction, in asthma, 85-86
Immobilizing behavior, in patient, 534-535
Immunization Practices Advisory Committee of the Center for Disease Control, tetanus and, 298, 298t-299t
Impedance plethysmography, 215
Inderal, *see* Propranolol hydrochloride
Indocin, *see* Indomethacin, for thrombus
Indomethacin, for thrombus, 216
Injection, site of, 277
Insect stings and bites, of hymenoptera species, 291-292
Insulin, for diabetic ketoacidosis, 77

Intermittent positive pressure breathing (IPPB)
    therapy, 86
  for croup, 138
  in near drowning, 99
  for pulmonary edema, 114
Interpolated PVB, 204
Intertrochanteric fracture, of hip, 319
Intestines, injuries to, 450-451
Intracranial pressure, increase in:
  Box theory and, 377
  clinical manifestations of, 462t
  and level of consciousness, 378
  and motor response, 378-379
  and other alterations, 379
  and pupillary response, 379
  and vital signs, 379
Intravenous pyelogram (IVP):
  in abdominal trauma, 443
  for urinary calculi, 244
  in urinary tract infection, 241
Intropin, see Dopamine
Intubation, endotracheal, 59-60, 59f
Iron, poisoning by, 498t
Irrigation:
  of ears, 335
  for minor wounds, 277
  in occular trauma, 343
  peritoneal, 441, 442f
Ischemia, 149
Isopropyl alcohol, poisoning by, 497t-498t
Isoproterenol:
  for atrioventricular junctional dysrhythmias, 202
  in cardiopulmonary arrest, 182t
  for heart blocks, 208-209
  for hypovolemic shock, 409t
  and IPPB therapy, 86
  for pulmonary embolus, 120
  for sinus dysrhythmias, 194
Isordil, see Isosorbide
Isosorbide:
  for CHF, 111
  for stable angina, 153
Isuprel, see Isoproterenol

Joint Commission on Accreditation of
    Hospitals (JCAH):
  and emergency care provision, 24
  and emergency department record, 33-34
  staff and equipment standards of, 36
Junctional escape beats, 202

Keflin, see Cephalothin, in septic shock
Kidney, injuries to, 449-450

Kirz rule, for wound irrigation, 276
Knee, injuries to, 320
Kocher method, for glenohumoral joint
    reduction, 311
Kussmaul respirations, 77
Kwell, see Gamma benzene hexachloride,
    for arthropod infestations

Labor, stages and phases of, 570t
Lacerations, nursing care for, 283
  facial, see Facial lacerations
  suturing and, 283-284
Lactic acid, arterial, 162t
Lanoxin, see Digoxin
Laparotomy, 449
Laryngitis, 129
Laryngotracheobronchitis, see Croup,
    subglottic
Lasix, see Furosemide
Lavage, see Irrigation
Left-sided heart failure, clinical manifestations
    of, 107-108, 107f
Legal terms, review of, 25-26
Levarterenol, see Norepinephrine
Level of consciousness (LOC):
  in coma, 70-71
  memory and, 365-366
Levophed, see Norepinephrine
Librium, see Chlordiazepoxide
    hydrochloride
Lidocaine hydrochloride:
  in cardiopulmonary arrest, 182t
  for facial lacerations, 335-336
  for minor wounds, 277
  for ventricular dysrhythmias, 205, 206
Life changes, 14, 15t
Life support, in cardiopulmonary arrest, 173t
Ligament, injury to, 325-326
Limb, trauma to, see Orthopedic trauma
Liver, injuries to, 448-449
Locked-in state, vs. coma, 74
Lumbar puncture (LP):
  in cerebrovascular accident, 232
  for coma patients, 76
  in hypertensive encephalopathy, 226
Lungs:
  contusions of, 427-428
  edema of, see Pulmonary edema
  embolus of, see Pulmonary embolus
  function tests of, 86
Lysergic acid diethylamide (LSD), poisoning
    by, 499t
"Lytic cocktail," for children, 277

Mafenide 10%, for burn wounds, 356t
Malignant hypertension, 219
Malignant hyperthermia, 545-546
Malpractice, 25
Mandibular fractures, 338
Mannitol:
 for brain decompression, 384-385
 in burn injury, 355
Marine creatures, bites and stings from, 295
Maxillary fracture, 339-340
Mechanical cell involvement, in cardiac chest pain, 151
Medications, dispensing of, 33
Melenemesis, 260
Memory, and level of consciousness, 365-366
Meningitis, in children, 479-481
Meningococcus, 479-481
Mental status examination, 532
Meperidine hydrochloride:
 for burn injury, 357
 for cholecystitis, 268
 for pancreatitis, 262
 for pediatric use, 336
 for urinary calculi, 244
Metabolic acidosis:
 in cardiogenic shock, 166
 status asthmaticus and, 90
Metaraminol:
 in cardiogenic shock, 163, 164t
 for insect stings, 292
Methadone:
 in heroin addiction, 517
 and opiate use, 527
Methanol, poisoning by, 497t
Methocarbamol, for black widow spider bites, 294
Methyldopa, renal function deterioration and, 229
Methylprednisolone:
 for brain decompression, 383
 for septic shock, 411
Methylprednisolone sodium succinate:
 for croup, 138
 for insect stings, 292
 in pulmonary contusions, 428
Metolazone, in heart failure, 228
Metronidazole, for vaginal infections, 576
Military antishock trouser (MAST), 179, 381-382
 in abdominal trauma, 445
 in hypovolemic shock, 402, 403f
Millipede, irritation caused by, 293
Missile injuries, nursing care for, 287-288
Mobitz I block, 207

Mobitz II block, 208-209
Morning after syndrome, 517
Morphine sulfate:
 for atrioventricular junctional dysrhythmias, 202
 for burn injury, 357
 in cardiogenic shock, 166
 for congestive heart failure, 109
 for pulmonary contusions, 428
 for pulmonary edema, 114
 for sympathetic stimulation reduction, 157
 for urinary calculi, 244
Motor function, in neurovascular alterations, 307
Motor response, in head and spine trauma, 368-369
 and increased intracranial pressure, 378-379
Multifocal PVBs, 204
Multiple trauma, 455-456, 458
 airway maintenance in, 459, 460t-461t
 bleeding and shock in, 459, 461-462
 consciousness level in, 462
 diagnostic studies in, 458-459
 digestive organ care in, 462-463
 emotional reaction to, 464-465
 excretory organ care in, 463-464
 fractures in, 464, 464t
 triage for, 456-458, 457t
Musculotendinous injury, 325-326
Myocardial conduction disturbances, 175
Myocardial contractility, enhancement of, 109
Myocardial depressant factor:
 burn injury and, 350
 in hypovolemic shock, 400
Myocardial hypoxia, etiology of, 191
Myocardial infarction, 147, 229
 cardiopulmonary arrest and, 176
 clinical manifestations of, 153t
 diagnostic studies for, 156
 dysrhythmia recognition and treatment in, 158
 initial stabilization of, 156-157
 pathophysiology of, 149-150, 150f
 preload and afterload reduction in, 158-159
 safe transportation in, 159
 sympathetic stimulation reduction in, 157-158
Myocardial muscle disease, 175
Myocardial rupture, 430-431
Myxedema, as cause of coma, 78-79

Naloxone:
 in chemical dependency, 523t
 for coma patients, 76
 respiratory depression and, 157, 336

INDEX

Narcan, see Naloxone
Nasal cannula, as oxygen delivery system, 66t
Nasogastric tube:
  in abdominal aneurysm, 251
  in bowel obstruction, 250
  in cardiopulmonary arrest, 184-185
  in cholecystitis, 268
  and gastric analysis, 257
  in GI bleeding, 261
Nasopharyngeal airway, 57
National Academy of Science, and "neglected epidemic," 596
National Center for Prevention and Control of Rape, 579
National Highway Safety Act, 4
Navane, see Thiothixine, in psychiatric emergency
Near drowning, 96-99
Nebcin, see Tobramycin sulfate, in septic shock
Neisseria gonorrhea, in sexually transmitted disease, 574-575
Neisseria meningitidis, and meningococcus, 479
Neomycin, for ocular trauma, 343
Nerves:
  of lower extremities, 316, 317f
  sensory patterns in hand, 316f
Neurovascular alterations, and orthopedic injury, 307-308
Newborn, intestinal obstructions in, 249
Nipride, see Sodium nitroprusside
Nitro-Bid paste, see Nitroglycerin
Nitroglycerin:
  for atrioventricular junctional dysrhythmias, 202
  for stable angina, 152, 153
  for vasodilation in infarction, 158
Nitrous oxide, 336
Nonacute patients, 40
  conditions of, 48t
Nonparoxysmal junctional tachycardia (NPJT), 202-203
Norepinephrine:
  in cardiogenic shock, 163, 164t
  for insect stings, 292
  sympathetic nervous system involvement and, 152
Nose:
  and cannula in oxygen delivery system, 66t
  fracture of, 337-338
Nursing flow sheet, 47
Nystatin vaginal suppositories, for *candida vulvovaginitis* infection, 576

Obstetrical problems, triage for, 560-561, 562t.
  See also Pregnancy; Vaginal bleeding
Ocular trauma:
  clinical manifestations of, 342
  discharge planning in, 343-344
  nursing care and related interventions, 342-343
  pathophysiology of, 341-342
Oculocephalic reflex, 370
Oculovestibular reflex, 370
Opiates, poisoning by, 496t
Orbital blow out fracture, 339
Orientation, and level of consciousness, 365
Organ donation, 31
Oropharyngeal airway, 56-57
Oropharynx, anatomy of, 139f
Orthopedic trauma, 319-320
  to ankle, 322
  bone structure and healing in, 308-309
  clavicular fracture in, 309-310
  discharge planning in, 326-329
  to elbow, 312-313
  to foot, 322-323
  to hip, 318-319
  to humerus, 311-312
  to knee, 320
  ligament and musculotendinous injuries in, 325-326
  neurovascular alterations and, 307-308
  nursing care measures in, 326
  to pelvis, 316-318, 317f
  soft tissue alterations and, 323-324
  shoulder injuries in, 310-311
  sprains and strains in, 324
  to tibia and fibula, 321-322
  triage for, 303-306, 306t
  to wrist, 314, 315f, 316f
  see also Fractures
Osteoporosis, 309
Otitis:
  external, 135-136
  media, 134-135
Otorrhea, 372
Ouabain, in CHF, 109, 199
Overdose:
  pupillary changes in, 500t
  and substance manifestations, 495t-499t
  triage for, 492-494, 501, 502t
  see also Poisoning
Oxygen:
  in cardiopulmonary arrest, 183t
  delivery systems for, 66t
  discharge planning and, 65, 67
  precautions for use of, 65

Oxygen (*Continued*)
  in status asthmaticus, 90
Oxygen-powered breathing devices, 66t
Oxygen reservoir mask, 66t

Pancreas, injuries to, 450-451
Pancreatitis, 262
  clinical etiologies of, 263t-265t
  signs and symptoms in, 266t
Paratonia, 368-369
Parkinsonism, 537
Parkland formula, *see* Ringer's lactate
Paroxysmal atrial tachycardia (PAT), 198-199
Pasteurella multocida, and wound infection, 297
Patient anxiety, 12-14
Patient perception, of emergency visit, 12-14
Patient transfers, 34-35
Pediatric patient, *see* Baby; Children
Pelvis:
  examination of, 561-563
  inflammatory disease of, 246-248
    in sexually transmitted diseases, 576-577
  injuries to, 316-318, 317f
Penetrating abdominal trauma, 438-439
  algorithm for, 444f
Penetrating cardiac trauma, 431-432
Penicillin:
  in abdominal trauma, 446
  burn injury and, 357
  for pelvic inflammatory disease, 248
  for streptococcal infection, 131
  see also Procaine penicillin
Pentobarbital, pediatric use of, 277
Peptic ulcer, *see* Gastric ulcer
Percussion, *see* Postural drainage and percussion
Pericardial tamponade, 429-430
Peritoneal lavage, in abdominal trauma, 441, 442f
Peritonitis, 246
Peritonsillar abscess, 129
Pertinent negatives, 43
Pertussis, 136-137
Pharyngitis, 128
Phenazopyridine hydrochloride, for urinary tract infection, 242
Phencyclidine (PCP), poisoning by, 498t-499t
Phenobarbitol:
  for cholecystitis, 268
  for seizures, 79
Phenoxybenzamine, for pheochromocytoma, 227

Phentolamine:
  for hypertensive crisis, 224t
  for pheochromocytoma, 227
Phenylbutazone, for thrombus, 216
Phenytoin, and seizures, 79, 385-386
Pheochromocytoma, 227-228
Phlebotomy, for pulmonary edema, 115
Pit vipers, bites from, 289-290
Placenta abruption and placenta previa, 566-567
Plasma components, in blood component therapy, 406t
Plasma derivatives, in blood component therapy, 407t
Plasma substitutes, in bowel obstruction, 250
Pneumomediastinum, following Heimlich maneuver, 64
Pneumothorax, 422-423
Poisoning:
  antidotes in, 504t-505t
  diagnostic studies for specific substances, 503t
  discharge planning in, 506-507
  nursing care and related interventions in, 501-504, 506
  pathophysiology of drug absorption in, 501
  pupillary changes in, 500t
  specific treatments for, 506t
  and substance manifestations, 495t-499t
  triage for, 492-494, 501, 502t
Polymyxin, for ocular trauma, 343
Polytrauma, *see* Multiple trauma
Positive end expiratory pressure (PEEP), 93
  in near drowning, 99
Postural drainage and percussion:
  for asthmatic patients, 87
  and chlorine gas inhalation, 93
Potassium chloride, for digitalis toxicity, 203
Potassium supplement, for anhidrotic heat exhaustion, 545-546
Povidone iodine, for burn wounds, 356
Prazosin, for CHF, 111
Preeclampsia, 228-229, 568-569
Pregnancy:
  bleeding in, *see* Vaginal bleeding
  hypertension and, 228-229, 567-569
  sexually transmitted disease and, 573
Pre-infarction syndrome, *see* Unstable angina pectoris
Premature atrial beat (PAB), 197-198
Premature junctional beat (PJB), 201-202
Premature ventricular beat (PVB), 203-205
Prickly heat, 545-546
Prinzmetal's angina, 147

INDEX

Probenecid:
  for pelvic inflammatory disease, 248, 577
  use with rape victims, 579
Procainamide for ventricular dysrhythmias, 205
Procaine hydrochloride, for minor wounds, 277
Procaine penicillin:
  for *neisseria gonorrhea* infection, 574
  for pelvic inflammatory disease, 577
  use with rape victims, 579
Prochlorperazine, in psychiatric emergency, 536
Prolixin, *see* Fluphenazine, in psychiatric emergency
Promethazine, for pediatric use, 336
Proparacaine, for ocular trauma, 343
Propoxyphene, for thrombus, 216
Propranolol hydrochloride:
  for atrial dysrhythmias, 199
  for pheochromocytoma, 228
  renal function deterioration and, 229
  for sinus tachycardia, 196
  for stable angina, 153
  for tachycardia in infarction, 157
Protamine, in anticoagulant therapy, 216
Proteinuria, 239
Protoscopy, for lower GI bleeding, 261
Psychiatric emergency:
  consent in, 35
  discharge planning in, 537
  and disruptive patients, 534
  and immobilized patient, 534-535
  medication therapy in, 536-537
  restraints in, 535-536
  and suicidal patient, 533-534
  symptoms associated with medical disorders, 531t
  triage for, 530-532, 533t
  and violent patient, 532-533
Psychological support, in spinal cord injury, 391-392
Public Law 93-154, 596
Pulmonary angiography, for pulmonary embolus, 120
Pulmonary contusions, 427-428
Pulmonary edema, 112
  airway maintenance in, 113
  clinical manifestations of, 112-113
  diagnostic studies in, 113
  discharge planning for, 116
  medication administration in, 114-115
  oxygen administration in, 113-114
  pathophysiology of, 112
  phlebotomy for, 115
  positioning in, 114
  promotion of physical and mental rest in, 115

rotating tourniquets for, 115-116
triage for, 104-105, 105t
Pulmonary embolus, 116-117, 117f
  anticoagulant therapy for, 121
  clinical manifestations of, 118-119
  diagnostic studies in, 119-120
  discharge planning for, 121-122
  fibrinolytic agents for, 121
  pathophysiology of, 117-118
  predisposition factors for, 118t
  supportive measures for, 120
  surgical intervention for, 121
  triage for, 104-105
  vasopressors for, 120
Pulmonary function tests (PFT), for asthmatic patient, 86
Puncture wounds, nursing care for, 286
Pupillary response:
  in head and spine trauma, 367-368
  and increased intracranial pressure, 379
  in overdose, 500t
Pyelonephritis, 240
Pyridium, *see* Phenazopyridine hydrochloride, for urinary tract infection

Quinidine, for atrial dysrhythmias, 198, 200

Rabies, 300
Radiation disaster, emergency department plan in, 592
Radiography, *see* X-ray studies
Radionuclide scanning, in abdominal trauma, 443
Radius, fracture of, 314
Rape, 29-30, 578-579
Reactive airway disease, *see* Asthma
Rebreathing mask, as oxygen delivery system, 66t
Records, in emergency department, 33-34, 47
Red blood cells, in blood component therapy, 405t
Reflexes, in head and spine trauma, 369-370
Regitine, *see* Phentolamine
Relaxation, 21
Reportable situations, 28-29
Rescue breathing, 179t. *See also* Airway maintenance
Respiratory emergency, triage for, 83-84, 85t
Restraints, use in psychiatric emergency, 535-536
Reticular activating system:
  coma and, 72
  and locked-in state, 74

Retrograde pyelogram, in abdominal trauma, 443
Retrograde pyelograph, in urinary tract infection, 241
Reye's syndrome:
  aspirin and, 471-472
  clinical manifestations of, 477, 478t
  nursing care and related interventions for, 478
  pathophysiology of, 476-477
Rhinitis, 127-128
Rhinorrhea, 372
Rhythmicity, 192
Ribs, fractured, 420-421
Right-sided heart failure, clinical manifestations of, 107f, 108
Rigid extension, 369
Rigid flexion, 369
Ringer's lactate:
  in abdominal aneurysm, 251
  in abdominal trauma, 441, 444
  in bowel obstruction, 250
  in burn injury, 354, 354f, 355
  for flail chest, 425
  for heat stroke, 550
Robaxin, *see* Methocarbamol, for black widow bites
Robert Wood Johnson Foundation, 4
Rocky Mountain Spotted Fever, 293
Root syndromes, 387
Rotating tourniquets, for pulmonary edema, 115-116
Rule of Nines, 351
Rupture, myocardial or major vessel, 430-431

Salicylates, poisoning by, 495t
Salter classification, of epiphyseal injuries, 309, 310f
Scorpion bites, care of, 293
Sedatives, poisoning by, 498t
Seizures:
  in children, 470
  coma and, 79
  in head and spine trauma, 385-386
  discharge planning and, 80
  drug and alcohol withdrawal and, 515
Sensory perception, in neurovascular alterations, 307-308
Septic shock:
  causes of, 408, 409t
  clinical manifestations of, 410
  diagnostic studies in, 410
  medications for, 411
  nursing care for, 410-411
  pathophysiology of, 408-410
  triage for, 396-397, 398t
Sexual abuse, of children, 487
Sexually transmitted diseases, 573-578
Shock:
  anaphylactic, 292
  burn, 349-350
  cardiogenic, *see* Cardiogenic shock
  hypovolemic, *see* Hypovolemic shock
  in multiple trauma, 461
  septic, *see* Septic shock
  spinal, 390
  toxic, 578
Shoulder injuries, 310-311
Sickle cell disease, 481-484
Sigmoidoscopy, for lower GI bleeding, 261
Silvadene, *see* Silver sulfadiazine 1%, for burn wounds
Silver nitrate 0.5%, for burn wounds, 356, 356t
Silver nitrate chlorhexidine digluconate 0.2%, 356t
Silver sulfadiazine 1%, for burn wounds, 356t
Sinus arrest, 196
Sinus bradycardia, 194
Sinus dysrhythmias, *see* Dysrhythmias, sinus
Sinusitis, 128
Sinus tachycardia, 195-196
Skin closure strips, 284
Snake bites, 289-291
SOAP format, in triage process, 42-44, 45t
Sodium bicarbonate:
  for burn injury, 357
  in cardiopulmonary arrest, 183t
  in hypovolemic shock, 40
  for metabolic acidosis, 166
  in septic shock, 411
Sodium nitroprusside:
  for abdominal aneurysm, 251
  in cardiogenic shock, 165t, 166
  in congestive heart failure, 111
  for hypertensive encephalopathy, 226-227
  for hypertensive crisis, 221, 223t
  for hypovolemic shock, 409t
Sodium sulfacetamide 10%, for ocular trauma, 343
Soft tissue:
  alterations in, 323-324
  injury to, 333-337
Solu-Cortef, *see* Hydrocortisone sodium succinate, for insect stings
Solu-Medrol, *see* Methylprednisolone sodium succinate

Spectinomycin:
  for *neisseria gonorrhea* infection, 575
  for pelvic inflammatory disease, 248
Speculum examination, of pelvis, 561-562
Spider bites, care of, 293-294
Spinal cord injuries, 386
  assessment of neck in, 388
  diagnostic studies in, 389-390
  respiratory and circulatory evaluation in, 387-388
  sensory evaluation in, 388-389, 389f
  motor ability in, 388
  nursing care and related interventions in, 390-392
  types of, 386-387
Spinal shock, nursing care for, 390
Spinal trauma, *see* Head and spine trauma
Spleen, injuries to, 448-449
Splenectomy, 449
Splints, 280
Sprain, 324
Sputum culture:
  in asthmatic patient, 86
  in bronchitis, 133
Stable angina pectoris, 147
  clinical manifestations of, 153t
  diagnostic studies for, 152
  discharge planning for, 154-155
  nursing care and related interventions, 152, 153
Stab wounds, care of, 287. See also Penetrating abdominal trauma; Penetrating cardiac trauma
Staphylococcus, skin infection by, 296-297
Staphylococcus aureus, and toxic shock syndrome, 578
Starling's law phenomenon, 166
State v. Amaniera, 1975, 31-32
Status asthmaticus, 87-88
  clinical manifestations of, 89
  diagnostic studies in, 89-90
  nursing care and related interventions for, 90
Statutory law, defined, 25
Stelazine, *see* Trifluoperazine
Sternum, fractures of, 421
Steroids:
  for asthmatic patients, 87
  for decompression of brain, 383
Stokes-Adams attacks, 209
Stimson method, for glenohumoral joint reduction, 311
Stomach, injuries to, 450-451
Stool analysis, for gastric bleeding, 257
Strain, 324

Strep throat, 128
Stress:
  and emergency department staff, 20-21
  and patient anxiety, 14
Stress fractures, of hip, 318-319
Stroke:
  cerebrovascular accident, *see* Cerebrovascular accident
  heat, 549-550, 551f
Substance abuse:
  commonly abused substances, 510, 510t
  discharge planning in, 526-527
  disposition following medical stabilization in, 525-526
  laboratory studies and clinical significance in, 522t
  nursing interventions in, 521-522, 524
  psychological intervention, 524-525
  rehabilitation rules of, 527
  triage for, 511-518, 519t
  see also Alcohol abuse; Chemical dependency; Drug abuse
Subtrochanteric fracture, of hip, 319
Subungual hematomas, 286
Suicidal patient, 533-534
  care of, 538
Sulf 10, *see* Sodium sulfacetamide 10%, for ocular trauma
Sulfamyelon, *see* Mafenide 10%, for burn wounds
Sulfisoxazole, for urinary tract infection, 242
Sulfisoxazole diolamine, for ocular trauma, 343
Susphrine, *see* Epinephrine
Sutures:
  considerations for, 283
  removal of, 284, 284t
  types of, 283-284
  for facial lacerations, 336
Symmetral, *see* Amantadine hydrochloride, parkinsonism
Sympathetic nervous system involvement, in cardiac chest pain, 151-152
Syncope, heat, 545-546

Tachycardia:
  in cardiogenic shock, 163
  sinus, 195-196
  ventricular, 205-206
Tagamet, *see* Cimetidine, for gastritis
Tamponade:
  cardiac, 462
  pericardial, 430
Tardive dyskinesia, 537
Telephone advice, 35

Temporal mandibular joint dislocations, 338
Tendon, injury to, 325-326
Tension pneumothorax, 422-423
Terbutaline, for asthmatic patients, 86
Tetanus:
  active immunity to, 298-299
  antitoxin, 300
  clostridium tetani, 297-298
  passive immunity to, 299-300
  prophylaxis for, 298, 299t
  toxoids, 298
    immunization schedules for, 298t-299t
Tetany, heat, 545-546
Tetracaine hydrochloride, for ocular trauma, 343
Tetracycline:
  for *chlamydia trachomatis* infection, 574
  for *neisseria gonorrhea* infection, 574
  for pelvic inflammatory disease, 577
  use with rape victims, 579
Thermal regulation, in neurologically injured patient, 382
Thiamine, for alcoholic ketosis, 78
Thiothixine, in psychiatric emergency, 536t
Thoracic injuries, 459, 460t-461t
Thorocotomy:
  in hemothorax, 424
  in pericardial tamponade, 430
Thorazine, *see* Chlorpromazine
Throat culture, 130
  for croup, 137
Thrombosis, cerebral, 231
Thrombus:
  triage for, 212-213, 213t
  venous and arterial, 213-216
Tibia, injuries of, 321-322
Ticar, *see* Ticarcillin, in septic shock
Ticarcillin, in septic shock, 412
Tick bites, care of, 293
Tobramycin sulfate, in septic shock, 412t
Tonsillitis, 128-129
Toxemia, 567-569
Toxic shock syndrome, 578
Toxic substance, ingestion of, 35
Tracheobronchial injuries, 426
Tracheostomy, 60-61
Tracheotomy, epiglottitis and, 141
Transfer, of patient, 34-35
Transient ischemic attack, 230
Transtracheal catheter ventilation, 60
Tranxene, *see* Clorazepate, in chemical dependency
Trauma, *see* Abdominal trauma; Chest trauma; Head and spine trauma; Multiple trauma; Ocular trauma; Orthopedic trauma
Treatment:
  consent for, 26-27
  refusal of, 28
Triage, 7, 39-40
  data assessment in, 43-44
  data collection in, 44-46
  in emergency department disaster plan, 591
  management plan in, 44
  objective data in, 43
  priority of care in, 46-47, 48t
  subjective data in, 42-43
    PQRST mnemonic in, 144, 145t
  systems of, 40-41
Trichomonas vaginalis, in sexually transmitted disease, 576
Tricyclics, poisoning by, 496t
Trifluoperazine, in psychiatric emergency, 536t
Trigeminy, in PVB, 204
Trimethaphan:
  for acute dissecting aortic aneurysm, 228
  for hypertensive crisis, 224t
Tylenol, *see* Acetaminophen

Ulceration, gastric, *see* Gastric ulcer
Ulna, fracture of, 314
Ultrasonography, in cholecystitis, 267-268
Uncal herniation, in head and spine trauma, 378f, 380
Unifocal PVBs, 204
Unstable angina pectoris, 147
  clinical manifestations of, 153t
  diagnostic studies for, 156
  dysrhythmia recognition and treatment in, 158
  initial stabilization of, 156-157
  pathophysiology of, 149
  preload and afterload reduction in, 158-159
  safe transportation in, 159
  sympathetic stimulation reduction in, 157-158
Unsuccessful resuscitation, emotional support following, 185-187
Upper respiratory infection:
  diagnostic studies in, 130
  discharge planning for, 131-132
  nursing care and related interventions in, 130-131
  pathophysiology and clinical manifestations of, 127-129
  triage for, 126-127, 127t
Uremia, as cause of coma, 78
Ureter, injuries to, 449-450
Urethra, injuries to, 449-450

INDEX

Urethritis, 240
Urinalysis:
 in cardiogenic shock, 162t
 in hypertensive crisis, 219
 from twenty-four hour collections, in pheochromocytoma, 227
 in urinary tract infection, 242
Urinary calculi, 243-244
Urinary tract infections, 238-239
 clinical manifestations of, 240-241
 diagnostic studies in, 241-242
 discharge planning in, 242-243
 nursing care and related interventions for, 242
 pathophysiology of, 239-240
 sources of, 240t
Urolithiasis, 243-244

Vagal stimulation, etiology of, 191
Vaginal bleeding:
 abortion and, 563-564
 ectopic pregnancy and, 564-565
 gestational trophoblastic disease and, 565-566
 placenta abruption and placenta previa and, 566-567
Vaginal infection, and sexually transmitted disease, 573-578
Valium, *see* Diazepam
Vanilmandelic acid (VMA), levels in pheochromocytoma, 227
Variant angina, 147
Vasoactive agents, for hypovolemic shock, 408, 409t
Vasodilator drugs:
 in cardiogenic shock, 165t, 166
 for congestive heart failure, 111
 for pulmonary edema, 115
 see also individual drug names
Vasopressor drugs:
 in cardiogenic shock, 163, 164t-165t
 for GI bleeding
 see also individual drug names
Venereal disease, 573-578
Venereal Disease Research Laboratories (VDRL) test, for pelvic inflammatory disease, 247
Venography, 215
Ventilation:
 and chlorine gas inhalation, 93
 transtracheal catheter, 60
 see also Airway maintenance; *individual technique names*
Ventilatory function tests, in bronchitis, 133
Ventricular dysrhythmias, *see* Dysrhythmias, ventricular

Ventricular fibrillation, 177, 206-207
Ventricular tachycardia, 205-206
Venturi mask, as oxygen delivery system, 66t
Verapamil, for atrial dysrhythmias, 199
Violent patient, 532-533
 care of, 537-538
Visual stimuli, and patient anxiety, 14
Vital signs:
 in head and spine trauma, 370-371
 increased intracranial pressure, 379
 normal pediatric, 469t
Volkmann's contracture, 313
Vomiting, in children, 474-476

Warfarin sodium:
 for pulmonary embolus, 121
 for thrombus, 216
Wenckebach block, 207
Wernicke-Korsakoff syndrome, 517
Wernicke's encephalopathy, 78
White blood cell (WBC) level:
 in asthmatic patient, 86
 in pharyngitis differential diagnosis, 130
Whooping cough, 136-137
Withdrawal, drug and alcohol, 515
 and delirium tremens, 517
 nursing interventions in, 524
Wilmington General Hospital v. *Manlove*, 24-25
Wound closure, approaches to, 278
Wound healing, physiology of, 273-276
Wound infections, 296
 from *clostridium botulism*, 297
 from *clostridium perfringens*, 297
 from *clostridium tetani*, *see* Tetanus, *clostridium tetani*
 from *pasteurella multocida*, 297
 rabies, 300
 from *staphylococcus*, 296-297
Wounds:
 in abdominal trauma, 443, 444f, 445f
 in burn injury, 355-357
 in chest trauma, 431-432
 gunshot, care of, 288-289
 minor:
  anesthesia administration, 276-278
  application of dressings, bandages and splints to, 278-280
  cleansing and irrigation of, 276
  debridement and closure of, 278
  discharge planning for, 280, 281f, 283
  other penetrating, care of, 288
  stab, care of, 288-289
  triage for, 271-273, 274t

Wringer injuries, 286
Wrist, injuries to, 314, 315f, 316, 316f

X-ray studies:
  in abdominal aneurysm, 251
  in abdominal trauma, 441-442
  for asthmatic patient, 86
  in bowel obstruction, 250
  for bronchitis, 133
  in cardiogenic shock, 162t
  in cardiopulmonary arrest, 177
  for coma patients, 74
  in congestive heart failure, 108
  for croup, 137
  in hypertensive crisis, 221
  for pulmonary edema, 113
  for pulmonary embolus, 119
  upper GI series, 256-257
  in urinary tract infection, 241

Zaroxolyn, *see* Metolazone, in heart failure
Zygomatic fracture, 339